Handbook of Chinese Herbal Medicine

Handbook of Chinese Herbal Medicine

Editor: Lydia Stephens

MURPHY & MOORE
www.murphy-moorepublishing.com

Murphy & Moore Publishing,
1 Rockefeller Plaza,
New York City, NY 10020, USA

Visit us on the World Wide Web at:
www.murphy-moorepublishing.com

ISBN: 978-1-63987-276-3 (Hardback)

Cataloging-in-Publication Data

Handbook of chinese herbal medicine / edited by Lydia Stephens.
p. cm.
Includes bibliographical references and index.
ISBN 978-1-63987-276-3
1. Herbs--Therapeutic use--China. 2. Medicine, Chinese. 3. Materia medica--China. I. Stephens, Lydia.
RM666.H33 H36 2022
615.321--dc23

Table of Contents

Preface

Chinese herbal medicine is a branch of traditional Chinese medicine. It involves the use of Chinese herbs for treating diseases. The most common method of Chinese herbal medicine is the preparation of decoction. Such a decoction includes nine to eighteen substances. These substances are classified as the main herbs or ancillary herbs. A decoction may also use some substances which cancel out the side effects or toxicity of herbs. These decoctions are later condensed and converted into a powdered or granular form. The most prominent herbs used in chines herbal medicine are wolfberry, astragalus, ginseng, cinnamon, dong quai, licorice, salvia, coptis, etc. This book is compiled in such a manner, that it will provide an in-depth knowledge about the theory and practice of Chinese herbal medicine. From theories to research to practical applications, case studies related to all contemporary topics of relevance to this field have been included herein. This book is a vital tool for all researching or studying this discipline as it gives incredible insights into emerging trends and concepts.

This book is a result of research of several months to collate the most relevant data in the field.

When I was approached with the idea of this book and the proposal to edit it, I was overwhelmed. It gave me an opportunity to reach out to all those who share a common interest with me in this field. I had 3 main parameters for editing this text:

1. Accuracy - The data and information provided in this book should be up-to-date and valuable to the readers.
2. Structure - The data must be presented in a structured format for easy understanding and better grasping of the readers.
3. Universal Approach - This book not only targets students but also experts and innovators in the field, thus my aim was to present topics which are of use to all.

Thus, it took me a couple of months to finish the editing of this book.

I would like to make a special mention of my publisher who considered me worthy of this opportunity and also supported me throughout the editing process. I would also like to thank the editing team at the back-end who extended their help whenever required.

Editor

1

Complete chloroplast genome of the medicinal plant *Amomum compactum*: gene organization, comparative analysis, and phylogenetic relationships within Zingiberales

Ming-li Wu[1,2], Qing Li[3], Jiang Xu[1] and Xi-wen Li[1*]

Abstract

Background: *Amomum compactum* is one of the basic species of the traditional herbal medicine amomi fructus rotundus, with great pharmacology effect. The system position of *A. compactum* is not clear yet, and the introduction of this plant has been hindered by many plant diseases. However, the correlational molecular studies are relatively scarce.

Methods: The total chloroplast (cp) DNA was extracted according to previous studies, and then sequenced by 454 GS FLX Titanium platform. Sequence assembly was complished by Newbler. Genome annotation was preformed by CPGAVAS and tRNA-SCAN. Then, general characteristics of the *A. compactum* cp genome and genome comparsion with three Zingiberaceae species was analyzed by corresponding softwares. Additionally, phylogenetical trees were reconstructed, based on the shared protein-coding gene sequences among 15 plant taxa by maximum parsimony (MP) and maximum likelihood (ML) methods.

Results: The *A. compactum* cp genome with a classic quadripartite structure, consisting of a pair of reverse complement repeat regions (IRa/IRb) of 29,824 bp, a large single copy (LSC, 88,535 bp) region as well as a small single copy (SSC, 15,370 bp) region, is 163,553 bp in total size. The total GC content of this cp genome is 36.0%. The *A. compactum* cp genome owns 135 functional genes, that 113 genes are unique, containing eighty protein-coding genes, twenty-nine tRNA (transfer RNA) genes and four rRNA (ribosomal RNA) genes. Codon usage of the *A. compactum* cp genome is biased toward codons ending with A/T. Total 58 SSR loci and 24 large repeats are detected in the *A. compactum* cp genome. Relative to three other Zingiberaceae cp genomes, the *A. compactum* cp genome exhibits an obvious expansion in the IR regions. In *A. compactum* cp genome, the *ycf1* pseudogene is 2969 bp away from the IRa/SSC border, whereas in other Zingiberaceae species, it is only 4–5 bp away from the IRa/SSC border. Comparative cp genome sequences analysis of *A. compactum* with other Zingiberaceae reveals that the gene order and gene content differ slightly among Zingiberaceae species. The phylogenetic analysis based on 67 protein-coding gene sequences supports the phylogenetic position of *A. compactum*.

Conclusions: The study has identified unique features of the *A. compactum* cp genome which would be helpful for us to understand the cp genome evolution and offer useful information for phylogenetics and further studies of this traditional medicinal plant.

*Correspondence: xwli@icmm.ac.cn
[1] Institute of Chinese Materia Medica, China Academy of Chinese Medical Sciences, Dongcheng District, Dongzhimen Nanxiaojie within 16, Beijing 100700, China
Full list of author information is available at the end of the article

Keywords: *Amomum compactum*, Chloroplast genome, SSR, Phylogeny, High-throughput sequencing technology

Background

Chloroplasts can provide necessary energy for plants growth as photosynthetic organelles, which also participate in other major life activities such as starch storage, sugar synthesis and many critical biological metabolic pathways. As circular DNA molecules, cp genomes mainly vary from 120 to 160 kb in size with a typical quadripartite organization in angiosperms [1]. Two reverse complement copies of IR region (20–28 kb) separate the whole cp genome into a LSC region (80–90 kb) and a SSC region (16–27 kb) [2]. In angiosperms, cp genomes usually encode approximately 80 unique proteins, 30 tRNAs and four rRNAs. Previous studies have corroborated that cp gene order, gene content, and genome organization are highly conserved in plants [3, 4]. Owing to the high conservation and monolepsis, cp genomes are widely used in species identification, phyletic evolution studies and genetic engineering. The availability of whole cp genomes has helped to resolve phylogenetic relationships among major clades of angiosperms with greater accuracy [5, 6]. Nevertheless, with the number of cp genomes increasing, gene losses, structural rearrangements and IR contractions/expansions have been reported, which can also be exploited for the reconstruction of plant phylogenies [7–9].

Amomum compactum (genus *Amomum*, family Zingiberaceae) is one of the basic species of the traditional Chinese medicine *amomi fructus rotundus*, which is mainly produced in Vietnam and Thailand and is cultivated as a medicinal plant in the Guangdong, Guangxi and Yunnan provinces of China with great pharmacology effect. However, bacterial wilt, damping-off, leaf spot and other major plant diseases have become a severe obstacle for the introduction of this plant. Many plants belonging to the Zingiberaceae family are used as important seasoning and medicinal plants, such as *Zingiber officinale*, *Amomum villosum*, *Curcuma longa*, *Zingiber mioga*, *Elettaria cardamomum*, and *Alpinia officinarum*. In addition, previous studies have shown that the efficacy, chemical composition and pharmacological effects among the five genera of Zingiberaceae are strongly correlated. It is of great significance and broad interest to investigate the genetic relationships of traditional Chinese medicinal plants to find alternative medicinal plants. With the number of whole cp genomes in the Zingiberaceae increasing, the cp genome sequences of other species in Zingiberaceae are becoming easier to be assembled. However, studies of amomi fructus rotundus are scarce both inside and outside China, especially molecular studies.

This study reports the assembly, annotation and structural analysis of *A. compactum* cp genome for the first time. And to reveal the structure of this cp genome, we compare the organization (IR expansion/contraction and divergent regions) of complete cp genomes between *A. compactum* and other Zingiberaceae species. We also provide the result of phylogenetic analyses on basis of 67 protein-coding gene sequences from *A. compactum* and 14 monocot cp genomes.

Methods

DNA extraction and sequencing

Fresh *A. compactum* leaves were acquired from cultivated bases in Guangdong Province, China. The total cp DNA was extracted from roughly 100 g of leaves through an improved method by Li et al. [10]. The quality of cp DNA was checked by Nanodrop-2000 spectrometer (Nanodrop Technologies, Wilmington, DE, USA), and agarose gel electrophoresis. Pure cp DNA was used for shotgun library construction with 454 GS FLX Titanium platform. The obtained SFF file was preprocessed by trimming short (L < 50 bp) and low-quality (Q < 20) reads. Trimmed reads were assembled using Newbler V2.6 (GS FLX De Novo Assembler Software). In order to verify the assembly, the four junctional regions were further confirmed by Sanger sequencing.

Genome assembly and annotation

Preliminary gene annotation of this cp genome was performed by CpGAVAS, a program available online (http://www.herbalgenomics.org/0506/cpgavas) [11]. The position of each gene was then manually corrected by Apollo [12] after alignment to the reference genomes by MEGA 5.0. In addition, according to start and stop codons, minor revisions were performed. The tRNAs were further confirmed by the online tool tRNAscan-SE with default settings (http://lowelab.ucsc.edu/tRNAscan-SE/). [13]. Then, the circular map of this cp genome was accomplished by OrganellarGenomeDRAW program (http://ogdraw.mpimp-golm.mpg.de/) [14]. Finally, the complete cp genome of *A. compactum* was submitted to NCBI GenBank database.

Sequence analyses

Relative synonymous codon usage (RSCU) values, which were used to research the features of variations in synonymous and nonsynonymous codon usage by disregarding the composition impact of amino acid, were determined using MEGA 6.0 [15]. Additionally, GC content and

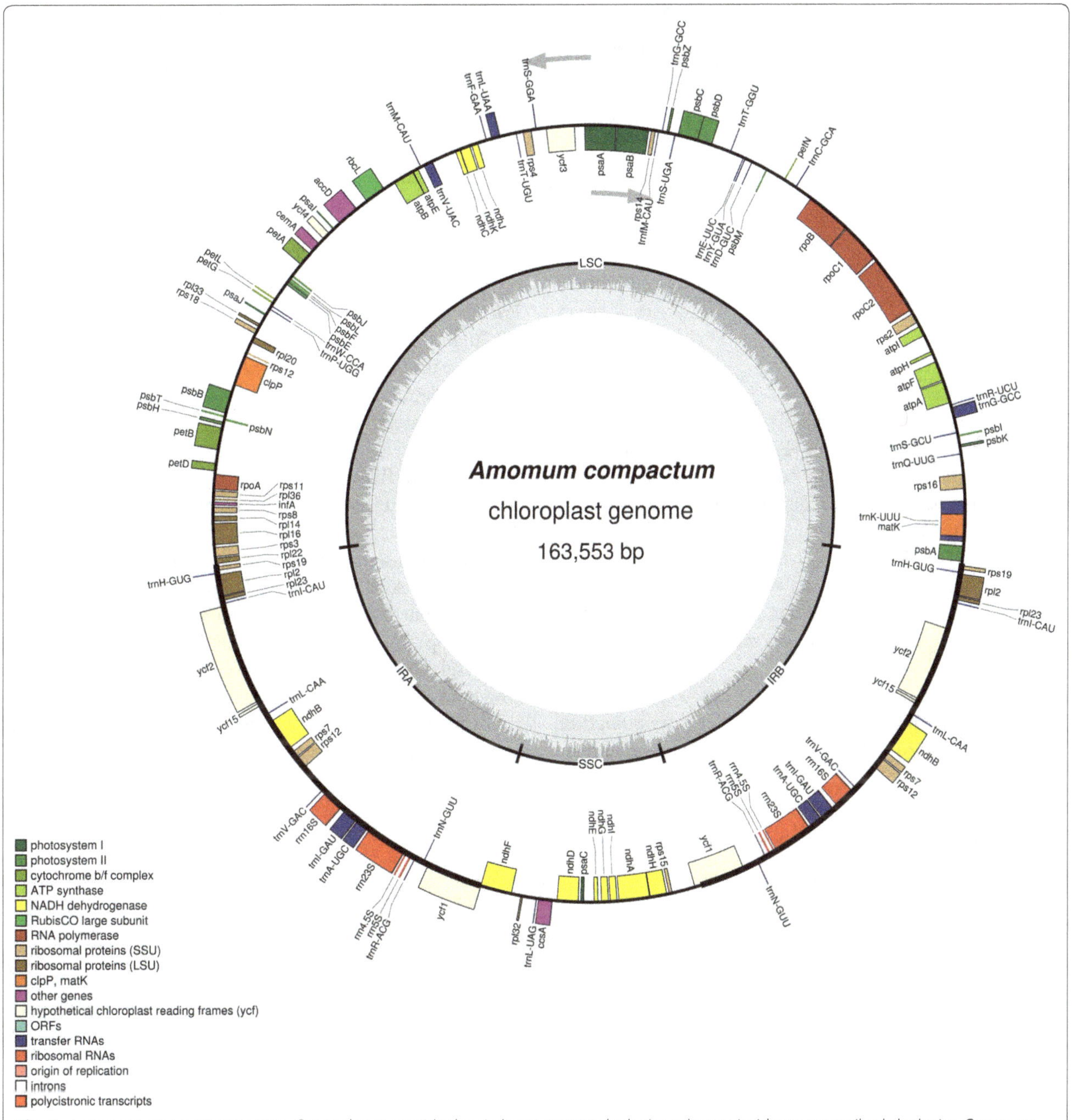

Fig. 1 *A. compactum* cp genome map. Genes drawn outside the circle are counterclockwise, whereas inside are transcribed clockwise. Genes are color-coded according to different functional groups. The darker gray represents GC content in the inner circle, conversely the lighter one represents AT content

codon usage were determined by MEGA 6.0. SSRs (simple sequence repeats) loci were detected by MISA software (http://pgrc.ipk-gatersleben.de/misa/), with following thresholds: ten, six, five, five, five, and five repeat units for mono-nucleotide, di-nucleotide, tri-nucleotide, tetra-nucleotide, penta-nucleotide, and hexa-nucleotide SSRs, respectively. To analyze the repeat structure, REPuter [16] (http://bibiserv.techfak.uni-bielefeld.de/reputer/) was performed to detect forward (direct) and palindromic (inverted) repeats in the cp genome. The minimum repeat unit was set to 30 bp in length, the identity of repeats was set to > 90%, and the Hamming distance equals three. All identified results were verified and redundant repeats were manually removed.

Table 1 Base composition in the *A. compactum* cp genome

	T(U)%	C%	A%	G%	Length (bp)
LSC	33.8	17.2	32.5	16.5	88,535
IR	28.8	19.8	30.1	21.3	29,824
SSC	34.3	15.6	35.9	14.2	15,370
Total	32.3	18.3	31.7	17.8	163,553
CDS	31.6	17.2	31.5	19.8	79,701
1st position	24	18.2	31.3	26.7	26,567
2nd position	32	20.2	30.0	17.4	26,567
3rd position	39	13.1	33.1	15.3	26,567

CDS protein-coding regions

Genome comparison

Pairwise alignments of several cp genome sequences were conducted by MUMmer [17], and the dot plots were drawn using a Perl script. The complete cp genomes of *A. compactum* and three other Zingiberaceae species (Additional file 1), *Curcuma flaviflora* (KR967361), *Curcuma roscoeana* (KF601574), and *Zingiber spectabile* (JX088661), were used for comparative analysis by mVISTA program (http://genome.lbl.gov/vista/index.shtml) [18] in Shuffle-LAGAN mode. *A. compactum* was set as the reference.

Phylogenomic analysis

To examine the phylogenetic position of *A. compactum*, 14 complete chloroplast genomes were downloaded from NCBI. The 67 shared protein-coding gene sequences were extracted using a Python script and aligned separately by ClustalW2. Phylogenetical trees were reconstructed based on 67 concatenated protein-coding gene sequences by MP and ML methods. The best-fitting model was filtrated by jModelTest 2.1.7 through the Akaike information criterion (AIC) [19]. The MP tree was reconstructed by PAUP ver. 4.0b10 [20] with a heuristic search, while ML analysis was calculated by RAxML-HPC 2.7.6.3 on XSEDE in the CIPRES Science Gateway (http://www.phylo.org/) with default parameters. Based on APGIII, *Fritillaria cirrhosa* was set as an outgroup. Both MP and ML analyses used 1000 bootstrap replicates.

The Minimum Standards of Reporting Checklist includes details of the experimental design, statistics, and resources used in this study.

Results and discussion

General characteristics of the *A. compactum* cp genome

The complete cp genome sequence of *A. compactum* is 163,553 bp in length with a obvious quadripartite structure (Fig. 1). A pair of inverted region (IR) with 29,824 bp in length partition the rest sequence into a LSC region (88,535 bp) and a SSC region (15,370 bp) (Table 1). The universal GC content of this cp sequence was 36.0%, which has been reported to act a significant role in evolution of genomic structures. Nevertheless, the overall GC content is unequally distributed across the cp genome,

Table 2 Gene content of the *A. compactum* cp genome

Gene category	Gene group	Gene name
Self-replication	rRNA genes	*rrn16*[c], *rrn23*[c], *rrn5*[c], *rrn4.5*[c]
	tRNA genes	*trnH-GUG*[c], *trnK-UUU*[a], *trnQ-UUG*, *trnS-GCU*, *trnC-GCA*, *trnD-GUC*, *trnY-GUA*, *trnE-UUC*, *trnR-UCU*, *trnT-GGU*, *trnS-UGA*, *trnG-GCC*[c], *trnfM-CAU*, *trnS-GGA*, *trnT-UGU*, *trnL-UAA*[a], *trnF-GAA*, *trnV-UAC*[a], *trnW-CCA*, *trnP-UGG*, *trnI-CAU*[c], *trnL-CAA*[c], *trnV-GAC*[c], *trnI-GAU*[a, c], *trnA-UGC*[a, c], *trnR-ACG*[c], *trnN-GUU*[c], *trnL-UAG*, *trnM-CAU*
	Small subunit of ribosome	*rps4*, *rps14*, *rps18*, *rps2*, *rps12*[b, c], *rps11*, *rps8*, *rps3*, *rps19*, *rps7*[c], *rps15*, *rps16*[a]
	Large subunit of ribosome	*rpl33*, *rpl20*, *rpl36*, *rpl14*, *rpl16*[a], *rpl22*, *rpl2*[a, c], *rpl23*[c], *rpl32*
	DNA dependent RNA polymerase	*rpoB*, *rpoC1*[a], *rpoC2*, *rpoA*
	Translational initiation factor	*infA*
Genes for photosynthesis	Subunits of NADH dehydrogenase	*ndhA*[a], *ndhB*[a, c], *ndhC*, *ndhD*, *ndhE*, *ndhF*, *ndhG*, *ndhH*, *ndhI*, *ndhJ*, *ndhK*
	Subunits of photosystem I	*psaA*, *psaB*, *psaC*, *psaI*, *psaJ*, *ycf3*[b], *ycf4*
	Subunits of photosystem II	*psbA*, *psbB*, *psbC*, *psbD*, *psbE*, *psbF*, *psbH*, *psbI*, *psbJ*, *psbK*, *psbL*, *psbM*, *psbN*, *psbT*, *psbZ*
	Subunits of cytochrome b/f complex	*petN*, *petA*, *petL*, *petG*, *petB*[a], *petD*
	Subunits of ATP synthase	*atpI*, *atpH*, *atpF*[a], *atpA*, *atpE*, *atpB*
	Large subunit of rubisco	*rbcL*
Genes of unknown function	Open reading frames (ORF, ycf)	*ycf1*, *ycf15*[c], *ycf2*[c]
	Pseudogenes	*ycf1*

[a] Gene with one intron

[b] Gene with two introns

[c] Gene with two copies

Table 3 Codon-anticodon recognition patterns and codon usage in the *A. compactum* cp genome

Amino acid	Codon	No.	RSCU	tRNA	Amino acid	Codon	Count	RSCU	tRNA
Phe	UUU	971	1.31		Tyr	UAU	811	1.57	
Phe	UUC	516	0.69	*trnF-GAA*	Tyr	UAC	221	0.43	*trnY-GUA*
Leu	UUA	892	1.96	*trnL-UAA*	Stop	UAA	48	1.66	
Leu	UUG	559	1.23	*trnL-CAA*	Stop	UAG	22	0.76	
Leu	CUU	567	1.25		His	CAU	519	1.6	
Leu	CUC	181	0.4		His	CAC	129	0.4	*trnH-GUG*
Leu	CUA	381	0.84	*trnL-UAG*	Gln	CAA	706	1.54	*trnQ-UUG*
Leu	CUG	151	0.33		Gln	CAG	210	0.46	
Ile	AUU	1146	1.47		Asn	AAU	989	1.55	
Ile	AUC	426	0.55	*trnI-GAU*	Asn	AAC	289	0.45	*trnN-GUU*
Ile	AUA	763	0.98	*trnI-CAU*	Lys	AAA	1114	1.49	*trnK-UUU*
Met	AUG	614	1	*trn(f)M-CAU*	Lys	AAG	383	0.51	
Val	GUU	521	1.45		Asp	GAU	875	1.64	
Val	GUC	159	0.44	*trnV-GAC*	Asp	GAC	192	0.36	*trnD-GUC*
Val	GUA	559	1.56	*trnV-UAC*	Glu	GAA	1125	1.53	*trnE-UUC*
Val	GUG	194	0.54		Glu	GAG	350	0.47	
Ser	UCU	598	1.74		Cys	UGU	232	1.56	
Ser	UCC	337	0.98	*trnS-GGA*	Cys	UGC	66	0.44	*trnC-GCA*
Ser	UCA	412	1.2	*trnS-UGA*	Stop	UGA	17	0.59	
Ser	UCG	182	0.53		Trp	UGG	452	1	*trnW-CCA*
Pro	CCU	442	1.62		Arg	CGU	365	1.37	*trnR-ACG*
Pro	CCC	202	0.74		Arg	CGC	86	0.32	
Pro	CCA	325	1.19	*trnP-UGG*	Arg	CGA	342	1.29	
Pro	CCG	120	0.44		Arg	CGG	113	0.43	
Thr	ACU	537	1.57		Arg	AGA	519	1.95	*trnR-UCU*
Thr	ACC	237	0.7	*trnT-GGU*	Arg	AGG	168	0.63	
Thr	ACA	433	1.27	*trnT-UGU*	Ser	AGU	430	1.25	
Thr	ACG	157	0.46		Ser	AGC	102	0.3	*trnS-GCU*
Ala	GCU	626	1.82		Gly	GGU	604	1.39	
Ala	GCC	203	0.59		Gly	GGC	141	0.33	*trnG-GCC*
Ala	GCA	434	1.26	*trnA-UGC*	Gly	GGA	714	1.65	
Ala	GCG	112	0.33		Gly	GGG	276	0.64	

RSCU relative synonymous codon usage

which is lowest in SSC region (29.8%) but highest in IR regions (41.1%), followed by LSC region (33.7%).

As shown in Fig. 1, the *A. compactum* cp genome totally encodes 135 functional genes, that 113 are unique, containing eighty protein-coding genes, twenty-nine tRNAs and four rRNAs (Table 2). Among the functional genes, all rRNAs, eight tRNAs and seven protein-coding genes are duplicated in IR regions. The LSC region includes 60 protein-coding genes and 21 tRNAs, whereas the SSC region includes 11 protein-coding genes and one tRNA gene. Among the protein-coding genes, 72 are single-copy, whereas eight are duplicated. Among the tRNA genes, 20 are single-copy genes and nine are duplicated. Among the 113 unique genes, 13 include one intron (eight protein-coding and five tRNAs) and three (*ycf3*, *clpP*, and *rps12*) include two introns (Table 2). Unusually, the *rps12* gene is trans-spliced, of which the 5′ end is situated in LSC region whereas two replicative 3′ ends are located in IRa and IRb regions respectively. What's more, the *ndhA* gene contains the longest intron region (1033 bp).

The protein-coding gene sequences are 79,701 bp in length, which comprise 26,567 codons. And the usage frequency of codon was counted and exhibited in Table 3. In protein-coding sequences (CDSs), the AT content are 55.3% at the first codon positions, 62.0% at the second codon positions and 72.1% at the third codon positions, respectively (Table 1). Most protein-coding genes in land plant cp genomes use the standard ATG as the initiation codon. However, in the *A. compactum* cp genome,

Table 4 Simple sequence repeats in the *A. compactum* cp genome

cpSSR ID	Repeat motif	Length (bp)	Start	End	Region	Annotation
1	(T)10	10	3975	3984	LSC	*trnK-UUU*
2	(A)10	10	4328	4337	LSC	
3	(TA)6	12	4900	4911	LSC	
4	(A)10	10	5287	5296	LSC	*rps16* intron
5	(A)11	11	6253	6263	LSC	
6	(TA)6	12	6609	6620	LSC	
7	(A)10	10	7204	7213	LSC	
8	(AT)6	12	7521	7532	LSC	
9	(A)10	10	7700	7709	LSC	
10	(T)12	12	8633	8644	LSC	
11	(A)13	13	14,885	14,897	LSC	
12	(T)10	10	17,474	17,483	LSC	
13	(A)10	10	19,831	19,840	LSC	*rpoC2*
14	(T)11	11	24,121	24,131	LSC	*rpoC1* intron
15	(A)10	10	28,802	28,811	LSC	
16	(A)15	15	29,013	29,027	LSC	
17	(A)11	11	30,868	30,878	LSC	
18	(T)10	10	35,129	35,138	LSC	
19	(TA)7	14	38,632	38,645	LSC	
20	(A)12	12	39,292	39,303	LSC	
21	(A)12	12	47,481	47,492	LSC	
22	(T)10	10	48,986	48,995	LSC	
23	(A)10	10	50,236	50,245	LSC	
24	(AT)7	14	50,395	50,408	LSC	
25	(T)10	10	51,829	51,838	LSC	
26	(T)11	11	52,709	52,719	LSC	
27	(ATA)5	15	54,345	54,359	LSC	
28	(A)11	11	54,562	54,572	LSC	
29	(T)10	10	58,778	58,787	LSC	
30	(T)11	11	59,269	59,279	LSC	
31	(A)12	12	60,919	60,930	LSC	
32	(T)10	10	61,621	61,630	LSC	
33	(AT)6	12	63,489	63,500	LSC	
34	(A)12	12	68,715	68,726	LSC	
35	(AT)10	20	69,266	69,285	LSC	
36	(T)10	10	70,716	70,725	LSC	
37	(A)10	10	72,600	72,609	LSC	*rps18*
38	(TA)7	14	74,094	74,107	LSC	*rps12* intron
39	(A)10	10	74,569	74,578	LSC	*clpP* intron
40	(T)11	11	74,845	74,855	LSC	*clpP* intron
41	(T)10	10	75,108	75,117	LSC	*clpP* intron
42	(T)10	10	75,572	75,581	LSC	*clpP* intron
43	(T)10	10	75,831	75,840	LSC	*clpP* intron
44	(A)10	10	79,177	79,186	LSC	
45	(AT)6	12	79,751	79,762	LSC	*petB* intron
46	(T)10	10	86,407	86,416	LSC	*rpl16* intron
47	(T)11	11	88,970	88,980	IRa	
48	(T)10	10	116,573	116,582	IRa	*ycf1*
49	(A)11	11	120,872	120,882	SSC	

Table 4 continued

cpSSR ID	Repeat motif	Length (bp)	Start	End	Region	Annotation
50	(T)11	11	121,055	121,065	SSC	
51	(A)11	11	128,865	128,875	SSC	*ndhA* intron
52	(T)10	10	129,188	129,197	SSC	*ndhA* intron
53	(AT)6	12	131,778	131,789	SSC	
54	(T)11	11	133,103	133,113	SSC	
55	(T)12	12	133,236	133,247	SSC	
56	(T)11	11	133,374	133,384	SSC	*ycf1*
57	(A)10	10	135,507	135,516	IRb	*ycf1*
58	(A)11	11	163,109	163,119	IRb	

Table 5 Long repeat sequences in *A. compactum* cp genome

ID	Repeat start 1	Type	Size (bp)	Repeat start 2	Mismatch (bp)	E value	Gene	Region
1	3990	P	34	3996	− 3	4.12E−06	*trnK-UUU* (intron)	LSC
2	8768	P	31	48,057	− 3	1.98E−04	IGS; *trnS-GGA*	LSC
3	10,522	F	30	39,347	− 3	7.15E−04	*trnG-GCC* (intron)	LSC
4	31,322	P	32	31,352	− 3	5.46E−05	IGS	LSC
5	32,991	F	30	33,020	− 3	7.15E−04	IGS	LSC
6	39,660	P	32	39,701	0	4.08E−10	IGS	LSC
7	41,551	F	58	43,775	− 3	7.54E−20	*psaB*; *psaA*	LSC
8	41,595	F	37	43,819	− 2	2.39E−09	*psaB*; *psaA*	LSC
9	63,481	P	31	126,101	− 3	1.98E−04	IGS	LSC; SSC
10	63,481	F	31	126,106	− 3	1.98E−04	IGS	LSC; SSC
11	63,487	F	32	69,264	− 3	5.46E−05	IGS	LSC
12	67,809	P	31	67,864	− 2	6.83E−06	IGS	LSC
13	71,632	F	30	71,659	0	6.53E−09	IGS	LSC
14	72,281	F	42	72,302	− 3	1.21E−10	*rps18*	LSC
15	91,249	F	46	91,299	− 1	2.10E−16	*trnI-CAU*; IGS	IRa
16	91,249	P	46	160,743	− 1	2.10E−16	*trnI-CAU*; IGS	IRa; IRb
17	91,299	P	46	160,793	− 1	2.10E−16	IGS	IRa; IRb
18	93,917	F	30	93,938	− 3	7.15E−04	*ycf2*	IRa
19	93,917	P	30	158,120	− 3	7.15E−04	*ycf2*	IRa; IRb
20	93,938	P	30	158,141	− 3	7.15E−04	*ycf2*	IRa; IRb
21	121,695	P	30	121,723	− 3	7.15E−04	IGS	SSC
22	158,122	F	30	158,143	− 3	7.15E−04	*ycf2*	IRb
23	160,743	F	46	160,793	− 1	2.10E−16	IGS	IRb
24	160,762	F	30	160,812	− 3	7.15E−04	IGS	IRb

F forward, *P* palindromic, *IGS* intergenic space

two genes use alternatives to ATG as start codon, as following: ATC for *ndhD* and ATA for *rpl2*. Relative synonymous codon usage (RSCU) is a statistics of uneven usage of synonymous and nonsynonymous codons in the coding sequences. An RSCU value < 1.00 indicates that the use of a codon is less frequent than expected, whereas a codon used more frequently will attain an RSCU value > 1.00. A total of 96.7% (29/30) of preferred synonymous codons, i.e., RSCU values > 1, end with A/U, whereas 90.6% (29/32) of non-preferred synonymous codons, i.e., RSCU values < 1, end with G/C. This codon usage pattern is similar with other reported cp genomes [21, 22], which might be driven by the high proportion of A/T. The usage of the start codon (ATG) and UGG (coding TRP) show no bias (RSCU value = 1).

Repeat and SSR analysis

SSRs are a class of tandemly repeated sequences that consists of 1–6 nucleotide repeat units. SSRs are important in plant typing and widely developed as molecular genetic markers for species identification. Total 58 SSRs loci were found in the *A. compactum* cp genome (Table 4), and 47 SSRs were only composed of A/T bases. Furthermore, 10 SSRs were composed of di-nucleotide (AT/TA) repeats, and one SSR was composed of trinucleotide (ATA) repeats. Obviously, the SSRs in the *A. compactum* cp genome were rich in A/T, which has been reported in many plant families [23–25]. Among these SSRs, 17 SSRs were situated in protein-coding genes and one was located in a tRNA gene. Furthermore, five were in coding regions and 12 in intronic regions. No tetra-, penta- or hexa-nucleotide repeats over 15 bp long was detected. REPuter allowed us to identify 24 repeats, including 13 forward and 11 palindromic repeats (Table 5). Almost all repeats were situated in the intronic and intergenic regions, although few of them were situated in protein-coding regions [26]. As reported in other genomes, the gene richest in repeats was *ycf2*, carrying two direct and two palindromic repeats.

IR expansion/contraction in the *A. compactum* cp genome

The variations of angiosperm cp genomes in length are mainly because of the contraction and expansion of boundary regions between the IR regions with single copy (SC) regions. A minute comparison of junctional regions between the IR and SC boundaries among *A. compactum*, *C. flaviflora*, *C. roscoeana*, and *Z. spectabile* is presented in Fig. 2. In addition, a size comparison of cp genome among the four Zingiberaceae species is shown in Additional file 2: Table S1. In spite of the alike lengths of IR regions in these four species (from 25,618 to 29,824 bp), few IR contractions/expansions were still detected. *rpl22*, *ycf1* and *rps19* pseudogenes with various lengths were situated in IRb/LSC or IRb/SSC boundaries. The borderline of the IRb/LSC junction was situated in left side of the *rps19* gene in examined cp genomes, except in *Z. spectabile*, which resulted from the contraction of the IRa region in the *Z. spectabile* cp genome. By contrast, the *ycf1* pseudogene was situated in the left side of the IRa-SSC border and was 4–5 bp away from the IRa-SSC borderline, except in the *A. compactum* cp genome. The size of the *ycf1* pseudogene was 918 bp in *A. compactum*, 1068 bp in *C. flaviflora* and *C. roscoeana*, and 924 bp in *Z. spectabile*. In addition, in the *A. compactum* cp genome, the *ycf1* pseudogene was 2969 bp away from the IRa-SSC borderline, that indicated the expansion of the IR region. The *trnH* gene was situated in LSC region, except in *Z. spectabile* cp genome, where it was situated in SSC region and was 136 bp away from the IRb-LSC borderline.

Comparison with other Zingiberaceae cp genomes

Three sequences representing the Zingiberaceae (*C. flaviflora*, *C. roscoeana* and *Z. spectabile*) were selected for comparison with *A. compactum*. Pairwise cp genome alignments between *A. compactum* and other three cp genomes regained a high degree of synteny (Additional file 3: Figure S1, Additional file 4: Figure S1

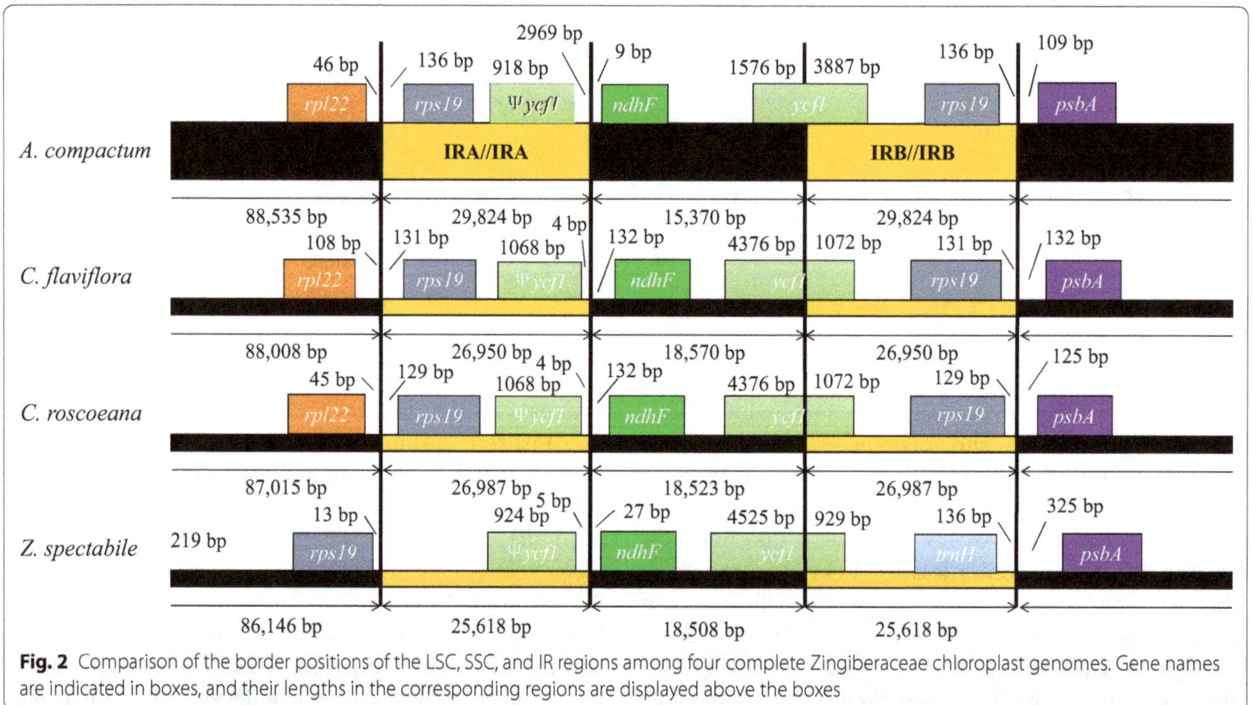

Fig. 2 Comparison of the border positions of the LSC, SSC, and IR regions among four complete Zingiberaceae chloroplast genomes. Gene names are indicated in boxes, and their lengths in the corresponding regions are displayed above the boxes

and Additional file 5: Figure S3). To detect the divergent regions in the cp genome, this study compared the sequence identities among four Zingiberaceae cp genomes by mVISTA, using the annotation of *A. compactum* as a reference. The multiple sequences alignment showed the coding regions are highly conserved, however the non-coding regions are divergent (Fig. 3). As an example, the intergenic sequences between the *trnT-GGU–psbD, rps16–trnQ-UUG, atpH–atpI, trnE-UUC–trnT-GGU, trnT-UGU–trnL-UAA, petA–psbL* and *psaC–ndhE* regions were highly divergent, parts of which have been also reported as divergent sequences in other plant. Obviously, the LSC region and SSC region were more divergent than IR regions.

Phylogenetic analysis

Cp genomes are widely employed in the study of evolution through phylogenetics. To examine the phylogenetic position of *A. compactum* and its relationship within Zingiberales, MP and ML phylogenetical analyses were performed based on 67 protein-coding gene sequences from 15 plant taxa, including *A. compactum*, as sequenced in the study. The total alignment was 51,452 bp in length. The results are presented in Figs. 4 and 5. The basic topologies were similar in the MP and ML analyses, but there were few differences. Bootstrap values were all extremely high, and nine of the 12 nodes with bootstrap values of ≥ 90% were found in MP tree, whereas eight of 12 nodes were found in ML tree with

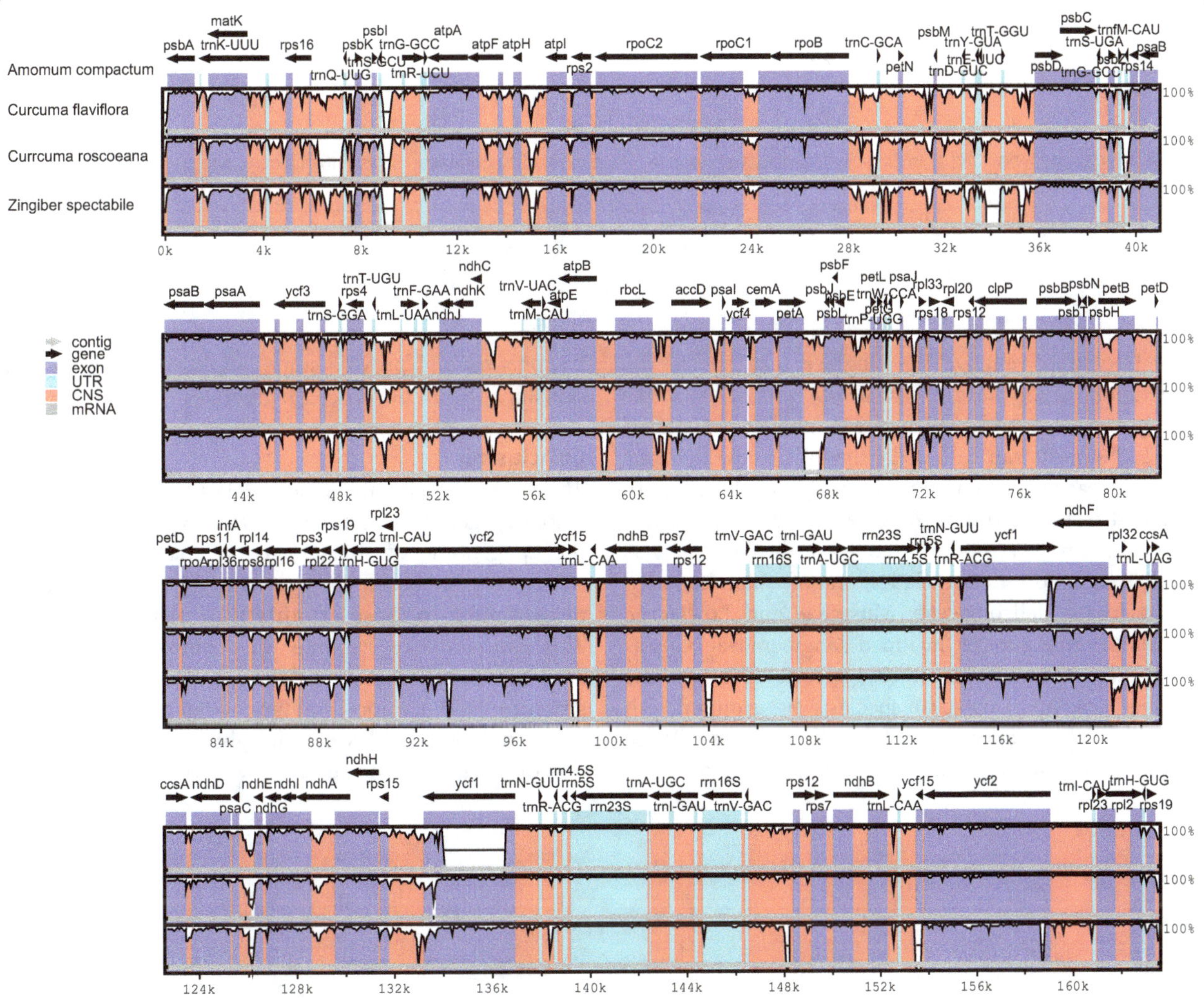

Fig. 3 Sequence comparison of the *A. compactum*, *C. flaviflora*, *C. roscoeana* and *Z. spectabile* cp genomes generated by mVISTA. Black lines designate regions of sequence identity by a 50% identity cutoff with *A. compactum*. Dashed rectangles indicate highly divergent regions of *A. compactum* compared with *C. flaviflora*, *C. roscoeana* and *Z. spectabile*

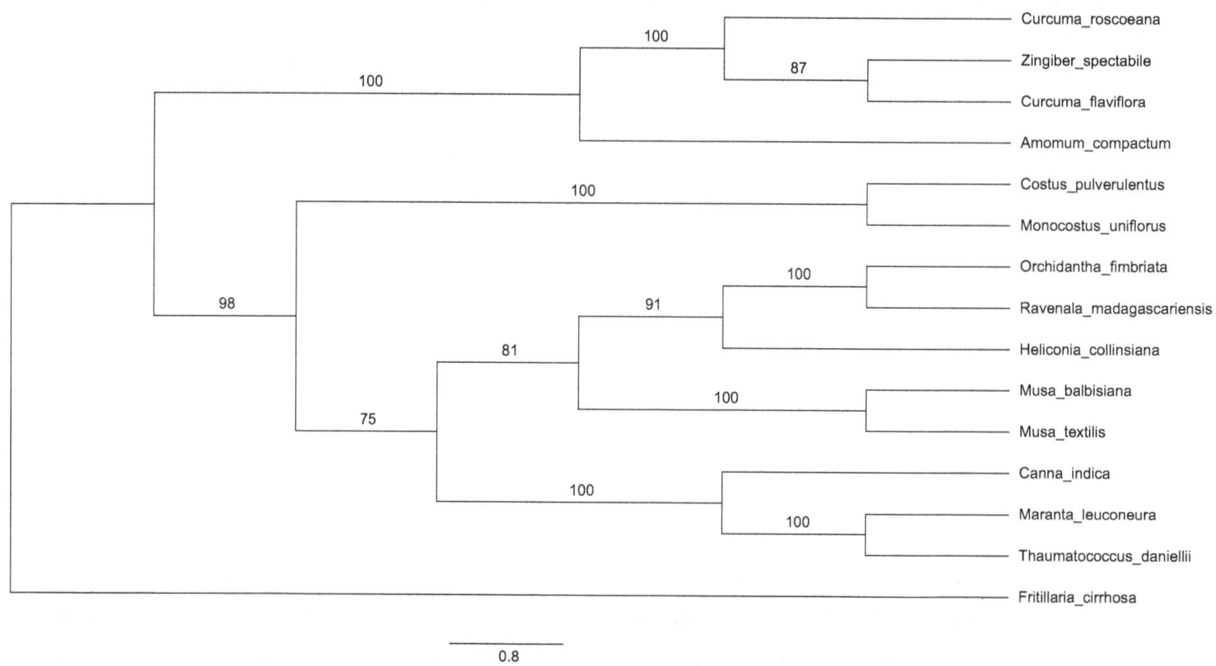

Fig. 4 MP phylogenetical tree of 15 Zingiberales species, on basis of 67 protein-coding gene sequences in the cp genomes. Bootstrap values are indicated upon the branches

100% bootstrap values. The Zingiberaceae species *A. compactum, C. flaviflora, C. roscoeana and Z. spectabile* were grouped in both MP and ML phylogenetic trees with 100% bootstrap values. In the MP trees, the four Zingiberaceae species composed a unique clade and were separated from the rest of Zingiberales with high bootstrap values in every node. By contrast, the ML tree was mainly separated into two clades, one of which included Strelitziaceae, Heliconiaceae, Musaceae and Lowiaceae species, whereas another included Zingiberaceae, Costaceae, Cannaceae and Marantaceae species. However, the Zingiberaceae and Costaceae species were grouped with a very low bootstrap value (15%) in the ML tree. These phylogenetic results strongly support the position of *A. compactum* and provide some helpful hints about relationships within the order Zingiberales.

Conclusion

The research assembled, annotated and analyzed the whole cp genome of *A. compactum*, which reveals that the cp genome of *A. compactum* shares a quadruple structure, gene order, GC content, and codon usage features, similar to those of other land plant cp genomes. This *Amomum* cp genome was compared with three available Zingiberaceae cp genomes, while the genome structure and composition are similar. Also phylogenetic analysis provides new insight into phyletic evolution of this genus. Our research will contribute to species

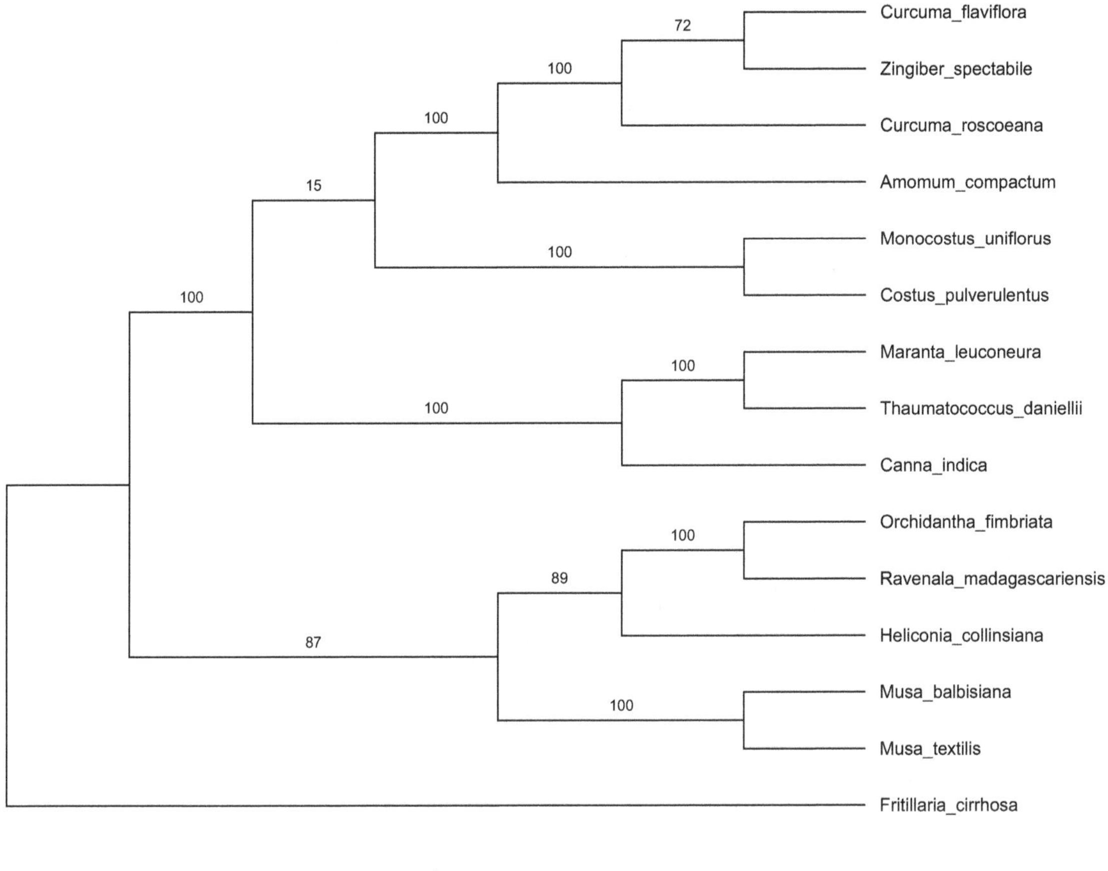

Fig. 5 ML phylogenetical tree of 15 Zingiberales species, on basis of 67 protein-coding gene sequences in the cp genome. Bootstrap values are indicated upon the branches

identification and evolutionary mechanisms required for the further study of *A. compactum.*

Additional files

Additional file 1. Minimum Standards of Reporting Checklist.

Additional file 2: Table S1. Size comparison of *A. compactum* cp genomic regions with those of 3 other Zingiberaceae cp genomes.

Additional file 3: Figure S1. Chloroplast genomic alignment between *A. compactum* and *C. flaviflora* (KR967361).

Additional file 4: Figure S2. Chloroplast genomic alignment between *A. compactum* and *C. roscoeana* (KF601574).

Additional file 5: Figure S3. Chloroplast genomic alignment between *A. compactum* and *Z. spectabile* (JX088661).

Abbreviations

cp: chloroplast; LSC: large single copy; SSC: small single copy; IR: inverted repeat; tRNA: transfer RNA; rRNA: ribosomal RNA.

Authors' contributions

XL and JX initiated the research, MW and QL drafted the paper and processed the data, XL supervised the task, the above authors analysed the results and reviewed the manuscript. All authors read and approved the final manuscript.

Author details

[1] Institute of Chinese Materia Medica, China Academy of Chinese Medical Sciences, Dongcheng District, Dongzhimen Nanxiaojie within 16, Beijing 100700, China. [2] Pharmacy Faculty, Hubei University of Chinese Medicine, No. 1, Huangjiahu West Road, Hongshan District, Wuhan 430065, Hubei, China. [3] Department of Pharmacy, Changzheng Hospital, Second Military Medical University, No. 415 Fengyang Road, Huangpu District, Shanghai 200003, China.

Acknowledgements

All authors thank Dr. Shi-Lin Chen for his helps on group discussion and manuscript polishing.

Competing interests

The authors declare that they have no competing interests.

Consent for publication
Not applicable.

Funding
This work is supported by the grants from the National Key Technology Support Program (2015BAI05B02) and from the China Academy of Chinese Medical Sciences Special Fund for Thirteen-five key research (ZZ10-007).

References

1. Bendich AJ. Circular chloroplast chromosomes: the grand illusion. Plant Cell Online. 2004;16:1661–6.
2. Chumley TW, Palmer JD, Mower JP, Fourcade HM, Calie PJ, et al. The complete chloroplast genome sequence of *Pelargonium hortorum*: organization and evolution of the largest and most highly rearranged chloroplast genome of land plants. Mol Biol Evol. 2006;23:2175–90.
3. Palmer JD. Plastid chromosomes: structure and evolution. In: Bogorad L, Vasil I, editors. Cell culture and somatic cell genetics of plants. San Diego: Academic Press; 1991. p. 5–53.
4. Raubeson LA, Jansen RK. Chloroplast genomes of plants. In: Henry RJ, editor. Plant diversity and evolution: genotypic and phenotypic variation in higher plants. Cambridge: CAB International; 2005. p. 45–68.
5. Jansen RK, Cai Z, Raubeson LA, Daniell H, dePamphilis CW, et al. Analysis of 81 genes from 64 plastid genomes resolves relationships in angiosperms and identifies genome-scale evolutionary patterns. Proc Natl Acad Sci. 2007;104:19369–74.
6. Givnish TJ, Ames M, McNeal JR, McKain MR, Steele PR, et al. Assembling the tree of the monocotyledons: plastome sequence phylogeny and evolution of Poales. Ann Mo Bot Gard. 2010;97:584–616.
7. Millen RS, Olmstead RG, Adams KL, Palmer JD, Lao NT, et al. Many parallel losses of infA from chloroplast DNA during angiosperm evolution with multiple independent transfers to the nucleus. Plant Cell Online. 2001;13:645–58.
8. Guisinger M, Chumley T, Kuehl J, Boore J, Jansen R. Implications of the plastid genome sequence of Typha (Typhaceae, Poales) for understanding genome evolution in Poaceae. J Mol Evol. 2010;70:149–66.
9. Downie SR, Palmer JD. Use of chloroplast DNA rearrangements in reconstructing plant phylogeny. In: Soltis PS, Soltis DE, Doyle JJ, editors. Molecular systematics of plants. New York: Chapman and Hall; 1992. p. 14–35.
10. Li X-W, Hu Z-G, Lin X-H, Li Q, Gao H-H, Luo G-A, et al. High-throughput pyrosequencing of the complete chloroplast genome of Magnolia officinalis and its application in species identification. Acta Pharm Sin. 2012;47:124–30.
11. Liu C, Shi LC, Zhu YJ, Chen HM, Zhang JH, Lin XH, et al. CpGAVAS, an integrated web server for the annotation, visualization, analysis, and GenBank submission of completely sequenced chloroplast genome sequences. BMC Genom. 2012;13:715.
12. Lewis SE, Searle SMJ, Harris N, Gibson M, Iyer V, Richter J, et al. Apollo: a sequence annotation editor. Genome Biol. 2002. https://doi.org/10.1186/gb-2002-3-12-research0082.
13. Lowe TM, Eddy SR. tRNAscan-SE: a program for improved detection of transfer RNA genes in genomic sequence. Nucleic Acids Res. 1997;25:0955–64.
14. Lohse M, Drechsel O, Kahlau S, Bock R. OrganellarGenomeDRAW—a suite of tools for generating physical maps of plastid and mitochondrial genomes and visualizing expression data sets. Nucl Acids Res. 2013;41(Web Server issue):W575.
15. Tamura K, Peterson D, Peterson N, Stecher G, Nei M, Kumar S. MEGA5: molecular evolutionary genetics analysis using maximum likelihood, evolutionary distance, and maximum parsimony methods. Mol Biol Evol. 2011;28:2731–9.
16. Kurtz S, Choudhuri JV, Ohlebusch E, Schleiermacher C, Stoye J, Giegerich R. REPuter: the manifold applications of repeat analysis on a genomic scale. Nucleic Acids Res. 2001;29:4633–42.
17. Kurtz S, Phillippy A, Delcher AL, Smoot M, Shumway M, Antonescu C, et al. Versatile and open software for comparing large genomes. Genome Biol. 2004;5:1–9.
18. Mayor C, Brudno M, Schwartz JR, Poliakov A, Rubin EM, Frazer KA, et al. VISTA: visualizing global DNA sequence alignments of arbitrary length. Bioinformatics. 2000;16:1046–7.
19. Posada D. jModelTest: phylogenetic model averaging. Mol Biol Evol. 2008;25:1253–6.
20. Swofford DL. PAUP*. Phylogenetic analysis using parsimony (*and other methods). Version 4.0b10. Sunderland: Sinauer Associates; 2003.
21. Tangphatsornruang S, Sangsrakru D, Chanprasert J, Uthaipaisanwong P, Yoocha T, Jomchai N, et al. The chloroplast genome sequence of mungbean (*Vigna radiata*) determined by high-throughput pyro-sequencing: structural organization and phylogenetic relationships. DNA Res. 2010;17:1–22.
22. Qian J, Song J, Gao H, Zhu Y, Xu J, Pang X, et al. The complete chloroplast genome sequence of the medicinal plant Salvia miltiorrhiza. PLoS ONE. 2013;8:e57607.
23. Yi D, Kim K. Complete chloroplast genome sequences of important oilseed crop *Sesamum indicum* L. PLoS ONE. 2012;7:e35872.
24. Melotto-Passarin D, Tambarussi E, Dressano K, De Martin V, Carrer H. Characterization of chloroplast DNA microsatellites from Saccharum spp. and related species. Genet Mol Res. 2011;10:2024–33.
25. Martin G, Baurens FC, Cardi C, Aury JM, D'Hont A. The complete chloroplast genome of banana (*Musa acuminata*, Zingiberales): insight into plastid monocotyledon evolution. PLoS ONE. 2013;8:e67350.
26. Yang Y, Dang YY, Li Q, Lu JJ, Li XW, Wang YT. Complete chloroplast genome sequence of poisonous and medicinal plant *Datura stramonium*: organizations and implications for genetic engineering. PLoS ONE. 2014;9(11):e110656.

2

Application of delayed luminescence method on measuring of the processing of Chinese herbal materials

Mengmeng Sun[1,5†], Wen-Te Chang[2†], Eduard Van Wijk[4,6], Min He[1], Roeland Van Wijk[4,6] and Mei Wang[1,3*]

Abstract

Background: Based on the principle of tradition Chinese medicine, the processing refers to various techniques that alter the overall properties of herbal materials to meet the requirements of therapeutic applications. However, the standards of quality control and scientific standard operation protocol for processing manufacturing are largely unknown and there is a huge demand for the development of scientific tools for evaluating the quality during and after the processing. The key challenge in evidence-based medicine is to characterize the processing of herbal materials from system-based perspective.

Methods: Delayed luminescence (DL) as a rapid, direct, systemic tool was used to characterize the properties of raw and processed materials of Rehmanniae radix and Ginseng radix et rhizome. Hyperbolic function was used to extract four parameters from DL curves of herbal materials. Statistical tools, including one-way analysis of variance and principal component analysis, were used to differentiate raw and processed herbal materials.

Results: Our results showed DL properties were able to reliably identify raw and processed materials of Rehmanniae radix and Ginseng radix et rhizoma, respectively. In addition, the results indicated that after four cycles of processing for Rehmanniae radix, there was no much significant change in DL parameters which resembles the results obtained from chemical analyses (after five cycles) using ^{1}HNMR and gas chromatography–mass spectrometry in previous studies.

Conclusion: DL may serve as a fast, robust and sensitive tool for evaluating processing on herbs and may be used as part of a comprehensive platform for assessing the quality of herbal materials.

Keywords: Delayed luminescence, Chinese herbal medicine, Processing, Quality control

Background

In Chinese herbal medicine (CHM), the processing refers to various techniques that alter the properties of herbal materials to meet the requirements of therapeutic applications [1, 2]. It includes basic methods such as removing impurities, washing, cutting, drying, as well as steaming, boiling, calcining and stir frying of herbal materials to increase solubility, remove unpleasant smells, reduce toxicity, decrease side-effects, enhance the pharmacological efficacy and stabilized, and modify the therapeutic property [1, 2]. Based on the principle of Chinese medicine, pharmaceutical actions of CHM are traditionally classified according to the patient's responses, resulting in descriptive properties of herbal materials such as taste and warm/cold [3]. Processing has a close relationship with the therapeutic properties. For example, according to Chinese medicine principle, raw Rehmanniae radix is considered to have "sweet and bitter" with "cold" properties and can be used to treat "heat" syndromes; but the processed Rehmanniae radix has been provided with "sweet" and "warm" properties and can be used to treat "cold" syndromes [4]. In addition, white Ginseng radix et

*Correspondence: M.wang@biology.leidenuniv.nl
†Mengmeng Sun and Wen-Te Chang contributed equally to this work
1 Leiden University European Center for Chinese Medicine and Natural Compounds, Institute of Biology, Leiden University, Sylviusweg 72, 2333 BE Leiden, The Netherlands
Full list of author information is available at the end of the article

rhizoma is considered to have the property "warm", but this property may be enhanced in its processed product named red Ginseng radix et rhizome [5]. The different therapeutic properties of these herbs are also recognized in the Chinese Pharmacopoeia 2015 to the extent that there are now separate monographs for raw and processed Rehmannie radix, as well as white and red Ginseng radix et rhizoma, reflecting their differences in therapeutic applications [5, 6]. Moreover, modern research has indicated that chemical components can be changed by processing and then may induce different therapeutic properties in these herbal materials [6, 7].

In current CHM practice, almost all the herbal materials are strictly required to be properly processed before using for therapeutic applications. Yet, the standards of quality control and scientific standard operation protocol for processing manufacturing are largely unknown and there is a huge demand for the development of scientific tools for fast, robust and sensitive measurements for evaluating the quality during and after the processing. There is a common concept to the processing of herbal materials in CHM: "obeying ancient processing methods" [1, 2]. For instance, the ancient method of "steam with rice wine nine times and dry nine times" was emphasized in the processing of Rehmanniae radix [4]. However, the ancient methods may not suit to modern industrial production and the processing methods for many herbal materials have been already changed [1, 2]. Since lack of objective criteria, non-unified standards are still existed in practice in different locations of China, and the technology of CHM processing mainly depends on the practitioner's experiences. Therefore, to develop the tools of quality control for herbal materials processing are urgently needed. As a conventional method, chemical analysis is the most common method and has provided many important information to help the quality assessment on CHM processing. For instance, Chang and colleagues have reported that the modification of therapeutic properties of processed Rehmanniae radix was related to the changes of metabolic profiling during the processing [4]. In addition, Raman, mid-infrared and near-infrared spectroscopy as non-destructive and fast measurement tools have been used to discriminated raw and processed plant materials [8–10]. Given the overall changes in CHM processing, comprehensive, systemic and rapid method for quality assessment of CHM processing are still worth to further investigate.

Recently, various luminescence related technologies are widely used in the mechanism of disease research and drug quality control [11–17]. Delayed luminescence (DL) is the long-term decay of weak photon emissions from materials following exposure to light with a wavelength of 400–800 nm [3]. DL provides a comprehensive method for measuring biological systems, including food quality and seed germination [18, 19]. Recently, we used DL to study the features of Chinese herbal materials. The results suggest that specific DL properties can be used to indicate differences in herbal materials prepared under different conditions, including the age of the herb, the grown environments [20, 21]. These differences in DL properties reflect variations in both the bioactive components contained in the herb and the therapeutic properties of herbal materials. Importantly, in our preliminary results, DL was used to distinguish the Acunitum roots (*Aconitum carmichaelii* Debx.) materials processed by different methods [21]. In this study, we measured DL between raw and processed Rehmanniae radix, as well as white and red Ginseng radix et rhizoma in order to further investigate the application of DL in the quality control of CHM processing. The results obtained from our DL measurements show DL properties can indicate the changes in processing of these herbal materials; therefore, DL can provide new insights into the processing of herbal medicines.

Methods

Information of experimental design and resources

The information regarding the experimental design, statistics, and resources used in this study are attached in the minimum standards of reporting checklist (Additional file 1).

Herbal materials

Raw roots of Rehmannia (*Rehmannia glutinosa* Libosch.) were provided by China Medical University (Taichung, Taiwan). For preparing processed Rehmanniae radix, the raw roots were dried in an oven at 55 °C, then the dried roots were soaked in yellow rice wine (Michiu, Taiwan Tobacco & Liquor Corp., Taipei, Taiwan) for 15 min, and steamed with water for 60 min. After that, the processed Rehmanniae radix was dried overnight at 55 °C [4]. This procedure was repeated for nine times to obtain processed Rehmanniae radix from one to nine cycles, respectively [4]. Roots and rhizomes of white and red Ginseng (*Panax Ginseng* C. A. Mey.) were purchased in five batches from TongRenTang Co., Ltd. (Beijing, China). The identities of all herbal samples were verified by Dr. Wen-Te Chang (China Medical University) and were deposited at China Medical University (Taichung, Taiwan).

Delayed luminescence

Sample preparation

Each herbal material was crushed using a model QE-100 grinder (Yili Company, Zhejiang Province, China) and passed through a standard sieve to obtain 150-μm particle. All the herbal materials were kept in a dark, light–tight box containing 35-mm silica gel (Boom BV, Meppel, the Netherlands) at room temperature for 16 h before DL measurements were conducted [21].

DL measurement

The procedure to perform DL measurements was described previously [21]. The equipment used to measure DL was provided from Meluna Research (Geldermalsen, the Netherlands) and included a photomultiplier tube (PMT) (type 9558QB; Electron Tubes Enterprises Ltd., Ruislip, UK) vertically positioned on a dark sample chamber kept at 22 °C. The PMT contains a cathode end (51 mm diameter) with sensitivity at 300–800 nm. The PMT was cooled to −25 °C in order to reduce the dark count rate to 10 counts per second. The DL signal was amplified using a type 9301 fast preamplifier (ORTEC, Oak Ridge, TN). Data were acquired using a personal computer containing a model 6602 counting card (National Instruments, Austin, TX).

Each Rehmanniae radix sample was used to prepare five 1-g samples. Each 1-g sample was placed in a Petri dish (35-mm diameter) and illuminated for 10 s using a model 284-2812 white halogen excitation source (Philips, Germany). For each 1-g sample, the DL signal was measured three consecutive times, resulting in a total of fifteen measurements in the five samples to examine the DL properties of that particular Rehmanniae radix. Each batch of Ginseng radix et rhizoma (1 g) was placed in a Petri dish and illuminated for 10 s using the same white halogen light source, then measured three consecutive times, and a total of fifteen measurements in five batches were used to examine the DL properties of that particular Ginseng materials. The DL decay signature was obtained by recording the number of photon counts in consecutive 0.05-s periods for a total of 60 s, yielding a total of 1200 data points.

Data processing and statistical analysis

The DL decay curve for each sample, measured over a 60-s period, was fitted to the following hyperbolic function [22]:

$$I_{(t)} = \frac{I_0}{\left(1 + \frac{t}{Tau}\right)^{Beta}}$$

$$T = \left(e^{\frac{1}{Beta}} - 1\right) \times Tau$$

where I_0 is the initial intensity of the DL curve, Beta is an index factor associated with the rate of DL decay, and Tau and T represents the DL characteristics and decay time, respectively [22]. The R package nnet (version 3.2.2) was used to perform the DL curve-fitting [23]. The average of each DL property from the fifteen measurements was calculated and used to represent the DL signature of each herbal material. One-way analysis of variance (ANOVA) with least significant difference (LSD) post hoc analysis was used to compare the DL properties between raw and processed Rehmanniae radix; differences were considered significant at $p < 0.05$. Principal component analysis (PCA) and Orthogonal projections to latent structures discriminant analysis (OPLS-DA) was used to indicate the level of discrimination between DL properties in Rehmanniae radix samples, using the tools provided in the MetaboAnalyst software package (http://www.metaboanalyst.ca) [24]. A two-tailed, unpaired Student's t test (SPSS version 23.0) was used to compare the DL properties between white and red Ginseng radix et rhizoma; differences were considered significant at $p < 0.05$.

Results

According to the ancient description for the processing of Rehmanniae radix, "steaming and drying for nine cycles", has been regarded as the standard method [4]. More scientific studies need to be established to understand the working principle of this type of processing. Previous studies suggested that differences in chemical profiles of processed Rehmanniae radix became smaller after five processing cycles (Additional file 2: Fig. S1) [4, 25, 26]. In this study, DL has been used to measure raw and processed Rehmanniae radix samples in order to investigate the processing approach. We pooled the data from fifteen measurements to plot DL decay curves in specific Rehmanniae radix samples. Figure 1 illustrates the different DL kinetics of Rehmanniae radix samples using a log–log scale (A linear scale in Additional file 3: Fig. S2). Raw Rehmanniae radix samples show significantly different DL curves compared with processed materials, and differences generally become smaller after multiple

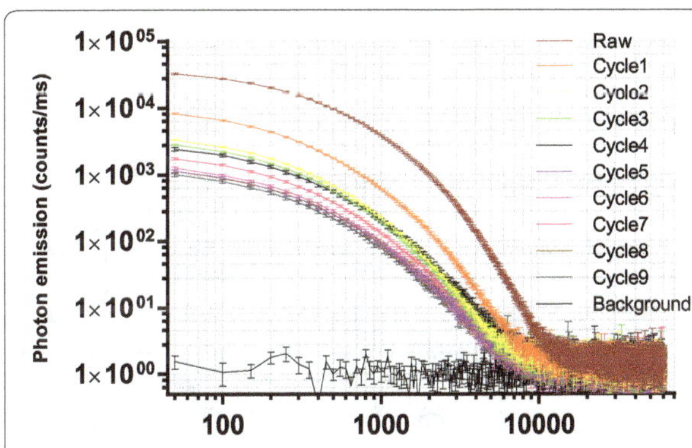

Fig. 1 DL decay curves for pooled samples from Rehmanniae radix samples. Data are plotted as the mean ± SEM. Note that the data are plotted on a log–log scale

processing. The DL spectra of Rehmanniae radix samples are illustrated using raw material as an example in Additional file 4: Fig. S3. Next, four parameters were derived from these DL curves, these four parameters were compared between all Rehmanniae radix samples using a one-way ANOVA. The results are summarized in Fig. 2. Figure 2 reveals that all four parameters (T, I_0, Beta and Tau) can be used to differentiate between raw and processed Rehmanniae radix samples. Only I_0 can be used to distinguish between cycle 1 and the other cycles in processed Rehmanniae radix samples. To further display the differences between processed Rehmanniae radix samples in DL properties, an unsupervised PCA approach was used to obtain a focused view of the variance in the four DL parameters. Figure 3a shows the PCA score plot using the four DL parameters in which PC1 and PC2 account for 64% and 27.3% of the total variance, respectively. This plot shows that the DL properties of the first three processed cycles and the last six processed cycles generally form distinct clusters, with the seventh processed cycle misclassified as belonging to the group on the left side of Fig. 3a. Therefore, a supervised clustering approach (OPLS-DA; Fig. 3b) was further performed to make the optimal separation. OPLS-DA evaluation with cross-validation revealed predictive accuracy of 0.88 and goodness-of-fit (R^2) of 0.93. The results obtained from the OPLS-DA analysis revealed a better classification effect compared to the results obtained from the PCA analysis. The data show that the differences in DL properties of processed Rehmanniae radix became smaller after the fourth processing cycle. Thus, DL shows similarities in identified effects to indicate the processing of Rehmanniae radix compared to chemical analyses (Additional file 2: Fig. S1) [4, 25, 26].

As a next step for further examination of the identification effects of DL in herbal materials processing, commercial white and red Ginseng radix et rhizoma were studied. The DL spectra of Ginseng samples are summarized in Additional file 4: Fig. S3. The significant differences in most DL parameters were found between white and red Ginseng radix et rhizome (Fig. 4), which

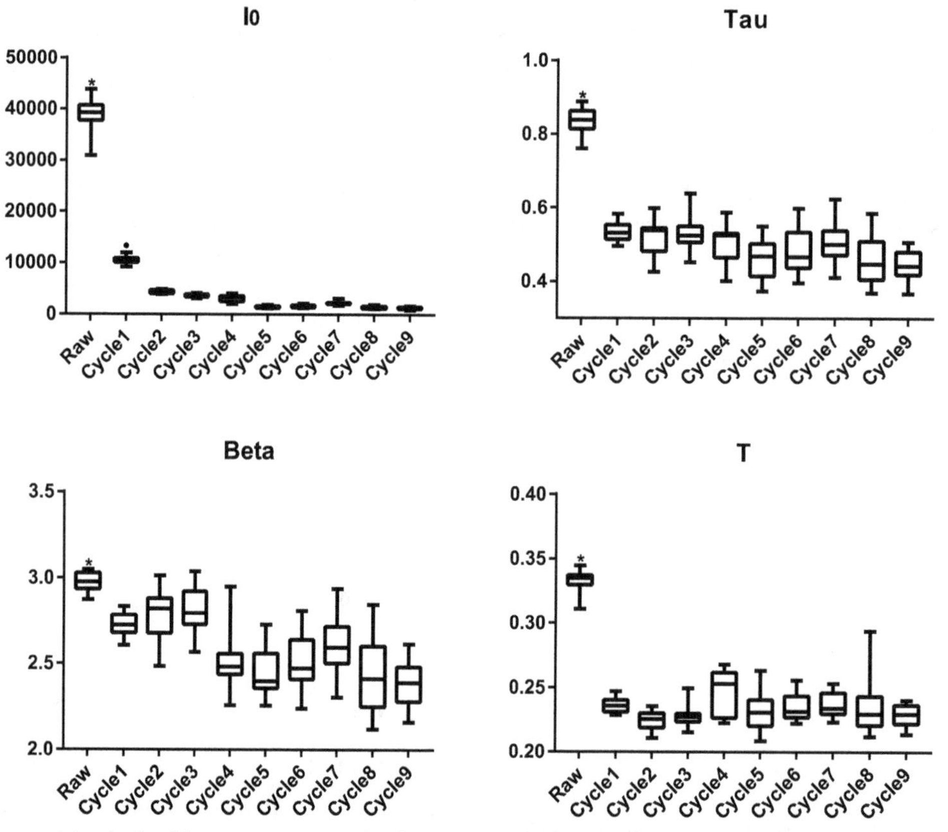

Fig. 2 Box plot summarizing the four DL properties measured in the Rehmanniae radix samples. I0 is the initial intensity of the DL curve, Beta is an index factor associated with the rate of DL decay, and Tau and T represents the DL characteristics and decay time, respectively. *$p < 0.05$ between raw material and all materials in processing cycles; ●$p < 0.05$ between material in processing cycle 1 and materials in the other processing cycles (one-way ANOVA with LSD)

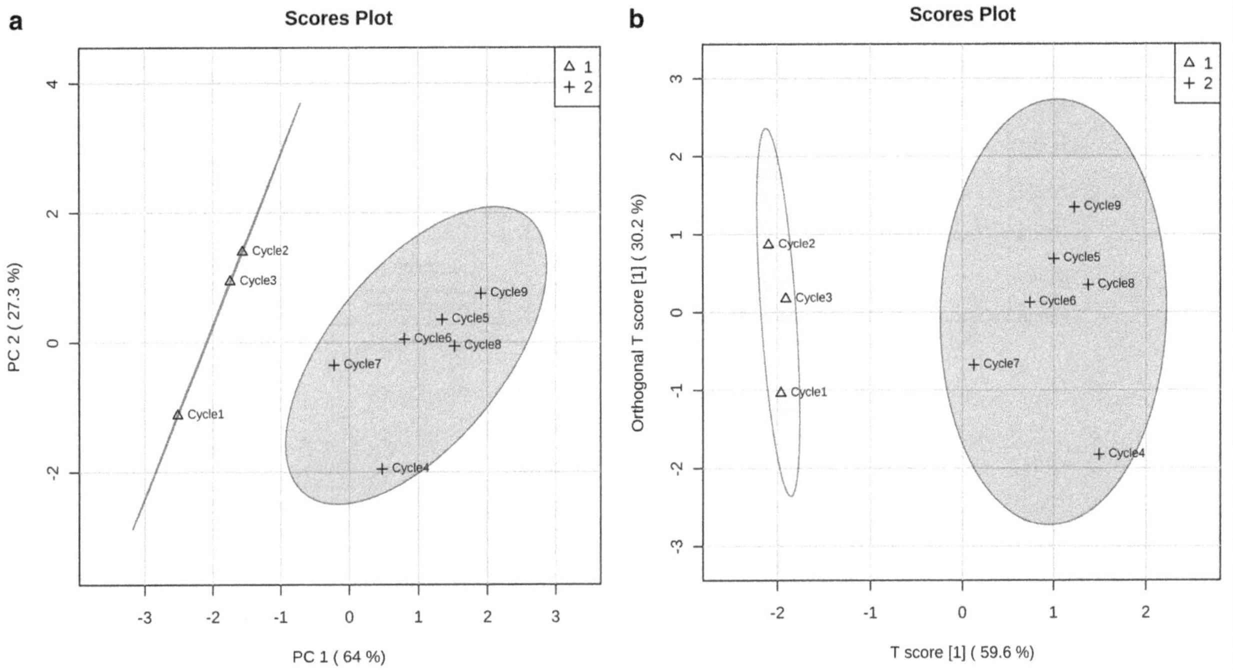

Fig. 3 PCA and OPLS-DA scores obtained from the DL data. **a** PCA and **b** OPLS-DA score plots of the DL data obtained from processed Rehmanniae radix samples, showing two separated clusters. The separated clusters were marked with a "△" (cluster 1) or a "+" (cluster 2) symbol, in which cycles 1–3 belongs to one cluster and cycles 4–9 belongs to another cluster

indicates DL may be suitable in measurements for more processed herbal materials.

Discussion

Our data indicates that DL may reflect the changes caused by processing in Rehmanniae radix and Ginseng radix et rhizoma. The molecular absorption of excitation energy determines the dynamics of the subsequent DL emission [27]. DL properties can be influenced by changes of molecular conformations and interactions such as forming of hydrogen bonds and carbon-to-nitrogen ratio [20, 21], resulting in the radiant transfer of energy from one excited molecule to another, causing a change in the herb's DL kinetics [3]. Processing can lead to significant chemical changes [28]. For example, Rehmanniae radix is rich in polysaccharides, which can be hydrolyzed to monosaccharides (e.g. galactose and glucose) during the processing [4]. In addition, the contents of catalpol, raffinose, and stachyose gradually decrease by processing in Rehmanniae radix [4]. Moreover, changes in concentration of acidic polysaccharides and structural conversions of ginsenosides are detected in white and red Ginseng radix et rhizome [6]. Since these primary and secondary metabolites in Rehmanniae radix and Ginseng radix et rhizoma can interact with molecular conformations and interactions in an overall level [29], the DL properties show significant changes during processing. Interestingly, DL properties of processed Rehmanniae radix can be classified in PCA and OPLS-DA analyses. It indicates that the DL characteristics became stable after the fourth processing cycle. This result is similar with previous chemical analyses which indicated that the chemical components were stable after the fifth processing cycle using plant metabolomics tools such as ^{1}HNMR and gas chromatography–mass spectrometry (GC–MS) [4, 25, 26]. Plant metabolomics provides a relatively comprehensive analysis of various compounds in biological systems based on specific platforms [30], and it has been considered as a suitable tool for herb quality control in a system level [31]. Similar to plant metabolomics, DL is a highly sensitive systemic measurement that reflects the overall properties of a biological system [32, 33]. Therefore, DL can provide a close approximation of the system level structures identified by using plant metabolomics. However, metabolomics analyses are not able to evaluate the entire integral profile of chemical components since diversity of various molecular and the limitation in measurement technology platforms. In contrast, DL can measure directly the herbal materials and reflect systemic properties of herbs. Therefore, combing DL properties and herbal metabolites may provide a comprehensive work platform which may reveal new insight into herbal quality control in the future.

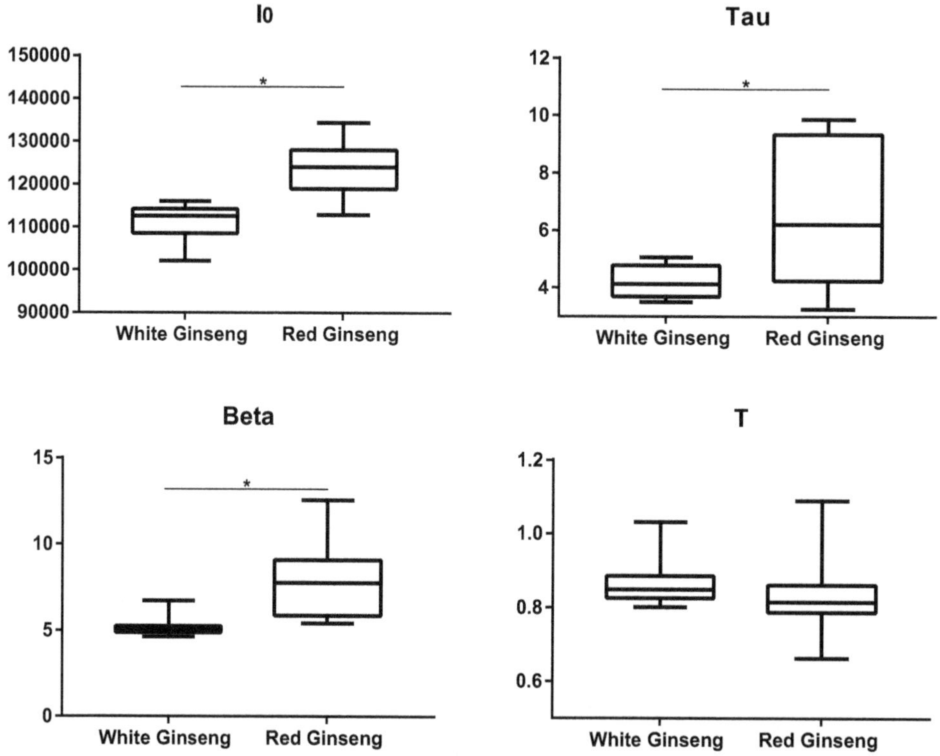

Fig. 4 Box plot summarizing the four DL properties measured in the Ginseng radix et rhizoma samples. *$p < 0.05$ (two-tailed, unpaired Student's t-test)

In the principle of Chinese medicine, the therapeutic actions of herbs are interpreted by a conceptual description of herbal properties such as taste and warm/cold etc. [3]. This type of description is based on practice experience which aiming the treatment of the human body as a whole [34, 35]. Therefore, based on the Chinese medicine's principle the therapeutic actions are modified after the processing procedure [5, 6]. Modern chemical and biological research may reveal the changes of metabolites after the processing and therefore the pharmacological effects [6]. However, the therapeutic effects of herbs are not simply related to the identified components, as other chemical compounds within herbs can combine synergistically with bioactive components to form overall therapeutic effects [36]. Therefore, comprehensive strategies should be considered in quality control of herbal materials processing to further explain the effects of processing on the pharmacological actions of herbs. In this aspect, to explore novel technology on quality assessment based on therapeutic effects is very important. DL measurement is a new tool, need further to explore for evaluating the changes of therapeutic properties caused by herbal processing. The results of this study provides a suitable foundation for follow-up studies. Further studies can include more herbs, and additional platforms for investigation the bioactivity of raw and processed herbal materials. In brief, DL is a new technique for studying CHM, thereby facilitating the move toward the comprehensive quality control in herbal materials processing.

Conclusion

The data presented in this article shows that DL properties from raw and processed herbal materials can be distinguished significantly. DL measurements show similar results to differentiate raw and processed Rehmanniae radix compared to chemical analysis using plant metabolomics [4, 25, 26]. The results indicate that after four cycles of processing for Rehmanniae radix, there is no much significant change in DL parameters which resembles the results obtained from chemical analysis (after five cycles). As multi-processing method has been recognized to treat raw Rehmanniae radix in both Chinese and Vietnamese pharmacopoeias [1], further research should be performed to validate whether DL can identify raw and processed Rehmanniae radix prepared under different processing methods. Since we are able to detect different DL characters in different processed Aconitum roots prepared using different methods [21], it is highly possible that different processing method will lead to different DL characteristic parameters, however, further confirmation for this predication required additional research. Finally, DL provides a rapid, direct, systemic tool for analyzing overall properties of herbal processing. It is a promising new technology to measure quality control in herbal materials [37].

Additional files

Additional file 1. Minimum standards of reporting checklist.

Additional file 2: Fig. S1. Dendrogram of the hierarchical cluster analysis of chemical profiles of raw and processed Rehmanniae radix samples. A–C indicates three independent batches of raw and processed Rehmanniae radix samples in previous study [4]. ^{1}HNMR and Fourier transform (FT)-mass spectrometry were used to obtain chemical profiles of these samples [4]. Chemical data of these samples was used to perform hierarchical cluster analysis (Distance Measure: Spearman; Clustering Algorithm: Ward).

Additional file 3: Fig. S2. DL decay curves for pooled samples from Rehmanniae radix samples. Data are plotted as the mean ± SEM. Note that the data are plotted on a linear scale.

Additional file 4: Fig. S3. Spectral distribution of DL emission of Rehmanniae radix and Ginseng radix et rhizome.

Abbreviations

DL: delayed luminescence; CHM: Chinese herbal medicine; ANOVA: one-way analysis of variance; LSD: least significant difference; PCA: principal component analysis; PLS-DA: orthogonal projections to latent structures discriminant analysis; GC–MS: gas chromatography–mass spectrometry.

Authors' contributions

MS and MW designed the study. MH, VWE and RWE conducted the statistical analyses. MS, WTC and MH drafted the manuscript and prepared tables and figures. MS, WTC, VWE and MW contributed to revisions of the manuscript. All authors read and approved the final manuscript.

Author details

[1] Leiden University European Center for Chinese Medicine and Natural Compounds, Institute of Biology, Leiden University, Sylviusweg 72, 2333 BE Leiden, The Netherlands. [2] Department of Chinese Pharmaceutical Sciences and Chinese Medicine Resources, College of Chinese Medicine, China Medical Univer sity, 91, Hsueh-Shih Road, Taichung 40402, Taiwan. [3] SU BioMedicine, Postbus 546, 2300 AM Leiden, The Netherlands. [4] Meluna Research, Koppelsedijk 1-a, 4191 LC Geldermalsen, The Netherlands. [5] Changchun University of Chinese Medicine, No. 1035, Boshuo Rd, Jingyue Economic Development District, Changchun 130117, China. [6] Sino-Dutch Centre for Preventive and Personalized Medicine, Gasthuislingelaan 33, 4002 AG Tiel, The Netherlands.

Acknowledgements

The authors thank Dr. Ping Sun for help and support with the herbal materials.

Competing interests

The authors declare that they have no competing interests.

Consent for publication

The manuscript is approved by all authors for publication.

Funding

Not applicable.

References

1. Zhao Z, Liang Z, Chan K, Lu G, Lee ELM, Chen H, Li L. A unique issue in the standardization of Chinese materia medica: processing. Planta Med. 2010;76(17):1975–86.
2. Wang M, Franz G. The role of the European Pharmacopoeia (Ph Eur) in quality control of traditional Chinese herbal medicine in European member states. WJTCM. 2015;1:5–15.
3. Sun M, Chang WT, Van Wijk E, He M, Koval S, Lin MK, Van Wijk R, Hankemeier T, van der Greef J, Wang M. Characterization of the therapeutic properties of Chinese herbal materials by measuring delayed luminescence and dendritic cell-based immunomodulatory response. Photochem Photobiol B Biol. 2017;168:1–11.
4. Chang WT, Choi YH, Van der Heijden R, Lee MS, Lin MK, Kong H, Kim HK, Verpoorte R, Hankemeier T, van der Greef J, Wang M. Traditional processing strongly affects metabolite composition by hydrolysis in Rehmannia glutinosa roots. Chem Pharm Bull. 2011;59(5):546–52.
5. Press China Chemical Industry. Pharmacopoeia of the People's Republic of China. Beijing: China Chemical Industry Press; 2015.
6. He M, Huang X, Liu S, Guo C, Xie Y, Meijer A, Wang M. The difference between white and red ginseng: variations in ginsenosides and immunomodulation. Planta Med. 2018. https://doi.org/10.1055/a-0641-6240.
7. Zhang RX, Li MX, Jia ZP. Rehmannia glutinosa: review of botany, chemistry and pharmacology. J Ethnopharmacol. 2008;117(2):199–214.
8. Schrader B, Klump HH, Schenzel K, Schulz H. Non-destructive NIR FT Raman analysis of plants. J Mol Struct. 1999;509(1–3):201–12.
9. Sun S, Chen J, Zhou Q, Lu G, Chan K. Application of mid-infrared spectroscopy in the quality control of traditional Chinese medicines. Planta Med. 2010;76(17):1987–96.
10. Xin N, Gu XF, Wu H, Hu YZ, Yang ZL. Discrimination of raw and processed *Dipsacus asperoides* by near infrared spectroscopy combined with least squares-support vector machine and random forests. Spectrochim Acta A Mol Biomol Spectrosc. 2012;89:18–24.
11. Lu L, Chan DSH, Kwong DW, He HZ, Leung CH, Ma DL. Detection of nicking endonuclease activity using a G-quadruplex-selective luminescent switch-on probe. Chem Sci. 2014;5(12):4561–8.
12. Lin S, Gao W, Tian Z, Yang C, Lu L, Mergny JL, Leung CH, Ma DL. Luminescence switch-on detection of protein tyrosine kinase-7 using a G-quadruplex-selective probe. Chem Sci. 2015;6(7):4284–90.
13. Vellaisamy K, Li G, Ko CN, Zhong HJ, Fatima S, Kwan HY, Wong CY, Kwong WJ, Tan W, Leung CH, Ma DL. Cell imaging of dopamine receptor using agonist labeling iridium (iii) complex. Chem Sci. 2018;9(5):1119–25.
14. Burke CS, Byrne A, Keyes TE. Targeting photo-induced DNA destruction by Ru (II) tetraazaphenathrene in live cells by signal peptide. J Am Chem Soc. 2018;140:6945–55.
15. Boyle KM, Barton JK. A family of Rhodium complexes with selective toxicity toward mismatch repair-deficient cancers. J Am Chem Soc. 2018;140(16):5612–24.
16. Liu JB, Yang C, Ko CN, Vellaisamy K, Yang B, Lee MY, Leung CH, Ma DL. A long lifetime iridium (III) complex as a sensitive luminescent probe for bisulfite detection in living zebrafish. Sensor Actuat B-Chem. 2017;243:971–6.
17. Ho NT, Desai D, Zaman MH. Rapid and specific drug quality testing assay for artemisinin and its derivatives using a luminescent reaction and novel microfluidic technology. Am J Trop Med Hyg. 2015;92(6):24–30.
18. Vesetova TV, Veselovsky VA, Rubin AB, Bochvarov PZ. Delayed luminescence of air-dry soybean seeds as a measure of their viability. Physiol Plant. 1985;65(4):493–7.
19. Triglia A, Malfa G, Musumeci F, Leonardi C, Scordino A. Delayed luminescence as an indicator of tomato fruit quality. J Food Sci. 1998;63(3):512–5.
20. Sun M, Li L, Wang M, van Wijk E, He M, van Wijk R, Koval R, Hankemeier T, van der Greef J, Wei S. Effects of growth altitude on chemical constituents and delayed luminescence properties in medicinal rhubarb. Photochem Photobiol B Biol. 2016;162:24–33.
21. Sun M, Wijk R, Wijk E, Wang M, Wietmarschen H, Hankemeier T, van der Greef J. Delayed luminescence: an experimental protocol for Chinese herbal medicines. Luminescence. 2016;31(6):1220–8.
22. Pang J, Yang M, Fu J, Zhao X, van Wijk E, Wang M, Liu Y, Zhou X, Fan H, Han J. Classification of Chinese herbs based on the cluster analysis of delayed luminescence. Luminescence. 2016;31(2):491–8.
23. Ihaka R, Gentleman R. R: a language for data analysis and graphics. J Comput Graph Stat. 1996;5(3):299–314.

24. Xia J, Wishart DS. Using MetaboAnalyst 3.0 for comprehensive metabolomics data analysis. Curr Protoc Bioinform. 1996;55:1–91.
25. Chang WT, Thissen U, Ehlert KA, Koek MM, Jellema RH, Hankemeier T, van der Greef J, Wang M. Effects of growth conditions and processing on *Rehmannia glutinosa* using fingerprint strategy. Planta Med. 2006;72(05):458–67.
26. Meng X, He M, Guo R, Duan R, Huo F, Lv C, Wang B, Zhang S. Investigation of the effect of the degree of processing of Radix Rehmanniae Preparata (Shu Dihuang) on Shu Dihuangtan carbonization preparation technology. Molecules. 2017. https://doi.org/10.3390/molecules22071193.
27. BarenboIm GM, DomanskiI AN, Turoverov KK. Luminescence of biopolymers and cells. Berlin: Springer; 1969.
28. Yu L, Sun SQ, Fan KF, Zhou Q, Noda I. Research on processing medicinal herbs with multi-steps infrared macro-fingerprint method. Spectrochim Acta A Mol Biomol Spectrosc. 2005;62(1–3):22–9.
29. Wink M. Modes of action of herbal medicines and plant secondary metabolites. Medicines. 2015;2(3):251–86.
30. Hall RD. Plant metabolomics: from holistic hope, to hype, to hot topic. New Phytol. 2006;169(3):453–68.
31. van der Kooy F, Maltese F, Choi YH, Kim HK, Verpoorte R. Quality control of herbal material and phytopharmaceuticals with MS and NMR based metabolic fingerprinting. Planta Med. 2009;75(7):763–75.
32. Brizhik L, Scordino A, Triglia A, Musumeci F. Delayed luminescence of biological systems arising from correlated many-soliton states. Phys Rev E. 2001;64(3):031902.
33. Popp FA, Yan Y. Delayed luminescence of biological systems in terms of coherent states. Phys Lett A. 2002;293(1–2):93–7.
34. Hassel CA, Hafner CJ, Soberg R, Adelmann J, Haywood R. Using Chinese medicine to understand medicinal herb quality: an alternative to biomedical approaches? Agric Hum Values. 2002;19(4):337–47.
35. Cheng JT. Drug therapy in Chinese traditional medicine. J Clin Pharmacol. 2000;40(5):445–50.
36. Li SP, Zhao J, Yang B. Strategies for quality control of Chinese medicines. J Pharm Biomed Anal. 2011;55(4):802–9.
37. Sun M. Development of personalized health monitoring using ultra-weak photon emission based on systems medicine concepts. Leiden: Leiden University; 2017.

3

Cellular stress response mechanisms of Rhizoma coptidis

Jin Wang, Qian Ran, Hai-rong Zeng, Lin Wang, Chang-jiang Hu and Qin-wan Huang*

Abstract

Rhizoma coptidis has been used in China for thousands of years with the functions of heating dampness and purging fire detoxification. But the underlying molecular mechanisms of Rhizoma coptidis are still far from being fully elucidated. Alkaloids, especially berberine, coptisine and palmatine, are responsible for multiple pharmacological effects of Rhizoma coptidis. In this review, we studied on the effects and molecular mechanisms of Rhizoma coptidis on NF-κB/MAPK/PI3K–Akt/AMPK/ERS and oxidative stress pathways. Then we summarized the mechanisms of these alkaloid components of Rhizoma coptidis on cardiovascular and cerebrovascular diseases, diabetes and diabetic complications. Evidence presented in this review implicated that Rhizoma coptidis exerted beneficial effects on various diseases by regulation of NF-κB/MAPK/PI3K–Akt/AMPK/ERS and oxidative stress pathways, which support the clinical application of Rhizoma coptidis and offer references for future researches.

Keywords: Rhizoma coptidis, Alkaloids, Pathways, Diseases

Background

Rhizoma coptidis has been historically well-used as a heat-clearing drug in China. There are many researches on Rhizoma coptidis, but most of them are only a small part of the whole molecular mechanisms. So we need to summarize these researches and find out some rules, which have guiding significance for the further research of Rhizoma coptidis. Modern pharmacological studies have demonstrated that Rhizoma coptidis possesses multiple properties, including neuroprotection [1], anti-inflammation [2–4], antioxygenation [5, 6], anti-cancer [7], anti-atherosclerosis [8], anti-diabetes [9] and anti-obesity [3], etc. These effects of Rhizoma coptidis are attributed to its alkaloid components, especially isoquinoline alkaloids [10]. We chose five isoquinoline alkaloids (berberine, coptisine, palmatine, jateorrhizine, epiberberine) and one aporphine alkaloid (magnoflorine) of Rhizoma coptidis as research goals (Fig. 1).

When the body is under external pressure, cells produce stress responses, defense reactions to resist pressure damage, including NF-κB, MAPK, Akt, AMPK, ERS and oxidative stress signaling pathways [11–14]. NF-κB pathways are associated with immunity, inflammation and cell survival. MAPK pathways refer to various cellular functions, including cell proliferation, differentiation and migration. Akt pathways have effects on apoptosis, protein synthesis, metabolism and cell cycle. AMPK pathways are energy regulation pathways. AMPK pathways inhibit biosynthetic pathways with energy consumption, such as protein, fatty acid and glycogen synthesis. ERS pathways are triggered by the unbalance of ER environment, including hypoxia, disturbance of Ca^{2+} homeostasis and glucose starvation. Oxidative stress pathways are caused by the imbalance of oxidation and antioxidation in body. Oxidative stress pathways regulate redox balance by Nrf2 and other ways.

The theory of traditional Chinese medicine is more from experience and inference, still lack of sufficient scientific basis, and cannot provide a modern scientific basis for overseas popularization and clinical use. Traditional Chinese medicine has multi-components, multi targets. Their complex components have different pharmacokinetic characteristics and complex interactions. The mechanism of Chinese medicine is complex and systematic. As a traditional Chinese medicine, Rhizoma coptidis

*Correspondence: hqwan2163@163.com
College of Pharmacy, Chengdu University of Traditional Chinese Medicine, No. 1166, Liutai Road, Wenjiang District, Chengdu 611137, China

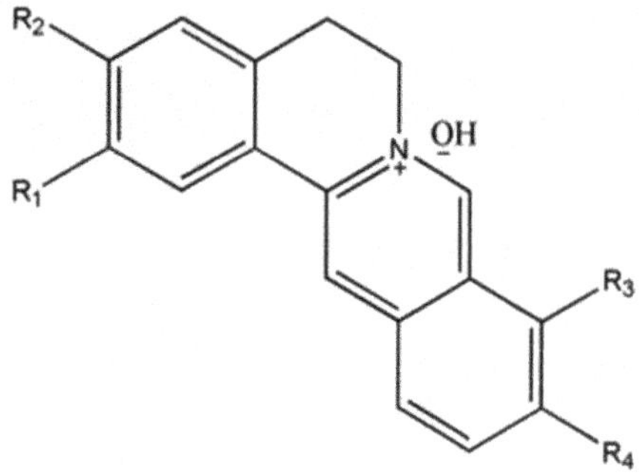

a

	R1	R2	R3	R4
Berberine	-OCH2O-		OMe	OMe
Coptisine	-OCH2O-		-OCH2O-	
Palmatine	OMe	OMe	OMe	OMe
Epiberberine	OMe	OMe	-OCH2O-	
Jatrorhizine	OH	OMe	OMe	OMe

b

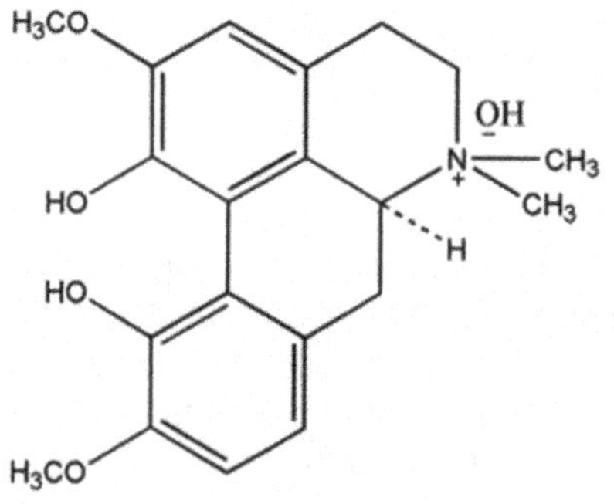

c

Fig. 1 Structures of alkaloids involved in this review. **a** The parent structure of main alkaloids in Rhizoma coptidis. **b** Substituents of the five isoquinoline alkaloids. **c** The molecular structure of magnoflorine

has excellent therapeutic effects on various diseases, but the underlying systematic molecular mechanisms are still far from being fully elucidated. In this review, we sorted out the relationship of Rhizoma coptidis among components, diseases and NF-κB/MAPK/PI3K/Akt/AMPK/ERS/oxidative stress pathways, systematically studying on how Rhizoma coptidis exerts beneficial effects to various diseases, which supported the clinical application of Rhizoma coptidis and provided references for the future researches.

The effects of Rhizoma coptidis on NF-κB/MAPK/PI3K–Akt/AMPK/ERS and oxidative stress pathways

Molecular mechanisms of Rhizoma coptidis inhibiting NF-κB pathways

NF-κB pathways, expressing in all nucleated cells, participate in various diseases by regulation of cellular immunity, proliferation, differentiation and apoptosis, etc. [15]. NF-κB pathways can be mainly activated by two pathways. The canonical pathways are triggered by TNF-α, IL-1β or viral infections. The activation of IKK and the degradation of IκB-α play key roles in the regulation of canonical pathways. TNF-α, IL-1β or LPS activate IKK and lead the degradation of IκB-α and p50/p65 NF-κB dimer entering the nucleus for DNA transcription [16]. In atypical pathways, the activation of NF-κB is shown to be independent from the phosphorylation of IKK and the degradation of IκB-α [17].

Rhizoma coptidis can regulate NF-κB pathways partly as Additional file 1: Table S1 and Fig. 2. Rhizoma coptidis regulates the NF-κB pathways as follows: (A) inhibition of the activity of membrane receptors, including TLR4, CD14; (B) inhibition of the phosphorylation of nuclear factor kappa-B kinase (IKK); (C) inhibition of the degradation of NF-κB inhibitor alpha (IκBα); (D) inhibition of activated NF-κB into the nucleus and its binding activity to DNA. Rhizoma coptidis exerts anti-inflammatory and anti-apoptotic effects through the above-mentioned ways, thereby has potential effects to diabetes, osteoarthritis, etc. Berberine reduces the levels of IL-1β, TNF-α in aortic sera and the mRNA expressions of NF-κBp65, iNOS, ICAM-1, IL-6 also reduced by inhibiting the migration of NF-κB to the nucleus in atherosclerotic mice [8, 18]. Coptisine reduces the expression of proinflammatory cytokines including TNF-α, IL-1β and IL-6 in ApoE−/− mice partly by inhibiting NF-κB activation [19].

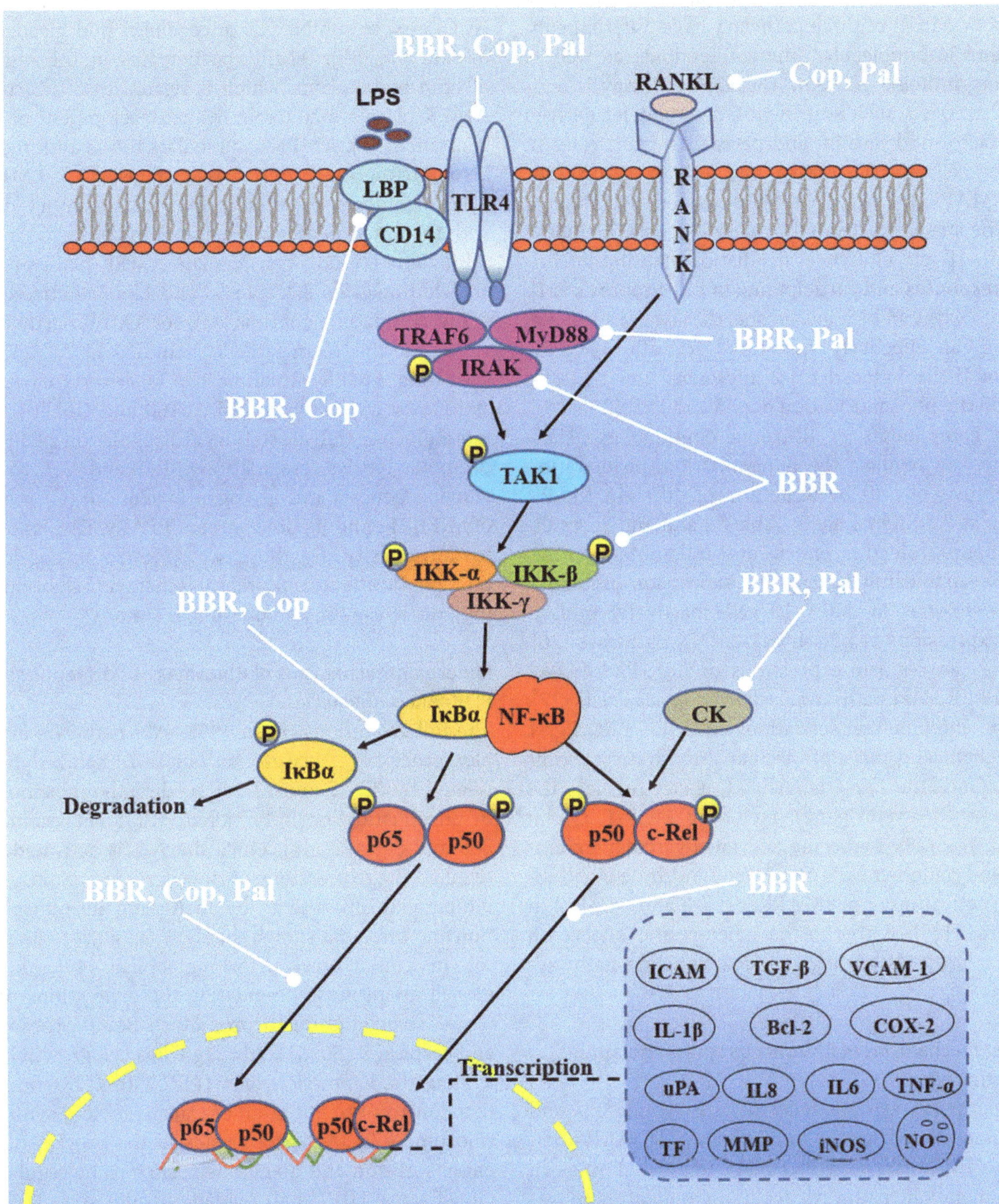

Fig. 2 Molecular mechanisms of Rhizoma coptidis on NF-κB pathways (—• indicates inhibition/reduction, arrow indicates promotion/stimulation). NF-κB pathways can be suppressed by Rhizoma coptidis at least four ways, including inhibition of the activity of membrane receptors (i.e., TLR4, CD14), inhibition of the phosphorylation of nuclear factor kappa-B kinase (IKK), inhibition of the degradation of NF-κB inhibitor alpha (IκBα), inhibition of activated NF-κB into the nucleus and its binding activity to DNA

Molecular mechanisms of Rhizoma coptidis inhibiting MAPK pathways

MAPK (Mitogen activated protein kinases) pathways play important roles in inflammatory response, cell proliferation, differentiation and apoptosis, etc., mainly through three pathways, ERK (extracellular regulated protein kinases), JNK (c-Jun N-terminal kinase) and p38 MAPK [20, 21]. The activations of MAPK pathways are very conservative. Each MAPK is activated by a specific MAPK kinase. MAPK are the pivots of each pathways.

MAPKK kinase (MAP3K or MKKK) and MAPK kinase (MAP2K or MKK) of three pathways have different substrates and intermolecular interconnections, as well as scaffolding proteins [22, 23]. The ERK pathway is activated by mitogen, such as growth factor, platelet-derived growth factor and insulin, and plays important roles in regulating cell growth, survival and differentiation. JNK and p38MAPK pathways weakly activated by mitogen, but can be strongly activated by stress signals, including TNF-α, IL-1β and ultraviolet irradiation, causing inflammatory responses and participating in cell apoptosis [24]. Three pathways can be adjusted specifically. For example, berberine can effectively inhibit the activation of ERK in LPS or IFN-γ induced BV-2 microglia, but it has no impact on the phosphorylation of p38 and JNK [25].

Active components of Rhizoma coptidis, especially berberine, can regulate the differentiation, proliferation and apoptosis of cells by inhibition of different MAPK pathways as Additional file 2: Table S2 and Fig. 3, resulting in neuroprotective effect, anti-inflammation, etc. Berberine significantly inhibits the expression of inflammatory cytokines in ARPE-19 cells partly by inhibiting the expressions of p38, ERK1/2, JNK pathways [26]. Berberine can regulate expressions of ERK/P38MAPK/JNK and PI3K–Akt pathways in thyroid cancer cells [27]. Berberine inhibits the activations of MEK/ERK/Egr-1 after mechanical damage of vascular smooth muscle cells in vitro. Once the Egr-1 is enabled, it can regulate the expressions of several genes, including MCP-1, Cyclin D1 and c-Fos [28]. Berberine alleviates vascular inflammation and remodels with metabolic syndrome by inhibiting the activation of p38MAPK, ATF-2 and MMP-2 in the arteries [29]. Berberine has therapeutic effects on diabetic neuropathy through MAPK signaling pathways [30].

Molecular mechanisms of Rhizoma coptidis regulating AMPK pathways

AMPK pathways exist in most of eukaryotic cells and metabolism related tissues and organs [31]. AMP-activated protein kinase (AMPK) plays important roles in multiple metabolic pathways, including regulating movement, nutrition and hormonal signals at cellular level, so as to control energy consumption and substrate utilization of whole body and maintain the balance of energy metabolism [32, 33]. AMPK promotes glucose uptake and transport by regulating the expression of GLUT4, including promoting GLUT4 translocation and unlocking GLUT4 gene expression [34, 35]. AS160 is a downstream target of AMPK. Phosphorylation of AS160 promotes the translocation of GLUT4 and glucose uptake [36]. PFK (6-phosphofructo-2-kinase) is a speed limiting enzyme of glycolysis. AMPK regulates the phosphorylation of PFK2 [37]. AMPK also can inhibit the activation of FAS, ACC, etc., to inhibit gluconeogenesis and glycogen formation [38, 39]. AMPK participates in the regulation of lipid metabolism, which is related to SREBP1C [40]. AMPK plays a major role in the development of insulin resistance [41]. AMPK can regulate the secretion of insulin and homeostasis of pancreatic β cells [42]. AMPK also plays significant roles in various inflammatory diseases with the function of anti-inflammation [43].

Rhizoma coptidis can regulate AMPK pathways partly as Additional file 3: Table S3 and Fig. 4. Active components of Rhizoma coptidis activate AMPK partly by activating the upstream targets, including LKB1 [25]. After activating AMPK, Rhizoma coptidis exerts its function as follows: (A) activation of AS160 and GLUT4 to promote glucose transportation; (B) regulation of PFK-2 to promote glycolysis; regulation of FAS and ACC to inhibit gluconeogenesis and glycogen formation; (C) inhibition of SREBP1c and its downstream PPARγ, FAS, and ACC1 to anti-obesity. By those ways, Rhizoma coptidis has therapeutic effects on cerebral ischemia [44], brain injury [45], diabetes [46], and obesity [47], etc.

Molecular mechanisms of Rhizoma coptidis regulating PI3K–Akt pathways

The full activations of the PI3K–Akt pathways are complex processes. Akt (protein kinase B) can be phosphorylated by PDK1 and PDK2, or directly phosphorylated by phosphatidylinositol 3′-kinase (PI3K) in residues Thr-308 and Ser-473 [48]. Once the Akt is activated, it can regulate the expressions of downstream factors. Akt can inhibit GSK-3β activity by increasing its phosphorylation and there has shown that GSK-3β plays an important role in cellular survival and metabolism [49]. Akt inhibits cell apoptosis by regulating the expressions of BAD (Bcl-2-associated death promoter), Bcl-2, procaspase-9, and caspase-9 [50, 51]. Akt regulates cell growth by controlling the expression of mTORC1 (mTOR complex 1) that controls the initiation of translation and synthesis of ribosome [52]. Akt participates in the process of nutrient absorption and metabolism, such as by regulation of GLUT4 and HIF-1α to mediate insulin stimulation and glucose absorption. Akt is also involved in angiogenesis and cell migration [53–56].

Rhizoma coptidis can regulate PI3K–Akt pathways partly as Additional file 4: Table S4 and Fig. 5. Berberine can be utilized to treat skin pigmentation and prevent cardiac dysfunction by regulating PI3K/Akt/GSK3 pathway [57, 58]. Berberine regulates cardiac fibroblast proliferation, collagen synthesis, cytokine secretion and induces the apoptosis of gastric cancer cells by Akt/mTOR/p70S6K pathway [59, 60]. Berberine protects endothelial progenitor cells from TNF-α by increasing

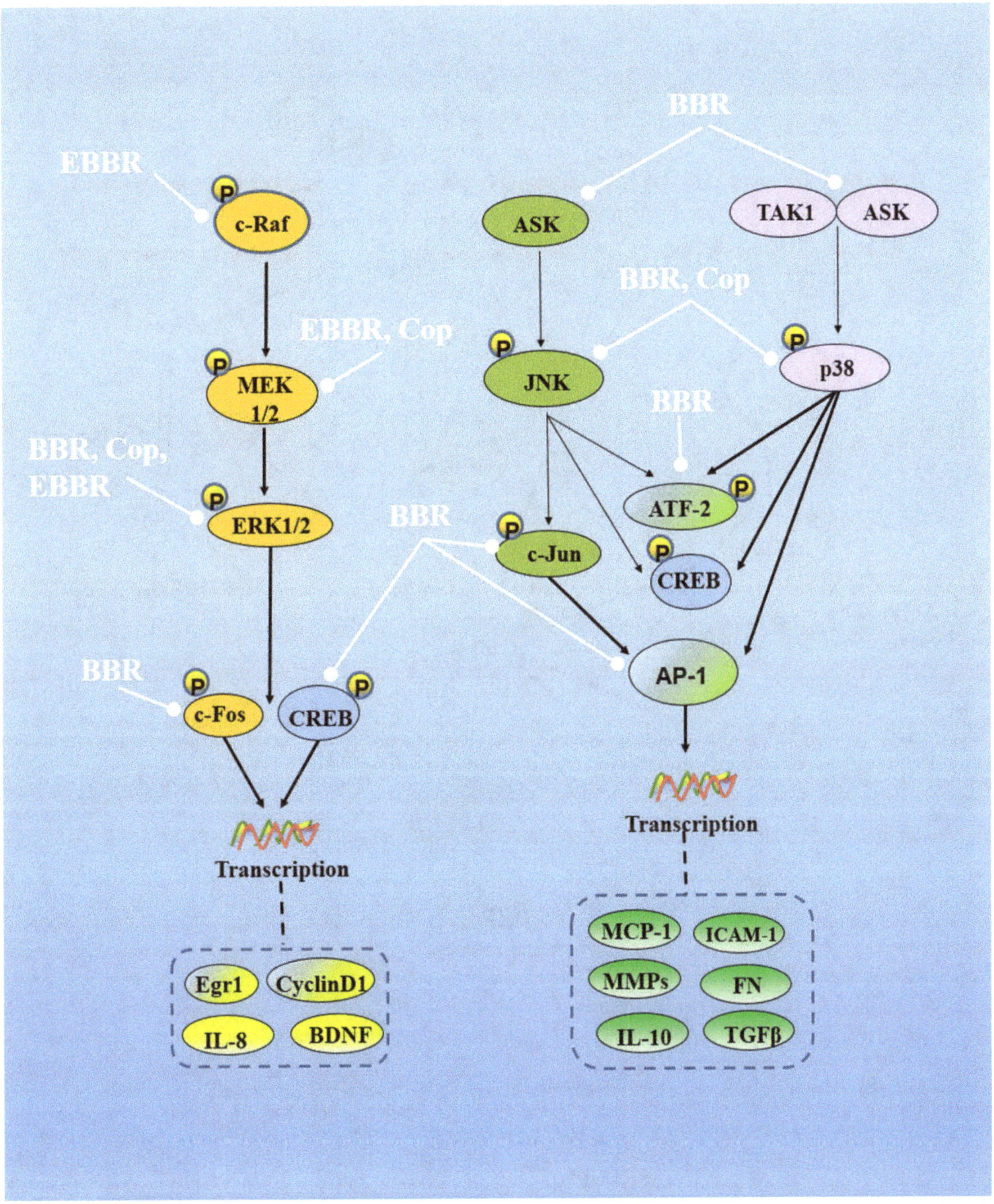

Fig. 3 Molecular mechanisms of Rhizoma coptidis on MAPK pathways (—• indicates inhibition/reduction, arrow indicates promotion/stimulation). Rhizoma coptidis can modulate MAPK pathways via several pathways, including ERK, JNK and p38 pathways. Three pathways can be adjusted specifically by Rhizoma coptidis. Through modulation of various MAPK pathways, Rhizoma coptidis suppresses inflammatory responses causing by TNF-α, IL-1β and ultraviolet irradiation and inhibits of apoptosis

the expressions of PI3K/Akt/eNOS [61]. PI3K–Akt pathways are widely expressed in the development of central nervous system [62]. BBR regulates the PI3K/Akt/GSK3β pathway at the early stage of neuronal polarization and promotes AMPK activation in low energy state to mediate the growth of neurite and affect the stability of cellular cytoskeleton [32]. Also, BBR induces the activation of PI3K/Akt/Nrf2 to protect dopaminergic SH-SY5Y neuron cells, NSC34 motoneuron cells and astrocytes [1, 63, 64].

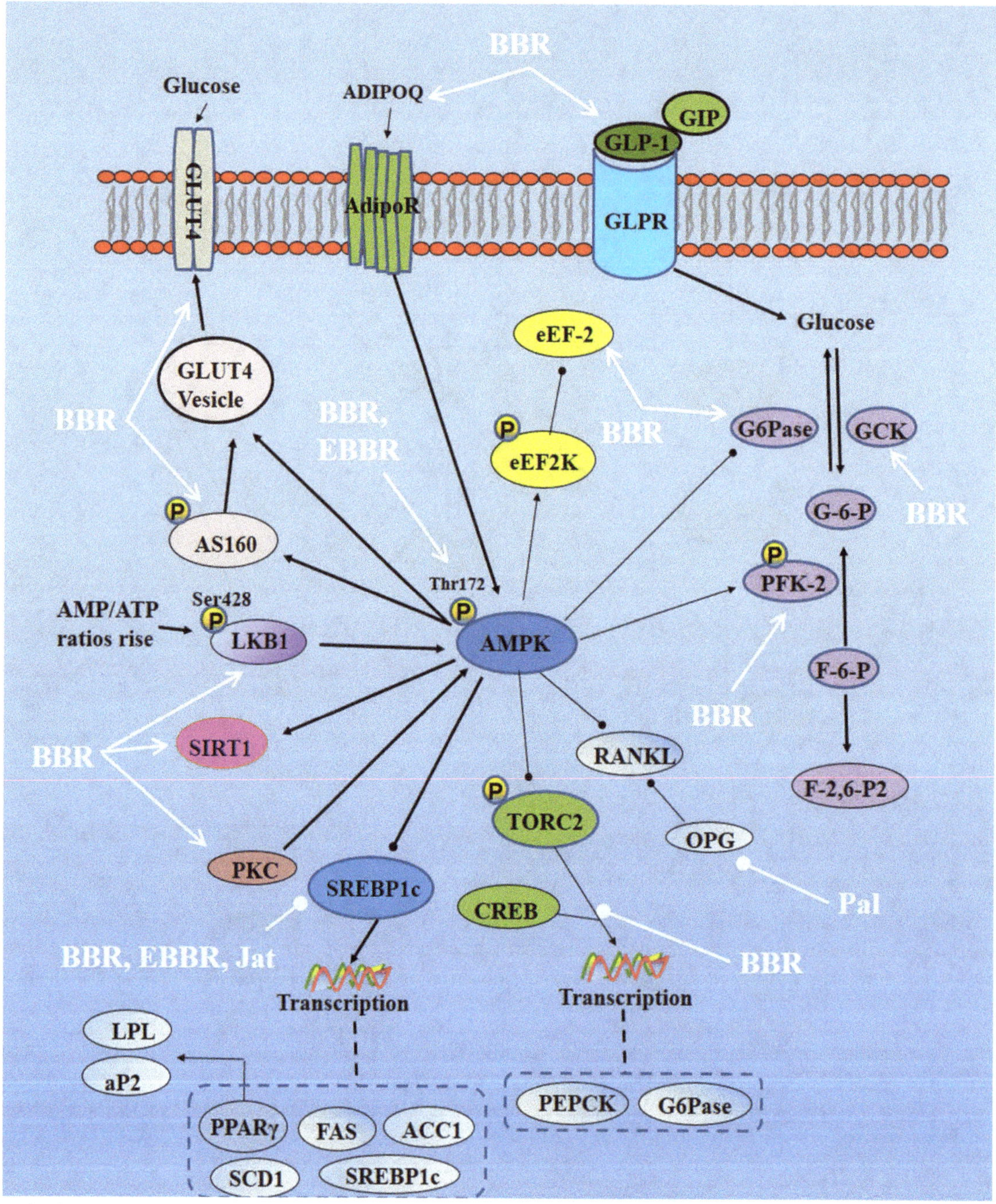

Fig. 4 Molecular mechanisms of Rhizoma coptidis on AMPK pathways (—• indicates inhibition/reduction, arrow indicates promotion/stimulation). Rhizoma coptidis can activate AMPK pathways via modulating upstream targets (i.e., LKB1). Once AMPK is activated, downstream signals of AMPK will be stimulated to demonstrate multiple biological effects, including anti-obesity, anti-diabetes, etc.

Molecular mechanisms of Rhizoma coptidis regulating ERS pathways

Endoplasmic reticulum (ER) is an important subcellular organelle that completes the protein folding and modification. When cells are subjected to intensive stimuli, such as oxygen deprivation, glucose starvation, disturbance of Ca^{2+} homeostasis, the endoplasmic reticulum will accumulate of unfolded/misfolded protein and induce endoplasmic reticulum stress (ERS). Then transcription factor 6 (ATF6), inositol-requiring protein-1 (IRE1) and PKR-like ER kinase (PERK) will be activated to reduce endoplasmic reticulum burden and maintain endoplasmic

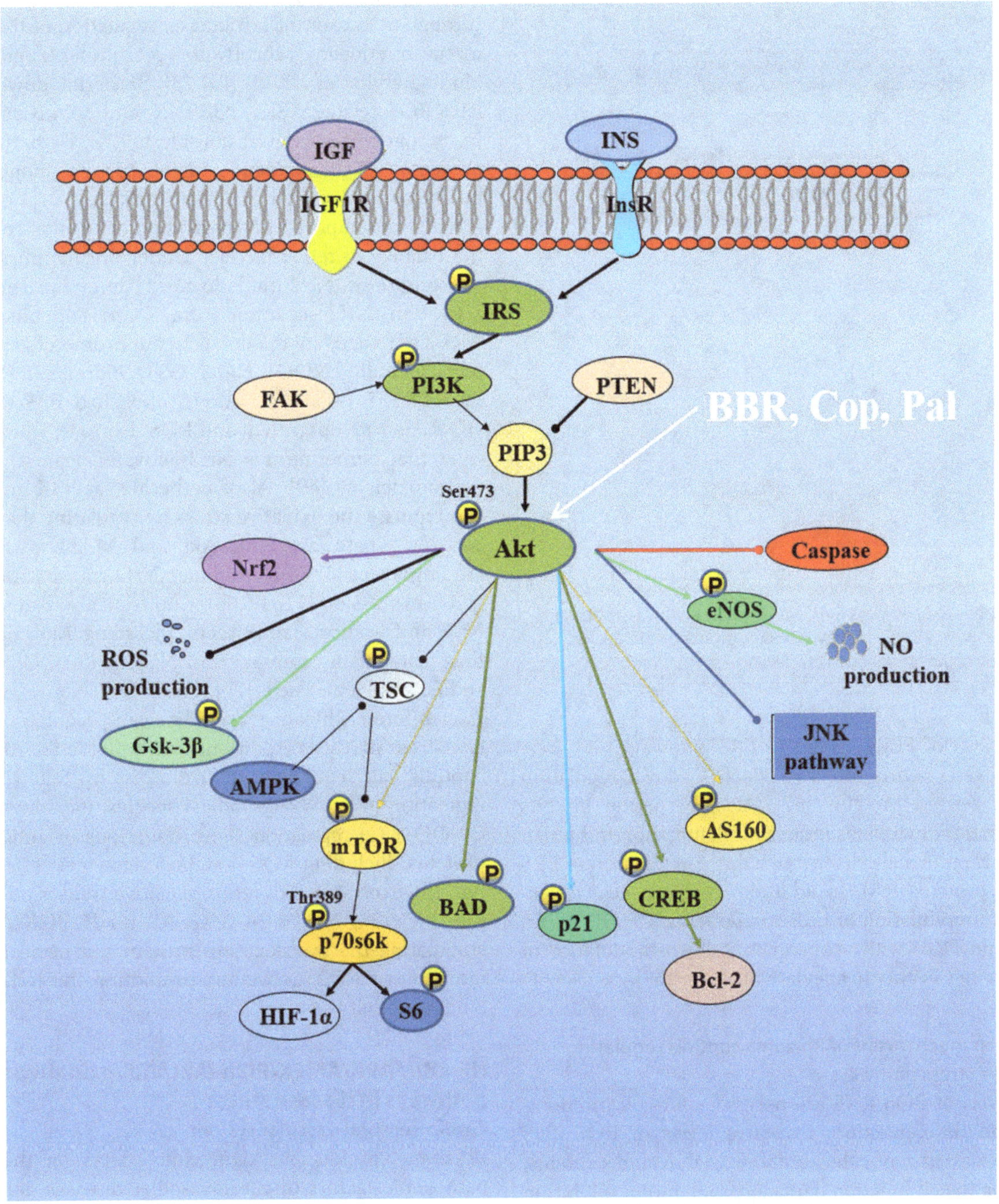

Fig. 5 Molecular mechanisms of Rhizoma coptidis on PI3K–Akt pathways (—• indicates inhibition/reduction, arrow indicates promotion/stimulation). By modulating upstream targets (i.e., IRS, PI3K), Rhizoma coptidis increases Akt ser473 phosphorylation. Once Akt is activated, downstream signals (i.e. GSK3β, mTOR, Nrf2) will be stimulated to demonstrate multiple biological effects, including decrease in oxidative stress, inhibition of apoptosis and suppression of inflammation

reticulum homeostasis [11, 65]. Recent studies have shown that ERS pathways play critical roles in the pathogenesis of obesity, insulin resistance and T2DM [66]. Berberine is localized both in the nucleus and ER [32]. Rhizoma coptidis, through down-regulation of proteins in ERS pathways, including PERK, IRE-1α, eIF2α and CHOP, has therapeutic effects on ER stress-associated diseases, including obesity, inflammation and diabetes (Additional file 5: Table S5; Fig. 6). Berberine protects HepG2 cells from ER stress damage by inhibiting the

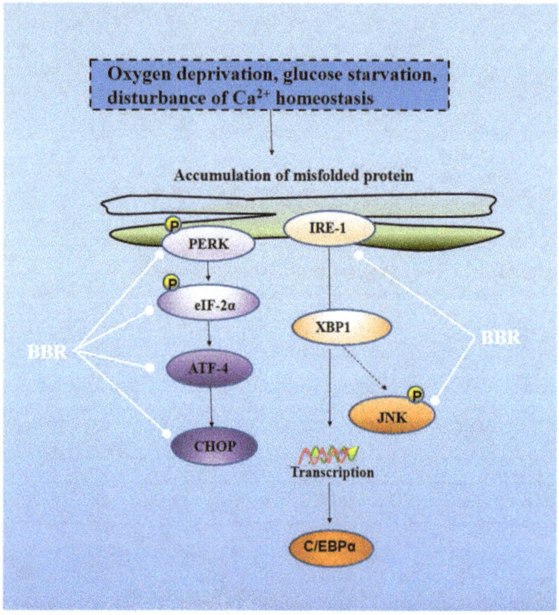

Fig. 6 Molecular mechanisms of Rhizoma coptidis on ERS pathways (—• indicates inhibition/reduction, arrow indicates promotion/stimulation). ERS pathways can be inhibited by Rhizoma coptidis at least two ways, including inhibition of the expression of IRE-1 and inhibition of the phosphorylation of PERK

expressions of PERK, eIF2α in ERS pathways [66]. Berberine exerts neuroprotective effects by down-regulation of ERS related proteins [67]. Also, berberine inhibits inflammatory cytokines induced inflammation in human intestinal epithelial cells through down-regulation of ERS related proteins [68]. In addition, berberine can selectively up-modulation of ERS components, CHOP, ATF3, ATF4 and TRB3 with a concomitant down-modulation of C/EBPα and PPARγ to alleviate ER stress [69].

Molecular mechanisms of Rhizoma coptidis regulating oxidative stress pathways

Low levels of ROS/RNS are necessary for cell proliferation and differentiation. Excessive levels of ROS/RNS directly destruct of cell membrane, DNA and proteins, resulting in cell function damage, proliferation inhibition and apoptosis [70]. ROS are radical species, including O^{2-}, H_2O, OH•, peroxylradicals, etc. RNS are radical species, including NO and $ONOO^-$, etc. [71, 72]. Under normal condition, antioxidant proteins, such as glutathione (GSH), ROS metabolic enzymes, including glutathione peroxidase, catalase and superoxide dismutase (SOD), are in balance. When this redox homeostasis is unbalanced, oxidative stress will be activated and participate in the occurrence and development of various diseases [72].

Oxidative stress interacts with other pathways [65]. NF-κB, MAPKs, AP-1, HIF, PI3K/Akt are redox-sensitive transcription factors. ROS activates NF-κB pathways through activation of IκB kinase, regulation of the chromatin remodeling, coactivator recruitment and DNA binding ability of NF-κB [72, 73]. Berberine down regulates ROS-related ASK1, p38/JNK, and NF-κB pathways in osteoarthritis synovial fibroblasts [74]. Berberine also prevents ROS dependent and JNK driven apoptosis in bone marrow mesenchymal stem cells [70].

Nrf2 is an important transcription factor that regulates the balance of redox in cells. Under normal physiological conditions, Nrf2 binds to Keap1 in cytoplasm. After activation, Nrf2 separates from Keap1 and binding to ARE site to activate the downstream promoters and proteins, including NQO1, HO-1, GST, thioredoxin [75, 76]. In SH-SY5Y cells, Nrf2 siRNA abolished BBR-induced HO-1, neurite outgrowth and ROS decrease, which indicates that berberine is a Nrf2 activator against glucose neurotoxicityas [49]. Also, berberine, a PI3K activator, can regulate the oxidative stress by regulating the PI3K–Akt–Nrf2 pathway. PI3K–Akt and MAPKs pathways are important for BBR to induce Nrf2 translocation and HO-1 expression [21, 49, 64]. Coptisine also can activate Nrf2 and its upstream targets, including Akt and JNK, thus to regulate expressions of NQO1, ROS, GSH SOD and GPx in HepG2 cells [77].

Therefore, Rhizoma coptidis can regulate oxidative stress partly as Additional file 6: Table S6. Rhizoma coptidis can regulate oxidative stress by following: (1) regulation of ROS/RNS radical species, including H_2O_2, $ONOO^-$; (2) regulation the productions of antioxidant proteins, including ROS metabolic enzymes; (3) regulation the expressions of redox-sensitive transcription factors, including NF-κB, MAPKs, AP-1, HIF, PI3K/Akt; (4) stimulating the translocation activity and nuclear accumulation of Nrf2, as well as promoting the Nrf2-DNA binding activity.

NF-κB/MAPK/AMPK/PI3K–Akt/ERS/oxidative stress pathways in disease states

Cardio-cerebral-vascular system

Rhizoma coptidis has significant effects on the main pathogenic factors of cardiovascular diseases, including anti-atherosclerosis, lipid lowering and anti-ischemia reperfusion injury. These properties have been attributed to alkaloid components of Rhizoma coptidis, including berberine, coptisine, palmatine, epiberberine, jatrorrhizine and magnoflorine [78, 79].

Ischemic–reperfusion injury

Rhizoma coptidis has therapeutic effects on ischemia–reperfusion injury by regulation of Akt/AMPK/p38/ERS/oxidative stress pathways as follows: (1) regulation of Ak/GSK3β/CREB as well as JNK/ERK1/2 to reduce ischemic brain injury [48]; (2) activation of PI3K–Akt, enhancement the accumulation of HIF-1α and promoting of HIF-1α mediated Sphk2 transcriptional to protect endogenous nerves [44]; (3) activation of AMPK, phosphorylation of Akt, thus exerting protective effects on the non-ischemic regions of the diabetic heart [80]; (4) activation of AMPK and PI3K–Akt–eNOS pathways to reduce myocardial apoptosis induced by ischemia/reperfusion in diabetic rats [81]; (5) regulation of lactate dehydrogenase (LDH), creatine phosphokinase (CK), superoxide dismutase and catalase (CAT) and other antioxidant enzyme activities [82]; (6) P38MAPK is crucial in myocardial ischemia and reperfusion [83]. Rhizoma coptidis also inhibits ischemia–reperfusion injury by blocking the activity of p38MAPK.

Obesity

Berberine, epiberberine, coptisine, palmatine, and magnoflorine can inhibit the lipid accumulation significantly in a dose-dependent manner in 3T3-L1 cells. They can down regulate the expression of adipocyte marker proteins, including C/EBP-α and PPAR-γ. The inhibition ability is as follows: coptisine > berberine > epiberberine > palmatine > magnoflorine [84].

AMPK and SREBP-1c are the main therapeutic targets for the treatment of metabolic diseases. AMPK is a kinase responsible for the phosphorylation of SREBP-1c in adipocytes. SREBP-1c is a transcription factor associated with the promoter region of a number of genes related to fat formation. SREBP-1c plays an important role in increasing triglyceride synthesis by increasing numbers of adipose producing genes related to FAS, also by promoting the expression of PPAR-γ [85]. Berberine can induce SREBP-1c phosphorylation by AMPK/Akt phosphorylation, thus inhibiting protein hydrolysate, nuclear translocation and DNA binding ability of SREBP-1c and reduce the expressions of lipogenic genes including FAS, LPL, PPAR-γ, C/EBP-α and ACC1 in a dose-dependent manner [85]. Epiberberine can inhibit lipid accumulation by regulating the expressions of AMPK/Akt and cellular differentiation mediated Raf/MEK1/ERK1/2, and then down regulating the main transcription factors of adipose formation, such as PPAR-c, C/EBP-α, SREBP-1c, and FAS in 3T3-L1 adipocytes [47]. Jatrorrhizine can also down regulate the expressions of SREBP-1c and FAS in the liver of high-fat diet-induced obesity mouse model [86].

Diabetes and its complications

Berberine, epiberberine, magnoflorine, palmatine, jatrorrhizine and coptisine have antidiabetic potential [87, 88]. Jatrorrhizine, palmatine and magnoflorine have potential therapeutic effects on diabetic complications such as retinopathy, cataract, neuropathy, and kidney disease [89].

Insulin resistance and glucose metabolism disorder

Rhizoma coptidis plays a therapeutic role in insulin resistance partly by regulating the TLR4/JNK/NF-κB pathways and Akt/AMPK/GLP-1/ERS pathways. In the insulin resistance models, Rhizoma coptidis acts on the TLR4/JNK/NF-κB inflammatory pathways and inhibits the activities of MCP-1, IL-6, TNF-α, JNK and NF-κB [9, 90–93]. AMPK also plays an important role in Rhizoma coptidis's treatments on diabetes [94]. Rhizoma coptidis up-regulates the expression of LKB1, AMPK and inhibits the translocation of TOCR2 into the nucleus in the liver of diabetic rats [46]. Berberine regulates the expression of GLUT4 in insulin-resistant cells with AMPK dependent and Akt independent ways. Akt is an important kinase that mediates glucose metabolism stimulated by insulin, and the deficiency of Akt can lead to glucose metabolism disorder. Rhizoma coptidis acts on Akt pathways by modifying IRS, phosphorylation of downstream Akt and activating PKC to improve insulin signaling cascade [66, 95, 96]. Protein kinase C (PKC) is expressed by the insulin receptor. Berberine can decrease insulin resistance by activating PKC, and inhibitor of PKC can eliminates InsR activation and InsR mRNA transcription induced by berberine [97]. IRS-1 is the principal link between inflammation and insulin resistance [95]. Berberine can improve the IRS-1 level in the brain and restore the expressions of GLUT1 and GLUT3 in the treatment of diabetic animals [98]. Berberine also improves insulin resistance in non-alcoholic fatty liver disease by regulating the expression levels of IRS-2 [95]. Akt induces GLUT translocation to the plasma membrane and regulates downstream targets involved in glycogen synthesis including GSK-3β and glucokinase [99]. Berberine activates Akt and GCK in liver and adipose tissue. The activity of GSK-3β in the liver was also inhibited by berberine [90, 96, 99]. Recent studies have shown that ERS play important roles in obesity, insulin resistance and T2DM. Rhizoma coptidis treats on insulin resistance partly by acting on the ERS pathways, including JNK, PERK, eIF2α and ORP150 to protect cells from ER stress injury [66].

Rhizoma coptidis also treats insulin resistance by activation of GLP-1. Berberine may regulate the secretion of GLP-1 by regulating AMPK [100]. GLP-1 plays an important role in stimulating glucose dependent insulin secretion, inhibiting glucagon release, promoting β cell proliferation, and gastric emptying and food intake [100]. Rhizoma coptidis can increase the expression of GLP in type 2 diabetic rats to stimulate glucose consumption and lower the levels of blood glucose [101]. Berberine also promotes the secretion of GLP-1 by activating TGR5 and bitterer receptor subtype TAS2R38. TGR5 plays an important role in regulating glycolipid metabolism, inhibiting inflammation, and improving kidney disease [101, 102].

Glucose transportation is the speed limiting step of glucose metabolism and can be activated in the peripheral tissue by two different ways: (1) IRS-1/PI3K signal transduction stimulated by insulin; (2) activation of muscle contraction through AMPK [103]. Berberine can improve glucose metabolism by insulin independent way in insulin sensitive cells including HepG2, C2C12, L6, 3T3-L1 cells [91, 104]. Berberine can increase the ratio of AMP/ATP and activate AMPK and Akt pathways to promote acute insulin mediated glucose transportation [101, 103].

Diabetic nephropathy

Diabetic nephropathy (DN) is one of the microvascular complications of diabetes and is the main cause of end-stage diabetes [105]. Oxidative stress, ERS and inflammation play important roles in the treatment of DN with Rhizoma coptidis. The levels of AGEs, P-PKC-β and TGF-β increased in injured kidneys. Berberine significantly reduced these levels, but the specific mechanisms remain to be further studied [106].

Rhizoma coptidis can treat diabetic nephropathy by AMPK/NF-κB/MAPK/Akt/oxidative stress/ERS pathways in diabetic nephropathy. (A) Under high glucose conditions in glomerular mesangial cells, berberine activates TGR5 and inhibits NF-κB/AP-1/MAPK pathways, decreasing the expressions of fibronectin (FN), ICAM-1, TGF-β1 and the phosphorylation levels of c-Jun/c-Fos [101, 107, 108]. High glucose can induce the over expressions of TGF-β1 in diabetic animals and patients, leading to renal fibrosis. However, berberine can reduce the expression of TGF-β1 by NF-κB pathways [108]. At the same time, berberine suppresses the p38MAPK pathways to inhibit the formation of fibronectin and collagen, which participate in renal fibrosis [105]. (B) Under high glucose conditions in renal tubular epithelial cells, berberine activates the PI3K/Akt pathways, reducing the expressions of apoptosis related proteins including Bax, cytochrome c, caspase3 and caspase9. Berberine also has effects on the oxidative stress pathways by reducing ROS production, promoting the expressions of GSH, SOD, Nrf2 and OH-1 to protect the renal tubular epithelial cells from apoptosis [75]. In dorsal root ganglion neurons, Berberine can reduce ROS production and rescue mitochondrial dysfunction induced by high glucose by increasing the expression of p-AMPK and Nrf2 [109]. (C) The sertoli cells arrange at the height of the glomerular basement membrane, and the lack of sertoli cells in regeneration is the main restriction of glomerular healing. Berberine can prevent Aldo induced sertoli cells injury and apoptosis by inhibiting the expressions of ERS related protein GRP78 and CHOP [110].

Discussion and conclusion

As a traditional Chinese medicine, Rhizoma coptidis is widely cultivated in China. It can be employed in infectious diseases, cardiovascular diseases, diabetes and so on. Its new efficacy is also constantly being discovered. In this paper, we summarized its mechanisms from the relationships of effective components, diseases and pathways. We found that various pharmacological effects of Rhizoma coptidis were due to its overall effects on multiple targets and pathways. The single component of the Rhizoma coptidis can act on several pathways at the same time. Multiple effective components of Rhizoma coptidis also play synergistic roles in pathways. In Osteoarthritis articular chondrocytes, berberine activates Akt/p70S6K/S6 pathway to promote protein synthesis, cell survival and matrix production, and also strongly induces differentiation through PI3K/Akt and p38 kinase pathway [111, 112]. Berberine also regulates the formation of osteoclasts through the negative feedback of AK1 and the activation of AMPK [113]. Coptisine inhibits NF-kB activation and the expression of COX-2, MMP-3, MMP-13 in Osteoarthritis articular chondrocytes [114]. Palmatine may attenuate osteoclast differentiation by inhibiting the expressions of OPG, RANK and RANKL [115, 116].

The related signaling pathways of Rhizoma coptidis are complex. It has been studied from the point of network pharmacology and revealed some mechanisms from the body system. But the activations of the corresponding biomarkers are caused by which components, which components regulate the networks or targets and whether there are synergistic/antagonistic effects between these components remain to be further studied. How to integrate the components, pharmacological actions and targets of Rhizoma coptidis is the focus and difficulty of future researches.

Therefore, in order to make full use of Rhizoma coptidis, we should use the modern technical means, such as the combination of the composition-activity relationship with metabolomics, to find the material basis and system mechanisms of Rhizoma coptidis. It will provide important bases for clinical application and comprehensive utilization of Rhizoma coptidis.

Additional files

Additional file 1: Table S1. The effects of Rhizoma coptidis on NF-κB pathways (↓indicates inhibition/reduction, ↑indicates increase).

Additional file 2: Table S2. The effects of Rhizoma coptidis on MAPK pathways (↓indicates inhibition/reduction, ↑indicates increase).

Additional file 3: Table S3. The effects of Rhizoma coptidis on AMPK pathways (↓indicates inhibition/reduction, ↑indicates increase).

Additional file 4: Table S4. The effects of Rhizoma coptidis on PI3K-Akt pathways (↓indicates inhibition/reduction, ↑indicates increase).

Additional file 5: Table S5. The effects of Rhizoma coptidis on ERS pathways (↓indicates inhibition/reduction, ↑indicates increase).

Additional file 6: Table S6. The effects of Rhizoma coptidis on Oxidative Stress pathways (↓indicates inhibition/reduction, ↑indicates increase).

Abbreviations

BBR: berberine; Cop: coptisine; Pal: palmatine; EBBR: epiberberine; Jat: jateorrhizine; Mag: magnoflorine; PI3K: phosphatidylinositol 3′-kinase; MyD88: myeloid differentiation primary response protein; IKK: inhibitor of nuclear factor kappa-B kinase; IκBα: NF-κB inhibitor alpha; TLR4: toll like receptor 4; LBP: lipopolysaccharide binding protein; CK: casein kinase; IRAK: interleukin 1 receptor associated kinase; ICAM-1: intercellular adhesion molecule-1; Bcl-2: B-cell lymphoma-2; VCAM-1: vascular cell adhesion molecule-1; u-PA: urokinase plasminogen activator; MMP: matrix metalloproteinase; RANKL: receptor activator for nuclear factor-κ B ligand; mTOR: mammalian target of rapamycin; MEK1/2: mitogen-activated protein kinase kinase 1/2; ASK1: apoptosis signal-regulating kinase 1; Egr1: early growth response protein-1; TAK1: TGFβ-activated kinase 1; MCP-1: monocyte chemoattractant protein-1; CREB: cAMP-response element binding protein; BDNF: brain-derived neurotrophic factor; FN: fibronectin; AP-1: activator protein-1; TGF-β1: transforming growth factor beta 1; ICAM-1: intercellular cell adhesion molecule-1; Cytc: cytochrome c; MMPs: matrix metalloproteinases; ATF-2: activating transcription factor-2; GLUT: glucose transporter; TORC2: CREB-regulated transcription co-activator 2; GCK: glucokinase; ADIPOQ: adiponectin; ACC: acetyl-CoA carboxylase; GLP-1: glucagon-like peptide-1; GIP: gastric inhibitory polypeptide; LKB1: liver kinase B1; PEPCK: phosphoenolpyruvate carboxykinase; G6Pase: glucose-6-phosphatase; eEF2: eukaryotic translation elongation factor 2; SREBP-1c: sterol regulatory element-binding transcription factor-1c; PPARγ: peroxisome proliferator-activated receptor γ; aP2: activating protein 2; LPL: lipoprotein lipase; FAS: fatty acid synthase; OPG: osteoprotegerin; SIRT1: sirtuin 1; IRS: insulin receptor substrate; InsR: insulin receptor; IGF-1: insulin-like growth factor-1; HIF-1α: hypoxia inducible factor-1α; ROS: reactive oxygen species; PTEN: phosphatidylinositol-3,4,5-trisphosphate 3-phosphatase and dual-specificity protein phosphatase; FAK: focal adhesion kinase; eIF2α: eukaryotic initiation factor 2α; IRE-1α: inositol-requiring enzyme-1α; CHOP: C/EBP homologous protein; C/EBPα: CCAAT/enhancer binding protein alpha; GRP78: glucose-regulated protein 78; ATF4: AMP-dependent transcription factor 4; Nrf2: nuclear factor-erythroid 2 related factor 2; HO-1: heme oxygenase-1; GSH: glutathione; SOD: superoxide dismutase; 8-OHdG: 8-hydroxy-2 deoxyguanosine; NQO1: NAD(P)H quinone dehydrogenase 1; MPO: myeloperoxidase; ONOO−: peroxynitrite anion; NOX: nicotinamide adenine dinucleotide phosphate-oxidase; GPx: glutathione peroxidase; STZ: streptozotocin.

Authors' contributions

QWH is corresponding author on the study. JW and QR contribute equally as first author and were responsible for collecting materials, writing the paper. HRZ and LW helped organizing the information and edited in the article pictures. CJH and QWH analyzed the article and made recommendations. All authors read and approved the final manuscript.

Acknowledgements

We are indebted to our alma mater, Chengdu University of Traditional Chinese Medicine for provided convenience in the collection of documents. Thanks for all the help from everyone in our lab. Thanks Hongyi Qi (*College of Pharmaceutical Sciences, Southwest University, Chongqing, China*) for critical reading of this manuscript and Wei Peng (*College of Pharmacy, Chengdu University of Traditional Chinese Medicine, Chengdu, China*) for helpful advice.

Competing interests

The authors declare that they have no competing interests.

Consent for publication

Not applicable.

Funding

This work is financially supported by the national Chinese medicine standardization project (Code: ZYBZH-Y-CQ-46); project of administration of traditional Chinese medicine of Sichuan province (Code: 2018JC011).

References

1. Hsu YY, et al. Berberine activates Nrf2 nuclear translocation and protects against oxidative damage via a phosphatidylinositol 3-kinase/Akt-dependent mechanism in NSC34 motor neuron-like cells. Eur J Pharm Sci. 2012;46(5):415–25.
2. Yan B, et al. Palmatine inhibits TRIF-dependent NF-kappaB pathway against inflammation induced by LPS in goat endometrial epithelial cells. Int Immunopharmacol. 2017;45:194–200.
3. Zou ZY, et al. Coptisine attenuates obesity-related inflammation through LPS/TLR-4-mediated signaling pathway in Syrian golden hamsters. Fitoterapia. 2015;105:139–46.
4. Gao MY, et al. Berberine inhibits LPS-induced TF procoagulant activity and expression through NF-kappaB/p65, Akt and MAPK pathway in THP-1 cells. Pharmacol Rep. 2014;66(3):480–4.
5. Zhao H, et al. Berberine suppresses gero-conversion from cell cycle arrest to senescence. Aging. 2013;5(8):623–36.
6. Yokozawa T, et al. Protective role of Coptidis Rhizoma alkaloids against peroxynitrite-induced damage to renal tubular epithelial cells. J Pharm Pharmacol. 2005;57(3):367–74.
7. Zhang Y, Liang Y, He C. Anticancer activities and mechanisms of heat-clearing and detoxicating traditional Chinese herbal medicine. Chin Med. 2017;12(1):20.
8. Feng M, et al. Comparative effect of berberine and its derivative 8-cetylberberine on attenuating atherosclerosis in ApoE(−/−) mice. Int Immunopharmacol. 2017;43:195–202.
9. Zhang DS, et al. Effect of berberine on the insulin resistance and TLR4/IKKbeta/NF-kappaB signaling pathways in skeletal muscle of obese rats with insulin resistance. J Sichuan Univ Med Sci Ed. 2015;46(6):827–31.
10. Meng FC, et al. Coptidis rhizoma and its main bioactive components: recent advances in chemical investigation, quality evaluation and pharmacological activity. Chin Med. 2018;13(1):13.
11. Kültz D. Molecular and evolutionary basis of the cellular stress response. Annu Rev Physiol. 2005;67(1):225–57.
12. Hardie DG, Ross FA, Hawley SA. AMPK: a nutrient and energy sensor that maintains energy homeostasis. Nat Rev Mol Cell Biol. 2012;13(4):251–62.
13. Simmons SO, Fan CY, Ramabhadran R. Cellular stress response pathway system as a sentinel ensemble in toxicological screening. Toxicol Sci. 2009;111(2):202–25.
14. Qi H, Li L, Ma H. Cellular stress response mechanisms as therapeutic targets of ginsenosides. Med Res Rev. 2017;38(4):625–54.
15. Oeckinghaus A, Hayden MS, Ghosh S. Crosstalk in NF-κB signaling pathways. Nat Immunol. 2011;12(8):695–708.

16. Gilmore TD. Introduction to NF-kappaB: players, pathways, perspectives. Oncogene. 2006;25(51):6680–4.
17. Esparza-López J, et al. Doxorubicin induces atypical NF-κB activation through c-Abl kinase activity in breast cancer cells. J Cancer Res Clin Oncol. 2013;139(10):1625–35.
18. Wan X, et al. Berberine ameliorates chronic kidney injury caused by atherosclerotic renovascular disease through the suppression of NFkappaB signaling pathway in rats. PLoS ONE. 2013;8(3):e59794.
19. Feng M, et al. The protective effect of coptisine on experimental atherosclerosis ApoE−/− mice is mediated by MAPK/NF-κB-dependent pathway. Biomed Pharmacother. 2017;93:721–9.
20. Nebreda AR, Porras A. p38 MAP kinases: beyond the stress response. Trends Biochem Sci. 2000;25(6):257–60.
21. Sun Z, Huang Z, Zhang DD. Phosphorylation of Nrf2 at multiple sites by MAP kinases has a limited contribution in modulating the Nrf2-dependent antioxidant response. PLoS ONE. 2009;4(8):e6588.
22. Morrison DK, Davis RJ. Regulation of MAP kinase signaling modules by scaffold proteins in mammals. Annu Rev Cell Dev Biol. 2003;19(19):91–118.
23. Enslen H, Davis RJ. Regulation of MAP kinases by docking domains. Biol Cell. 2001;93(1–2):5–14.
24. Kyriakis JM, Avruch J. Mammalian mitogen-activated protein kinase signal transduction pathways activated by stress and inflammation. Physiol Rev. 2001;81(2):807–69.
25. Lu DY, et al. Berberine suppresses neuroinflammatory responses through AMP-activated protein kinase activation in BV-2 microglia. J Cell Biochem. 2010;110(3):697–705.
26. Wang Q, et al. Effect of berberine on proinflammatory cytokine production by ARPE-19 cells following stimulation with tumor necrosis factor-alpha. Invest Ophthalmol Vis Sci. 2012;53(4):2395–402.
27. Li L, et al. Berberine could inhibit thyroid carcinoma cells by inducing mitochondrial apoptosis, G0/G1 cell cycle arrest and suppressing migration via PI3K-AKT and MAPK signaling pathways. Biomed Pharmacother. 2017;95:1225–31.
28. Liang KW, et al. Berberine suppresses MEK/ERK-dependent Egr-1 signaling pathway and inhibits vascular smooth muscle cell regrowth after in vitro mechanical injury. Biochem Pharmacol. 2006;71(6):806–17.
29. Li XX, et al. Berberine attenuates vascular remodeling and inflammation in a rat model of metabolic syndrome. Biol Pharm Bull. 2015;38(6):862–8.
30. Zhou J, et al. Neuroprotective effect of berberine is mediated by MAPK signaling pathway in experimental diabetic neuropathy in rats. Eur J Pharmacol. 2016;774:87–94.
31. Carling D, et al. AMP-activated protein kinase: nature's energy sensor. Nat Chem Biol. 2011;7(8):512–8.
32. Lu J, et al. Berberine regulates neurite outgrowth through AMPK-dependent pathways by lowering energy status. Exp Cell Res. 2015;334(2):194–206.
33. Steinberg GR, Kemp BE. AMPK in health and disease. Physiol Rev. 2009;89(3):1025–78.
34. Lee JO, et al. Metformin regulates glucose transporter 4 (GLUT4) translocation through AMP-activated protein kinase (AMPK)-mediated Cbl/CAP signaling in 3T3-L1 preadipocyte cells. J Biol Chem. 2012;287(53):44121–9.
35. Miyamoto L, et al. Effect of acute activation of 5′-AMP-activated protein kinase on glycogen regulation in isolated rat skeletal muscle. J Appl Physiol. 2007;102(3):1007–13.
36. Schweitzer GG, Arias EB, Cartee GD. Sustained postexercise increases in AS160 Thr642 and Ser588 phosphorylation in skeletal muscle without sustained increases in kinase phosphorylation. J Appl Physiol. 2012;113(12):1852–61.
37. Arden C, et al. A role for PFK-2/FBPase-2, as distinct from fructose 2,6-bisphosphate, in regulation of insulin secretion in pancreatic beta-cells. Biochem J. 2008;411(1):41–51.
38. Cantó C, Auwerx J. AMP-activated protein kinase and its downstream transcriptional pathways. Cell Mol Life Sci CMLS. 2010;67(20):3407–23.
39. Chen MH, Lin CH, Shih CC. Antidiabetic and antihyperlipidemic effects of *Clitocybe nuda* on glucose transporter 4 and AMP-activated protein kinase phosphorylation in high-fat-fed mice. Evid Based Complement Altern Med. 2014;2014(10):981046.
40. Diraison F, et al. Over-expression of sterol-regulatory-element-binding protein-1c (SREBP1c) in rat pancreatic islets induces lipogenesis and decreases glucose-stimulated insulin release: modulation by 5-aminoimidazole-4-carboxamide ribonucleoside (AICAR). Biochem J. 2004;378(3):769–78.
41. Fujii N, et al. Ablation of AMP-activated protein kinase α2 activity exacerbates insulin resistance induced by high-fat feeding of mice. Diabetes. 2008;57(11):2958–66.
42. Viollet B, et al. Targeting the AMPK pathway for the treatment of type 2 diabetes. Front Biosci. 2009;14(9):3380–400.
43. Salt IP, Palmer TM. Exploiting the anti-inflammatory effects of AMP-activated protein kinase activation. Expert Opin Investig Drugs. 2012;21(8):1155–67.
44. Zhang Q, et al. Berberine preconditioning protects neurons against ischemia via sphingosine-1-phosphate and hypoxia-inducible factor-1α. Am J Chin Med. 2016;44(5):927–41.
45. Chen M, et al. Berberine protects homocysteic acid-induced HT-22 cell death: involvement of Akt pathway. Metab Brain Dis. 2015;30(1):137–42.
46. Jiang SJ, et al. Berberine inhibits hepatic gluconeogenesis via the LKB1-AMPK-TORC2 signaling pathway in streptozotocin-induced diabetic rats. World J Gastroenterol. 2015;21(25):7777–85.
47. Choi JS, et al. Anti-adipogenic effect of epiberberine is mediated by regulation of the Raf/MEK1/2/ERK1/2 and AMPKalpha/Akt pathways. Arch Pharm Res. 2015;38(12):2153–62.
48. Pires ENS, et al. Berberine was neuroprotective against an in vitro model of brain ischemia: survival and apoptosis pathways involved. Brain Res. 2014;1557:26–33.
49. Hsu YY, Tseng YT, Lo YC. Berberine, a natural antidiabetes drug, attenuates glucose neurotoxicity and promotes Nrf2-related neurite outgrowth. Toxicol Appl Pharmacol. 2013;272(3):787–96.
50. Datta SR, et al. Akt phosphorylation of BAD couples survival signals to the cell-intrinsic death machinery. Cell. 1997;91(2):231–41.
51. Cardone MH, et al. Regulation of cell death protease caspase-9 by phosphorylation. Science. 1998;282(5392):1318–21.
52. Saito Y, et al. Dysfunctional gastric emptying with down-regulation of muscle-specific microRNAs in *Helicobacter pylori*-infected mice. Gastroenterology. 2011;140(1):189–98.
53. Lum JJ, et al. The transcription factor HIF-1α plays a critical role in the growth factor-dependent regulation of both aerobic and anaerobic glycolysis. Genes Dev. 2007;21(9):1037–49.
54. Morbidelli L, Donnini S, Ziche M. Role of nitric oxide in the modulation of angiogenesis. Curr Pharm Des. 2003;9(7):521–30.
55. Zhou GL, et al. Opposing roles for Akt1 and Akt2 in Rac/Pak signaling and cell migration. J Biol Chem. 2006;281(47):36443–53.
56. Liu LZ, et al. Berberine modulates insulin signaling transduction in insulin-resistant cells. Mol Cell Endocrinol. 2010;317(1–2):148–53.
57. Song YC, et al. Berberine regulates melanin synthesis by activating PI3K/AKT, ERK and GSK3beta in B16F10 melanoma cells. Int J Mol Med. 2015;35(4):1011–6.
58. Chang W, et al. Berberine treatment prevents cardiac dysfunction and remodeling through activation of 5′-adenosine monophosphate-activated protein kinase in type 2 diabetic rats and in palmitate-induced hypertrophic H9c2 cells. Eur J Pharmacol. 2015;769:55–63.
59. Ai F, et al. Berberine regulates proliferation, collagen synthesis and cytokine secretion of cardiac fibroblasts via AMPK-mTOR-p70S6K signaling pathway. Int J Clin Exp Pathol. 2015;8(10):12509–16.
60. Yi T, et al. Akt signaling is associated with the berberine-induced apoptosis of human gastric cancer cells. Nutr Cancer. 2015;67(3):523–31.
61. Xiao M, et al. Berberine protects endothelial progenitor cell from damage of TNF-alpha via the PI3K/AKT/eNOS signaling pathway. Eur J Pharmacol. 2014;743:11–6.
62. Ryder J, Su Y, Ni B. Akt/GSK3beta serine/threonine kinases: evidence for a signalling pathway mediated by familial Alzheimer's disease mutations. Cell Signal. 2004;16(2):187–200.
63. Chen JH, et al. Berberine induces heme oxygenase-1 up-regulation through phosphatidylinositol 3-kinase/AKT and NF-E2-related

factor-2 signaling pathway in astrocytes. Int Immunopharmacol. 2012;12(1):94–100.
64. Bae J, et al. Berberine protects 6-hydroxydopamine-induced human dopaminergic neuronal cell death through the induction of heme oxygenase-1. Mol Cells. 2013;35(2):151–7.
65. Fulda S, et al. Cellular stress responses: cell survival and cell death. Int J Cell Biol. 2010;2010(2010):214074.
66. Wang ZS, et al. Berberine reduces endoplasmic reticulum stress and improves insulin signal transduction in Hep G2 cells. Acta Pharmacol Sin. 2010;31(5):578–84.
67. Li HY, et al. Berberine improves diabetic encephalopathy through SIRT1/ER stress pathway in db/db mice. Rejuvenation Res. 2017. https://doi.org/10.1089/rej.2017.1972.
68. Hao X, et al. Berberine ameliorates pro-inflammatory cytokine-induced endoplasmic reticulum stress in human intestinal epithelial cells in vitro. Inflammation. 2012;35(3):841–9.
69. Pham TP, Kwon J, Shin J. Berberine exerts anti-adipogenic activity through up-regulation of C/EBP inhibitors, CHOP and DEC2. Biochem Biophys Res Commun. 2011;413(2):376–82.
70. Zhang W, et al. Berberine protects mesenchymal stem cells against hypoxia-induced apoptosis in vitro. Biol Pharm Bull. 2009;32(8):1335–42.
71. Brüne B. The intimate relation between nitric oxide and superoxide in apoptosis and cell survival. Antioxid Redox Signal. 2005;7(3–4):497–507.
72. Trachootham D, et al. Redox regulation of cell survival. Antioxid Redox Signal. 2008;10(8):1343–74.
73. Gloire G, Piette J. Redox regulation of nuclear post-translational modifications during NF-kappaB activation. Antioxid Redox Signal. 2009;11(9):2209–22.
74. Liu SC, et al. Berberine attenuates CCN2-induced IL-1beta expression and prevents cartilage degradation in a rat model of osteoarthritis. Toxicol Appl Pharmacol. 2015;289(1):20–9.
75. Zhang X, et al. Berberine activates Nrf2 nuclear translocation and inhibits apoptosis induced by high glucose in renal tubular epithelial cells through a phosphatidylinositol 3-kinase/Akt-dependent mechanism. Apoptosis. 2016;21(6):721–36.
76. Itoh K, et al. An Nrf2 small Maf heterodimer mediates the induction of phase II detoxifying enzyme genes through antioxidant response elements. Biochem Biophys Res Commun. 1997;236(2):313–22.
77. Hu YR, et al. Activation of Akt and JNK/Nrf2/NQO1 pathway contributes to the protective effect of coptisine against AAPH-induced oxidative stress. Biomed Pharmacother. 2017;85:313–22.
78. Tan HL, et al. Rhizoma coptidis: a potential cardiovascular protective agent. Front Pharmacol. 2016;7:362.
79. He K, Kou S, Zou Z, et al. Hypolipidemic effects of alkaloids from rhizoma coptidis in diet-induced hyperlipidemic hamsters. Planta Med. 2016;82(08):690–7.
80. Zhang X, et al. Neuroprotection of early and short-time applying berberine in the acute phase of cerebral ischemia: up-regulated pAkt, pGSK and pCREB, down-regulated NF-kappaB expression, ameliorated BBB permeability. Brain Res. 2012;1459:61–70.
81. Chen K, et al. Berberine reduces ischemia/reperfusion-induced myocardial apoptosis via activating AMPK and PI3K-Akt signaling in diabetic rats. Apoptosis. 2014;19(6):946–57.
82. Youngmin K, et al. Palmatine from Coptidis rhizoma reduces ischemia reperfusion-mediated acute myocardial injury in the rat. Food Chem Toxicol. 2009;47(8):2097–102.
83. Ashraf MI, et al. A p38MAPK/MK2 signaling pathway leading to redox stress, cell death and ischemia/reperfusion injury. Cell Commun Signal CCS. 2014;12(1):6.
84. Choi JS, et al. *Coptis chinensis* alkaloids exert anti-adipogenic activity on 3T3-L1 adipocytes by downregulating C/EBP-alpha and PPAR-gamma. Fitoterapia. 2014;98:199–208.
85. Jang J, et al. Berberine activates AMPK to suppress proteolytic processing, nuclear translocation and target DNA binding of SREBP-1c in 3T3-L1 adipocytes. Mol Med Rep. 2017;15(6):4139–47.
86. Yang W, et al. Jatrorrhizine hydrochloride attenuates hyperlipidemia in a high-fat diet-induced obesity mouse model. Mol Med Rep. 2016;14(4):3277–84.
87. Choi JS, et al. Protein tyrosine phosphatase 1B inhibitory activity of alkaloids from Rhizoma Coptidis and their molecular docking studies. J Ethnopharmacol. 2015;171:28–36.
88. Patel MB, Mishra S. Hypoglycemic activity of alkaloidal fraction of *Tinospora cordifolia*. Phytomedicine. 2011;18(12):1045–52.
89. Patel MB, Mishra S. Isoquinoline alkaloids from *Tinospora cordifolia* inhibit rat lens aldose reductase. Phytother Res. 2012;26(9):1342–7.
90. Ye L, et al. Inhibition of M1 macrophage activation in adipose tissue by berberine improves insulin resistance. Life Sci. 2016;166:82–91.
91. Zhao W, et al. Nandinine, a derivative of berberine, inhibits inflammation and reduces insulin resistance in adipocytes via regulation of AMP-kinase activity. Planta Med. 2017;83(3–04):203–9.
92. Wang Y. Attenuation of berberine on lipopolysaccharide-induced inflammatory and apoptosis responses in beta-cells via TLR4-independent JNK/NF-kappaB pathway. Pharm Biol. 2013;52(4):532–8.
93. Zhu L, Han J, Yuan R, et al. Berberine ameliorates diabetic nephropathy by inhibiting TLR4/NF-κB pathway. Biol Res. 2018;51(1):9.
94. Wang Y, et al. Berberine prevents hyperglycemia-induced endothelial injury and enhances vasodilatation via adenosine monophosphate-activated protein kinase and endothelial nitric oxide synthase. Cardiovasc Res. 2009;82(3):484–92.
95. Xing LJ, et al. Berberine reducing insulin resistance by up-regulating IRS-2 mRNA expression in nonalcoholic fatty liver disease (NAFLD) rat liver. Eur J Pharmacol. 2011;668(3):467–71.
96. Lou T, et al. Berberine inhibits inflammatory response and ameliorates insulin resistance in hepatocytes. Inflammation. 2011;34(6):659–67.
97. Kong WJ, et al. Berberine reduces insulin resistance through protein kinase C-dependent up-regulation of insulin receptor expression. Metabolism. 2009;58(1):109–19.
98. Sandeep MS, Nandini CD. Influence of quercetin, naringenin and berberine on glucose transporters and insulin signalling molecules in brain of streptozotocin-induced diabetic rats. Biomed Pharmacother. 2017;94:605–11.
99. Xie X, et al. Berberine ameliorates hyperglycemia in alloxan-induced diabetic C57BL/6 mice through activation of Akt signaling pathway. Endocr J. 2011;58(9):761–8.
100. Yu Y, et al. Modulation of glucagon-like peptide-1 release by berberine: in vivo and in vitro studies. Biochem Pharmacol. 2010;79(7):1000–6.
101. Yang Z, et al. Berberine attenuates high glucose-induced fibrosis by activating the G protein-coupled bile acid receptor TGR5 and repressing the S1P2/MAPK signaling pathway in glomerular mesangial cells. Exp Cell Res. 2016;346(2):241–7.
102. Yu Y, et al. Berberine induces GLP-1 secretion through activation of bitter taste receptor pathways. Biochem Pharmacol. 2015;97(2):173–7.
103. Cheng Z, et al. Berberine-stimulated glucose uptake in L6 myotubes involves both AMPK and p38 MAPK. Biochim Biophys Acta. 2006;1760(11):1682–9.
104. Chang W, et al. Berberine improves insulin resistance in cardiomyocytes via activation of 5′-adenosine monophosphate-activated protein kinase. Metabolism. 2013;62(8):1159–67.
105. Liu W, et al. Berberine reduces fibronectin and collagen accumulation in rat glomerular mesangial cells cultured under high glucose condition. Mol Cell Biochem. 2009;325(1–2):99–105.
106. Qiu YY, Tang LQ, Wei W. Berberine exerts renoprotective effects by regulating the AGEs-RAGE signaling pathway in mesangial cells during diabetic nephropathy. Mol Cell Endocrinol. 2017;443:89–105.
107. Lan T, et al. Berberine attenuates high glucose-induced proliferation and extracellular matrix accumulation in mesangial cells: involvement of suppression of cell cycle progression and NF-kappaB/AP-1 pathways. Mol Cell Endocrinol. 2014;384(1–2):109–16.
108. Lan T, et al. Berberine suppresses high glucose-induced TGF-beta1 and fibronectin synthesis in mesangial cells through inhibition of sphingosine kinase 1/AP-1 pathway. Eur J Pharmacol. 2012;697(1–3):165–72.
109. Yerra VG, et al. Adenosine monophosphate-activated protein kinase modulation by berberine attenuates mitochondrial deficits and redox imbalance in experimental diabetic neuropathy. Neuropharmacology. 2017;131:256.
110. Wang B, et al. Berberine improved aldo-induced podocyte injury via inhibiting oxidative stress and endoplasmic reticulum stress pathways both in vivo and in vitro. Cell Physiol Biochem. 2016;39(1):217–28.
111. Yu SM, et al. Berberine induces dedifferentiation by actin cytoskeleton reorganization via phosphoinositide 3-kinase/Akt and p38 kinase pathways in rabbit articular chondrocytes. Exp Biol Med (Maywood). 2016;241(8):800–7.

112. Zhao H, et al. Berberine ameliorates cartilage degeneration in interleukin-1beta-stimulated rat chondrocytes and in a rat model of osteoarthritis via Akt signalling. J Cell Mol Med. 2014;18(2):283–92.
113. Lee YS, et al. AMP kinase acts as a negative regulator of RANKL in the differentiation of osteoclasts. Bone. 2010;47(5):926–37.
114. Zhou K, et al. Coptisine prevented IL-beta-induced expression of inflammatory mediators in chondrocytes. Inflammation. 2016;39(4):1558–65.
115. Ishikawa S, et al. Influence of palmatine on bone metabolism in ovariectomized mice and cytokine secretion of osteoblasts. In Vivo. 2015;29(6):671–7.
116. Hanada R, et al. RANKL/RANK—beyond bones. J Mol Med. 2011;89(7):647–56.

4

Anticancer drug discovery from Chinese medicinal herbs

Mu-Yang Huang[1†], Le-Le Zhang[1†], Jian Ding[2] and Jin-Jian Lu[1*]

Abstract

Cancer is still presenting a serious threat to human health worldwide. The understanding of the complex biology of cancer and the development of oncotherapy have led to increasing treatment approaches such as targeted therapy and immunotherapy. Chinese medicinal herbs have attracted considerable attention due to their potential anticancer effects. Some natural products or formulae from Chinese medicinal herbs with directly or indirectly anticancer effects have been reported. In this article, we summarized the current progression on development of anticancer drugs from Chinese medicinal herbs, toward providing ideas for further development and application of Chinese medicinal herbs in cancer therapy.

Keywords: Chinese medicinal herbs, Anticancer, Drug discovery, Natural products, Formulae

Background

Cancer is a high-morbidity and high-mortality disease, which presents a serious threat to human health. According to the global cancer statistics, there was millions of new cancer cases and deaths occur around the world. The statistics also predicted that the number of new cancer cases will constantly increase in the future [1–3]. However, the complexity and covertness of cancer always make it difficult to diagnose at the incipient stage of disease. Cancer often develops into the advanced stage when the patient is diagnosed with neoplastic disease, which extremely augments treatment difficulties. Chemotherapy and radiotherapy are still commonly conventional approaches for treatment of patients harboring advanced cancer [4]. In the past decades, scientists have gained in-depth understanding about the complex biology of cancer [5], which improves the cancer treatment significantly. Recently, targeted therapy and immunotherapy have also been proposed and made a hit [6, 7]. Besides, some complementary or alternative therapies including Chinese medicinal herbs are applied to supplement clinical treatment [8, 9].

Chinese medicinal herbs with multi-target and multi-level function characteristics have earned increasing attention in the fields of cancer prevention and treatment [10]. Studies have shown that some Chinese medicines as well as many classical formulae exhibit prominent anticancer effects and have potentials to supplement cancer treatment [11, 12]. Arsenic trioxide (As_2O_3), a toxic Chinese medicines, has been successfully applied in the clinical treatment for patients of acute promyelocytic leukemia [13]. In addition, clinical case reports have presented that some formulae, including PHY906 based on Huang-Qin-Tang (黃芩湯), can improve the life quality of patients and exert synergetic effects with conventional drugs [14]. Chinese medicinal herbs are potential candidates to be developed as new anticancer drugs. In this article, we summarize the current progression of anticancer drug development from Chinese medicinal herbs and discuss some drug discovery strategies, toward providing ideas for their further development and application in the field of cancer therapy.

Development of natural products

Natural products with potential anticancer effects

Natural products represent a rich source with remarkable chemical diversity for discovery and development of new

*Correspondence: jinjianlu@umac.mo; jinjian.lu@163.com
†Mu-Yang Huang and Le-Le Zhang contributed equally to this work
[1] State Key Laboratory of Quality Research in Chinese Medicine, Institute of Chinese Medical Sciences, University of Macau, 7014, N22, Avenida da Universidade, Taipa, Macao, China
Full list of author information is available at the end of the article

drugs [15]. The development of modern technologies has broadened the cognition of chemical components of Chinese medicinal herbs. A large number of natural products isolated and identified from Chinese medicinal herbs have been investigated for their anticancer potential [16]. Drug screening is an indispensable step during drug discovery. In consideration of the huge amounts of natural products from Chinese medicinal herbs, preliminary screening using rational and efficient screening models are highly desirable for drug discovery. Over the past decades, some important anticancer agents were discovered based on classical phenotypic screening (function-first), and some were developed from general target-based screening (target-first) [17]. For example, the famous chemotherapeutic drugs including cisplatin and taxanes, were discovered via cytotoxic phenotype investigation and followed by the identification of their mechanisms of molecular actions [18–20]. Some others were developed from target-based discovery, such as epothilone (target tubulin) and temozolomide (target DNA) [21, 22]. Similarly, most of the previous reported natural products with anticancer potential were discovered based on the classical targets screening or the main "criterion" of cytotoxicity profiling. However, few of the natural products reported in the literature has progressed into further clinical evaluation ultimately, leading to the suspect and argument about the rationality and efficiency of these classical models. Along with the better understanding of tumor biology, targeted therapy (BCR-ABL, EGFR, VEGFR, HER2, mTOR, c-Met, etc.) and immunotherapy (CTLA-4, PD-1/PD-L1, etc.) have shown exciting anticancer effects in clinic recently. In this case, we wonder whether natural products isolated from Chinese medicinal herbs can also regulate some important signaling pathways to exert anticancer effects. Magnolol (Fig. 1a), a component isolated from *Magnoliae Officinalis Cortex*, was reported to possess anticancer effects against human breast cancer via inhibiting EGFR signaling pathways [23]. Another study showed that oleanolic acid (Fig. 1b), distributed in many Chinese medicines, exerted inhibition effect against tumor angiogenesis via suppression of STAT3 and Hedgehog pathways [24]. It is well known that various of Chinese medicinal herbs may have potentials to regulate immune system. Discovery of anticancer agents regulating relative immune checkpoints represents another considerable strategy. Recently, researchers have found that curcumin (Fig. 1c), isolated from *Curcumae Longae Rhizoma*, decreased PD-L1 expression and then sensitize the cancer cells to anti-CTLA4 therapy [25]. Those studies suggested that natural products from Chinese medicinal

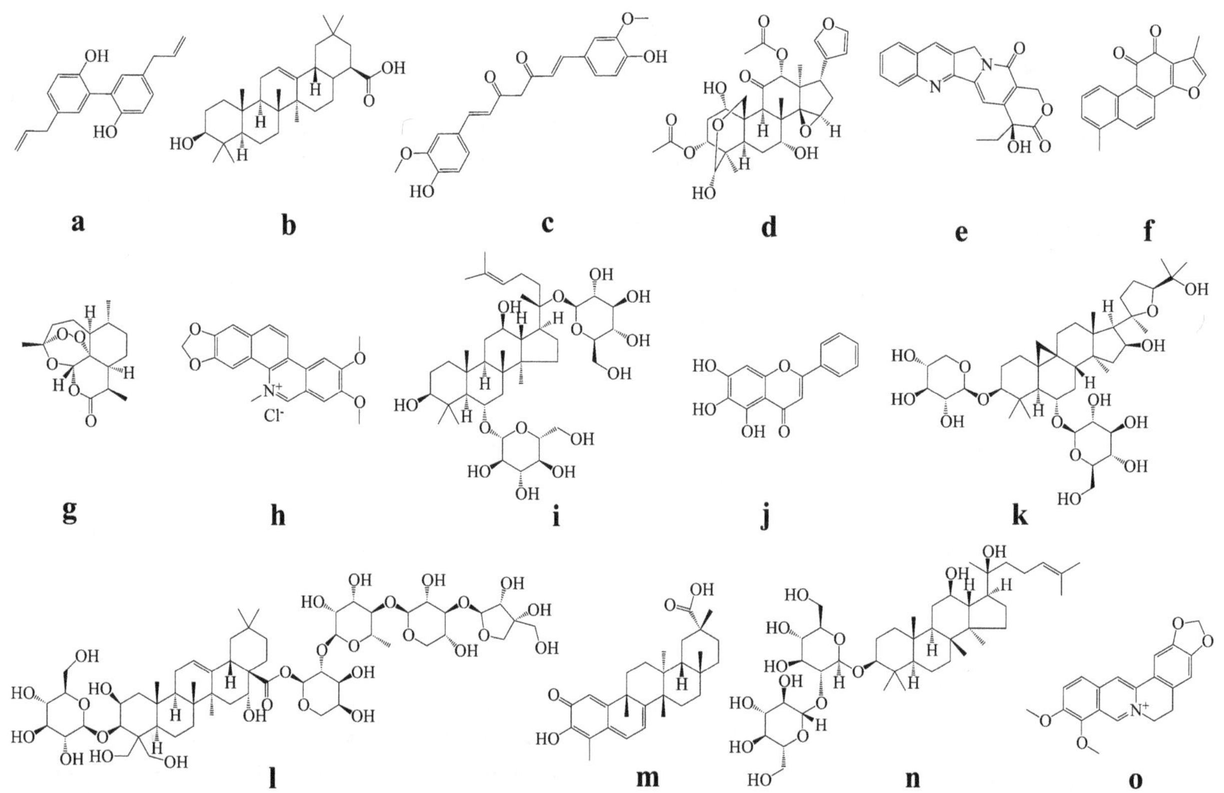

Fig. 1 Chemical structures of the natural products. **a** magnolol; **b** oleanolic acid; **c** curcumin; **d** toosendanin; **e** camptothecin; **f** tanshinone I; **g** artemisinin; **h** nitidine chloride; **i** ginsenoside Rg1; **j** baicalein; **k** astragaloside IV; **l** platycodin D; **m** celastrol; **n** ginsenoside Rg3; **o** berberine

herbs have potentials to regulate some essential signals in cancer cells. Targeting or regulating these proteins/pathways can serve as an accessible drug development strategy, highlighting the need of more specific screening models. Beside the widely used target-based screening, phenotypic screening is another important approach in drug discovery, especially when the specific target or mechanism of action is unclear. With the deeper understanding of cancer biology, more and more phenotypic screening models based on relative disease status such as cell migration, invasion, epithelial-mesenchymal transition (EMT) and stemness, also were established and applied for drug discovery. Tumor cells undergoing EMT exhibit stem-like properties, escape from immune surveillance, and generate resistance to apoptosis and antitumor drugs, and several clinical trials have documented the efficacy of the EMT inhibitory agents as potential anticancer candidates [26]. A study showed that toosendanin (Fig. 1d), isolated from *Toosendan Fructus*, could reverse the transforming growth factor β-induced EMT and morphological change in pancreatic cancer cells and then inhibit the disease progression [27]. Apart from the 'classic' cancer phenotypes in vitro, non-cell-autonomous phenotypes such as immune evasion, induction of tumor promoting inflammation and angiogenesis involve cell–cell interactions that are challenging to model and screen in vitro [28]. Taken together, with the increasing discovery of potential therapeutic targets and better understanding of disease process, drug screening platforms remain to be further developed and innovated to obtain lead compounds accurately.

Based on the efficient drug screening, plenty of compounds with potential anticancer effects can be obtained. Lots of natural compounds, including terpenoids, quinones, alkaloids, saponins, coumarins, etc., have been proven to have potential anticancer effects [29–33]. Nevertheless, many natural products which possess superior effects in vitro may not show satisfying results in vivo, owing to their non-specific effect, adverse reactions in vivo, poor solubility or other drug-like properties. Structural modification is a powerful tool to further improve the efficacy of drug candidates and the drug-like properties [34]. For example, camptothecin (Fig. 1e) is a famous natural product isolated from *Camptotheca Acuminata* with good anticancer effects, but its poor solubility and severe side effects lead to many limitations, while its derivatives (structural modification) like topotecan, irinotecan, and belotecan, have been successfully proven in clinic [35, 36]. Recently, study showed that novel nitrogen-enriched derivatives with better anticancer effect and drug-like properties was discovered from structural modification of tanshinone I (Fig. 1f) purified from *Salviae Miltiorrhizae Radix Et Rhizoma* [37]. Beside the anticancer drugs, a series of efficient and diversity oriented artemisinin (Fig. 1g) derivatives with various biological activities have been developed based on the antimalarial agent artemisinin, further proved the importance of structural modification [38, 39]. Furthermore, efforts toward efficient structural modification and total synthesis of bioactive agents have resulted in development of various new synthetic methods such as "Click chemistry", which may be employed in development of natural products [40].

Beside the chemical structural modification, pharmaceutical method represents another powerful tool to improve medicine safety and drug-like properties. For instance, drug delivery system like antibody–drug conjugate method can enhance therapeutic effects or reduce side effects in some cases. Lidamycin is one of the most potent antitumor agents but causes adverse effects. Antibody–drug conjugate system successfully reduced the side effects caused by lidamycin [41], which set an example for toxic Chinese medicinal herbs development. Other pharmaceutical methods including nanoparticle technology and micelle preparation also have been documented to further improve the solubility and stability of compounds [42]. For example, poor delivery and stability of artemisinin reduce the anticancer effect, but both can be improved by encapsulating artemisinin into nano drug delivery systems. Recently, cucurbit[7]uril, an emerging pharmaceutical excipient was proposed as to improve various properties of drug molecules or active pharmaceutical ingredients. Supramolecular formulation of nitidine chloride (Fig. 1h), a compound from *Zanthoxyli Radix*, by cucurbit[7]uril significantly alleviated its hepatotoxicity and improved its anticancer activity [43]. Totally, based on the preliminary drug screening and evaluation, specific pharmaceutical methods should be taken into consideration in allusion to the characteristics of relative drug candidates.

Combination therapy

As a complementary or alternative therapy, Chinese medicinal herbs in combination with other drugs serve as a promising strategy [44, 45]. Many investigations on combination therapy have been conducted to overcome the problems that appear during clinical cancer treatment, including side effects, drug resistance, and unsatisfactory treatment outcomes, etc. The strategies of combination therapy which can increase therapeutic efficacy or minimizing toxicity have been highlighted [46], and combination therapy is proposed to be a feasible strategy for Chinese medicinal herbs development.

Adverse drug reactions are common in some conventional cancer treatment, such as chemotherapy and radiotherapy. They may threaten the health of patients and offset the therapeutic benefits of anticancer drugs. Some natural products with effects of anti-inflammation, immune regulation, or toxicity reduction may possess potentials to be developed as adjuvant agents to relieve the side effects during the treatment. Combination therapy with Chinese medicinal herbs has been documented to reduce the toxicity induced by chemotherapy and improve the survival quality of patients [47]. For instance, a study has shown that ginsenoside Rg1 (Fig. 1i), isolated from *Ginseng Radix Et Rhizoma*, can alleviate cisplatin-induced hepatic injury in mice [48]. A number of natural products, such as *Scutellariae Radix* derived baicalein (Fig. 1j) and *Astragali Radix* derived astragaloside IV (Fig. 1k), were demonstrated to relieve the doxorubicin-induced cardiotoxicity [49–51]. Those evidences indicate that side effects induced by the conventional therapy can possibly be alleviated by Chinese medicinal herbs.

Beside alleviating the side effects, combination strategy with Chinese medicinal herbs also exhibit promising potential to improve the therapeutic efficacy, which may be a good choice for some clinical cases wherein patients cannot benefit from monotherapy. Combination of targeted therapy with chemotherapy has been applied in clinic and achieved a good response in some patients [52]. Similarly, natural products isolated from Chinese medicinal herbs also have been demonstrated to exert synergistic effects with other anticancer drugs. Studies have found that platycodin D (Fig. 1l), isolated from *Platycodonis Radix*, remarkably enhanced the antiproliferative effects of AKT and mTOR inhibitors [53, 54]. The anticancer efficacy of TRAIL/APO-2L was dramatically improved by celastrol (Fig. 1m), a natural product purified from *Tripterygium wilfordii*, both in vitro and in vivo [55]. Combination of cisplatin with dihydroartemisinin, a derivative of artemisinin, significantly decreased tumor size in lung carcinoma xenografted mice model via downregulation of VEGFR [56]. Synergistic effect of Dan-Shen-Injection (丹参注射液) was reported when combined with chemotherapy or antiangiogenic therapy [57]. Therefore, combination therapy with Chinese medicinal herbs is a good strategy for enhancing the anticancer effects. As mentioned above, although immunotherapy has achieved great success, only a minority of patients could respond to PD-1/PD-L1 antibodies. We hypothesize that some Chinese medicinal herbs with immunoregulation effects may sensitize patients to immunotherapy.

Additionally, identification of natural products to overcome drug resistance represents another important strategy since drug resistance lead to treatment failure in clinic and remains an obstacle in cancer therapy [58]. Aside from discovering new alternative drugs, scientists have also devoted to find combination strategies to overcome drug resistance. It is reported that various types of mechanisms such as overexpression of some transporters, activation of bypass signaling, and emergence of EMT would lead to drug resistance during cancer treatment [59, 60]. One strategy is to screen natural products that can potentially prevent or delay resistance of tumor to relative drugs. A study has shown that ginsenoside Rg3 (Fig. 1n), purified from *Ginseng Radix Et Rhizoma*, provides a new regimen to delay acquired resistance of EGFR tyrosine kinase inhibitors and ultimately improves median progression-free survival and overall response rate in advanced non-small cell lung cancer patients [61]. For the patients with acquired resistance, overcoming the resistant status or re-sensitizing the therapeutic effects serve as another strategy. A study suggested that *Coptidis Rhizoma* derived berberine (Fig. 1o), which has been widely used in intestinal infection treatment, sensitized the therapeutic effect of cisplatin in the cisplatin-resistant ovarian cancer cells through the miR-93/PTEN/AKT signaling pathway [62].

Development of Chinese medicinal formulae

Formulae are the main forms of Chinese medicines used in clinic, which also play an essential role in cancer therapy. Numerous formulae have been recorded, but the working mechanisms for most of them remain unknown. Clinically, they are often used in combination with conventional drugs to achieve a synergistic anticancer effect or to reduce the side effects. For example, the formula Xue-Fu-Zhu-Yu-Tang (血府逐瘀湯) decreased the tumor weight by enhancing the immune function in the tumor-bearing mice, and the combinational use of Xue-Fu-Zhu-Yu-Tang increased the effect of chemotherapy [63, 64]. The Sheng-Mai-Yin (生脈飲) can relieve the myocardial toxicity caused by doxorubicin [65]. However, the difficulties of quality control (QC) and mechanism study still represent the main obstacles for the development and clinical usage of Chinese medicinal formulae.

QC is a critical step in Chinese medicinal herbs' development, since the quality standard is essential to ensure the safety and efficacy. Recently, technologies for the QC of Chinese medicinal herbs have made great progress, while many problems, such as single QC markers and lack of biological effect evaluation, still need to be improved. Active ingredient or high-content component-based QC is unitary and lack of association with pharmaceutical/biological effects, which make it difficult to evaluate the comprehensive quality of complicated formulae. In this case, a more comprehensive QC pattern is required to guarantee the reproducibility and efficacy in formulae development. PHY906, an adjuvant based on a 1800 year-old formula called Huang-Qin-Tang showed potential to increase the therapeutic index of cancer treatment in several studies [66–68]. The development of PHY906 gave a paradigm of comprehensive QC pattern in formulae exploitation, indicating that both chemical analysis and pharmacology/biology evaluation are important. For chemical analysis, more and more efficient and accurate approaches like chromatographic fingerprint technique are used to analyze the components in Chinese medicines. For instance, 162 compounds in Ji-Tong-Ning-Tablet (脊痛寧片) were detected via an UPLC-Q–TOF–MS method, which significantly improved its QC [69]. Besides, pharmacokinetic metabolites also play essential roles in the prediction and management of therapeutic effects, which can be detected by serum pharmacochemistry methods or metabonomics methods. Study showed that 22 absorbed prototypes and 16 metabolites of Da-Bu-Yin-Wan (大補陰丸) were successfully analyzed from rats' serum after the administration of Da-Bu-Yin-Wan [70]. Apart from chemical analysis, the pharmacological or biological effects should be taken into consideration for QC. Appropriate biological assays based on pharmacological or biological effects and mechanisms of the formulae might improve their QC [71]. In total, to ensure the reliability and uniformity of Chinese medicinal formulae in anticancer drug development and clinical usage, both chemical analysis and pharmacology/biology evaluation based comprehensive patterns of QC need to be further developed.

Mechanism study is another bottleneck for the development of Chinese medicinal formulae, due to complicated components, multi-target effects, complicated interaction with organisms, etc. The traditional 'one target, one drug' mechanism study mode is unsuitable for the development of formulae. Along with the application of multi-omics, systems biology and network pharmacology have been developed rapidly and offer promising potential in the mechanism study of formulae. Realgar-Indigo naturalis (複方磺黛片) is an effective formula used for the treatment of acute promyelocytic leukemia. The systems biology strategy based on the molecular, cellular, and organism levels evaluation in vitro and in vivo has been successfully used in its mechanism study, which demonstrated that Realgar-Indigo naturalis formula intensified degradation of promyelocytic leukemia-retinoic acid receptor alpha oncoprotein, increased reprogramming of myeloid differentiation regulators, and enhanced G0/G1 arrest in acute promyelocytic leukemia cells [72]. Similarly, the network pharmacology approach was also successfully applied to clarify the possible therapeutic mechanisms of Liu-Wei-Di-Huang-Wan (六味地黄丸). The results indicated that the effects of Liu-Wei-Di-Huang-Wan on the "Yin deficiency" pattern in Chinese medicine was mediated by maintaining homeostasis in the endocrine system, the immune system and metabolism [73]. Recently, a concept of integrated pharmacology was proposed and used in the mechanism study of formulae, which integrated many subjects such as chemistry, pharmacokinetics, pharmacology, computational science and so on. Based on the integrated pharmacology, the multi-target and multi-component mechanism of Wen-Dan-Tang (溫膽湯), a Chinese herbal formula for treatment of metabolic syndrome, has been thoroughly studied. Six peroxisome proliferators-activated receptors were predicted as targets that exhibited strong binding affinities with 217 active ingredients of Wen-Dan-Tang [74]. Taken together, these approaches provide new insights into the mechanism study of anticancer formulae as well as further discovery of anticancer drugs from Chinese medicinal herbs.

Discussion

To date, a number of Chinese medicinal herbs (both natural products and formulae) have been documented to possess anticancer activities through various potential mechanisms (Fig. 2). Meanwhile, some of the Chinese medicinal herbs can improve the therapeutic outcomes of patients when used in combination with conventional anticancer drugs due to the presence of synergetic effects, alleviation of side effects, or delaying/overcoming of drug resistance. This manuscript summarizes the anticancer drug development strategies from Chinese medicinal herbs (Fig. 3). Although abundant work about Chinese medicinal herbs have been carried out in the past decades, several points still need to be taken into consideration for future development. Firstly, an effective QC is crucial to ensure the safety and efficacy of Chinese medicinal herbs, especially for formulae. Since numerous factors influence the effects of Chinese medicinal herbs, a more comprehensive QC pattern is required. Aside from some rising chemical analysis methods, such as chromatographic fingerprint and multi-component quantification [75, 76], pharmacology/biology evaluation is needed. Secondly, although Chinese medicinal herbs and formulae have been widely used in clinic, especially in China, the working mechanisms for most of them still remain to be clarified. The better understanding of the involved mechanisms will promote the discovery of more potential anticancer compounds or formulae. Thirdly, many natural products have been extensively studied and proven to exhibit anticancer effects in vitro, while showing poor activity in vivo. Such limitations may be caused by their poor bioavailability or toxicity. Thus, the implementation of some chemical and pharmaceutical methods is necessary during drug development. For those which have been proven safe and effective in vitro and in vivo, clinical trials can be considered under a good quality control. Fourthly, previous investigations mainly focused on

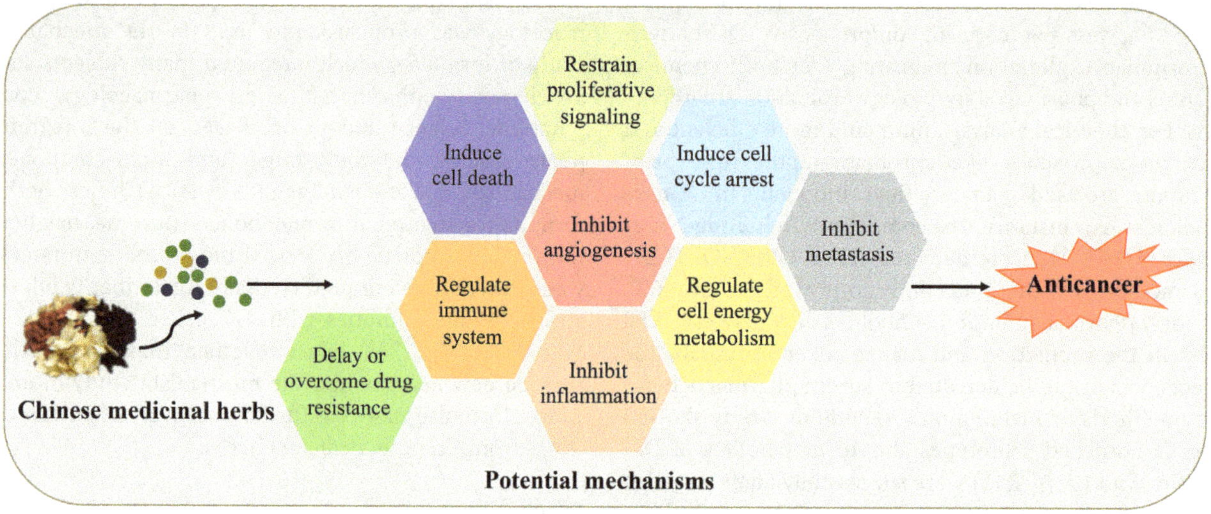

Fig. 2 Potential anticancer mechanisms of Chinese medicinal herbs

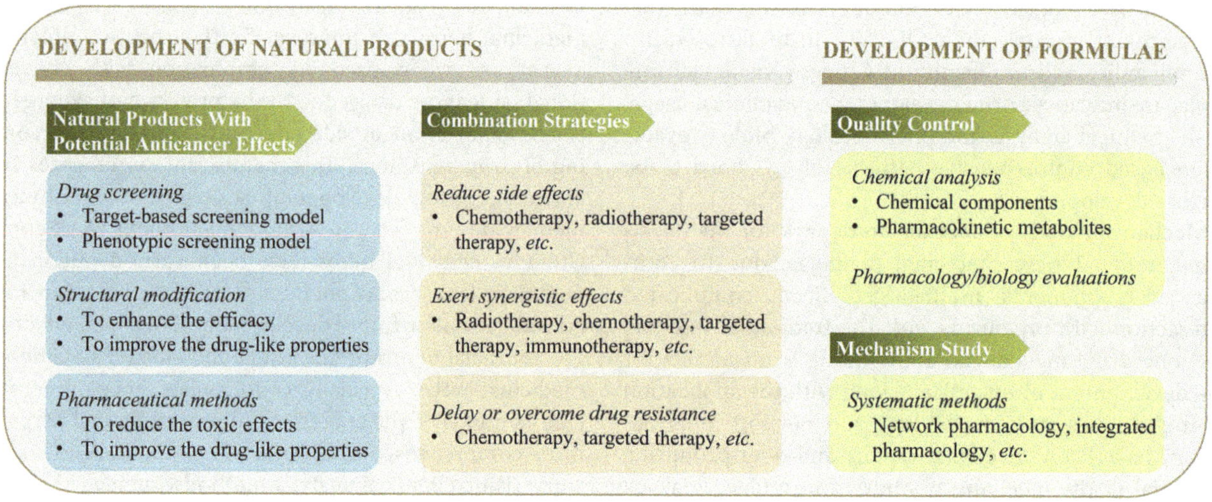

Fig. 3 Anticancer drug development strategies from Chinese medicinal herbs

the natural products which show high contents in Chinese medicinal herbs owing to the limitation of chemical analysis and isolation technologies. However, beside those high-content compounds, there are still many low-content components existing in Chinese medicinal herbs, which also presents a huge resource for drug development. With the development of more and more advanced chemical analysis technologies and screening models, those low-content compounds can be purified and identified for drug discovery. Fifthly, the microbiota of healthy human is in a state of dynamic equilibrium, and a recent study indicated that the imbalance of microbiota would be associated with various types of diseases including cancer [77]. Microbiota can not only promote the occurrence and development of tumor, but also exhibit inhibitory effect against tumor development in some cases [78, 79]. Meanwhile, it was reported that microbiota was associated with the effects of immunotherapy such as anti-CTLA4 and anti-PD-L1 therapy [80, 81]. We wonder whether the anticancer effects of some Chinese medicinal herbs are related with the regulation of microbiota. Last but not least, in recent years, artificial intelligence technology has been introduced into the field of drug discovery and applied in almost all aspects of drug development, such as drug screening and target predicting [82]. Considering the complexity of Chinese medicinal herbs, application of artificial intelligence technology may promote the development of anticancer drugs from Chinese medicinal herbs.

Conclusion

Chinese medicinal herbs provide abundant resource library for drug development. It is extensively potential to discover more anticancer drugs from both natural products and traditional formulae. In this review, we documented the current progression on development of anticancer drugs from Chinese medicinal herbs including the natural products and formulae, along with the defects and obstacles remain to be overcome. A series of drug development strategies and technical approaches that suitable for discovery and development of anticancer drugs from Chinese medicinal herbs have been summarized and discussed. Totally, anticancer drug discovery from Chinese medicinal herbs still need a lot of hard work.

Abbreviations

As_2O_3: arsenic trioxide; EGFR: epidermal growth factor receptor; VEGFR: vascular endothelial growth factor receptor; HER2: human epidermal growth factor 2; mTOR: mechanistic target of rapamycin kinase; PD-1/PD-L1: programmed cell death 1/programmed cell death ligand 1; CTLA-4: cytotoxic T-lymphocyte associated antigen 4; EMT: epithelial-mesenchymal transition; TRAIL/APO-2L: tumor necrosis factor α (TNF-α)–related apoptosis-inducing ligand; QC: quality control; UPLC-Q–TOF–MS: ultra-performance liquid chromatography combined with quadrupole time of flight mass spectrometry.

Authors' contributions

MYH and LLZ drafted the manuscript. JD and JJL conceived and designed the review. All authors read and approved the final manuscript.

Author details

[1] State Key Laboratory of Quality Research in Chinese Medicine, Institute of Chinese Medical Sciences, University of Macau, 7014, N22, Avenida da Universidade, Taipa, Macao, China. [2] Division of Anti-tumor Pharmacology, State Key Laboratory of Drug Research, Shanghai Institute of Materia Medica, Chinese Academy of Sciences, Shanghai, China.

Acknowledgements

This work was supported by the Science and Technology Development Fund, Macao S.A.R (176/2017/A3); the Research Fund of University of Macau (MYRG2018-00165-ICMS, MYRG2015-00091-ICMS-QRCM, and MYRG2015-00101-ICMS-QRCM).

Competing interests

The authors declare that they have no competing interests.

Consent for publication

All of authors consent to publication of this work in Chinese Medicine.

Funding

The Science and Technology Development Fund, Macao S.A.R (176/2017/A3); the Research Fund of University of Macau (MYRG2018-00165-ICMS, MYRG2015-00091-ICMS-QRCM, and MYRG2015-00101-ICMS-QRCM).

References

1. Torre LA, Bray F, Siegel RL, Ferlay J, Lortet-Tieulent J, Jemal A. Global cancer statistics, 2012. CA Cancer J Clin. 2015;65:87–108.
2. Siegel RL, Miller KD, Jemal A. Cancer statistics, 2016. CA Cancer J Clin. 2016;66:7–30.
3. Chen W, Zheng R, Baade PD, Zhang S, Zeng H, Bray F, et al. Cancer statistics in China, 2015. CA Cancer J Clin. 2016;66:115–32.
4. Arruebo M, Vilaboa N, Saez-Gutierrez B, Lambea J, Tres A, Valladares M, et al. Assessment of the evolution of cancer treatment therapies. Cancers. 2011;3:3279–330.
5. Hanahan D, Weinberg RA. Hallmarks of cancer: the next generation. Cell. 2011;144:646–74.
6. Chae YK, Pan AP, Davis AA, Patel SP, Carneiro BA, Kurzrock R, et al. Path toward precision oncology: review of targeted therapy studies and tools to aid in defining "Actionability" of a molecular lesion and patient management support. Mol Cancer Ther. 2017;16:2645–55.
7. Dustin ML. Cancer immunotherapy: killers on sterols. Nature. 2016;531:583–4.
8. Judson PL, Abdallah R, Xiong Y, Ebbert J, Lancaster JM. Complementary and alternative medicine use in individuals presenting for care at a comprehensive cancer center. Integr Cancer Ther. 2017;16:96–103.
9. Carmady B, Smith CA. Use of Chinese medicine by cancer patients: a review of surveys. Chin Med. 2011;6:22.
10. Liu J, Wang S, Zhang Y, Fan HT, Lin HS. Traditional Chinese medicine and cancer: history, present situation, and development. Thorac Cancer. 2015;6:561–9.
11. Hsiao WL, Liu L. The role of traditional Chinese herbal medicines in cancer therapy—from TCM theory to mechanistic insights. Planta Med. 2010;76:1118–31.
12. Zhang Y, Liang Y, He C. Anticancer activities and mechanisms of heat-clearing and detoxicating traditional Chinese herbal medicine. Chin Med. 2017;12:20.
13. Gill H, Yim R, Lee HKK, Mak V, Lin SY, Kho B, et al. Long-term outcome of relapsed acute promyelocytic leukemia treated with oral arsenic trioxide-based reinduction and maintenance regimens: a 15-year prospective study. Cancer. 2018;124:2316–26.
14. Rockwell S, Grove TA, Liu Y, Cheng YC, Higgins SA, Booth CJ. Preclinical studies of the Chinese Herbal Medicine formulation PHY906 (KD018) as a potential adjunct to radiation therapy. Int J Radiat Biol. 2013;89:16–25.
15. Katz L, Baltz RH. Natural product discovery: past, present, and future. J Ind Microbiol Biotechnol. 2016;43:155–76.
16. Tan W, Lu J, Huang M, Li Y, Chen M, Wu G, et al. Anti-cancer natural products isolated from chinese medicinal herbs. Chin Med. 2011;6:27.
17. Swinney D. Phenotypic vs. target-based drug discovery for first-in-class medicines. Clin Pharmacol Ther. 2013;93:299–301.
18. Siddik ZH. Cisplatin: mode of cytotoxic action and molecular basis of resistance. Oncogene. 2003;22:7265–79.
19. Crown J, O'leary M. The taxanes: an update. Lancet. 2000;355:1176–8.
20. Johnson RK. Screening methods in antineoplastic drug discovery. J Natl Cancer Inst. 1990;82:1082–3.
21. Rowinsky EK, Calvo E. Novel agents that target tublin and related elements. Semin Oncol. 2006;33:421–35.
22. Newlands E, Stevens M, Wedge S, Wheelhouse R, Brock C. Temozolomide: a review of its discovery, chemical properties, pre-clinical development and clinical trials. Cancer Treat Rev. 1997;23:35–61.
23. Lee DH, Szczepanski MJ, Lee YJ. Magnolol induces apoptosis via inhibiting the EGFR/PI3K/Akt signaling pathway in human prostate cancer cells. J Cell Biochem. 2009;106:1113–22.
24. Li L, Lin J, Sun G, Wei L, Shen A, Zhang M, et al. Oleanolic acid inhibits colorectal cancer angiogenesis in vivo and in vitro via suppression of STAT3 and Hedgehog pathways. Mol Med Rep. 2016;13:5276–82.
25. Lim SO, Li CW, Xia W, Cha JH, Chan LC, Wu Y, et al. Deubiquitination and stabilization of PD-L1 by CSN5. Cancer Cell. 2016;30:925–39.
26. Colak S, ten Dijke P. Targeting TGF-β signaling in cancer. Trends Cancer. 2017;3:56–71.
27. Pei Z, Fu W, Wang G. A natural product toosendanin inhibits epithelial-mesenchymal transition and tumor growth in pancreatic cancer via deactivating Akt/mTOR signaling. Biochem Biophys Res Commun. 2017;493:455–60.

28. Moffat JG, Rudolph J, Bailey D. Phenotypic screening in cancer drug discovery—past, present and future. Nat Rev Drug Discov. 2014;13:588.
29. Huang M, Lu JJ, Huang MQ, Bao JL, Chen XP, Wang YT. Terpenoids: natural products for cancer therapy. Expert Opin Investig Drugs. 2012;21:1801–18.
30. Lu JJ, Bao JL, Wu GS, Xu WS, Huang MQ, Chen XP, et al. Quinones derived from plant secondary metabolites as anti-cancer agents. Anticancer Agents Med Chem. 2013;13:456–63.
31. Lu JJ, Bao JL, Chen XP, Huang M, Wang YT. Alkaloids isolated from natural herbs as the anticancer agents. Evid Based Complement Altern Med. 2012;2012:485042.
32. Xu XH, Li T, Fong CM, Chen X, Chen XJ, Wang YT, et al. Saponins from Chinese medicines as anticancer agents. Molecules. 2016;21:1326.
33. Venkata Sairam K, Gurupadayya BM, Chandan RS, Nagesha DK, Vishwanathan B. A review on chemical profile of coumarins and their therapeutic role in the treatment of cancer. Curr Drug Deliv. 2016;13:186–201.
34. Yao H, Liu J, Xu S, Zhu Z, Xu J. The structural modification of natural products for novel drug discovery. Expert Opin Drug Discov. 2017;12:121–40.
35. Li QY, Zu YG, Shi RZ, Yao LP. Review camptothecin: current perspectives. Curr Med Chem. 2006;13:2021–39.
36. Sriram D, Yogeeswari P, Thirumurugan R, Ratan Bal T. Camptothecin and its analogues: a review on their chemotherapeutic potential. Nat Prod Res. 2005;19:393–412.
37. Ding C, Tian Q, Li J, Jiao M, Song S, Wang Y, et al. Structural modification of natural product tanshinone I leading to discovery of novel nitrogen-enriched derivatives with enhanced anticancer profile and improved drug-like properties. J Med Chem. 2018;61:760–76.
38. Lu P, Zhang FC, Qian SW, Li X, Cui ZM, Dang YJ, et al. Artemisinin derivatives prevent obesity by inducing browning of WAT and enhancing BAT function. Cell Res. 2016;26:1169–72.
39. Efferth T. Beyond malaria: the inhibition of viruses by artemisinin-type compounds. Biotechnol Adv. 2018. https://doi.org/10.1016/j.biotechadv.2018.01.001.
40. Ma N, Wang Y, Zhao BX, Ye WC, Jiang S. The application of click chemistry in the synthesis of agents with anticancer activity. Drug Des Dev Ther. 2015;9:1585–99.
41. Wang R, Li L, Zhang S, Li Y, Wang X, Miao Q, et al. A novel enediyne-integrated antibody-drug conjugate shows promising antitumor efficacy against CD30(+) lymphomas. Mol Oncol. 2018;12:339–55.
42. Xu W, Xing FJ, Dong K, You C, Yan Y, Zhang L, et al. Application of traditional Chinese medicine preparation in targeting drug delivery system. Drug Deliv. 2015;22:258–65.
43. Li W, Yin H, Bardelang D, Xiao J, Zheng Y, Wang R. Supramolecular formulation of nitidine chloride can alleviate its hepatotoxicity and improve its anticancer activity. Food Chem Toxicol. 2017;109:923–9.
44. Qi F, Zhao L, Zhou A, Zhang B, Li A, Wang Z, et al. The advantages of using traditional Chinese medicine as an adjunctive therapy in the whole course of cancer treatment instead of only terminal stage of cancer. Biosci Trends. 2015;9:16–34.
45. Qi F, Li A, Inagaki Y, Gao J, Li J, Kokudo N, et al. Chinese herbal medicines as adjuvant treatment during chemo- or radio-therapy for cancer. Biosci Trends. 2010;4:297–307.
46. Cheng YC, Tsai MY, Chen CJ, Hung YC. Combination therapy of traditional Chinese medicine and Western medicine to treat refractory polymyositis: a case report. J Altern Complement Med. 2015;21:304–6.
47. Chen S, Flower A, Ritchie A, Liu J, Molassiotis A, Yu H, et al. Oral Chinese herbal medicine (CHM) as an adjuvant treatment during chemotherapy for non-small cell lung cancer: a systematic review. Lung Cancer. 2010;68:137–45.
48. Gao Y, Chu S, Shao Q, Zhang M, Xia C, Wang Y, et al. Antioxidant activities of ginsenoside Rg1 against cisplatin-induced hepatic injury through Nrf2 signaling pathway in mice. Free Radic Res. 2017;51:1–13.
49. Yu J, Wang C, Kong Q, Wu X, Lu JJ, Chen X. Recent progress in doxorubicin-induced cardiotoxicity and protective potential of natural products. Phytomedicine. 2018;40:125–39.
50. Sahu BD, Kumar JM, Kuncha M, Borkar RM, Srinivas R, Sistla R. Baicalein alleviates doxorubicin-induced cardiotoxicity via suppression of myocardial oxidative stress and apoptosis in mice. Life Sci. 2016;144:8–18.
51. Jia Y, Zuo D, Li Z, Liu H, Dai Z, Cai J, et al. Astragaloside IV inhibits doxorubicin-induced cardiomyocyte apoptosis mediated by mitochondrial apoptotic pathway via activating the PI3K/Akt pathway. Chem Pharm Bull. 2014;62:45–53.
52. Pirker R, Pereira JR, Szczesna A, Von Pawel J, Krzakowski M, Ramlau R, et al. Cetuximab plus chemotherapy in patients with advanced non-small-cell lung cancer (FLEX): an open-label randomised phase III trial. Lancet. 2009;373:1525–31.
53. Li T, Chen X, Chen X, Ma DL, Leung CH, Lu JJ. Platycodin D potentiates proliferation inhibition and apoptosis induction upon AKT inhibition via feedback blockade in non-small cell lung cancer cells. Sci Rep. 2016;6:37997.
54. Li T, Chen X, Dai XY, Wei B, Weng QJ, Chen X, et al. Novel Hsp90 inhibitor platycodin D disrupts Hsp90/Cdc37 complex and enhances the anticancer effect of mTOR inhibitor. Toxicol Appl Pharmacol. 2017;330:65–73.
55. Zhu H, Ding WJ, Wu R, Weng QJ, Lou JS, Jin RJ, et al. Synergistic anti-cancer activity by the combination of TRAIL/APO-2L and celastrol. Cancer Invest. 2010;28:23–32.
56. Bhaw-Luximon A, Jhurry D. Artemisinin and its derivatives in cancer therapy: status of progress, mechanism of action, and future perspectives. Cancer Chemother Pharmacol. 2017;79:451–66.
57. Guan Z, Lan H, Chen X, Jiang X, Li Z, Yu X, et al. Synergistic effects and mechanism of Danshen injection in combination with chemotherapy and antiangiogenic therapy for colon cancer. Int J Clin Exp Med. 2017;10:6437–44.
58. Holohan C, Van Schaeybroeck S, Longley DB, Johnston PG. Cancer drug resistance: an evolving paradigm. Nat Rev Cancer. 2013;13:714–26.
59. Gottesman MM. Mechanisms of cancer drug resistance. Annu Rev Med. 2002;53:615–27.
60. Singh A, Settleman J. EMT, cancer stem cells and drug resistance: an emerging axis of evil in the war on cancer. Oncogene. 2010;29:4741–51.
61. Li Y, Wang Y, Niu K, Chen X, Xia L, Lu D, et al. Clinical benefit from EGFR-TKI plus ginsenoside Rg3 in patients with advanced non-small cell lung cancer harboring EGFR active mutation. Oncotarget. 2016;7:70535.
62. Chen Q, Qin R, Fang Y, Li H. Berberine sensitizes human ovarian cancer cells to cisplatin through miR-93/PTEN/Akt signaling pathway. Cell Physiol Biochem. 2015;36:956–65.
63. Qi YB, Wu JH, Liu BY, Zhang DS. Effects of Xue Fu Zhu Yu decoction on immune function of tumor-bearing mice. Modern Prev Med. 2005;5:446–8.
64. Lu XF. Experimental study on the effects of chemotherapy combined with Xuefu Zhuyu decoction polysaccharide on transplanted tumor in rats. Mod J Integr Tradit Chin West Med. 2008;16:2446–7.
65. Zhang K, Zhang J, Wang X, Wang L, Pugliese M, Passantino A, et al. Cardioprotection of Sheng Mai Yin a classic formula on adriamycin induced myocardial injury in Wistar rats. Phytomedicine. 2018;38:1–11.
66. Liu SH, Cheng YC. Old formula, new Rx: the journey of PHY906 as cancer adjuvant therapy. J Ethnopharmacol. 2012;140:614–23.
67. Lam W, Bussom S, Guan F, Jiang Z, Zhang W, Gullen EA, et al. The four-herb Chinese medicine PHY906 reduces chemotherapy-induced gastrointestinal toxicity. Sci Transl Med. 2010;2:45ra59.
68. Lam W, Jiang Z, Guan F, Huang X, Hu R, Wang J, et al. PHY906(KD018), an adjuvant based on a 1800-year-old Chinese medicine, enhanced the anti-tumor activity of Sorafenib by changing the tumor microenvironment. Sci Rep. 2015;5:9384.
69. Gao D, Wang B, Huo Z, He Y, Polachi N, Lei Z, et al. Analysis of chemical constituents in an herbal formula Jitong Ning Tablet. J Pharm Biomed Anal. 2017;140:301–12.
70. Li X, Sun H, Zhang A, Liu Z, Zou D, Song Y, et al. High-throughput LC–MS method for the rapid characterization of multiple chemical constituents and metabolites of Da-Bu-Yin-Wan. J Sep Sci. 2017;40:4102–12.
71. Tilton R, Paiva AA, Guan JQ, Marathe R, Jiang Z, van Eyndhoven W, et al. A comprehensive platform for quality control of botanical drugs (PhytomicsQC): a case study of Huangqin Tang (HQT) and PHY906. Chin Med. 2010;5:30.
72. Wang L, Zhou GB, Liu P, Song JH, Liang Y, Yan XJ, et al. Dissection of mechanisms of Chinese medicinal formula Realgar-Indigo naturalis as an effective treatment for promyelocytic leukemia. Proc Natl Acad Sci USA. 2008;105:4826–31.
73. Liang X, Li H, Li S. A novel network pharmacology approach to analyse traditional herbal formulae: the Liu-Wei-Di-Huang pill as a case study. Mol BioSyst. 2014;10:1014–22.

74. Chen M, Yang F, Yang X, Lai X, Gao Y. Systematic understanding of mechanisms of a Chinese herbal formula in treatment of metabolic syndrome by an integrated pharmacology approach. Int J Mol Sci. 2016;17:2114.
75. Li SP, Zhao J, Yang B. Strategies for quality control of Chinese medicines. J Pharm Biomed Anal. 2011;55:802–9.
76. Liang Y, Xie P, Chau F. Chromatographic fingerprinting and related chemometric techniques for quality control of traditional Chinese medicines. J Sep Sci. 2010;33:410–21.
77. Hall AB, Tolonen AC, Xavier RJ. Human genetic variation and the gut microbiome in disease. Nat Rev Genet. 2017;18:690–9.
78. Li J, Sung CY, Lee N, Ni Y, Pihlajamaki J, Panagiotou G, et al. Probiotics modulated gut microbiota suppresses hepatocellular carcinoma growth in mice. Proc Natl Acad Sci USA. 2016;113:E1306–15.
79. Peuker K, Muff S, Wang J, Kunzel S, Bosse E, Zeissig Y, et al. Epithelial calcineurin controls microbiota-dependent intestinal tumor development. Nat Med. 2016;22:506–15.
80. Vetizou M, Pitt JM, Daillere R, Lepage P, Waldschmitt N, Flament C, et al. Anticancer immunotherapy by CTLA-4 blockade relies on the gut microbiota. Science. 2015;350:1079–84.
81. Sivan A, Corrales L, Hubert N, Williams JB, Aquino-Michaels K, Earley ZM, et al. Commensal Bifidobacterium promotes antitumor immunity and facilitates anti-PD-L1 efficacy. Science. 2015;350:1084–9.
82. Schneider G. Automating drug discovery. Nat Rev Drug Discov. 2018;17:97–113.

5

Wnt5a mediates the effects of Bushen Huoxue decoction on the migration of bone marrow mesenchymal stem cells in vitro

Wei Shen[1†], Hui Luo[1†], Liangliang Xu[2], Zhifang Wu[1], Hongtai Chen[1], Yamei Liu[3], Lijuan Yu[3], Liuchao Hu[1], Bin Wang[1*] and Yiwen Luo[1*]

Abstract

Background: Bushen Huoxue decoction (BHD) has a significant effect on fracture rehabilitation, yet its underlying mechanism is still unknown. The purpose of this study was to explore whether BHD promotes bone marrow mesenchymal stem cell (BMSC) migration through the Wnt5a signalling pathway.

Methods: BHD was extracted by petroleum, and its composition was analysed. Cell viability in the presence of various concentrations of BHD for 24, 48 and 72 h was measured using a Cell Counting Kit-8 assay. Transwell assays and wound healing assays were used to observe the migration ability of BMSCs. Lentiviral vectors were used to knock down Wnt5a. Polymerase chain reaction and Western blot analyses were used to further compare Wnt5a signalling components at the mRNA and protein levels between groups.

Results: BHD treatment groups showed increased migration ability and Wnt5a expression. Knocking down Wnt5a using a lentivirus significantly inhibited the effects of BHD, which implies that BHD promotes BMSC migration ability through activation of Wnt5a.

Conclusions: BHD can enhance BMSC migration, possibly by activating Wnt5a signalling.

Keywords: Fracture, Bushen Huoxue decoction, Bone marrow mesenchymal stem cell, Migration, Wnt5a

Background

Bone fracture can severely impact a patient's quality of life. Many patients suffer from fractures, which are both costly and require extensive time to heal. Bone fracture healing is a remarkably complex repair process which is similar to the embryonic development [1]. Delayed union or poor fracture healing poses a serious threat to the quality of life of patients. Bone fractures are repaired by two mechanisms: direct and indirect bone repair. Indirect fracture healing is initiated by an immediate inflammatory response, which results in the recruitment of bone marrow mesenchymal stem cells (BMSCs) to the injury site. Condensation is the pivotal stage in the development of skeletal and other mesenchymal tissues. It occurs when a previously dispersed population of cells gathers together to differentiate into a single cell/tissue type such as cartilage, bone, muscle [2]. BMSCs subsequently differentiate into chondrocytes, which produce cartilage and form a callus [3]. Bone formation begins when mesenchymal cells form condensations involving different cellular processes (migration, adhesion, proliferation, and growth) [2]. By identifying relevant cytokines and chemokines released from the bone injury region, BMSCs in niches can be activated and migrate to the injury region [4]. Therefore, intervening measures can accelerate BMSC migration processes and may contribute to bone repair.

Wnt signalling pathways can be divided into two categories: canonical (Wnt/β-catenin-dependent) pathways and non-canonical pathways. Non-canonical Wnt

*Correspondence: wangbin1973@163.com; gzzyydxlyw@126.com
†Wei Shen and Hui Luo contributed equally to this work
[1] Department of Traumatology, The Third Affiliated Hospital of Guangzhou University of Traditional Chinese Medicine, 22 Jiangnan-Xi Road, Guangzhou 510240, Guangdong, People's Republic of China
Full list of author information is available at the end of the article

signalling pathways include the Wnt/PCP and Wnt/protein kinase C (PKC)-Ca^{2+} pathways [5]. Both pathways are linked to cell adhesion and movement [6, 7]. Wnt5a activates the latter pathways [6, 8, 9] and is closely associated with cell motility and invasion [10].

Bushen Huoxue decoction (BHD) has been used to treat craniocerebral diseases and ovarian diseases [11–13] and is helpful for treating bone diseases such as osteoarthritis and osteoporosis [14, 15]. BHD was first described by Zhuquan Zhao in the Qing Dynasty. Since then, it has been widely used in patients with fractures, especially elderly patients. According to traditional Chinese medicine, BHD can promote blood circulation, help alleviate swelling at the fracture site and accelerate bone repair. Studies demonstrated that BHD treated group could obviously promote differentiation, proliferation and mineralization of osteoblasts through activation of Wnt/β-catenin signaling pathway and can also improve cartilage metabolism in experimental rabbits and possesses osteo-chondric protective effects in antagonizing peroxidation injury [16, 17]. In our previous study, we compared the migration ability of BMSCs treated with BHD extracted with four different solvents (petroleum ether, ethyl acetate, absolute alcohol and water). We found that BHD extracted with petroleum induced the greatest improvement in cell migration in a dose-dependent manner [18]. However, the underlying mechanism is still unknown. The purpose of this study was to explore this unknown mechanism. We hypothesized that BHD promotes cell migration ability by activating Wnt5a.

Methods

The minimum standards of reporting checklist contains details of the experimental design, and statistics, and resources used in this study (Additional file 1).

BHD preparation and detection of herbal ingredients

Eleven Chinese herbs (Radix Rehmanniae 18 g, Semen Cuscutae 18 g, Fructus Psoraleae 18 g, Eucommia ulmoides 6 g, Fructus Corni 6 g, Herba Cistanches 6 g, Fructus Lycii 6 g, Radix Angelicae Pubescentis 6 g, Radix Angelicae Sinensis 6 g, Myrrha 6 g, and Flos Carthami 3 g) were purchased from The Third Affiliated Hospital of Guangzhou University of Chinese Medicine. After drying for 24 h and being pulverized into powder, the total herbs were wrapped with filter paper and transferred to a Soxhlet apparatus. The components were extracted using the Soxhlet extraction method in petroleum [19]. The extract was concentrated by rotary evaporation and plaster precipitation, and the product was weighed. One gram was dissolved in petroleum and analysed by gas chromatography–mass spectrometry (GC–MS). The remaining product was dissolved in dimethylsulfoxide and filtered through a 0.22-μm syringe filter (Millex-GP, USA) before use. The concentration of the storage solution was 400 μmol/ml and was diluted to the needed concentration before use.

BMSC isolation and culture

This study was approved by the Animal Care and Use Committee of Guangzhou University of Traditional Chinese Medicine. BMSCs were isolated from Sprague–Dawley rats (male, 4 weeks old, 60–80 g) in a sterile environment (n = 30). Rats were euthanized by carbon dioxide inhalation. The bone marrow of the bilateral femoral and tibial shafts was flushed out with serum-free low-glucose Dulbecco's modified Eagle's medium (DMEM) to obtain a single-cell suspension. The obtained bone marrow solution was centrifuged at 1200 rpm for 6 min, the supernatant liquid was removed, and the cell pellets were resuspended in glucose-DMEM supplemented with 10% foetal bovine serum, 1% β-mercaptoethanol and 1% penicillin and streptomycin (all from Gibco, USA). The medium was discarded after 24 h of primary culture and then changed once every 3 days. On day 4, the non-adherent cells were washed out with phosphate-buffered saline (PBS), and the adherent cells were further expanded until reaching 80% confluence. Cells were digested with a 0.25% trypsin solution and observed under an inverted microscope. The digestion was terminated by addition of low-glucose DMEM containing 10% serum when cells became round and detached. A single-cell suspension was prepared and subcultured at a ratio of 1:2. The medium was changed several times to obtain pure BMSCs. Cells from passages 3 to 5 were used in the study.

Osteoblast and adipocyte differentiation

BMSCs were cultured and seeded in 6-well plates in L-DMEM containing 10% FBS and 1% penicillin–streptomycin for 24 h. The medium was replaced by osteoblast media or adipocyte media when cells became confluent. The osteoblast media contained 10^{-8} M dexamethasone, 10 mM β-glycerophosphate and 0.05 mM L-ascorbic acid (all from Sigma-Aldrich, MO, USA), while the adipocyte media contained 10^{-6} M dexamethasone, 0.5 mM isobutylmethylxanthine, 100 μM indomethacin and 10 mg/l insulin (all from Sigma-Aldrich, MO, USA). The medium was changed every 3 days. On the 21st day, alizarin red and oil red O staining were performed to observe the differentiation of BMSCs.

Characterization of BMSCs

Cells were harvested by trypsin, resuspended in cold PBS, and then incubated with the corresponding FITC/PE-conjugated antibodies for the stem cell markers CD-90,

CD-44, the endothelial marker CD-34, and the haematopoietic marker CD-45. Cells were analysed using a BD FACSCanto flow cytometer.

Detection of cell proliferation

BMSCs were inoculated at 2×10^5/ml in 96-well culture plates (approximately 2000 cells in 100 μl of medium per well). Then, 100 μl of serum-free medium was added, and cells were starved for 12 h. The medium was replaced with complete medium containing different concentrations of BHD (0, 1, 10, 25, 50, 100 and 150 μg/ml). Ten microlitres of CCK8 dye was add to each well after 24, 48 h, and cells were cultured for an additional 3 h. The absorbance was recorded at a wavelength of 450 nm using a microplate reader to determine the level of proliferation in each well (n = 6).

Scratch wound healing assay

BMSCs were seeded in 6-well plates and cultured until 95% confluence. The medium was displaced by serum-free L-DMEM for 12 h. A scratch wound was created with a micropipette tip. The cells were treated with different concentrations of BHD (0, 25, 50, 100, and 150 μg/ml), and the scratch area was observed under a phase contrast microscope and photographed (n = 6).

Cell migration assay

Cell migration ability was evaluated using in Transwell plates with a pore size of 8 μm (Corning Costar, Cambridge). Cells were digested and resuspended at 1×10^5/ml in serum-free medium in the upper chamber. The upper chamber was then loaded with 8×10^4 BMSCs in 200 μl serum-free medium. After culturing in an incubator for 2 h, the lower chamber was loaded with 700 μl complete medium containing different concentrations of BHD. The plates were incubated at 37 °C in 5% CO_2 for 10 h. The upper surface of the membrane was then gently scraped using a cotton swab to remove the non-migrated cells and washed with PBS. The membrane was then fixed in 4% paraformaldehyde for 30 min, followed by staining with Giemsa stain. Migrated cells were observed and photographed under a phase contrast microscope. The number of migrated cells was determined by averaging five random fields per well (n = 6).

Lentivirus transfection

To obtain BMSCs with silenced Wnt5a expression, BMSCs were cultured and transfected with Wnt5a-specific short hairpin RNA (sh-Wnt5a) lentiviral vectors. Green fluorescent protein (GFP) was expressed in the lentiviruses and was used to evaluate BMSC transduction efficiency. The transfection efficiency was tested by quantitative RT-PCR. Transfections were performed in BMSCs with a multiplicity of infection (MOI) of 6:1, following the manufacturer's instructions. Lentiviral vectors were purchased from GeneChem (Shanghai, China). The medium containing lentiviral vectors was replaced with complete medium after 12 h.

Real-time PCR analysis

Total RNA was extracted from BMSCs using TRIzol reagent (Invitrogen, Carlsbad, CA, USA) according to the manufacturer's instructions. The RNA concentration was measured using an ultraviolet spectrophotometer (BioSpec-nano). cDNA was produced from the total RNA using PrimeScript RT Master Mix (TaKaRa, Tokyo, Japan). Primer sequences are shown in Table 1. The expression levels of Wnt5a, PKC, JNK and CaMKII were analysed. The ΔΔCt method was used to calculate the expression of mRNAs relative to GAPDH. All steps were performed under RNase-free conditions.

Western blotting

For Western blotting, we used RIPA buffer (Boston BioProducts, Ashland, MA, USA) to extract the total protein of BMSCs. The protein concentration was measured by a BCA Protein Assay kit (Pierce, Rockford, IL, USA). Equivalent masses of protein samples (30 μg) were separated by 10% SDS-PAGE and electrophoretically transferred onto PVDF membranes (Millipore, Billerica, MA, USA). The PVDF membranes were blocked in TBST containing 5% skim milk for 1 h and then incubated with mouse anti-Wnt5a (1:1000, Abcam), rabbit anti-SAPK/JNK (1:1000, CST), rabbit anti-CaMKII (1:1000 CST), mouse anti-PKC (1:1000, Millipore) and rabbit anti-GAPDH (1:4000, Abcam) primary antibodies overnight at 4 °C. The membranes were washed in TBST and incubated with a corresponding secondary antibody for 1 h at room

Table 1 List of primer sequences for RT-PCR

Primer name	Sequence	Product length (bp)
WNT5A forward	5′-CGAAGACGGGCATCAAAGA-3′	97
WNT5A reverse	5′-TGCATCACCCTGCCAAAGA-3′	
JNK forward	5′-GGAGCGAACTAAGAATGGCG-3′	106
JNK reverse	5′-CATGTCATTGACAGACGGCG-3′	
CaMKII forward	5′-ATGGATGGAAATGGAATGCC-3′	102
CaMKII reverse	5′-CCCCGAACGATGAAAGTGAA-3′	
PKC forward	5′-AAGGTGGTCCACGAGGTGAA-3′	100
PKC reverse	5′-TTCCAATGCCCCAGATGAAG-3′	
GAPDH forward	5′-AGGGCTGCCTTCTCTTGTGA-3′	110
GAPDH reverse	5′-AACTTGCCGTGGGTAGAGTCA-3′	

temperature. Bands were visualized using an enhanced chemiluminescence kit according to the manufacturer's protocol.

Statistical analysis

Data are presented as the mean ± SD. One-way ANOVA was used for multiple comparisons. A value of $P < 0.05$ was considered statistically significant.

Results

Analysis of the herbal formula: BHD chemical ingredients

BHD extracted with petroleum ether was sent to the Chinese National Analytical Center, Guangzhou, and was analysed by GC–MS. A total of 45 peaks were shown in GC/MS spectrum. Standard analytical procedures were used for screening of ingredients. The spectrum of components was compared with spectrum stored in the NIST library version. The eluted compounds were characterized on the basis of their molecular formula, structure, retention time, and peak % area. A total of 21 distinct peaks are reflected. Twelve constituents were found in the fingerprint (Fig. 1) and are summarized in Table 2.

Table 2 Chemical components of BHD

No.	Identification	Peak % area
1.	δ-Elemene	0.19
2.	α-Copaene	0.16
3.	Caryophyllene	0.19
4.	β-selinene	0.29
5.	Caryophyllene oxide	0.74
6.	Curzerenone	3.21
7.	Unknown ingredient	1.72
8.	3-Butylphthalide; 3-butyl-1(3*H*)-isobenzofuranone	5.22
9.	Isopsoralen	2.43
10.	Psoralen	2.32
11.	Unknown ingredient	1.25
12.	Unknown ingredient	2.57
13.	Unknown ingredient	1.59
14.	Unknown ingredient	2.63
15.	Bakuchiol	34.92
16.	Osthole	18.54
17.	Unknown ingredient	3.28
18.	Decursin	1.87
19.	Unknown ingredient	0.99
20.	Unknown ingredient	2.73
21.	Unknown ingredient	0.95

Identification of BMSCs

BMSCs were cultured and passaged until passage 3. They showed a fusiform cell morphology (Fig. 2a, b), and cells had both osteogenic (Fig. 2c) and adipogenic differentiation ability (Fig. 2d). BMSC surface markers were analysed by flow cytometry. The cells were positive for CD90 (98.63%) and CD44 (98.48%) but negative for CD34 (0.25%) and CD45 (0.25%) (Fig. 2e), which morphologically and immunophenotypically demonstrated that the cells were BMSCs.

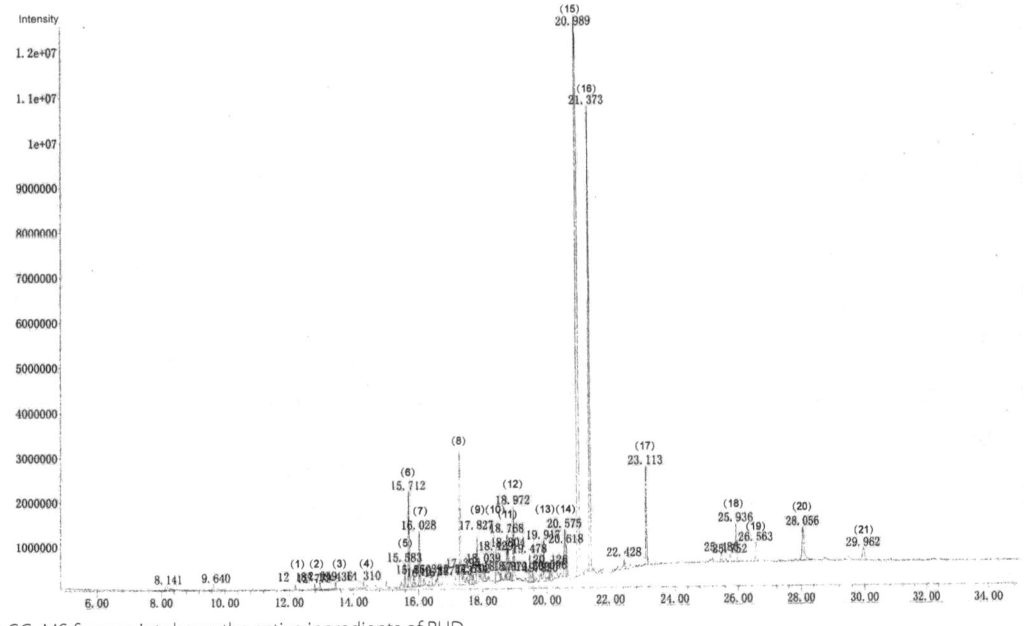

Fig. 1 The GC–MS fingerprint shows the active ingredients of BHD

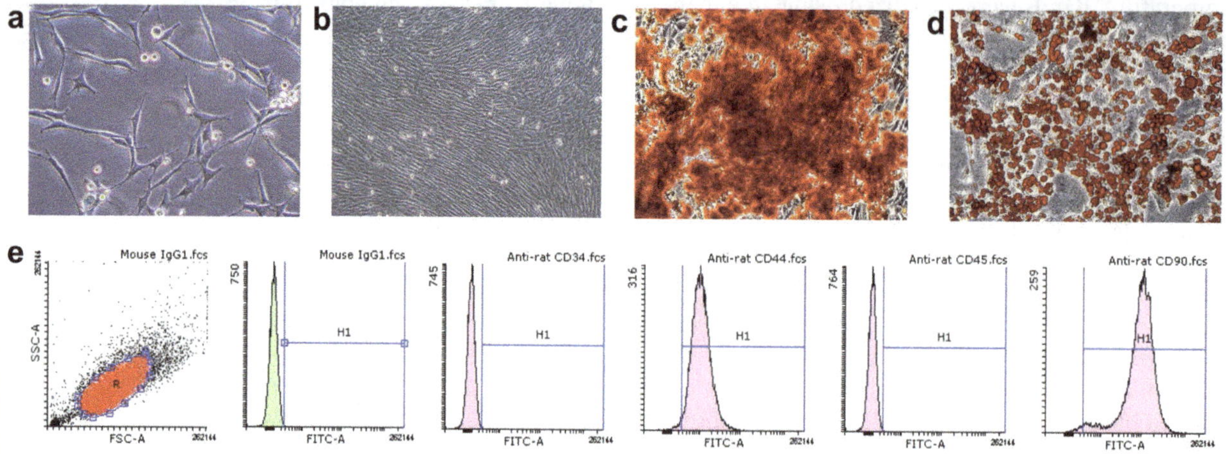

Fig. 2 **a** BMSCs exhibited a fusiform cell morphology. **b** BMSCs at passage 3 and 95% confluence. **c** Alizarin red staining shows that the cells were capable of osteogenesis. **d** Oil red O staining shows that cells were also adipogenic. **e** Cells were positive for CD-44, and CD-90 and negative for CD-34 and CD-45

Treatment of BMSCs with different concentrations of BHD

As shown in Fig. 3, cell viability peaked when BMSCs were treated with 100 μg/ml BHD for 24 h and 48 h (Fig. 3). These results show that low-dose BHD is not toxic to cells and can promote cell proliferation within 48 h of treatment.

Silencing Wnt5a inhibits BMSC migration

Different concentrations of BHD (150, 100, 50, 25 μg/ml) were added to the lower chamber of the Transwell plate, and migrated cells were counted after staining and photographing. Treated groups showed a significant acceleration of BMSC migration compared with that in the control group, especially in the 100 μg/ml BHD group (Fig. 4a). The scratch wound healing assay showed comparable results (Fig. 4b). To observe whether BHD could activate Wnt5a expression, BMSCs were transduced with sh-Wnt5a. After transfection by lentiviral vectors (Fig. 5a), sh-Wnt5a and sh-scrambled BMSCs were harvested and compared regarding Wnt5a expression. sh-Wnt5a BMSCs exhibited significantly reduced Wnt5a expression (Fig. 5c). Then, a Transwell assay was performed to compare their migration ability with the 100 μg/ml BHD group (Fig. 5b), and the data showed that silencing Wnt5a significantly inhibited the migration of BMSCs (Fig. 5d).

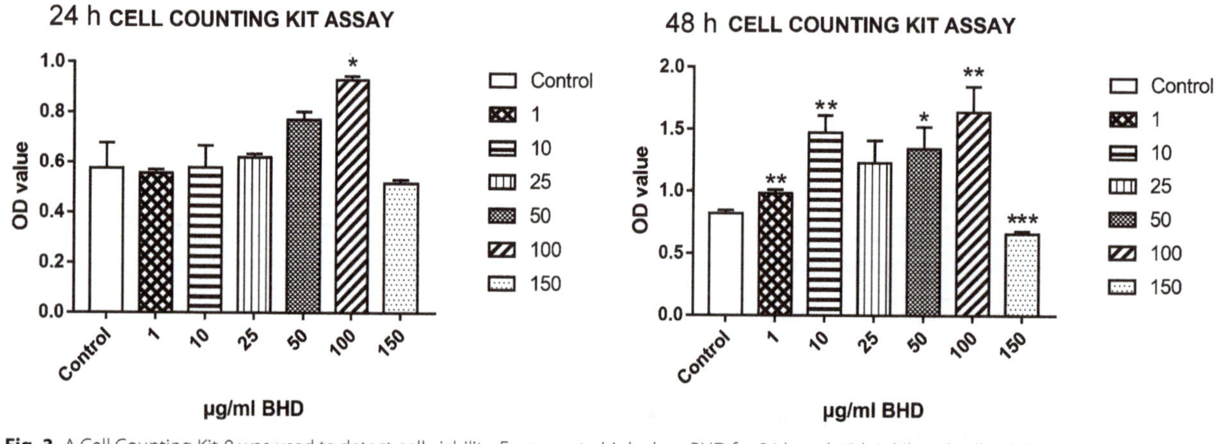

Fig. 3 A Cell Counting Kit-8 was used to detect cell viability. Exposure to high-dose BHD for 24 h and 48 h inhibited cell viability. Treatment with 100 μg/ml BHD increased cell viability at 24 h and 48 h. $^{*}P < 0.05$, $^{**}P < 0.01$, $^{***}P < 0.0001$ for the treatment groups vs. the control group (n = 6)

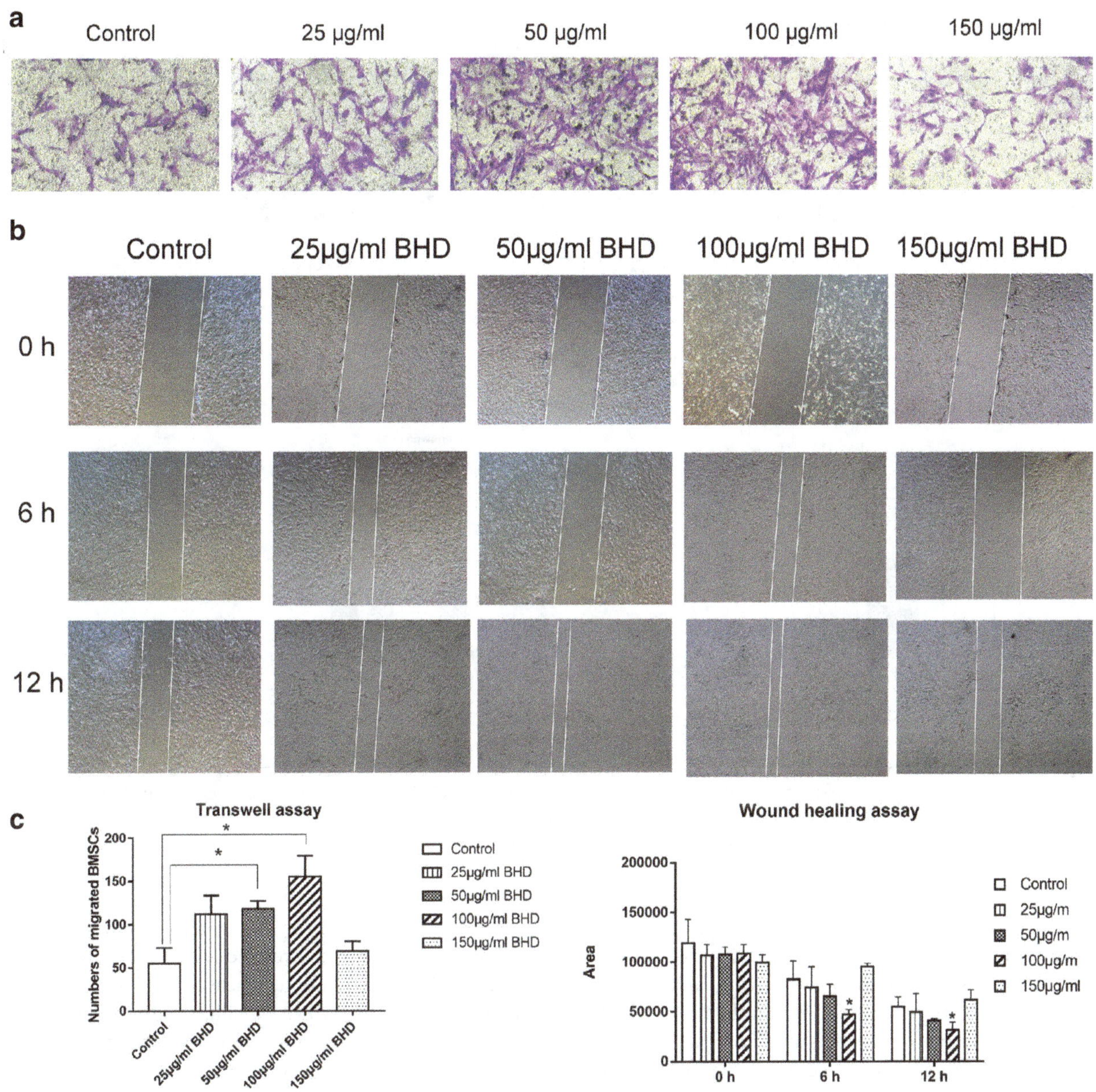

Fig. 4 BHD-treated groups showed a stronger migration ability, especially the 100 μg/ml BHD group. **a** Transwell assays showed that BHD enhanced cell migration ability. **b** Dynamic migration in the scratch wound healing assay. BMSCs treated with 100 μg/ml BHD showed outstanding performance with regard to healing speed. **c** The data for transwell assay and wound healing assay. *$P < 0.05$ for the treatment groups vs. the control group

BHD activates Wnt5a-related gene expression

To determine whether BHD can active Wnt5a, we treated BMSCs with 100 μg/ml BHD. Wnt5a, SAPK/JNK and CaMKII expression were all significantly increased at the mRNA level (Fig. 6a).

Western blot analysis

Comparable results at the protein level were observed in Western blot analyses of Wnt5a, SAPK/JNK, CaMKII and PKC. The data showed a parallel result to the mRNA data, which indicates that BHD can act on Wnt5a and upregulate its signalling proteins, SAPK/JNK, CaMKII and PKC (Fig. 6b).

Discussion

BHD has been used to promote fracture healing by doctors of traditional Chinese medicine since it was described by Zhuquan Zhao in the Qing Dynasty.

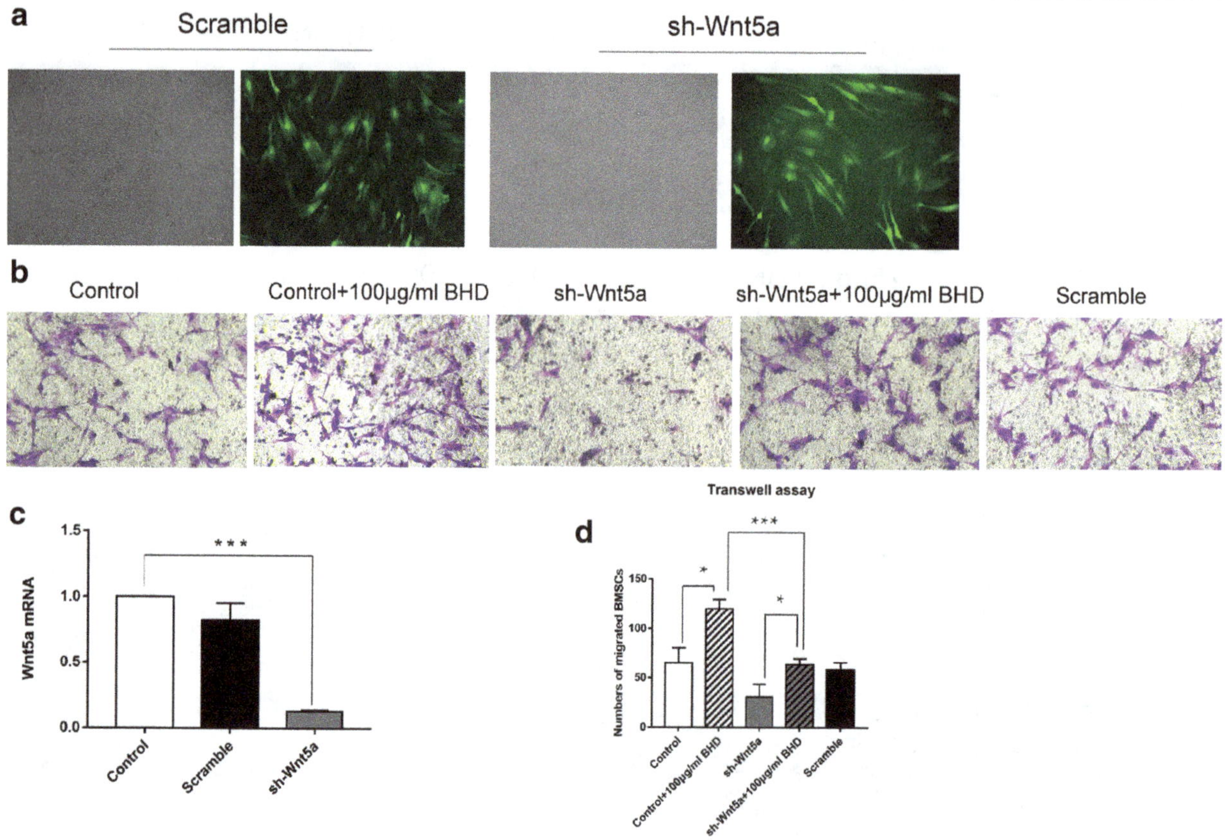

Fig. 5 Silencing Wnt5a inhibited BMSC migration. **a** Green fluorescent protein was used to demonstrate transfection efficiency. The cells were successfully transfected by Wnt5a-specific short hairpin RNA (sh-Wnt5a) lentiviral vectors. **b** Cell migration ability was promoted by 100 µg/ml BHD in both the control and sh-Wnt5a groups. Silencing Wnt5a reduced cell migration ability. **c** The efficiency of shRNA activity was analysed by real-time PCR. The expression of Wnt5a was significantly reduced. **d** The data for transwell assay $^{*}P < 0.05$, $^{***}P < 0.0001$

Because of its curative effect on fracture healing, it currently remains widely used in China as a complementary treatment for fractures. Fracture patients who receive conservative treatment in China are more likely to use BHD. Many researchers in China have observed its effect in patients with various types of fractures. Despite its long history of successful use, the underlying mechanism by which BHD promotes fracture healing is still unknown. In this study, we hypothesized that BHD enhances BMSC migration through activating the Wnt5a signalling pathway to facilitate bone healing. BHD contains 11 herbs, and after decoction, additional active ingredients were obtained. The main components of BHD are shown in Table 2. Several studies have shown a correlation between BHD components and bone diseases, mainly regarding fracture healing. Bakuchiol, the main ingredient of BHD, was shown to exhibit oestrogenic activity in both in vivo and in vitro models [20, 21]. Sunyer et al. found that oestrogen exerted bone-protective effects [22], which may contribute to fracture repair. Bakuchiol also exhibits anti-microbial, anti-inflammatory, anti-oxidative, anti-osteoporosis, and anti-depression or anti-stress activities [23]. Osthole has been widely studied in bone diseases because it may activate the β-catenin–BMP-2 signalling pathway to regulate osteoblast differentiation in vitro [24]. Zhang et al. demonstrated that osthole promotes the progression of repair by enhancing intracartilaginous ossification [25].

Many studies on the involvement of the Wnt pathway in the process of bone repair have been reported [26], and most are associated with the canonical Wnt/β-cat pathway. However, few studies have found a role for a non-canonical Wnt pathway, such as that of Wnt5a, in regulating the migration of BMSCs. The Wnt5a pathways are classified into nine categories, e.g., Wnt5a/planar cell polarity (PCP) signalling, Wnt5a/Ca^{2+} signalling, and Wnt5a/atypical PKC signalling [27]. The Wnt/PCP pathway has been linked to Wnt5a in vertebrates and can regulate cell migration and intercalation [6]. The Wnt/PCP pathway starts a signalling cascade that eventually leads to JNK activating the final transcription factor c-JUN (AP1) [5, 6]. Activation of the Wnt5a pathway can induce

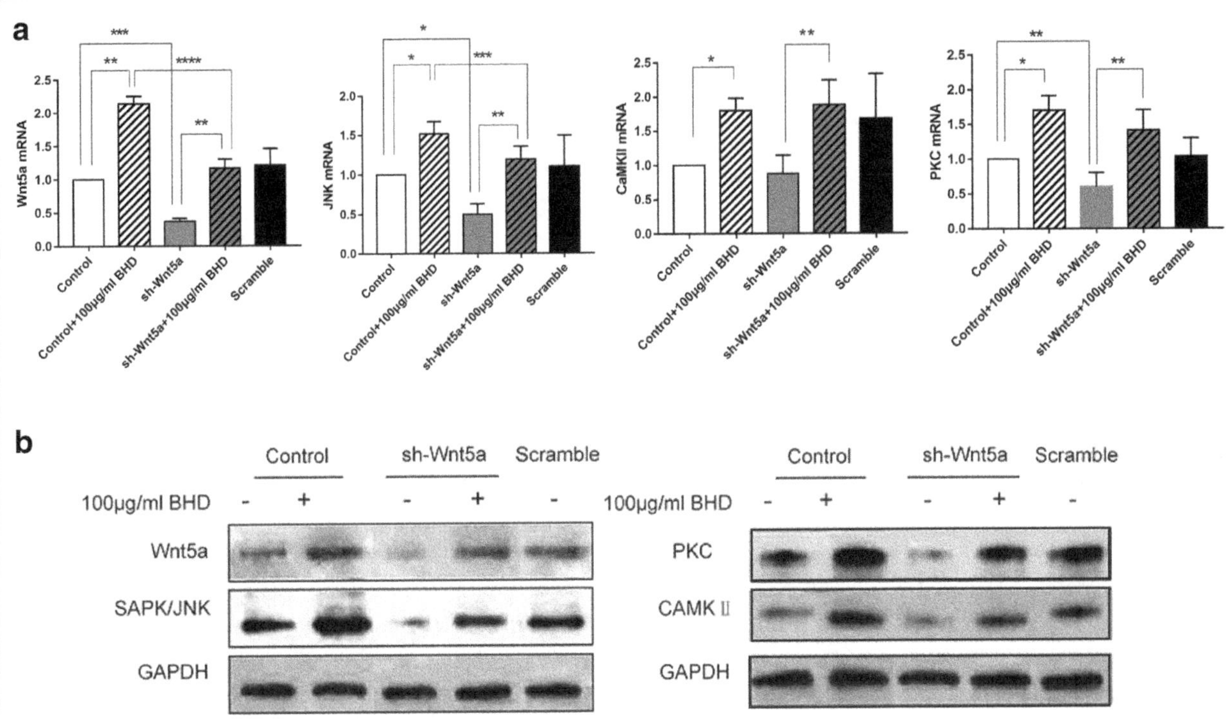

Fig. 6 BHD activates Wnt5a and its associated pathway. **a** mRNA expression of Wnt5a, JNK, PKC and CaMKII. $*P < 0.05$, $**P < 0.01$, $***P < 0.0001$. **b** Expression levels of Wnt5a, SAPK/JNK, PKC and CaMKII in all groups. The data show that BHD upregulated Wnt5a, SAPK/JNK, PKC and CaMKII

the release of calcium from intracellular stores and the upregulation of target proteins (PKC). In this study, we found that BHD-treated BMSCs showed better migration in the control group than in the sh-Wnt5a group. The expression of Wnt5a, PKC, CaMKII, and SAPK/JNK showed similar trends at the mRNA and protein levels, which indicates that BHD activates the Wnt5a/PCP and Wnt5a/PKC-Ca^{2+} pathways to enhance BMSC migration capacity.

Conclusion

Bone fracture healing is a unique physiologic process which the migration of BMSCs is essential during the inflammatory and hematoma stages. From ancient times to the present, herbs have played an important role in the treatment of diseases in China and have achieved remarkable results. With the development of modern medicine, especially surgical techniques, Chinese herbal medicine treatments can often play a supplementary role in clinical treatment. For example, BHD aids in healing bone fractures. In the present study, we investigated the effect of BHD on BMSC migration and found that BHD promoted BMSC migration through activation of the Wnt5a signalling pathway. Further research is needed to determine which herbal ingredient is responsible for this improvement in the curative effect.

Abbreviations

BHD: Bushen Huoxue decoction; BMSCs: bone marrow mesenchymal stem cells; Wnt5a: Wnt family member 5a; PCP: planar cell polarity; JNK: c-Jun N-terminal kinase; CaMKII: calcium–calmodulin-dependent protein kinase II; PKC: protein kinase C; GC–MS: gas chromatography–mass spectrometry; DMEM: Dulbecco's modified Eagle's medium; BCA: bicinchoninic acid; PBS: phosphate-buffered saline; TBST: tris-buffered saline plus Tween 20; SDS-PAGE: sodium dodecylsulfate–polyacrylamide gel electrophoresis; GFP: green fluorescent protein.

Authors' contributions

WS completed the Transwell assays and the scratch wound healing assays and drafted the manuscript. HL participated in lentivirus transfection, PCR, and Western blot experiments. LX modified the manuscript. YL, BW, YL conceived of the study and performed the statistical analysis. ZW prepared BHD. HC tested cell viability. LH and LY helped to make figures. All authors read and approved the final manuscript.

Author details

[1] Department of Traumatology, The Third Affiliated Hospital of Guangzhou University of Traditional Chinese Medicine, 22 Jiangnan-Xi Road, Guangzhou 510240, Guangdong, People's Republic of China. [2] Key Laboratory of Orthopaedics & Traumatology, The First Affiliated Hospital of Guangzhou University of Chinese Medicine, Guangzhou 510000, Guangdong, People's Republic of China. [3] Department of Diagnostics of Chinese Medicine, School of The Basic Medicine, Guangzhou 510006, Guangdong, People's Republic of China.

Acknowledgements

The authors would like to thank Prof Fengxue Zhang and Dongfeng Chen for the warm welcome into the research centre of basic integrative medicine of Guangzhou University of Chinese Medicine and the positive working environment.

Competing interests

The authors declare that they have no competing interests.

Consent for publication

Not applicable.

Funding

This work was supported by the National Natural Science Foundation of China (Nos. 81473699, 81503593, 81273783) and the Natural Science Foundation of Guangdong Province (CN) (2016A030313649, 2016A030310289).

References

1. Ferguson C, Alpern E, Miclau T. Does adult fracture repair recapitulate embryonic skeletal formation? Mech Dev. 1999;87:57–66.
2. Hall BK. All for one and one for all: condensations and the initiation of skeletal development. BioEssays. 2000;22:138–47.
3. Fazzalari NL. Bone fracture and bone fracture repair. Osteoporos Int. 2011;22:2003–6.
4. Ye X. Effects of hyperlipidemia and cardiovascular diseases on proliferation, differentiation and homing of mesenchymal stem cells. Curr Stem Cell Res Ther. 2017;12:377–87.
5. Kikuchi A, Yamamoto H, Sato A. New insights into the mechanism of Wnt signaling pathway activation. Int Rev Cell Mol Biol. 2011;291:21–71.
6. Simons M. Planar cell polarity signaling: from fly development to human disease. Annu Rev Genet. 2008;42:517–40.
7. Veeman MT, Axelrod JD. A second canon. Functions and mechanisms of beta-catenin-independent Wnt signaling. Dev Cell. 2003;5:367–77.
8. Sheldahl LC, Park M, Malbon CC. Protein kinase C is differentially stimulated by Wnt and Frizzled homologs in a G-protein-dependent manner. Curr Biol. 1999;9:695–8.
9. Slusarski DC, Yang-Snyder J, Busa WB. Modulation of embryonic intracellular Ca^{2+} signaling by Wnt-5a. Dev Biol. 1997;182:114–20.
10. Weeraratna AT, Jiang Y, Hostetter G, et al. Wnt5a signaling directly affects cell motility and invasion of metastatic melanoma. Cancer Cell. 2002;1:279–88.
11. Ye S, Gu Y, Xu Y, et al. Bushen Huoxue decoction improves cognitive decline in rats with cerebral hypoperfusion. Mol Med Rep. 2014;10:1635–41.
12. Huang C, Song K, Ma W, et al. Immunomodulatory mechanism of Bushen Huoxue Recipe alleviates cyclophosphamide-induced diminished ovarian reserve in mouse model. J Ethnopharmacol. 2017;208:44–56.
13. Li M, Yang HM, Luo DX, et al. Multi-dimensional analysis on Parkinson's disease questionnaire-39 in Parkinson's patients treated with Bushen Huoxue Granule: a multicenter, randomized, double-blinded and placebo controlled trial. Complement Ther Med. 2016;29:116–20.
14. Zhang R, Chen K, Lu D, et al. Study on efficacy of "bushen huoxue liquid" in male rats with osteoporosis induced by dexamethasone and its mechanism. Zhong Yao Cai. 2003;26:347–9.
15. Xu B, Jin HT, Wang XF, et al. Effects of serum of Bushen Huoxue prescription (Chinese characters) on classic Wnt/β-catenin signaling pathways of osteoblasts. Zhongguo Gu Shang. 2015;28:553–8.
16. Yuan Q, Kan WB, Song PF, et al. Influence of Bushen Huoxue decoction on beta-catenin, MMP-7 of synoviocytes in rats with knee osteoarthritis. Zhongguo Gu Shang. 2012;25:761–5.
17. Liu W, Wu YH, Liu XY, et al. Metabolic regulatory and anti-oxidative effects of modified Bushen Huoxue decoction on experimental rabbit model of osteoarthritis. Chin J Integr Med. 2013;19:459–63.
18. Luo YW, Wang B, Wu ZF, et al. Study of extracts from Bushen Huoxue Tang on promoting migration of rat bone marrow mesenchymal stem cells in vitro and expression of CXCR4. Trad Chin Drug Re Clin Pharmacol. 2016;03-0356-06:1003–9783.
19. Luque de Castro MD. Soxhlet extraction: past and present panacea. J Chromatogr A. 2010;1217:2383–9.
20. Xin D, Wang H, Yang J, et al. Phytoestrogens from *Psoralea corylifolia* reveal estrogen receptor-subtype selectivity. Phytomedicine. 2010;17:126–31.
21. Lim SH, Ha TY, Ahn J. Estrogenic activities of *Psoralea corylifolia* L. seed extracts and main constituents. Phytomedicine. 2011;18:425–30.
22. Sunyer T, Lewis J, Collin-Osdoby P. Estrogen's bone-protective effects may involve differential IL-1 receptor regulation in human osteoclast-like cells. J Clin Invest. 1999;103:1409–18.
23. Li L, Chen X, Liu CC, et al. Phytoestrogen bakuchiol exhibits in vitro and in vivo anti-breast cancer effects by inducing s phase arrest and apoptosis. Front Pharmacol. 2016;7:128.
24. Tang DZ, Hou W, Zhou Q, et al. Osthole stimulates osteoblast differentiation and bone formation by activation of beta-catenin-BMP signaling. J Bone Miner Res. 2010;25:1234–45.
25. Zhang Z, Leung WN, Li G, et al. Osthole promotes endochondral ossification and accelerates fracture healing in mice. Calcif Tissue Int. 2016;99:649–60.
26. Monroe DG, McGee-Lawrence ME, Oursler MJ. Update on Wnt signaling in bone cell biology and bone disease. Gene. 2012;492:1–18.
27. Zhu N, Qin L, Luo Z, et al. Challenging role of Wnt5a and its signaling pathway in cancer metastasis (review). Exp Ther Med. 2014;8:3–8.

6

Development of models for classification of action between heat-clearing herbs and blood-activating stasis-resolving herbs based on theory of traditional Chinese medicine

Zhao Chen[1,2], Yanfeng Cao[1,2], Shuaibing He[1] and Yanjiang Qiao[1,2*]

Abstract

Background: Action (*"gongxiao"* in Chinese) of traditional Chinese medicine (TCM) is the high recapitulation for therapeutic and health-preserving effects under the guidance of TCM theory. TCM-defined herbal properties (*"yaoxing"* in Chinese) had been used in this research. TCM herbal property (TCM-HP) is the high generalization and summary for actions, both of which come from long-term effective clinical practice in two thousands of years in China. However, the specific relationship between TCM-HP and action of TCM is complex and unclear from a scientific perspective. The research about this is conducive to expound the connotation of TCM-HP theory and is of important significance for the development of the TCM-HP theory.

Methods: One hundred and thirty-three herbs including 88 heat-clearing herbs (HCHs) and 45 blood-activating stasis-resolving herbs (BAHRHs) were collected from reputable TCM literatures, and their corresponding TCM-HPs/actions information were collected from Chinese pharmacopoeia (2015 edition). The Kennard–Stone (K–S) algorithm was used to split 133 herbs into 100 calibration samples and 33 validation samples. Then, machine learning methods including supported vector machine (SVM), k-nearest neighbor (kNN) and deep learning methods including deep belief network (DBN), convolutional neutral network (CNN) were adopted to develop action classification models based on TCM-HP theory, respectively. In order to ensure robustness, these four classification methods were evaluated by using the method of tenfold cross validation and 20 external validation samples for prediction.

Results: As results, 72.7–100% of 33 validation samples including 17 HCHs and 16 BASRHs were correctly predicted by these four types of methods. Both of the DBN and CNN methods gave out the best results and their sensitivity, specificity, precision, accuracy were all 100.00%. Especially, the predicted results of external validation set showed that the performance of deep learning methods (DBN, CNN) were better than traditional machine learning methods (kNN, SVM) in terms of their sensitivity, specificity, precision, accuracy. Moreover, the distribution patterns of TCM-HPs of HCHs and BASRHs were also analyzed to detect the featured TCM-HPs of these two types of herbs. The result showed that the featured TCM-HPs of HCHs were cold, bitter, liver and stomach meridians entered, while those of BASRHs were warm, bitter and pungent, liver meridian entered.

Conclusions: The performance on validation set and external validation set of deep learning methods (DBN, CNN) were better than machine learning models (kNN, SVM) in sensitivity, specificity, precision, accuracy when predicting the actions of heat-clearing and blood-activating stasis-resolving based on TCM-HP theory. The deep learning

*Correspondence: yjqiao@263.net
[2] Research Center of TCM Information Engineering, Beijing University of Chinese Medicine, Yangguang South Avenue, Fangshan District, Beijing 102488, China
Full list of author information is available at the end of the article

classification methods owned better generalization ability and accuracy when predicting the actions of heat-clearing and blood-activating stasis-resolving based on TCM-HP theory. Besides, the methods of deep learning would help us to improve our understanding about the relationship between herbal property and action, as well as to enrich and develop the theory of TCM-HP scientifically.

Keywords: Heat-clearing herbs (HCHs), Blood-activating stasis-resolving herbs (BASRHs), Machine learning, Deep learning, Herbal property, Traditional Chinese medicine (TCM)

Background

Traditional Chinese medicines (TCM) is one of the great herbal medicine systems worldwide, which plays an important role in current health care system in many countries. In the view of TCM theory, Yin-yang and five-elements theory is the central theory, which is used to explain how the world and body work [1]. The action of TCM is the high recapitulation for its therapeutic and health-preserving effect under the guidance of TCM theory [2]. TCM-HP, is the basic property of TCM and the high recapitulation of its functional characteristics [2]. The classic concept of TCM-HPs defines four fundamental characters (cold, cool, warm and hot), five fundamental tastes (salty, sour, bitter, sweet and pungent), four toxic states (toxic, nontoxic, very toxic, and slightly toxic), 12 meridians (bladder, spleen, large intestine, stomach, small intestine, liver, lung, heart, kidney, gallbladder, xin bao or pericardium and san jiao) [3]. TCM-HP also provides strong evidence to guide the clinical application of TCM. Many bioinformatics and pharmacological approaches were applied to study TCM-HP [1, 4, 5]. The research on the relationship between TCM-HP and action has been our great concern in the field of TCM.

The strategy of studying the relationship between TCM-HP and action have changed over the past decades. TCM-HP can not only be limited to a single property, but also need to be considered as a whole [6]. An Apriori algorithm was employed for producing association rules that described the intrinsic relationships between herbal property (qi, flavor and their combinations) and herbal efficacy [7]. However, the confirmed 120 resulting rules were dispersed and single property research could hardly characterize the whole effects of TCM. Hence the four fundamental characters, five fundamental tastes, and meridians need to be as a whole. Only in this way could we reveal the relationship between action and herbal property [8]. Multidimensional property of TCM is inherent basis of multiple action and is a collection of many herbal properties that determine the characteristics for efficiency of TCM [6]. Subsequently, property combination patterns for TCM [9–11] were proposed to reveal the relationship of TCM-HP and action from a holistic view of TCM.

Machine learning and deep learning methods have been widely applied in pharmaceutical research [12–17]. In life sciences, machine learning is often used to explain phenomena that are not completely theoretically understood [13]. Deep learning allows computational models that are composed of multiple processing layers to learn representations of data with multiple levels of abstraction [18].

Research on TCM-HP and action is helpful to discover the inherent relation between TCM-HP and action of TCM [7], which can illustrate the connotation holistic view of TCM-HP theory.

TCM-HP and action of TCM are both summary of clinical practices, so the classification of actions based on the holistic concept of TCM-HP is consistent with clinical practices. Machine learning methods have been applied to TCM researches with some success, for instance, for the TCM syndrome classification [19, 20], the relationship of TCM-HP and action [1, 3, 12, 13, 21–26].

In this work, 88 HCHs and 45 BASRHs were collected as our research objects and four different artificial intelligence methods were used to develop the classification models of TCM actions based on TCM-HP theory. In order to ensure robustness, these four constructed classification models (kNN, SVM, CNN, DBN) were tested with external validation set, including 15 HCHs and 5 BASRHs.

Heat clearing herbs, which tend to have cold characters, have been found to produce some combination of antimicrobial [27], anti-toxic [28], anti-inflammatory [29, 30], antipyretic [28], antioxidant [27, 31], platelet aggregation inhibition, sedative, immunomodulatory [32], and hepatoprotective activities [33]. The HCHs own anti-inflammatory and antimicrobial effects, and their potential mechanisms of action contributing to their anti-inflammatory and antimicrobial activity may be related to their action of removing heat and counteracting toxicity [34]. *Radix Salviae Miltiorrhizae* (*Dan Shen*) is an example of BASRHs, and the compound Tanshinone IIA isolated from it could be a promising agent to improve blood viscosity and microcirculation and to prevent cardiovascular diseases [35]. Salvianolic acid B is clinically effective because of its ability to change the gene expression profile of endothelial cells thereby preventing vascular events [36]. The Blood-Activating and Stasis-Resolving herb—Chuanxiong Hort may treat headache and has potential to be an agent for treating headache [37]. Because of the important clinical significance of these two kinds of typical TCM, they can lay the foundation for elucidating the relationship between TCM-HP and action.

Methods

Selection of HCHs and BASRHs

A total of 133 well established HCHs and BASRHs, given in Additional file 4: Table S1, were collected from reputable TCM literatures [38, 39], which were composed of 88 HCHs and 45 BASRHs. Their TCM-HPs and actions were collected from Chinese pharmacopoeia (2015 edition). External validation set (Additional file 4: Table S1) including 15 HCHs and 5 BASRHs were collected from a reputable TCM literature [39].

Digital representation of TCM and feature selecting for TCM-HPs

The classic concept of TCM herbal properties (TCM-HPs) defines four fundamental characters (cold, cool, neutral, warm and hot), five fundamental tastes (salty, sour, bitter, sweet and pungent), four toxic states (toxic, nontoxic, very toxic, and slightly toxic), and 12 meridians (bladder, spleen, large intestine, stomach, small intestine, liver, lung, heart, kidney, gallbladder, xin bao or pericardium and san jiao) [3]. With the continuous understanding of TCM-HP, the TCM-HPs of bland and astringent were added into five fundamental tastes in Chinese pharmacopoeia (2015 edition), and it would further enrich and develop TCM-HP theory. Four toxic states were considered the toxic effects of TCM, and the toxic action will cause injury of organs and tissues, functional impairment, pathological changes and even death [2]. So in this research, we only considered the relationship between TCM actions and TCM-HPs (four fundamental character, five fundamental tastes, 12 meridians).

TCM-HPs are thus divided into three classes: character (C), taste (T), meridian (M) for this research and there are totally 24 TCM-HPs in the class of C, T, M, respectively. The 24 herbal properties can be further divided into 5, 7 and 12, which fall into C, T and M, respectively, as shown in Table 1. This study is based on the holism concept of TCM-HP to determine the classification for actions of TCM. Other 3 herbal properties (neutral, bland, astringent) were added based on classic concept of TCM-HPs. The strength of each TCM-HP is not considered, as this study is a qualitative one. The value of a specific TCM-HP is 1 if the herb possesses the corresponding property, and it is 0 if the herb does not possess the property [3].

For instance, the heat-clearing herb Huang Qin (*Scutellariae Radix*) has cold character, bitter taste; lung, gallbladder, spleen, large intestine and small intestine meridians entered. So the TCM-HP vector of Huang Qin (*Scutellariae Radix*) is $\mathbf{V} = [V_1,V_2,V_3,V_4,V_5,V_6,V_7,V_8,V_9,V_{10},V_{11},V_{12},V_{13},V_{14},V_{15},V_{16},V_{17},V_{18},V_{19},V_{20},V_{21},V_{22},V_{23},V_{24}] = [1,0,0,0,0,0,1,0,0,0,0,0,0,0,1,1,0,0,1,1,0,1,0,0]$ according to the order in Table 1.

Traditional machine learning and deep learning methods

Machine learning explores the study and construction of algorithms that can learn from and make predictions on data [40]. The field of machine learning, which aims to build model from an example training set of input observations, and then make data-driven predictions or decisions expressed as outputs. The methods of machine learning hold promise to enable computers to assist humans in the analysis of large, complex data sets [41], and they are not following strictly static program instructions. Machine learning methods have been applied to a broad range of areas within genetics and genomics [7], drug discovery [42–44], medicinal and biomedical properties identification [45, 46], tracking literature [47],

Table 1 Chinese herbs properties' binarization table of some HCHs and BASRHs

CHMs	V_1	V_2	V_3	V_4	V_5	V_6	V_7	V_8	V_9	V_{10}	V_{11}	V_{12}	V_{13}	V_{14}	V_{15}	V_{16}	V_{17}	V_{18}	V_{19}	V_{20}	V_{21}	V_{22}	V_{23}	V_{24}
Zu Ye	1	0	0	0	0	0	0	1	1	1	0	0	0	1	0	0	0	0	0	1	1	0	0	0
Qin Pi	1	0	0	0	0	0	1	0	0	0	1	0	1	0	0	0	0	0	1	0	0	1	0	0
Lian Qiao	1	0	0	0	0	0	1	0	0	0	0	0	0	1	0	1	0	0	0	1	0	0	0	0
Zhi Zi	1	0	0	0	0	0	1	0	0	0	0	0	0	1	0	1	0	0	0	0	0	0	0	1
Qing Hao	1	0	0	0	0	0	1	0	1	0	0	0	1	0	0	0	0	0	1	0	0	0	0	0
Huang Qin	1	0	0	0	0	0	1	0	0	0	0	0	0	0	1	1	0	0	1	1	0	1	0	0
Dan Shen	1	0	0	0	0	0	1	0	0	0	0	0	1	1	0	0	0	0	0	0	0	0	0	0

V_1: cold, V_2: cool, V_3: neutral, V_4: warm, V_5: hot, V_6: sour, V_7: bitter, V_8: sweet, V_9: pungent, V_{10}: bland, V_{11}: astringent, V_{12}: salty, V_{13}: liver, V_{14}: heart, V_{15}: spleen, V_{16}: lung, V_{17}: kidney, V_{18}: xin bao or pericardium, V_{19}: gallbladder, V_{20}: small intestine, V_{21}: stomach, V_{22}: large intestine, V23: bladder, V24: san jiao, respectively, each of which includes 5, 7 and 12 TCM-HPs. The total number of unique TCM-HP vector for all TCM is $5 + 7 + 12 = 24$

cancer risk prediction and diagnosis [48], wind power prediction [49], etc.

However, the success of machine learning systems often requires a large amount of labeled data which is expensive to obtain and significant manual feature engineering. These feature representations are often hand-designed, require significant amounts of domain knowledge and human labor, and do not generalize well to new domains [50].

Deep learning (DL), a concept closely associated with artificial neutral networks (ANNs), is in principle the learning of layered concepts. Thus, a model could describe higher and lower-level concepts at different layers of its structure [51]. Deep learning discovers intricate structure in large data sets by using the back propagation algorithm to indicate how a machine should change its internal parameters that are used to compute the representation in each layer from the representation in the previous layer [46]. Deep learning had been applied in adapting advanced neural network architectures for pharmaceutical research [14, 15, 52], predicting drug-induced liver injury (DILI) [17]. While deep learning and particularly unsupervised deep learning is still in its infancy, particularly in biological applications [53]. Moreover, deep learning network predicted drug property and activity with a relative accuracy improvement of approximately 14% over Merck's in-house systems and resulted in an article in The New York Times [50, 54].

The research of TCM-HP will be accelerated by using the deep learning methods, which will promote the intelligent study of TCM-HP. With the deep neural network architectures, we can excavate the underlying regularities and rules from the data recorded in ancient literature. As it is well-known that the data of traditional Chinese medicine is highly nonlinear, it is an inevitable trend to find out the inherent rules by using deep neural network (Fig. 1).

Supported vector machine (SVM)

The support vector machine (SVM) is based on the statistical learning theory of VC dimension (Vapnik–Chervonenkis Dimension) and the risk structure of the minimum principle [55–58] and is also one of the most popular and successful binary classification methods. Its basic idea is to find a hyperplane in the feature space which separates the training data perfectly into two classes [59]. Moreover, SVM is a classier that performs classification tasks by constructing hyperplanes in a multidimensional space that separates cases of different class labels [60]. Least square support vector machine (LS-SVM) is an extension of standard support vector machines and it changes the error of optimization from first order into secondary order which covers a problem of solving quadratic programming into a problem of solving a set of linear equations [61, 62]. The method has been applied widely in biomedicine [63, 64].

K-nearest neighbor (KNN)

K-nearest neighbor algorithm is the most widely used classification and clustering algorithm. The k-nearest neighbors (kNN) algorithm is one of the simplest machine-learning methods to understand and explain, and the principle being that an instance is classified by a majority vote of its neighbors [65]. It provides a simple

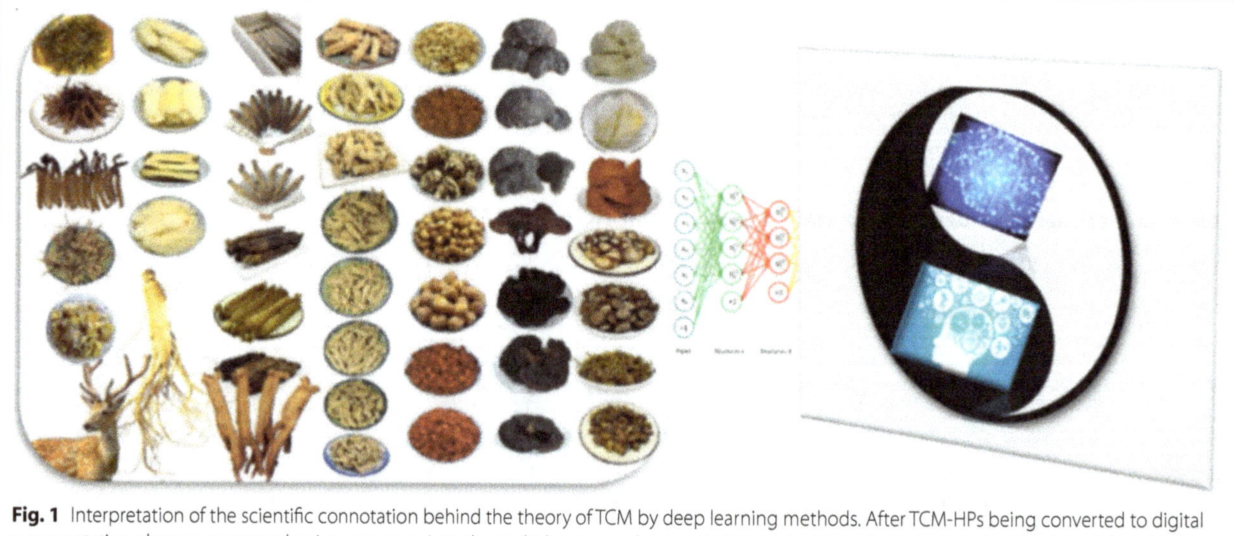

Fig. 1 Interpretation of the scientific connotation behind the theory of TCM by deep learning methods. After TCM-HPs being converted to digital representation, they were entered as input vectors into the multi-layer neural networks. The output layer is the action classification with multiple processing layers to learn representations of TCM-HPs. We can excavate the underlying regularities and rules between TCM-HPs and actions with the deep neural networks architectures

and intuitive rule for pattern discrimination, which has resulted in its extensive use in a variety of applications and gains a high classification rate [66, 67].

Each test sample is predicted to belong to the class most commonly found amongst its k closest neighbors, where k is a positive integer (Fig. 2). The Chinese herbal action classification is typically based on TCM-HP. TCM-HP is described as position vectors in the feature space that is usually of high dimensionality. Neighbors are identified on the basis of distance in the feature space. This is usually taken to be the Euclidean distance, though other metrics such as the Jaccard distance could be used. The minimum distance between the vectors gives the closest neighbor, so it is predicted that it belongs to the same class with the test object which the testing samples in the dataset are assigned to the class target value by a majority of its k nearest neighbor in the training set [68].

The Euclidean distance is often used to measure the similarity between two samples and more generally the distance between two p-dimensional vectors [69–71]. So the distance between these two TCM-HP vectors is computed as the length of the difference TCM-HP vector $\mathbf{V_r} - \mathbf{V_s}$, denoted by

$$d(V_r, V_s) = |V_r - V_s| = \sqrt{(V_{r_1} - V_{s_1})^2 + (V_{r_2} - V_{s_2})^2 \cdots + (V_{r_{24}} - V_{s_{24}})^2}$$

where $\mathbf{V_r}$, $\mathbf{V_s}$ denotes the vectors of TCM **r** and **s**. The 24 TCM-HPs were considered as 24-dimensional vectors

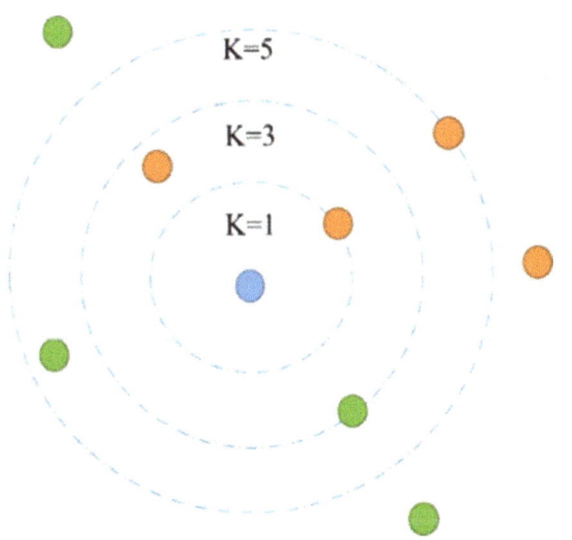

Fig. 2 Illustration of a kNN classification model. For k = 3, the blue one will be assigned to the red class, this time by a 2-1 vote; however, the blue one will be classified into the green class by a 3–2 majority. The 24 TCM-HPs were considered as 24-dimensional vectors and Euclidean distance were used to compute any two Chinese herbal vectors distance. Chinese herbal actions classification are typically based on TCM-HPs and we can classify the two kinds herbs based on 24-dimensional vectors with the kNN

and Euclidean distance were used to compute any two Chinese herbal vectors distance.

Deep belief network (DBN)

The deep belief network (DBN) is a neural network constructed from many layers of probabilistic model called restricted Boltzmann machines (RBMs) [72, 73].The training process of DBN can be achieved layer-by-layer from low to high layer to train these multilayer RBMs. Each RBM layer is trained by using the previous layer's hidden units (h) as input/visible units (v). Moreover, one RBM has a single layer of hidden units which are not connected to each other and have undirected, symmetrical connections to a layer of visible units. Contrastive divergence [74] based pre-training of these RBM layers is carried out to initialize the weights of DBN. Then, using the gibbs sampling method, the unbiased sample set could be got.

Hinton et al. [73] used complementary priors and derived a fast, greedy algorithm that could learn deep, directed belief networks one layer at a time, provided the top two layers form an undirected associative memory. The fast, greedy algorithm was used to initialize a slower learning procedure that fine-tunes the weights using a contrastive version of the wake-sleep algorithm.

In order to solve the problem of scaling full-sized, high-dimensional in images recognition, multiresolution deep belief networks [75] and convolutional deep belief networks [76] were constructed. In this research, the TCM-HP vectors were considered as input V_k, and the action classification was considered as output label as given in Fig. 3.

Convolutional neutral network (CNN)

Convolutional networks combine three architectural ideas to ensure some degree of shift and distortion invariance local receptive fields, shared weights or weight replication and sometimes spatial or temporal subsampling. Convolutional process is the biologically inspired variant of multilayer perceptions (MLPs), which exploits the spatially local correlation by enforcing a local connectivity pattern [77, 78]. The classical convolutional network is composed of alternating layers of convolution and pooling (i.e. subsampling). The aim of the first convolutional layer is to extract patterns found within local regions of the input images that are common throughout the dataset [79].

In CNN, convolution layer is regarded as features extraction layer and each feature map is a mapping plane in feature map layer. The fully connected layers aggregate the local information learned in the convolutional layers to do class discrimination and fully-connected network like DNNs, each hidden activation h_i is computed

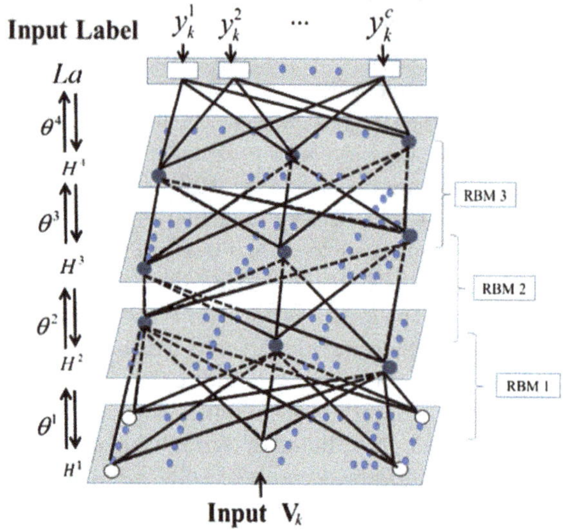

Fig. 3 Schematic representation of a DBN. The number of layer and the number of units on each layer in the scheme are only examples. In this research, the TCM-HPs vectors were considered as input V_k, and the action classification was considered as output label to train these multilayer RBMs

by multiplying the entire input **V** by weights **W** in that layer [80]. The weights **W** are then shared across the entire input space, as indicated in Fig. 4. In our research, 24 TCM-HPs were entered as input vectors, convolution and pooling operations were then made for each TCM-HP.

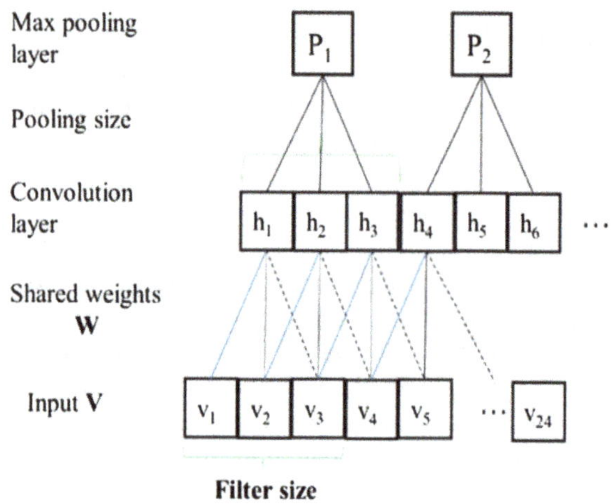

Fig. 4 Diagram showing a typical convolutional network architecture consisting of a convolutional and max-pooling layer. In CNN, convolution layer is regarded as features extraction layer and each feature map is a mapping plane in feature map is a mapping plane in feature map layer. In our research, 24 TCM-HPs were entered as input vectors, convolution and pooling operations were then made for each TCM-HPs

Methods for evaluating prediction performance of deep learning and traditional machine learning methods

For a binary classification exercise, predictions can be classed as true positives (TP), false positives (FP), true negatives (TN), and false negatives (FN). Cross-validation is also a popular strategy, and still allows models to be tested on data unseen in their generation.

As in the case of all discriminative methods, the performance of deep learning and traditional machine learning methods can be evaluated by the quantity of true positive or TP (correctly classified HCHs), true negative or TN (correctly classified BASRHs), false positive or FP (BASRHs falsely classified as HCHs), and false negative or FN (HCHs falsely classified as BASRHs) respectively. Sensitivity (P+), SEN = TP/(TP + FN) and specificity (P−), SPE = TN/(TN + FP) are the prediction accuracy for HCHs and BASRHs, respectively. The overall prediction accuracy, ACC = [(TP + TN)/(TP + TN + FP + FN)], and precision, PRE = TP/(TP + FP). The overall prediction accuracy and precision are used to measure the overall prediction performance.

The minimum standards of reporting checklist contains details of the experimental design, and statistics, and resources used in this study (Additional file 1).

Results

Distribution patterns of TCM-HPs of two kinds of herbs and their characteristics

According to holistic view of the TCM-HPs, the properties of 88 known HCHs are predominantly cold characters, bitter taste; liver and stomach meridians entered, respectively, which are given in Fig. 5. The properties of 45 known BASRHs are predominantly warm characters,

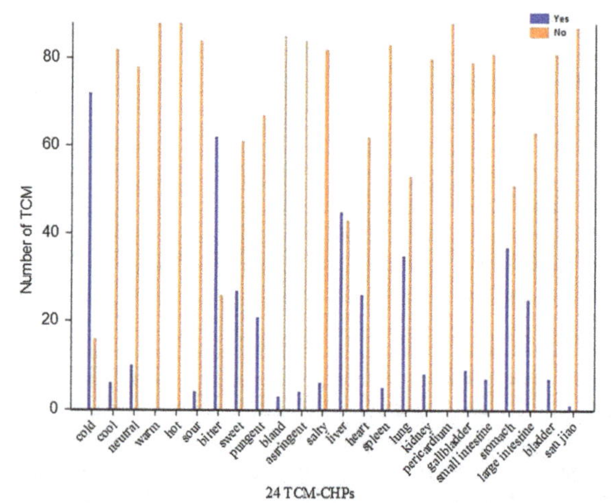

Fig. 5 The TCM-HPs distribution of 88 HCHs. 'Yes' represents the herbs have the TCM-HP, and 'No' represents the herbs do not have this TCM-HP

bitter and pungent taste; liver meridian entered, respectively, which are given in Fig. 6.

Figures 5, 6 showed the common distribution patterns of two kinds of herbs were bitter taste; liver meridian entered.

The TCM-HP rates of HCHs and BARSHs were compared as given in Fig. 7. From the herbal properties rate distribution, we knew that significant TCM-HP of BASRHs are bitter, pungent; liver entered and their rates were 66.7, 44.4, 93.3%, respectively. The prominent TCM-HP features were cold (81.8%), bitter (70.5%); liver (51.1%) and stomach (42.0%) entered in the 88 HCHs. Both of bitter and heart property rates in the two types of herbs were close proximity. However, the absolute value of differences for seven TCM-HP rates between HCHs and BASRH differed considerably as given in Table 2. If thirty percent of absolute value of difference was considered as setting value, the TCM-HP features were cold, warm character; spleen, liver and stomach meridians entered. Cold (81.8%)-bitter (70.5%)-liver (51.1%) combination could distinguish HCHs from BASRHs and warm (35.6%)-bitter (72.73%)/pungent (44.4%)-liver (93.3%) combination could distinguish BASRHs from HCHs.

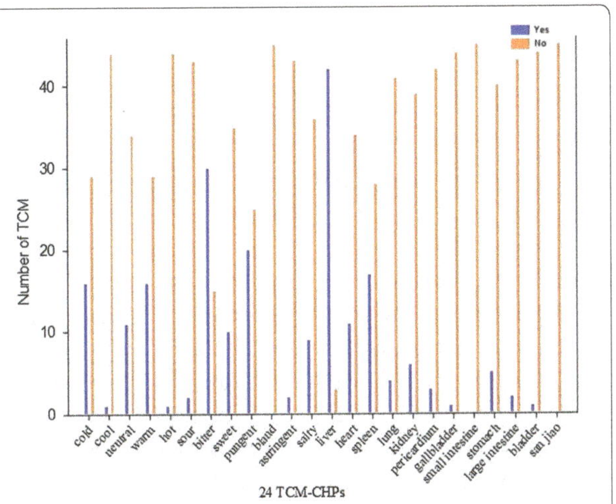

Fig. 6 The TCM-HPs distribution of 45 BASRHs. 'Yes' represents the herbs have the TCM-HP, and 'No' represents the herbs do not have this TCM-HP

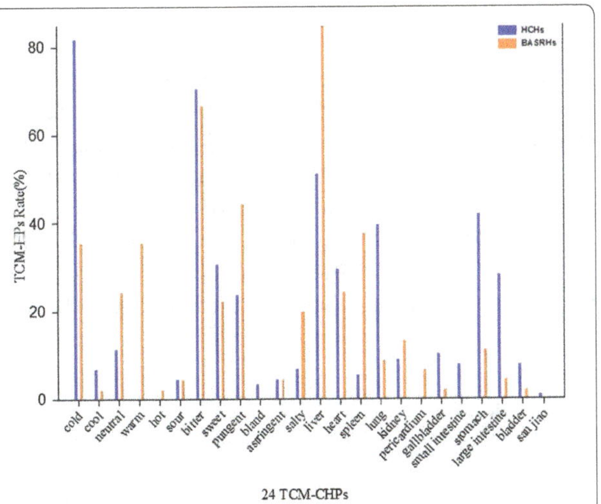

Fig. 7 The TCM-HPs rate distribution of 88 HCHs and 45 BASRHs. TCM-HPs rate denotes that percentage of the HCHs (BASRHs) with the same TCM-HP in the total number of HCHs (BASRHs)

Models analysis of TCM-HPs for distinguishing HCHs from BASRHs

A cross-validation study was conducted to determine whether the traditional machine learning method SVM is able to separate HCHs and BASRHs based on their TCM-HPs. In this research, a SVM on the calibration set was constructed with setting coef 0 to 10, the highest number of polynomial kernel functions to 1. Polynomial was chosen as kernel function of this model and set tenfold cross validation when training this model. The sensitivity for the SVM model was 94.4%, and the specificity for this model was 72.4%, respectively. The overall prediction accuracy was 88.0%. The results on the validation set and external validation set were given in Table 3.

The best overall accuracy by kNN method was achieved 72.7% with $k = 4$ using the Euclidean distance on validation set and achieved 85.0% on external validation set.

A 100 hidden units RBM were constructed in this research, with setting batchsize to 5, learning rate to 2. After 10,000 iterations, the results showed that its sensitivity, specificity, precision, accuracy were 100.00, 100.0, 100.0, 100.0% on the validation set. On the external validation set, the same result were obtained with this DBN model.

Table 2 Seven TCM-HP rates of HCHs and BASRHs and their absolute values of difference between HCHs and BASRHs

TCM-HPs	HP rates of HCHs (%)	HP rates of BASRHs (%)	Absolute value of difference (%)
Cold	81.8	24.24	62.65
Warm	0.00	35.6	35.6
Pungent	23.9	44.4	20.5
Liver	51.1	93.3	42.2
Spleen	5.7	37.8	32.1
Stomach	42.0	11.1	30.9
Large intestine	28.4	4.4	24.0

Table 3 Binary classification results with traditional machine learning and deep learning methods

Data set	Type of models	Sensitivity (%)	Specificity (%)	Precision (%)	Accuracy (%)
Calibration set	SVM	94.4	72.4	89.3	88
	DBN	/	/	/	/
	kNN	91.5	75.9	90.3	87
	CNN	/	/	/	/
Validation set	LS-SVM	82.4	81.3	82.4	81.8
	DBN	100	100	100	100
	kNN	82.4	62.5	70.0	72.7
	CNN	100	100	100	100
External validation set	SVM	93.3	75.0	87.5	85.0
	DBN	100	100	100	100
	kNN	86.7	80.0	92.9	85.0
	CNN	100	100	100	100

In this research, we trained a 2 convolution layers and 2 subsampling layers convolutional neural network with setting batchsize to 5, learning rate to 0.001. In the first convolution layer, we set 3 output units and 2 kernels; and in the second convolution layer, we set 6 output units and 2 kernels. After 10,000 iterations, the model's sensitivity, specificity, precision, accuracy were 100.00, 100.0, 100.0, 100.0% on the validation set and the external validation set.

The two deep learning method DBN, CNN achieved 100.0% accuracy on the validation set and external validation set than two other traditional machine learning methods was given in Table 3. It illustrated that deep learning methods had stronger predictive ability than two machine learning methods. These results also suggest that HCHs and BASRHs can be separated by deep learning and traditional machine learning methods based on their TCM-HPs with different accuracy and precision.

Discussion

The herbal properties distribution of HCHs and BASRHs showed their differences on TCM-HPs. The TCM-HPs of 88 known HCHs are predominantly cold, bitter; liver and stomach meridians entered. The TCM-HPs of 45 known BASRHs are predominantly warm, bitter, pungent; liver meridian entered. The traditional machine learning methods and deep learning methods were adopted to construct the actions classification models based on the TCM-HP theory. The traditional machine learning methods SVM and kNN achieved 87.5, 92.9% overall prediction accuracy on external validation set. Furthermore, deep learning method DBN, CNN achieved 100.0% overall prediction accuracy. Two Chinese herbs (San Qi, Yin Xing Ye) were falsely classified as HCHs and Yu Gan Zi were falsely classified as BASRHs using SVM methods. In kNN model, two herbs (Niu Huang, Yin Xian Ye) were classified as HCHs and Yu Gan Zi (*Phyllanthus emblica* L.) was classified as BASRHs. Error classification CHMs with SVM and kNN on external validation set were given in Tables 4, 5.

The 4 falsely classified CHMs using the traditional machine learning method SVM and kNN have the same characteristic in common—sweet. Furthermore, they are mostly liver and heart meridians entered. These results suggested that deep learning method DBN and CNN are capable of dividing known HCHs from known BASRHs and the TCM-HPs of the known HCHs contain useful information for distinguishing them from BASRHs.

Table 4 Error classification CHMs with SVM and kNN on external validation set

Category of CHMs	Type of models	Accuracy (%)	Error classification CHMs
HCHs and BASRHs	SVM	85.0	Yu Gan Zi (*Phyllanthus emblica* L.), San Qi (*Notoginseng radlx Et Rhizoma*), Yin Xian Ye (*Ginkgo folium*)
	kNN	85.0	Niu Huang (*Bovis calculus*), Yu Gan Zi (*Phyllanthus emblica* L.), Yin Xian Ye (*Ginkgo folium*)

Table 5 The herbal property of error classification CHMs

Error classification CHMs	TCM-HPs
Yu Gan Zi (*Phyllanthus emblica* L.)	Cool; sour, sweet, astringent; spleen, lung, stomach meridian entered
San Qi (*Notoginseng Radlx Et Rhizoma*)	Warm, bitter, sweet, liver and stomach meridian entered
Yin Xing Ye (*Ginkgo folium*)	Neutral, bitter, sweet, astringent; heart, lung meridian entered
Niu Huang (*Bovis calculus*)	Cool, sweet; heart, liver meridians entered

Conclusions

With deep learning methods and machine methods, we could understand the nonlinear relationship between TCM-HPs and actions. Moreover, the deep learning classification models would had better accuracy and generalization ability than machine learning in predicting actions of TCMs based TCM-HP theory. The distribution patterns of TCM-HPs between HCHs and BASRHs were analysed. HCHs were mainly cold, bitter; liver and stomach meridians entered. BASRHs are predominantly warm, bitter, pungent; liver meridian entered, respectively. Traditional machine learning and deep learning methods classification studies showed that HCHs could be distinguished from BASRHs based on TCM-HP theory.

Future work for elucidating the regularity of TCM formula compatibility using the deep learning methods based on TCM-HP theory was on going. This work will contribute to more specific and deeper understanding of the traditional Chinese medicine system. The expectation is that we can utilize the deeper regularity to guide the discovery of TCM, drug design and clinical treatment in the future.

Abbreviations

TCM: traditional Chinese medicine; HPs: herbal properties; TCM-HPs: traditional Chinese medicine herbal properties; SVM: supported vector machine; kNN: k-nearest neighbor; DBN: deep belief network; CNN: convolutional neutral network; HCHs: heat-clearing herbs; BASRHs: blood-activating stasis-resolving herbs; DILI: drug-induced liver injury; DL: deep learning; ML: machine learning.

Authors' contributions

ZC and YJQ substantial contributions to the conception or design of the work. YFC and SBH analysis and interpretation of data for the work. CZ and YFC writes all the codes. YJQ drafting the work and revising it critically for important intellectual content. ZC and YJQ final approval of the version to be published. All authors read and approved the final manuscript.

Author details

[1] School of Chines Materia Medica, Beijing University of Chinese Medicine, Yangguang South Avenue, Fangshan District, Beijing 102488, China. [2] Research Center of TCM Information Engineering, Beijing University of Chinese Medicine, Yangguang South Avenue, Fangshan District, Beijing 102488, China.

Acknowledgements

This work is supported and sponsored by the Natural Science Foundation of China (No. 81430094) and 2013 Co-operation Programs of Beijing Municipal Education Commission: Research on data fusion supporting platform of BT/IT/CT for traditional Chinese medicine.

Competing interests

The authors declare that they have no competing interests.

Consent for publication

All of authors consent to publication of this study in *Journal of Chinese Medicine.*

Funding

This work was supported by 2013 Co-operation Programs of Beijing Municipal Education Commission: Research on data fusion supporting platform of BT/IT/CT for traditional Chinese medicine; National Natural Science Foundation of China (No. 81430094).

References

1. Liang F, Li L, Wang ML, Niu XY, Zhan JP, He XJ, Yu CY, Jiang M, Lu AP. Molecular network and chemical fragment-based characteristics of medicinal herbs with cold and hot properties from Chinese medicine. J Ethnopharmacol. 2013;148(3):770–9.
2. Zhang T. Chinese materia medica. Beijing: High Education Press; 2008.
3. Ung CY, Li H, Kong CY, Wang JF, Chen YZ. Usefulness of traditionally defined herbal properties for distinguishing prescriptions of traditional Chinese medicine from non-prescription recipes. J Ethnopharmacol. 2007;109(1):21–8.
4. Zhang YL, Wang Y, Qiao YJ. Research on material base of TCM property based on pharmaco-phore. World Sci Technol. 2009;11(5):735–8.
5. Zhou J, Xie G, Yan X. Encyclopedia of traditional Chinese medicines. Isolat Compound AB. 2011;1:455.
6. Liang Q, Xie M. Identification of herbal properties from pharmaceutical multidimensional. Shanghai J Trad Chin Med. 2007;41:45–6 **(In Chinese)**.
7. Jin R, Lin Z, Xue C, Zhang B. An improved association-mining research for exploring TCM-HP theory: based on data of the Shennong's classic of materia medica. Chin J Integr Med. 2013;11:352–65.
8. Xiao B, Wang Y, Qiao YJ. Study on the Relationship between Chinese Herbal Nature and Function. Chin J Inf Tradit Chin Med. 2011;18(1):31–3 **(In Chinese)**.
9. Sun J, Zhang BX, Yan SR. Study on self-similarity of property combination mode of traditional Chinese medicines. China J Chin Mater Med. 2014;39(13):2378–81 **(In Chinese)**.
10. Hu Y, Sun J, Wang Y. Property combination patterns of traditional Chinese medicines. J Tradit Chin Med Sci. 2016;3(2):110–5.
11. Hu Y, Dong F, Wang Y, Qiao YJ. In silico method for studying property combination of traditional Chinese herbs. J Tradit Chin Med Sci. 2016;3(1):37–40.
12. Ung CY, Li H, Cao ZW. Are herb-pairs of traditional Chinese medicine distinguishable from others? Pattern analysis and artificial intelligence classification study of traditionally defined herbal properties. J Ethnopharmacol. 2007;111(2):371–7.
13. Balfer J. Development and interpretation of machine learning models for drug discovery [D]. Universitäts-und Landesbibliothek Bonn, Bonn; 2015.
14. Aliper A, Plis S, Artemov A, Ulloa A, Mamoshina P, Zhavoronkov A. Deep learning applications for predicting pharmacological properties of drugs and drug repurposing using transcriptomic data. Mol Pharm. 2016;13(7):2524–30.
15. Gawehn E, Hiss JA, Schneider G. Deep learning in drug discovery. Mol Inform. 2016;35(1):3–14.
16. Unterthiner T, Mayr A, Klambauer G, Steijaert M, Wegner JK, Ceulemans H, Hochreiter S. Deep learning as an opportunity in virtual screening. In: Proceedings of the deep learning workshop at NIPS. 2014.

17. Xu Y, Dai Z, Chen F, Gao S, Pei J, Lai L. Deep learning for drug-induced liver injury. J Chem Inf Model. 2015;55(10):2085–93.
18. LeCun Y, Bengio Y, Hinton G. Deep learning. Nature. 2015;521(7553):436–44.
19. Li GZ, Sun S, You M, Wang YL, Liu GP. Inquiry diagnosis of coronary heart disease in Chinese medicine based on symptom-syndrome interactions. Chin Med. 2012;7(1):9.
20. Yang, XB, Liang ZH, Zhang G, Luo YJ, Yin J. A classification algorithm for TCM syndromes based on P-SVM. In: IEEE Proceedings of 2005 international conference on machine learning and cybernetics. 2005; 6:3692–7.
21. Zhao YL, Wang JB, Xiao XH, Zhao HP, Zhou CP, Zhang XR, Jia L. Study on the cold and hot properties of medicinal herbs by thermotropism in mice behavior. J Ethnopharmacol. 2011;133(3):980–5.
22. Fusheng Z, Xiaoping L, Xushijie C, Jiannan C, Quanlin CHEN. Methodology for modeling on TCM-HP theory. World Sci Technol. 2009;11(2):229–33.
23. Shang E, Ye L, Fan X, Tang Y, Duan J. Discovery of association rules between TCM properties in drug pairs by association mining between datasets and probability tests. World Sci Technol. 2010;12(3):377–82.
24. Yao MC, Yuan YM, Ai L. Data mining and its application in the modernization of traditional Chinese medicine and traditional Chinese pharmacy. J Beijing Univ Tradit Chin Med. 2002;25(5):20–3 **(In Chinese)**.
25. Yao MC, Qiao YJ, Yuan YM, Ai L. Basis on artificial neural network method Chinese herbal function-efficacy classification research. China J Chin Mater Medica. 2003;28(7):689–91 **(In Chinese)**.
26. Yao MC, Zhang YL, Yuan YM. Study on the prediction of the effect attribution of the deficiency-nourishing drugs based on the quantification of TCM drug properties. J Beijing Univ Tradit Chin Med. 2004;27:7–18 **(In Chinese)**.
27. Sieniawska E, Baj T, Los R, Skalicka-Wozniak K, Malm A, Glowniak K. Phenolic acids content, antioxidant and antimicrobial activity of *Ligusticum mutellina* L. Nat Prod Res. 2013;27:1108–10.
28. China medical science and technology press. Pharmacopoeia of the People's Republic of China. 2015th ed. Beijing: China medical science and technology press; 2015.
29. Or TCT, Yang CLH, Law AHY, Li JCB, Lau ASY. Isolation and identification of anti-inflammatory constituents from *Ligusticum chuanxiong* and their underlying mechanisms of action on microglia. Neuropharmacology. 2011;60:823–31.
30. Huang J, Lu X, Zhang C, Lu J, Li G, Lin R, et al. Anti-inflammatory ligustilides from *Ligusticum chuanxiong* Hort. Fitoterapia. 2013;91:21–7.
31. Jeong JB, Ju SY, Park JH, Lee JR, Yun KW, Kwon ST, Jeong HJ. Antioxidant activity in essential oils of *Cnidium officinale* makino and *Ligusticum chuanxiong* hort and their inhibitory effects on DNA damage and apoptosis induced by ultraviolet B in mammalian cell. Cancer Epidemiol. 2009;33(1):41–6.
32. Bell CM, Simmonds MS, Appiah SS, Howes MJR. Plant substances as alternatives for animal products in traditional medicines. Report submitted to the Department for Environment Food and Rural Affairs. 2006.
33. Jiang WY. Therapeutic wisdom in traditional Chinese medicine: a perspective from modern science. Trends Pharmacol Sci. 2005;26(11):558–63.
34. Muluye RA, Bian Y, Alemu PN. Anti-inflammatory and antimicrobial effects of heat-clearing chinese herbs: a current review. J Tradit Complement Med. 2014;4(2):93–8.
35. Maione F, De Feo V, Caiazzo E, De Martino L, Cicala C, Mascolo N. Tanshinone IIA, a major component of Salvia milthorriza Bunge, inhibits platelet activation via Erk-2 signaling pathway. J Ethnopharmacol. 2014;155(2):1236–42.
36. Shi CS, Huang HC, Wu HL, Kuo CH, Chang BI, Shiao MS, Shi GY. Salvianolic acid B modulates hemostasis properties of human umbilical vein endothelial cells. Thromb Res. 2007;119(6):769–75.
37. Peng C, Xie X, Wang L, Guo L, Hu T. Pharmacodynamic action and mechanism of volatile oil from Rhizoma Ligustici Chuanxiong Hort. on treating headache. Phytomedicine. 2009;16(1):25–34.
38. Gao XM. Chinese materia medica. Beijing: China Press Tradit Chin Med; 2007.
39. Yan ZH. Chinese materia medica. Beijing: People's Medical Publishing House; 2014.
40. Kohavi R, Provost F. Glossary of terms. Mach Learn. 1998;30(2–3):271–4.
41. Libbrecht MW, Noble WS. Machine learning applications in genetics and genomics. Nat Rev Genet. 2015;16(6):321–2.
42. Giguère S, Laviolette F, Marchand M, Tremblay D, Moineau S, Liang X, Corbeil J. Machine learning assisted design of highly active peptides for drug discovery. Plos Comout Biol. 2015;11(4):e1004074.
43. Raccuglia P, Elbert KC, Adler PD, Falk C, Wenny MB, Mollo A, Norquist AJ. Machine-learning-assisted materials discovery using failed experiments. Nature. 2016;533(7601):73–6.
44. Zhang S. Application of machine leaning in drug discovery and development. Chemo-informatics and advanced machine learning perspectives: complex computational methods and collaborative techniques: complex computational methods and collaborative techniques. 2010. p. 235.
45. Jones DE, Ghandehari H, Facelli JC. A review of the applications of data mining and machine learning for the prediction of biomedical properties of nanoparticles. Comput Methods Program Biomed. 2016;132:93–103.
46. Nazarenko DV, Kharyuk PV, Oseledets IV, Rodin IA, Shpigun QA. Machine learning for LC–MS medicinal plants identification. Chemomet Intell Lab Syst. 2016;156:174–80.
47. Bornstein AT, McLoughlin MH, Aguilar J, Wong WS, Solomon BD. Tracking medical genetic literature through machine learning. Mol Genet Metab. 2016;118(4):255–8.
48. Asri H, Mousannif H, Moatassime HA, Noel T. Using machine learning algorithms for breast cancer risk prediction and diagnosis. Procedia Comput Sci. 2016;83:1064–9.
49. Heinermann J, Kramer O. Machine learning ensembles for wind power prediction. Renew Energ. 2016;89:671–9.
50. LeCun Y, Bengio Y, Hinton G. Deep learning. Nature. 2016;521(7553):436–44.
51. Mitchell JBO. Machine learning methods in chemoinformatics. Wires Comput Mol SCI. 2014;4(5):468–81.
52. Unterthiner T, Mayr A, Klambauer G, Steijaert M, Wegner JK, Ceulemans H, Hochreiter S. Deep learning as an opportunity in virtual screening. In: Proceedings of the deep learning workshop at NIPS. 2014. p. 27.
53. Mamoshina P, Vieira A, Putin E, Zhavoronkov A. Applications of deep learning in biomedicine. Mol Pharm. 2016;13(5):1445–54.
54. Markoff J. Scientists see promise in deep-learning programs. New York Times. 2012.
55. Bousquet O, Boucheron S, Lugosi G. Introduction to statistical learning theory. Advanced lectures on machine learning. Heidelberg: Springer; 2004. p. 169–207.
56. Pednault EPD. Statistical learning theory. New York: IBM Thomas J. Watson Research Division; 1997.
57. Vapnik VN, Vapnik V. Statistical learning theory. New York: Wiley; 1998.
58. Vapnik VN. An overview of statistical learning theory. IEEE Trans Neural Netw. 1999;10(5):988–99.
59. Utkin LV, Chekh AI, Zhuk YA. Binary classification SVM-based algorithms with interval-valued training data using triangular and Epanechnikov kernels. Neur Netw. 2016;80:53–66.
60. Santhanam T, Padmavathi MS. Application of K-means and genetic algorithms for dimension reduction by integrating SVM for diabetes diagnosis. Procedia Comput Sci. 2015;47:76–83.
61. Zhang N, Shetty D. An effective LS-SVM based approach for surface roughness prediction in machined surfaces. Neurocomputing. 2016;198:35–9.
62. Duolin W, Guihe Q, Jinnan D, Shuai Y. LS-SVM based human recognition on automotive active safety system. Heidelberg: In Mechanical Engineeering and Technology. Springer; 2012. p. 75–80.
63. Guyon I, Weston J, Barnhill S, Vapnik V. Gene selection for cancer classification using support vector machines. Mach Learn. 2002;46(1–3):389–422.
64. de Oliveira FSS, de Carvalho FAO, Silva AC, de Paivaa AC, Gattass M. Classification of breast regions as mass and non-mass based on digital mammograms using taxonomic indexes and SVM. Comput Biol Med. 2015;57:42–53.
65. Ma J, Sheridan RP, Liaw A, Dahl GE, Svetnik V. Deep neural nets as a method for quantitative structure-activity relationships. J Chem Inf Model. 2015;55(2):263–74.

66. Remus JJ, Morton KD, Torrione PA, Tantum SL, Collins LM. Comparison of a distance-based likelihood ratio test and k-nearest neighbor classification methods. In: IEEE workshop on machine learning for signal processing. 2008. p. 362–7.
67. Fukunaga K, Hostetler LD. k-Nearest-neighbor Bayes-risk estimation. IEEE Trans Inf Theory. 1975;21(3):285–93.
68. Supardi NZ, Mashor MY, Harun NH, Bakri FA, Hassan R. Classification of blasts in acute leukemia blood samples using k-nearest neighbour. In: IEEE international colloquium on signal processing and its applications. 2012. p. 461–5.
69. Khoa NM, Viet DT, Hieu NH. Classification of power quality disturbances using wavelet transform and K-nearest neighbor classifier. In: 2013 IEEE international symposium on industrial electronics (ISIE). 2013. p. 1–4.
70. Li X, Xiang C. Correlation-based K-nearest neighbor algorithm. In: IEEE international conference on software engineering and service science. 2012. p. 185–7.
71. Peterson LE. K-nearest neighbor. Scholarpedia. 2009;4(2):1883.
72. Bengio Y, Lamblin P, Popovici D, Larochelle H. Greedy layer-wise training of deep networks. Adv Neural Inf Process Syst. 2007;19:153.
73. Hinton GE, Osindero S, Teh YW. A fast learning algorithm for deep belief nets. Neural Comput. 2006;18(7):1527–54.
74. Hinton GE. Training products of experts by minimizing contrastive divergence. Neural Comput. 2002;14(8):1771–800.
75. Tao QQ, Zhan S, Li XH, Kurihara T. Robust face detection using local CNN and SVM based on kernel combination. Neurocomputing. 2016;211:98–105.
76. Lee H, Grosse R, Ranganath R, Ng AY. Unsupervised learning of hierarchical representations with convolutional deep belief networks. Commun ACM. 2011;54(10):95–103.
77. Zhang W, Qu C, Ma L, Guan J, Huang R. Learning structure of stereoscopic image for no-reference quality assessment with convolutional neural network. Pattern Recogn. 2016;59:176–87.
78. Hubel DH, Wiesel TN. Receptive fields and functional architecture of monkey striate cortex. J Physiol. 1968;195(1):215–43.
79. Zeiler MD, Fergus R. Stochastic pooling for regularization of deep convolutional neural networks. arXiv preprint arXiv. 2013. p. 1301.
80. Sainath TN, Mohamed AR, Kingsbury B, Ramabhadran B. Deep convolutional neural networks for LVCSR. In: 2013 IEEE international conference on acoustics, speech and signal processing. 2013. p. 8614–18.

7

Characterization and anti-tumor activity of a polysaccharide isolated from *Dendrobium officinale* grown in the Huoshan County

Yuan Wei[1], Linwei Wang[1], Dujun Wang[1], Dan Wang[1], Chongwei Wen[1], Bangxin Han[2] and Zhen Ouyang[1*]

Abstract

Background: Polysaccharides are carbohydrate chains composed of linked monosaccharide units. Accumulating studies report that polysaccharides isolated from *Dendrobium officinale* have a variety of functions. However, the composition and anti-tumor activity of *D. officinale* grown in the Huoshan area are largely unknown.

Methods: A polysaccharide (DOPA-1) was isolated from *D. officinale* by hot water extraction and ethanol precipitation, followed by purification via DEAE-cellulose and Sephadex G-100 chromatography. DOPA-1 was analyzed by infrared and nuclear magnetic resonance and then characterized by periodate oxidation and Smith degradation. The anti-tumor activity of DOPA-1 was then tested in HepG-2 cells.

Results: Our results show that DOPA-1 is mainly comprised of mannose, glucose, and galactose at a molar ratio of 1:0.42:0.27 and has an average molecular weight of 2.29×10^5 Da. Additionally, DOPA-1 inhibited HepG-2 cell growth in a dose-dependent manner. DOPA-1-treated HepG-2 cells also had increased reactive oxygen species (ROS) levels and decreased mitochondrial membrane potential. Furthermore, apoptosis was observed in DOPA-1-treated HepG-2 cells along with Bcl-2 downregulation and Bax upregulation at the protein level.

Conclusions: Our findings suggest that DOPA-1 induces apoptosis in tumor cells via altered mitochondrial function, ROS production, and altered apoptosis-related protein expression. This bioactive polysaccharide could, therefore, potentially be further developed as an anti-tumor adjuvant drug.

Keywords: *Dendrobium officinale*, Huoshan area, Polysaccharide characterization, Anti-tumor effect, Apoptosis

Background

Dendrobium officinale Kimura et Migo is a rare and endangered perennial orchid found in South and Southeast Asia. It is valued for its medicinal uses, including the treatment of fatigue, night sweats, fever, infantile convulsion, palpitations, and dizziness, and has been utilized in traditional Chinese medicine for more than 1000 years [1]. *D. officinale* grown in the Huoshan area, Anhui province of China, is recognized by its ability to grow in extremely harsh conditions. It is also considered to be the top grade of *D. officinale* by many researchers [2].

*Correspondence: zhenouyang@ujs.edu.cn
[1] School of Pharmacy, Jiangsu University, 301 Xuefu Road, Zhenjiang 212013, Jiangsu, China
Full list of author information is available at the end of the article

Polysaccharides are one of the main bioactive substances of many fungi, algae, and higher plants [3]. They are polymeric carbohydrate molecules composed of long chains of monosaccharide units. Polysaccharides play manifold roles and have broad activities in biochemical reaction, with an immense potential in healthcare and food industries, due to their therapeutic effects [4]. Accumulating evidence has shown that polysaccharides isolated from natural plants are nontoxic and have a variety of functions including inhibition of tumor cell proliferation [5], induction of tumor cell apoptosis [6], enhancement of immunity [7], and cellular protection from oxidative stress [8]. In addition, polysaccharides have also been found to reduce multidrug resistance and could potentially be applied as adjuvant drugs for chemotherapy [9].

In recent years, special attention has been paid to polysaccharides from *D. officinale* [10], as they have been reported to have significant anti-tumor [11], anti-oxidative [12], immunomodulatory [13], and blood sugar reducing [14] effects. Furthermore, the combination of *D. officinale* polysaccharides and recombinant interleukin (IL)-2 appears to be particularly effective at significantly enhancing PB-LAK cytotoxicity [15]. However, while polysaccharide content and activity have been evaluated in *D. officinale* samples from various origins, those of *D. officinale* from the Huoshan area have yet to be fully characterized, particularly with regards to their composition and anti-tumor activity.

In the present study, we isolated and purified a unique polysaccharide sample from *D. officinale* from the Huoshan are (designated DOPA-1) and then characterized its structure as well as its anti-tumor activities in HepG-2 cells. To the best of our knowledge, this is the first time this promising bioactive polysaccharide has been evaluated with regards to its composition and anti-tumor mechanisms.

Methods

Chemicals and reagents

Dendrobium officinale samples grown in the Huoshan area were provided by Tian-Xia-Ze-Yu Biological Technology Development Co., Ltd. (Huoshan County, Anhui, China). These samples were verified by Prof. Zhen Ouyang prior to being cut into small pieces no more than 3 mm in size.

Fetal bovine serum (FBS) and Dulbecco's modified Eagle's medium (DMEM) were obtained from Gibco (Grand Island, NY, USA). Standard monosaccharides (D-glucose, D-xylose, D-galactose, L-rhamnose, D-mannose, and D-arabinose), DEAE-52 cellulose, Sephadex G-100, dimethyl sulfoxide (DMSO), 3-(4,5-dimethylthiazol-2-yl)-2,5-diphenyltetrazolium bromide (MTT), 5-fluorouracil (5-FU), propidium iodide (PI), trypsin, JC-1, and the Annexin V-FITC/PI apoptosis detection kit were obtained from Sigma Aldrich (St. Louis, MO, USA). The Bax, Bcl-2, and β-actin antibodies were obtained from Santa Cruz Biotechnology (Santa Cruz, CA, USA). The DCFH-DA reactive oxygen species (ROS) assay and LDH cytotoxicity assay kits were purchased from Beyotime Institute of Biotechnology (Jiangsu, China). HepG-2 cells were provided by the Cell Bank of the Chinese Academy of Sciences (Shanghai, China). All other chemical reagents were of analytical grade. The Minimum Standards of Reporting Checklist contains details of the experimental design, and statistics, and resources used in this study.

Extraction and isolation

The components of *D. officinale* (20 g) were extracted three times with distilled water (400 mL × 3) for 2 h at 90 °C. The filtrate was combined and concentrated to 20 mL using a rotary evaporator at 60 °C. The concentrated supernatant was then evaporated under reduced pressure and precipitated by adding 95% ethanol until the total ethanol concentration reached 85%. The samples were subsequently stored at 4 °C overnight. The precipitate was collected following centrifugation (4000 rpm, 15 min), dissolved in distilled water, and lyophilized to obtain the crude polysaccharides. The crude polysaccharides were then deproteinized using the enzyme-Sevag method [16]. After the crude polysaccharides were dissolved in distilled water and fractionated on DEAE-52 cellulose, they were successively eluted with distilled water and an NaCl gradient (0.1–0.3 M) at 1.0 mL/min. The carbohydrate content of each fraction (10 mL/each) was monitored at 490 nm using the phenol–sulfuric acid method [17]. The obtained eluates were then combined, concentrated, dialyzed, lyophilized, and subjected to further purification on a Sephadex G-100 column. The fractions were subsequently combined and lyophilized to obtain a purified polysaccharide sample. The major fraction with only one main peak was lyophilized and named DOPA-1.

Homogeneity, molecular weight, and monosaccharide composition analysis

The homogeneity and molecular weight of DOPA-1 was determined with high performance liquid chromatography (HPLC) using a TSK-GEL G-4000 PWXL column (7.8 × 300 mm, column temperature 30 °C) and a Waters alliance refractive index detector (RID, detection temperature 30 °C). Prior to injection, the sample was filtered through a 0.45 μm membrane. Then, 10 μL of DOPA-1 (1.0 mg/mL) was injected into the HPLC column and eluted with distilled water at a flow rate of 0.45 mL/min. Dextrans of varying molecular weight (10, 40, 70, 500, and 2000 kDa) were used to establish a standard curve.

The monosaccharide composition of the purified DOPA-1 was measured by gas chromatography (GC). Briefly, 10 mg of the polysaccharides were hydrolyzed in a sealed glass tube with 5 mL of 2 M sulfuric acid at 100 °C for 8 h. The acid was then neutralized with barium carbonate. Next, the hydrolysate was acetylated with 10 mg of hydroxyl-amine hydrochloride in 1 mL of pyridine for 30 min at 90 °C. After cooling to 20–25 °C, 1 mL of acetic anhydride was added and further incubated for 30 min at 90 °C. Following cooling, the corresponding aldononitrile acetate derivatives were obtained and the corresponding monosaccharides (rhamnose, arabinose, xylose, mannose, glucose, and galactose) were then analyzed.

Infrared spectrum analysis

DOPA-1 (1.0 mg) was ground with KBr (100 mg) and pressed into a pellet. The Fourier transform infrared (FT-IR) spectra were recorded with an FT-IR spectrometer (Nicolet Nexus 470 FT-IR, USA) at a frequency range of 4000–500 cm^{-1}.

Nuclear magnetic resonance (NMR) spectroscopy

DOPA-1 (30 mg) was dissolved in 99.9% deuterium oxide (0.5 mL). The sample was then freeze-dried three times. The ^{1}H NMR spectra was recorded with a Bruker DRX-400 NMR spectrometer (Bruker, Rheinstetten, Germany) at 25 °C. Data processing was performed using standard Bruker XWIN-NMR software.

Periodate oxidation and Smith degradation

DOPA-1 (25 mg) was oxidized in 0.030 M $NaIO_4$ (25 mL) in the dark for 120 h and the absorption was monitored every 12 h with a UV spectrophotometer at 223 nm until a constant absorption value was achieved. $NaIO_4$ consumption was quantitatively measured using the UV spectrophotometric method [18] and the yield of formic acid was titrated with 0.01 M NaOH. Ethylene glycol (2 mL) was added to remove excess periodate. The periodate product was dialyzed and reduced with $NaBH_4$ (40 mg) for 24 h at room temperature. The product was then neutralized to pH 6.0–7.0 with acetic acid. Following dialysis and lyophilization, the product was finally hydrolyzed with 2 M trifluoroacetic acid (3 mL) at 110 °C for 6 h and the hydrolysate was subjected to GC analysis.

Cell culture and treatment

HepG-2 cells were cultured in DMEM medium supplemented with 10% (v/v) heat-inactivated FBS, 100 U/mL penicillin, and 100 μg/mL streptomycin in a humidified incubator at 37 °C with 5% CO_2. The medium was refreshed 2–3 times/week.

MTT cytotoxicity assay

A colorimetric MTT assay was performed to assess cell viability as previously described [19]. Briefly, HepG-2 cells were seeded in a 96-well plate at a concentration of 2.0×10^4 cells/well in 100 μL of medium. Following incubation at 37 °C for 24 h to allow adherence, the cells were treated with different concentrations (50, 100, 200, and 400 μg/mL) of DOPA-1 for 24 h. 5-FU (50 μg/mL) was used as a positive control, while untreated cells were used as a negative control. Following treatment, the medium in each well was removed and 100 μL of MTT (1 mg/mL) was added and incubated at 37 °C for 4 h. Next, the supernatant was aspirated and the crystal violet generated by viable cells was dissolved with 100 μL of DMSO. The absorbance was measured at 570 nm using a microplate reader.

LDH assay

Cell injury was quantitatively assessed by the measurement of lactate dehydrogenase (LDH). Cells were seeded in 96-well plates. After treatments, a LDH cytotoxicity assay kit (Beyotime, Jiangsu, China) was used to measure the released LDH. Briefly, 100 μl of culture medium was collected from each well. The absorbance of the medium was measured at 490 nm wavelength in an automatic microplate reader. Blank absorbance was subtracted from insult LDH values.

Determination of ROS levels

A DCFH-DA probe is the most common and sensitive tool for detecting intracellular ROS levels [20]. Logarithmic growth phase HepG-2 cells were digested, counted, and seeded in a 96-well culture plate at a density of 4×10^4 cells/well in 100 μL of medium. After the cells were treated with DOPA-1 for 24 h, the cells were washed twice with phosphate buffered saline (PBS) and incubated with 10 μM of DCFH-DA diluted in serum-free medium at 37 °C for 30 min. The fluorescence intensity was detected with a fluorescence microplate reader at an excitation wavelength of 488 nm and emission wavelength of 525 nm.

Determination of mitochondrial membrane potential (MMP)

JC-1 is a well-known fluorescent dye used to detect MMP. Following cell treatment, the culture medium was removed and the JC-1 dye (2.5 μg/mL) was added. After incubation at 37 °C for 10 min in the dark, the cells were washed twice with PBS. The fluorescence intensity was detected with a fluorescence microplate reader at an excitation wavelength of 488 nm and emission wavelength of 525/590 nm. The changes in MMP were then observed by fluorescence microscopy.

Flow cytometry

The rate of apoptosis was determined by cellular staining with Annexin V-FITC and PI [21]. Briefly, the treated cells (4×10^5 cells/mL) were washed twice with ice cold PBS and resuspended in 100 μL of 1× binding buffer. Next, 5 μL of Annexin V-FITC and 5 μL of PI were added and incubated for 10 min in the dark. The cells were then analyzed with a flow cytometer (Guava easyCyte, Merck Millipore, USA).

Western blotting analysis

Following treatment with DOPA-1 (50, 100, 200, and 400 μg/mL) for 24 h, HepG-2 cells were washed twice with ice-cold PBS and centrifuged at 12,000*g* for 10 min at 4 °C. After adding lysis buffer, the cells were incubated on ice for 20 min. The protein concentration of the supernatant was determined with a BCA protein assay kit. Proteins were separated by sodium dodecyl sulfate (SDS) polyacrylamide gel electrophoresis and then transferred onto a 0.45-μm polyvinylidene fluoride (PVDF) membrane. Subsequently, the membrane was blocked in blocking buffer (0.3 g bovine serum albumin [BSA], 20 mL PBS + Tween 20 [PBST], and 5% non-fat milk) for 2 h at room temperature, followed by incubation with the Bcl-2 (1:1000), Bax (1:1000), or β-actin (1:2000) primary antibodies overnight at 4 °C. The membranes were then washed three times with PBST (15 min each) and incubated with the appropriate secondary antibody (1:2000) for 2 h. Finally, the proteins were visualized with the ECL detection reagent and analyzed using a Chemi Doc XRS imaging system (Bio-Rad, CA, USA).

Statistical analysis

All experiments were performed in triplicate and the data were expressed as the mean ± standard deviation (SD). All statistical analyses were performed using GraphPad Prism 5. Analysis of variance (ANOVA) was used to compare the groups; $p < 0.05$ was considered a statistically significant difference.

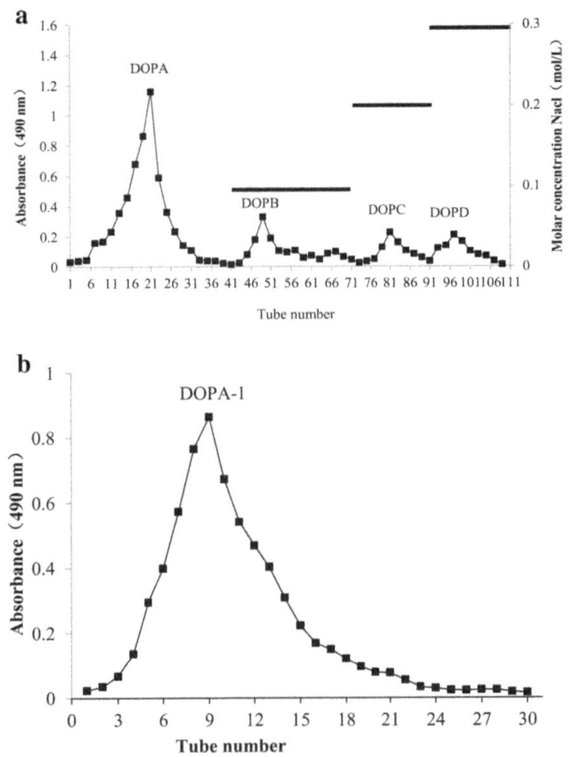

Fig. 1 Polysaccharide isolation and purification. **a** Elution profiles of the crude polysaccharide isolated from *D. officinale* grown in the Huoshan area using a DEAE-52 column. **b** Gel filtration chromatography was performed with a Sephadex G-100 column

Results

Isolation and purification of DOPA-1

The polysaccharide extracts from *D. officinale* were obtained by hot water extraction, 95% ethanol precipitation, and lyophilization resulting in an off-white floccule with a yield of 4.25%. The crude polysaccharides were deproteinized, eluted with distilled water, and then successively separated on DEAE cellulose-52 and Sephadex G-100 columns (Fig. 1). The main fraction eluted with distilled water (DOPA-1) was collected for further structural analysis.

Homogeneity, molecular weight, and monosaccharide composition analysis

The homogeneity, molecular weight, and monosaccharide composition of the purified polysaccharides were determined using HPLC and GC. DOPA-1 showed a single and symmetrically sharp peak at a retention time of 13.789 min (Fig. 2a), illustrating the homogenous nature of this polysaccharide. The average molecular weight of DOPA-1 was determined to be 2.29×10^5 Da based on the calibration data established with standard dextrans. The GC profiles show that DOPA-1 mainly consists of mannose, glucose, and galactose at a molar ratio of 1:0.42:0.27 (Fig. 2b).

Structural characterization of DOPA-1

The FT-IR spectra of DOPA-1 (Fig. 3a) exhibits the characteristic broad and intense absorption peaks at 3386 and 1027 cm^{-1} that are due to the stretching vibrations and deformation vibrations of the hydroxyl group, respectively. The signal at 2929 cm^{-1} has been attributed to the CH stretching vibration, while the signal at 1425 cm^{-1} is distinctive of a CH deformation vibration. The characteristic absorption of C=O (–NHCOCH3) was observed at 1645 cm^{-1}. The small band at 1380 cm^{-1} has been attributed to the presence of C=O (–COOH) stretching and the absorptions observed between 1300 and 1000 cm^{-1} indicate the presence of pyranose rings.

In an ^{1}H NMR spectrum, the anomeric proton signals of a sugar moiety are based on its conformation, α or β. Most of the signals attributed to α-anomeric pro-

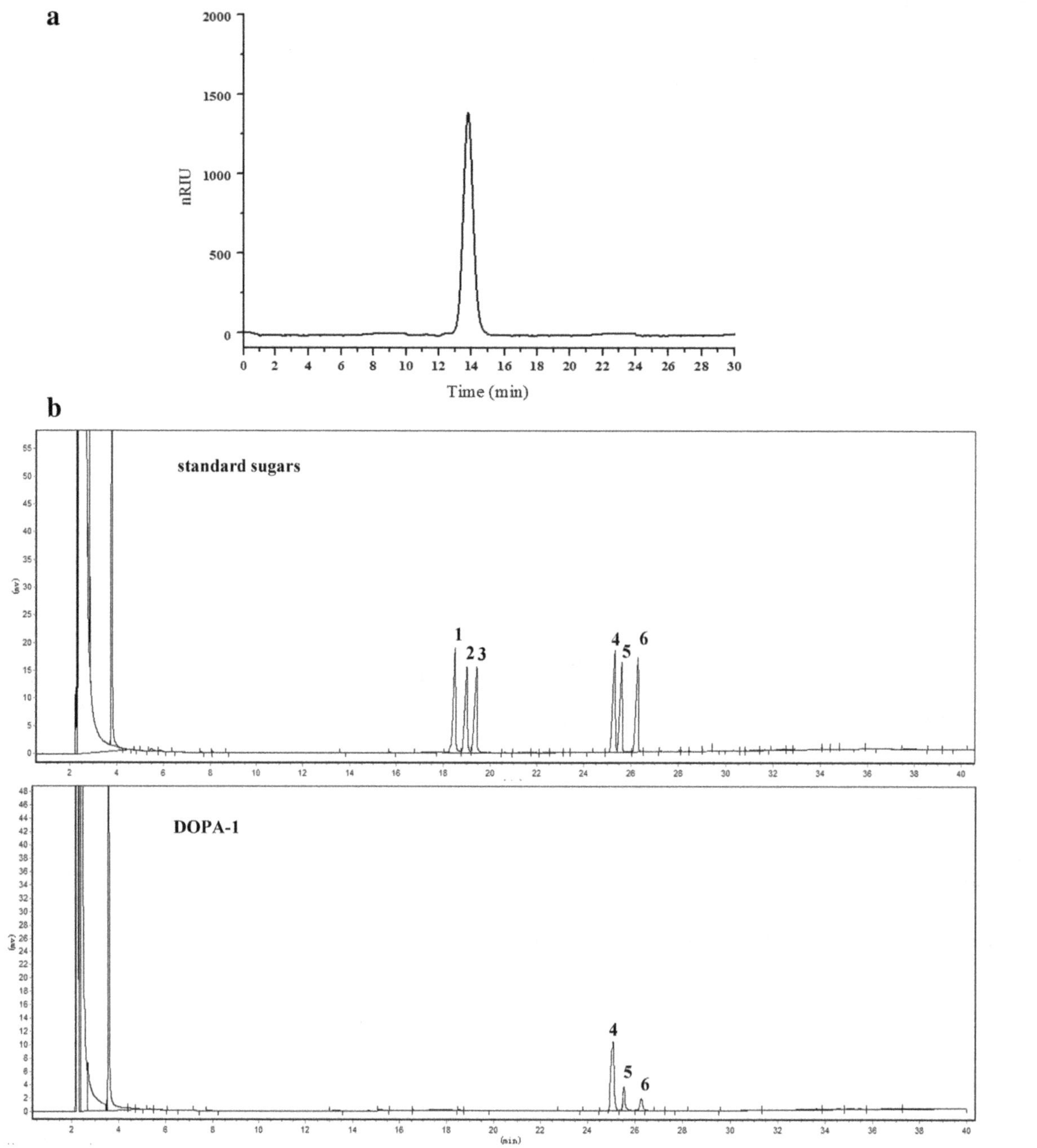

Fig. 2 Polysaccharide homogeneity, molecular weight, and monosaccharide composition analysis. **a** HPLC chromatogram of DOPA-1. **b** Monosaccharide composition GC analysis showing the peaks for (1) rhamnose, (2) arabinose, (3) xylose, (4) mannose, (5) glucose, and (6) galactose

tons usually resonate between 5 and 6 ppm, while the signals belonging to the β-anomeric protons resonate between 3 and 5 ppm. Thus, the signal at 5.24 ppm in the ^{1}H NMR spectrum of DOPA-1 indicates the presence of a pyranose residue containing an anomeric proton in the α-configuration (Fig. 3b). In addition, the signals resonating between 3.22 and 4 ppm indicate the existence of a β-type glycosidic linkage in DOPA-1.

Periodate oxidation and Smith degradation

The results of the periodate oxidation reaction show that 0.065 mmol $NaIO_4$ was consumed and 0.004 mmol formic acid was generated from DOPA-1, suggesting that an average of 1 mol of hexose residues (the molecular weight of each hexose residue multiplied by 180) consumed 0.389 mol periodate while generating 0.024 mol formic acid. The molar ratio of the

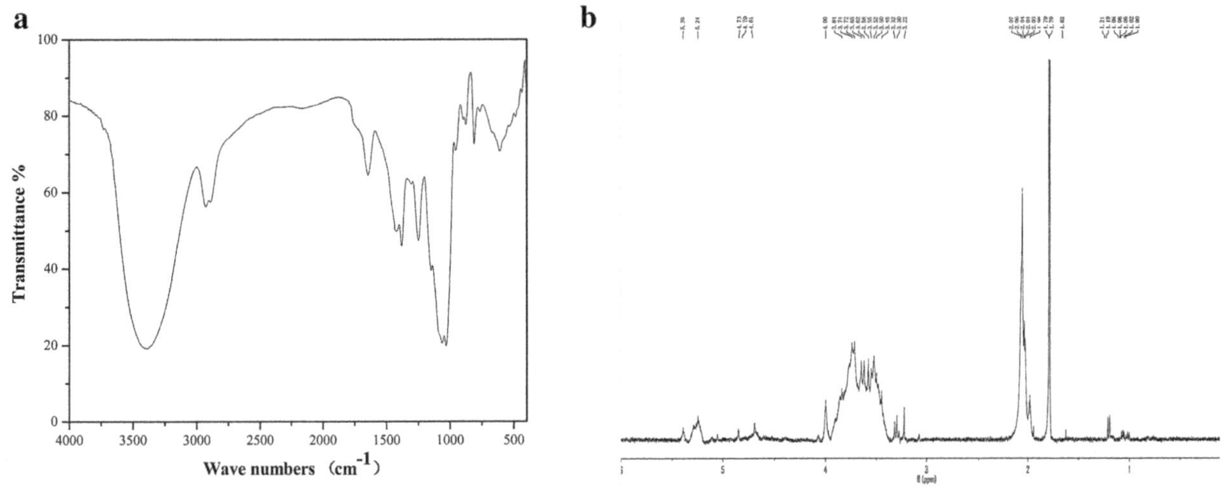

Fig. 3 Structural characterization of DOPA-1. **a** FT-IR and **b** ^{1}H NMR spectrum of DOPA-1

hexose residues, sodium periodate consumption, and formic acid generation was 1:0.389:0.024. Thus, it can be inferred that the 1→6 linkage residues or the non-reducing end groups of the (1→) linkage in DOPA-1 account for approximately 2.4%, while 34.1% of the residues are likely connected with 1→2 or 1→4 linkages. Approximately 63.5% of the residues are linked by 1→3 linkages. Furthermore, GC analysis of the Smith degradation reaction products detected glycerol and mannose at a molar ratio of 1.32:1. The presence of undegraded mannose indicates that DOPA-1 is composed primarily of 1→3 linkages, while glycerol detection implies the presence of 1→2 or 1→6 linkages in DOPA-1. As no erythritol was found, it can be deduced that there are no 1→4 linkages. Taken together, the results of these analyses highlight the existence of 1→3, 1→2, and 1→6 linkages in the main or branched chains of DOPA-1 (Fig. 4).

DOPA-1 cytotoxicity in HepG-2 cells

In this study, the effect of increasing concentrations of DOPA-1 (50, 100, 200, and 400 μg/mL) on HepG-2 cell growth was determined using an MTT assay. Notably, DOPA-1 cytotoxicity increased significantly ($p < 0.05$) in a dose-dependent manner (Fig. 5a). In fact, cell viability following treatment with 50, 100, 200, and 400 μg/mL DOPA-1 for 24 h was 94.51, 85.37, 71.63, and 46.76%, respectively, compared to the 5-FU-treated positive control group (52.4%). The LDH release level increased significantly ($p < 0.05$) in a dose-dependent manner (Fig. 5b), with the release viability was 13.67, 20.10, 26.67, and 31.32%, respectively, compared to the 5-FU-treated positive control group (38.65%). The effects of DOPA-1 toxicity were approximately consistent between the two assays. Those results indicated that DOPA-1 inhibits HepG-2 cell growth in vitro.

Effects of DOPA-1 on ROS production

The production of excess intracellular ROS can induce apoptosis. Thus, ROS generation in DOPA-1-treated HepG-2 cells was detected by DCFH-DA staining. As highlighted by the increasing fluorescence intensity in Fig. 6, ROS content increased with increasing DOPA-1 concentration in the treated cells. The ROS levels were significantly higher (for all but the lowest DOPA-1 concentration) than those in the untreated control cells. These results suggest that DOPA-1 induces apoptosis in HepG-2 cells via increased intracellular oxidative stress.

Effects of DOPA-1 on mitochondrial function in HepG-2 cells

Many studies have shown that mitochondria play an important role in apoptosis as well as ROS generation and that changes in MMP can be observed early in the apoptotic signaling cascade [22]. In the untreated controls cells, the fluorescence enzyme marker was mostly red, while green fluorescence was weak, indicating that the mitochondrial membrane was intact and MMP was relatively high (Fig. 7). However, the green fluorescence gradually increased, while the red fluorescence gradually weakened when treated with increasing DOPA-1 concentrations. This shift in fluorescent color signifies increased mitochondrial membrane permeability and decreased MMP as DOPA-1 concentration increased.

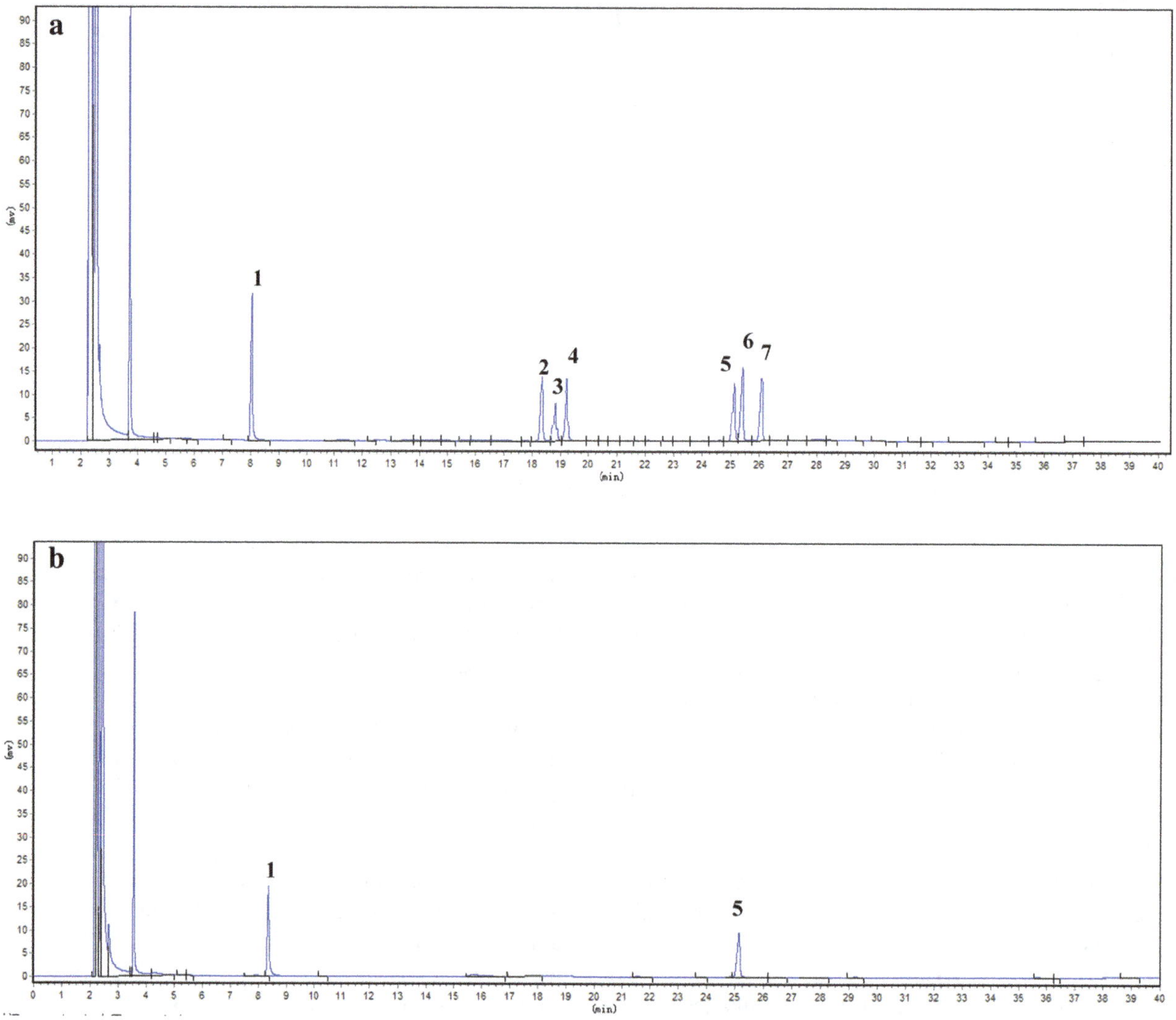

Fig. 4 GC chromatogram of DOPA-1 products following Smith degradation. The chromatograms show the peaks for **a** standard sugars and **b** DOPA-1. This includes peaks for (1) rhamnose, (2) arabinose, (3) xylose, (4) mannose, (5) glucose, and (6) galactose

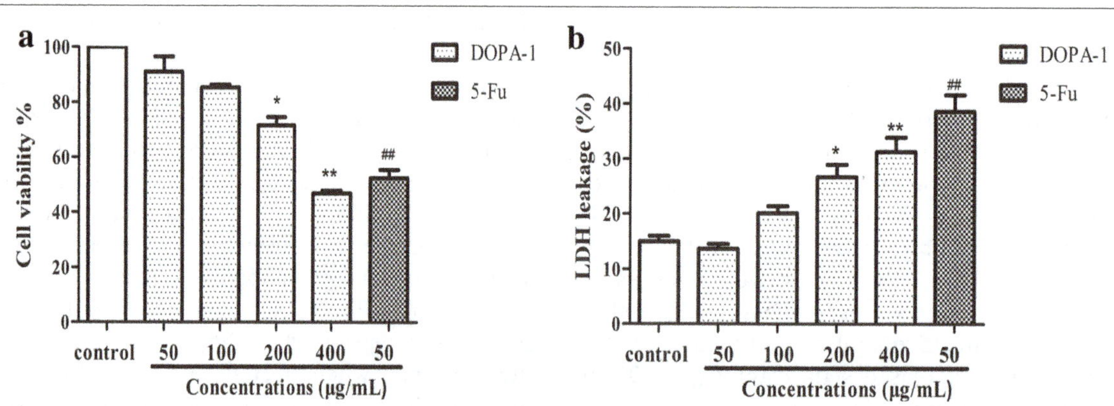

Fig. 5 DOPA-1 decreases HepG-2 cell viability. **a** Cell viability was assessed by MTT assay. **b** LDH release assay. The cells were treated with different concentrations of DOPA-1 for 24 h. Data are presented as the mean ± SD of three independent experiments. $^{*}p < 0.05$, $^{**}p < 0.01$, $^{\#\#}p < 0.01$, compared to the control

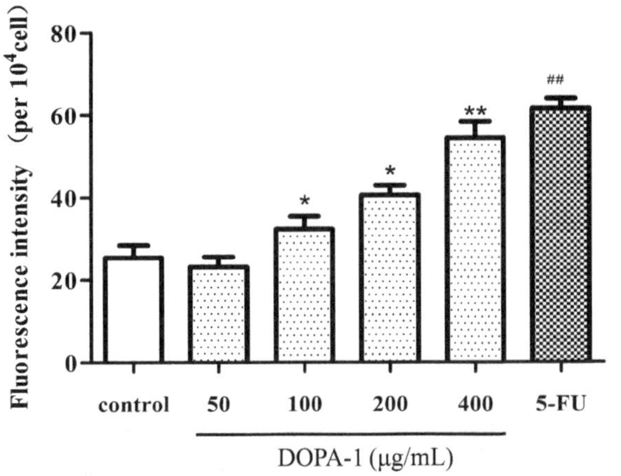

Fig. 6 DOPA-1 treatment increases intracellular ROS production in HepG-2 cells. Data are presented as the mean ± SD of three independent experiments. $^*p<0.05$, $^{**}p<0.01$, $^{\#\#}p<0.01$, compared to the control

Indeed, the mitochondrial membrane appeared to be almost entirely disrupted at the highest DOPA-1 concentration. The results of this analysis suggest that DOPA-1-induced apoptosis and increased ROS production are likely related to mitochondrial dysfunction.

Detection of apoptosis by flow cytometry

In order to examine the rate of apoptosis, Annexin VFITC/PI double staining was used in association with flow cytometry. As shown in Fig. 8A, the rate of apoptosis observed in cultures treated with 50, 100, 200, or 400 μg/mL DOPA-1 was 16.98, 19.82, 24.58, and 40.29%, respectively. Thus, similar to our earlier data, apoptosis increased in a dose-dependent manner and was significantly higher in the DOPA-1-treated groups than in the control group (11.0%).

Effects of DOPA-1 on apoptosis-related protein expression

In this analysis, we focused on the protein expression of both anti- and pro-apoptotic factors in DOPA-1-treated HepG-2 cells. The expression of the anti-apoptotic protein Bcl-2 gradually decreased with increasing DOPA-1 concentration, while expression of the pro-apoptotic protein Bax gradually increased (Fig. 8B). This Bax/Bcl-2 ratio is known to be an important factor in regulating apoptosis. Following treatment with 50, 100, 200, or 400 μg/mL of DOPA-1 for 24 h, the Bax/Bcl-2 ratio gradually increased and the excess Bax formed homodimers, leading to cell apoptosis. While the full underlying mechanism still requires additional investigation, these data imply that DOPA-1-induced HepG-2 cell apoptosis is likely regulated by the expression of apoptosis-related proteins including Bax and Bcl-2.

Discussion

Polysaccharides are carbohydrate chains of monosaccharides that are connected through glycosidic bonds. It is widely accepted that polysaccharide activity varies depending on its structure [23]. Thus, the type of glycosidic bonds in the polysaccharide backbone is a key factor in determining the functional effects of polysaccharides. For example, the presence of β-(1→3) linkages in the main chain of the glucan and additional β-(1→6) branch points have been shown to be necessary for anti-tumor activity [24]. Indeed, a previous study showed that the polysaccharide fractions of *Agaricus blazei* fruiting bodies have high anti-tumor activity and that their main glucan linkages are β-(1→6) and β-(1→3) [25]. In the present study, DOPA-1 appears to contain (1→3), (1→2), and (1→6) linkages in the main or branch chains, suggesting that it may account for the observed anti-tumor activity.

Previous studies have shown that elevated ROS levels may be involved in anti-tumor drug-induced cell death [26]. ROS are a group of oxygenated compounds produced during exogenous oxidation and intracellular aerobic metabolism [27]. Oxidative stress occurs when the rate at which ROS are cleared by the intracellular anti-oxidant system is slower than the rate at which they are produced [28]. High concentrations of ROS are known to upregulate proapoptotic protein expression, regulate the conformation of adenine nucleotide translocator protein in the inner mitochondrial membrane, and induce mitochondrial membrane permeability. ROS-mediated oxidative stress also reduces MMP, further activating cytochrome c and other apoptosis-inducing factors. As the mitochondrial membrane becomes more permeable, intracellular ROS will continue to rise, until tumor cell apoptosis is induced [29, 30]. Our results showed that DOPA-1 treatment increases intracellular ROS levels, as well as mitochondrial membrane permeability. Treatment also decreased MMP. These findings suggest that ROS and changes in the mitochondrial membrane play a significant role in the mechanism of DOPA-1 during cancer cell apoptosis.

In addition to ROS and mitochondrial function, we also evaluated the effects of DOPA-1 treatment on apoptosis-related protein expression. As a major modulator of apoptosis, the Bcl-2 protein family controls the release of mitochondrial apoptosis-inducing factors [31], which can be divided into pro-apoptotic proteins (such as Bax, Bak, and Bid) and anti-apoptotic proteins (such as Bcl-2, Bcl-xL, and Bcl-w) [32]. In this study, we found that DOPA-1 decreases Bcl-2 expression, while increasing Bax expression in HepG-2 cells. Thus, while the full mechanism underlying the anti-tumor effects of DOPA-1 still needs to be evaluated, these data suggest that this polysaccharide promotes HepG-2 cell apoptosis by regulating the expression of apoptosis-related proteins.

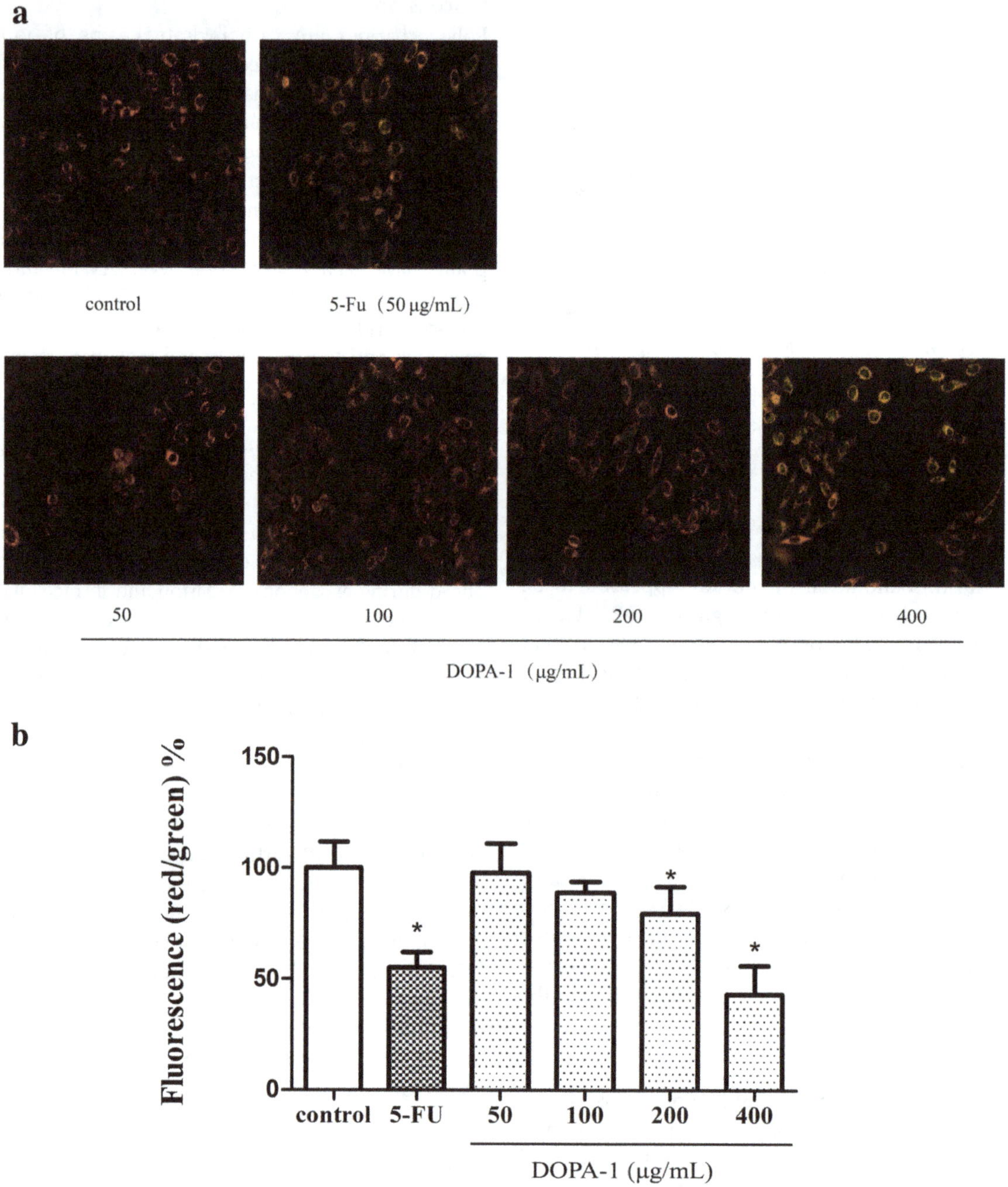

Fig. 7 Treatment with DOPA-1 alters mitochondrial function in HepG-2 cells. **a** Fluorescence micrographs of HepG-2 cells stained with JC-1. Changes in cell morphology were observed under ×200 magnification. **b** Quantitative analysis of MMP in HepG-2 cells. Data are expressed as the fluorescence ratio of red to green and are presented as the mean ± SD of three independent experiments. $^{*}p < 0.05$, compared to the control

Notably, a polysaccharide recently isolated from *D. officinale* showed immune-modulating activity [33], and a novel heteroxylan isolated from the same plant had potential on anti-angiogenesis activities [34]. Those polysaccharides had different molecular weights and compositions compared to DOPA-1. It would be of great interest to further investigate if the three polysaccharides from the same plant have synergistic effects on anti-tumor activities.

Conclusions

In this present study, we isolated, purified, and characterized a water-soluble polysaccharide from *D. officinale* grown in the Huoshan area, DOPA-1. To the best of our knowledge, this is the first time DOPA-1 has been evaluated with regards to its composition and anti-tumor mechanisms. This neutral homogeneous polysaccharide has an average molecular weight of

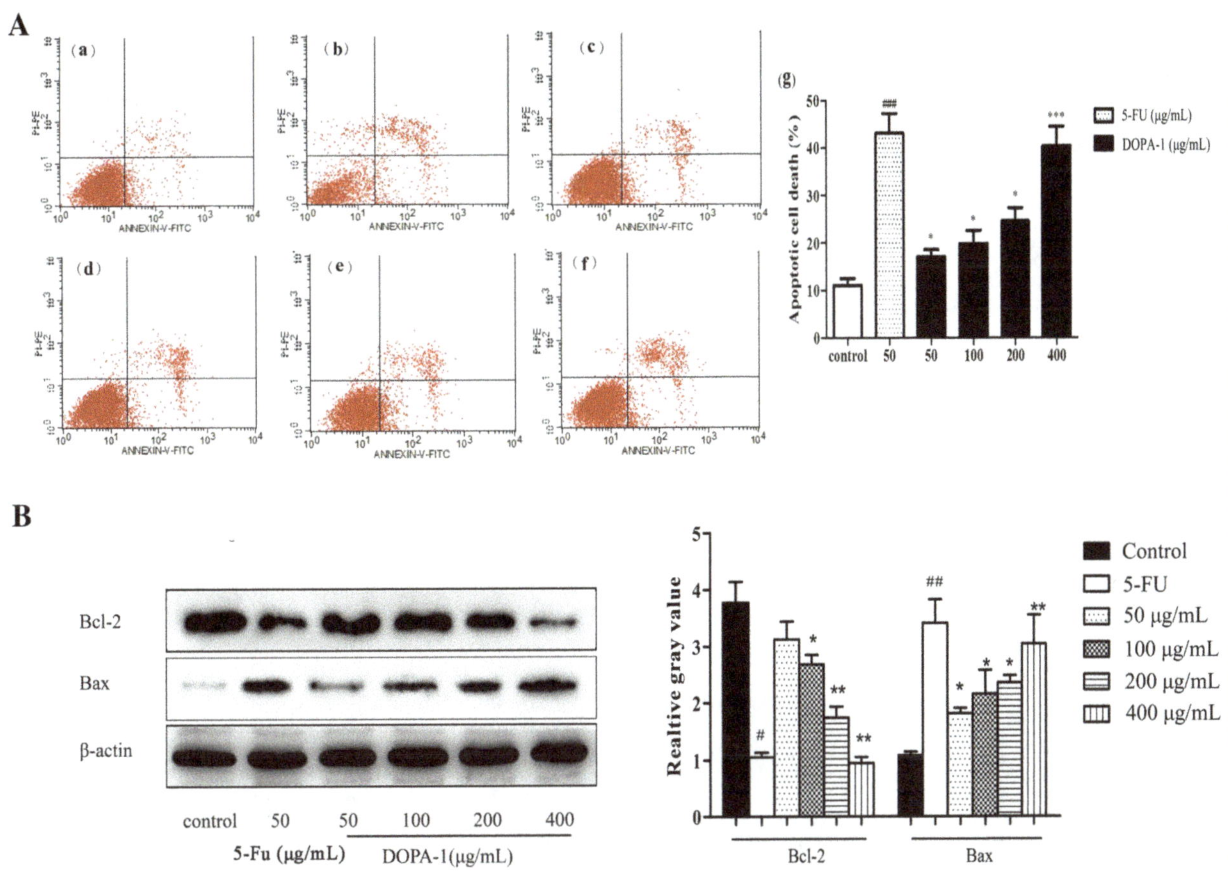

Fig. 8 DOPA-1 treatment induces dose-dependent HepG-2 cell apoptosis. **A** Flow cytometric analysis of HepG-2 cell apoptosis with Annexin V-FITC and PI labeling. Subpanels: (a) untreated control group, (b) 50 μg/mL 5-FU, (c) 50 μg/mL DOPA-1, (d) 100 μg/mL DOPA-1, (e) 200 μg/mL DOPA-1, (f) 400 μg/mL DOPA-1, and (g) the calculated apoptotic rate for each treatment group. **B** Western blotting analysis and quantitation of Bax and Bcl-2 expression. Data are presented as the mean ± SD of three independent experiments. $^{*}p < 0.05$, $^{**}p < 0.01$, $^{***}p < 0.001$, $^{\#}p < 0.05$, $^{\#\#}p < 0.01$, compared to the blank control group

2.29×10^5 Da and appears to be composed of mannose, glucose, and galactose at a molar ratio of 1:0.42:0.27. DOPA-1 inhibits in vitro tumor cell growth in a dose-dependent manner. The DOPA-1-mediated mechanism underlying tumor cell death involves ROS-induced mitochondrial dysfunction, namely increased membrane permeability and decreased MMP. Furthermore, DOPA-1-induced apoptosis also appears to be related to the downregulation of Bcl-2 protein expression and upregulation of Bax protein expression. In summary, this study provides insight into the composition and structure of the polysaccharides of *D. officinale* grown in the Huoshan area and highlights their distinct anti-tumor effects. This potent bioactive component could, therefore, potentially be further developed and used as an anti-tumor adjuvant drug.

Abbreviations

DOPA-1: *D. officinale* polysaccharide; FBS: fetal bovine serum; MTT: 3-(4,5-dimethylthiazol-2-yl)-2,5-diphenyltetrazolium bromide; DMEM: Dulbecco's modified Eagle's medium; 5-FU: 5-fluorouracil; PI: propidium iodide; DMSO: dimethyl sulfoxide; ROS: reactive oxygen species; HPLC: high performance liquid chromatography; RID: refractive index detector; FT-IR: Fourier transform infrared; NMR: nuclear magnetic resonance; TFA: trifluoroacetic acid; GC: gas chromatography; PBS: phosphate buffered saline; MMP: mitochondrial membrane potential; SDS: sodium dodecyl sulfate; PVDF: polyvinylidene fluoride; BSA: bovine serum albumin; PBST: PBS + Tween 20; SD: standard deviation; ANOVA: analysis of variance.

Authors' contributions

Study design and conception: ZOY; data collection and data analysis: YW, LWW, and DW; data interpretation: CWW and DJW; manuscript drafting: YW and LWW; critical revision of the manuscript: BXH and ZOY. All authors read and approved the final manuscript.

Author details

[1] School of Pharmacy, Jiangsu University, 301 Xuefu Road, Zhenjiang 212013, Jiangsu, China. [2] School of Biological and Pharmaceutical Engineering, West Anhui University, Lu'an 237012, China.

Acknowledgements

We gratefully acknowledge the National Natural Science Foundation of China, China Agriculture Research System, and National Key Research and Development Project for funding support.

Competing interests

The authors declare that they have no competing interests.

Consent for publication

All of authors consent to publication of this study in Journal of BMC-Chinese Medicine.

Funding

This work was supported by the National Natural Science Foundation of China (Nos. 81573529, 81072985, 81373480), China Agriculture Research System (CARS-21) and National Key Research and Development Project (2017YFC1700701).

References

1. Zhao P, Wang W, Feng FS, Wu F, Yang ZQ, Wang WJ. High-frequency shoot regeneration through transverse thin cell layer culture in Dendrobium Candidum Wall Ex Lindl. Plant Cell Tissue Organ Cult. 2007;90:131.
2. Wang K, Sui DJ, Wang CS, Yang L, Ouyang Z, Chen NF, et al. Protective effects of five different types of Dendrobium on CCl4-induced liver injury in mice. China J Chin Mater Medica. 2017;42:1945.
3. Li Q, Niu Y, Xing P, Wang C. Bioactive polysaccharides from natural resources including Chinese medicinal herbs on tissue repair. Chin Med. 2018;13:7.
4. Cao YJ, Pu ZJ, Tang YP, Shen J, Chen YY, Kang A, et al. Advances in bio-active constituents, pharmacology and clinical applications of rhubarb. Chin Med. 2017;12:36.
5. Lee CT, Kuo HC, Chen YH, Tsai MY. Current advances in the biological activity of polysaccharides in Dendrobium with intriguing therapeutic potential. Curr Med Chem. 2018;24:1.
6. Ji YB, Dong F, Gao SY, Zou X. Apoptosis induced by *Capparis spionosa* polysaccharide in human HepG2. Chin Tradit Herb Drugs. 2008;39:1364–7.
7. Shen CY, Zhang WL, Jiang JG. Immune-enhancing activity of polysaccharides from *Hibiscus sabdariffa* Linn. via MAPK and NF-kB signaling pathways in RAW264.7 cells. J Funct Foods. 2017;34:118–29.
8. Olatunji OJ, Yan F, Olatunji OO, Jian T, Yuan W, Zhen O, et al. Polysaccharides purified from *Cordyceps cicadae* protects PC12 cells against glutamate-induced oxidative damage. Carbohydr Polym. 2016;153:187–95.
9. Li F, Luo P, Liu H. A potential adjuvant agent of chemotherapy: sepia ink polysaccharides. Mar Drugs. 2018;16:485.
10. Huang K, Li Y, Tao S, Wei G, Huang Y, Chen D, et al. Purification, characterization and biological activity of polysaccharides from *Dendrobium officinale*. Molecules. 2016;21:701.
11. He TG, Yang LT, Li YR. Physicochemical properties and antitumor activity of polysaccharide DCPP1a-1 from suspension-cultured protocorms of Dendrobium candidum. Nat Prod Res Dev. 2007;19:410–4.
12. Luo QL, Tang ZH, Zhang XF, Zhong YH, Yao SZ, Wang LS, et al. Chemical properties and antioxidant activity of a water-soluble polysaccharide from *Dendrobium officinale*. Int J Biol Macromol. 2016;89:219–27.
13. He TB, Huang YP, Yang L, Liu TT, Gong WY, Wang XJ, et al. Structural characterization and immunomodulating activity of polysaccharide from *Dendrobium officinale*. Int J Biol Macromol. 2016;83:34–41.
14. Chen Y, Yang JK. Research progress of treatment of traditional Chinese medicine for liver cancer. J Liaoning Univ Trad Chin Med. 2010;4:951.
15. Luo HL, Cai TY, Chen QL, Huang MQ, Mei CE, Li YQ. Enhancement of *Dendrobium candidum* polysaccharide on killing effect of LAK cells of umbilical cord blood and peripheral blood of cancer patients in vitro. Chin J Cancer. 2000;19:1124–6.
16. Zha XQ. Polysaccharides in *Laminaria japonica* (LP): extraction, physicochemical properties and their hypolipidemic activities in diet-induced mouse model of atherosclerosis. Food Chem. 2012;134:244–52.
17. Bai R, Yuling MA, Zhang P, Wang YP, Li YD, Hu FD. Content determination of saccharide in polysaccharides containing galacturonic acid by phenol-sulfuric acid method combined with calibration factor method. Chin Pharm. 2017;28:2974–8.
18. Shi J, Cheng C, Zhao H, Jing J, Gong N, Lu W. In vivo anti-radiation activities of the Ulva pertusa polysaccharides and polysaccharide-iron(III) complex. Int J Biol Macromol. 2013;60:341–6.
19. Mosmann T. Rapid colorimetric assay for cellular growth and survival: application to proliferation and cytotoxicity assays. J Immunol Methods. 1983;65:55.
20. Son YO, Lee JC, Hitron JA, Pan J, Zhang Z, Shi X. Cadmium induces intracellular Ca^{2+}- and H_2O_2-dependent apoptosis through JNK- and p53-mediated pathways in skin epidermal cell line. Toxicol Sci Off J Soc Toxicol. 2010;113:127.
21. Ma L, Qin C, Wang M, Gan D, Cao L, Ye H, et al. Preparation, preliminary characterization and inhibitory effect on human colon cancer HT-29 cells of an acidic polysaccharide fraction from *Stachys floridana* Schuttl. ex Benth. Food Chem Toxicol. 2013;60:269–76.
22. Smiley ST, Reers M, Mottola-Hartshorn C, Lin M, Chen A, Smith TW, et al. Intracellular heterogeneity in mitochondrial membrane potentials revealed by a J-aggregate-forming lipophilic cation JC-1. Proc Natl Acad Sci USA. 1991;88:3671–5.
23. Nie S, Cui SW, Xie M, Phillips AO, Phillips GO. Bioactive polysaccharides from *Cordyceps sinensis*: isolation, structure features and bioactivities. Bioact Carbohydr Diet Fibre. 2013;1:38–52.
24. Wasser SP. Medicinal mushrooms as a source of antitumor and immunomodulating polysaccharides. Appl Microbiol Biotechnol. 2002;60:258–74.
25. Mizuno T, Hagiwara T, Nakamura T, Ito H, Shimura K, Sumiya T, et al. Antitumor activity and some properties of water-soluble polysaccharides from "Himematsutake", the fruiting body of Agavicus blazei Murill. Agric Biol Chem. 1990;54:2889–96.
26. de Keizer PL, Burgering BM, Dansen TB. Forkhead box o as a sensor, mediator, and regulator of redox signaling. Antioxid Redox Signal. 2011;14:1093–106.
27. Seo JY, Kim SK, Nguyen PH, Lee JY, Tung P, Sung SH, et al. Chemical constituents from a Gynostemma laxumand their antioxidant and neuroprotective activities. Chin Med. 2017;12:15.
28. Jia WX, Choi YT, Lau BS, Leung WN, Ng CF, Chan CW. Gastrodia and Uncaria (tianma gouteng) water extract exerts antioxidative and antiapoptotic effects against cerebral ischemia in vitro and in vivo. Chin Med. 2016;11:27.
29. Rottenberg H, Hoek JB. The path from mitochondrial ROS to aging runs through the mitochondrial permeability transition pore. Aging Cell. 2017;16:943–55.
30. Ploner C, Kofler R, Villunger A. Noxa: at the tip of the balance between life and death. Oncogene. 2008;27(Suppl 1):S84.
31. Fong Y, Tang CC, Hu HT, Fang HY, Chen BH, Wu CY, et al. Inhibitory effect of trans-ferulic acid on proliferation and migration of human lung cancer cells accompanied with increased endogenous reactive oxygen species and Î^{2}-catenin instability. Chin Med. 2016;11:45.
32. Hata AN, Engelman JA, Faber AC. The BCL-2 family: key mediators of the apoptotic response to targeted anti-cancer therapeutics. Cancer Discov. 2015;5:475–87.
33. Xie SZ, Liu B, Zhang DD, Zha XQ, Pan LH, Luo JP. Intestinal immunomodulating activity and structural characterization of a new polysaccharide from stems of *Dendrobium officinale*. Food Funct. 2016;7:2789.
34. Yue H, Liu Y, Qu H, Ding K. Structure analysis of a novel heteroxylan from the stem of *Dendrobium officinale* and anti-angiogenesis activities of its sulfated derivative. Int J Biol Macromol. 2017;103:533–42.

8

Siegesbeckia pubescens Makino inhibits Pam_3CSK_4-induced inflammation in RAW 264.7 macrophages through suppressing TLR1/TLR2-mediated NF-κB activation

Wei Sang[1†], Zhangfeng Zhong[1,4†], Kegang Linghu[1], Wei Xiong[1], Anfernee Kai Wing Tse[5], Wai San Cheang[1], Hua Yu[1,2,3,6*] and Yitao Wang[1,7*]

Abstract

Background: *Siegesbeckia pubescens* Makino (SP) is one of the important plant origins for the anti-inflammatory Chinese herbal medicine of Siegesbeckiae Herba. The current investigations indicated that the anti-inflammatory effects of SP were associated with the toll-like receptors (TLRs)-mediated nuclear factor-κB (NF-κB) and the mitogen-activated protein kinase (MAPK) signaling pathways.

Methods: Raw 264.7 macrophages were pretreated with the 50% ethanol extract of SP (SPE, 50–200 μg/mL) and then co-treated with Pam_3CSK_4 (200 ng/mL) for another 12 h. The inhibitory effect of SPE on Pam_3CSK_4-stimulated NO release and post-inflammatory cytokines secretions were determined using Griess reagent and Elisa kits, respectively. The influence of SPE on NF-κB and MAPKs signaling relevant proteins was measured by Western blotting analysis, while the intracellular nitric oxide (NO) generation and NF-κB/p65 nuclear translocation were determined using Leica TCS SP8 laser scanning confocal microscope. Moreover, the effect of SPE on luciferase reporter gene in NF-κB-luc DNA transfected raw 264.7 cells was determined using the Dual-Glo luciferase assay system kit.

Results: SPE dose-dependently (50–200 μg/mL) attenuated Pam_3CSK_4-induced NO release, post-inflammatory cytokines (IL-6, TNF-α and MCP-1) secretions and intracellular NO generation in raw 264.7 cells. Biologically, SPE suppressed Pam_3CSK_4-induced expressions of cyclooxygenase-2 (COX-2), inducible nitric oxide synthase (iNOS), phosphorylation of NF-κB/p65 and IκBα, but did not significantly show effect on the proteins involved in MAPKs signaling (p38, ERK and JNK). The results were further confirmed by NF-κB-luc reporter gene assay and p65 nuclear translocation assay.

Conclusions: In conclusion, SPE ameliorated Pam_3CSK_4-induced inflammation in raw 264.7 cells through suppressing TLR 1/2-mediated NF-κB activation.

Keywords: *Siegesbeckia pubescens* Makino, Pam_3CSK_4, Inflammation, Toll-like receptor 1/2, NF-κB

*Correspondence: bcalecyu@umac.mo; ytwang@umac.mo
†Wei Sang and Zhangfeng Zhong contributed equally to this work
[6] Institute of Chinese Medical Sciences, University of Macau, Room 8008, Building N22, Avenida da Universidade, Taipa, Macao SAR, China
[7] Institute of Chinese Medical Sciences, University of Macau, Room 1050, Building N22, Avenida da Universidade, Taipa, Macao SAR, China
Full list of author information is available at the end of the article

Background

Inflammation is an innate (non-specific) immune response and plays an important role in the physiological defense in response to various trauma or infection to the body [1]. An appropriate inflammatory response is necessary for the organism's healing potential and facilitates tissue repair. However, an excessive or prolonged response might cause continuously damage to the body and induce many chronic diseases, organ dysfunction or organ failure [2, 3]. Therefore, an effective means of modulating systemic inflammation is beneficial for patients with chronic inflammatory autoimmune diseases, such as rheumatoid arthritis and diabetic nephropathy.

In the past decades, numerous studies indicated that transcription factors NF-κB target genes were involved in the occurrence and progress of various inflammations [4–8]. Activation of NF-κB stimulated macrophage recruitment and maturation, as well as the further production of pro-inflammatory cytokines and chemokines, such as tumor necrosis factor (TNF)-α, interleukin (IL)-1β, IL-6, monocyte chemoattractant protein (MCP)-1, and so on [9, 10]. Subsequently, the secreted inflammatory mediators further accelerated the degree of inflammation and the development of diseases [11]. On the other hand, being a family of transmembrane receptors closely related to the innate immune response [12], toll-like receptors (TLRs) (TLR1–TLR10 for human TLRs) present different functions on regulating inflammatory signaling and mediators based on their capacity to recognize the host derived agonists mostly released from the damaged cells or tissues during the progression of the diseases [13–16]. In triacyl lipoprotein-induced inflammations, the activation of NF-κB signaling pathways and production of various pro-inflammatory cytokines through TLR1/TLR2 (a heterodimer of TLR1 and TLR2) activation have been investigated and reported [17–20]. Therefore, targeting TLR1/TLR2 heterodimer-induced inflammation might be the potential therapeutic approach for such inflammatory diseases.

Siegesbeckia pubescens Makino (SP) is one of the plant origins of the traditional Chinese herbal medicine of Siegesbeckiae Herba, which has been widely used for various inflammatory diseases in China from the Tang dynasty. Currently, the chemical analysis indicated that SP mainly contained diterpenoids [21], sesquiterpenoids [22], flavonoids [23], glycosides [24] and some other constituents [25]. Moreover, the SP extracts or derived components were investigated to present various pharmacological activities such as anti-inflammatory [22, 26, 27], anti-allergic [28], and anti-cancer effects [29, 30]. The anti-inflammatory activity of SP was demonstrated to be related to its suppression on lipopolysaccharide (LPS)-induced nitric oxide (NO) [26] and inflammatory mediators [31] productions via NF-κB inactivation [32]. However, in our preliminary studies, the 50% ethanol extract of SP has been observed to have better activity against Pam_3CSK_4-(a specific TLR1/TLR2 agonist) than LPS-induced NO production in RAW 264.7 macrophages. In this study, the potential mechanisms of SP on Pam_3CSK_4-induced inflammation were further investigated and reported.

Methods

The Minimum Standards of Reporting Checklist contains details of the experimental design, and statistics, and resources used in this study (Additional file 1).

Chemical and reagents

Rutin, kirenol and darutoside (the purities of all standards were higher than 98% by HPLC analysis) were purchased from Chengdu Pufei De Biotech Co., Ltd. (Chengdu, China). Hoechst 33342, 3-(4, 5-dimethylthiazol-2-yl)-2,5-diphenyltetrazolium bromide (MTT) and Griess reagent were purchased from Sigma Chemicals Ltd. (St. Louis, MO, USA). Milli-Q water was prepared using a Milli-Q system (Millipore, MA, USA).

Dulbecco's modified eagle medium (DMEM) and fetal bovine serum (FBS) were purchased from Gibco (Carlsbad, CA, USA). Pam_3CSK_4 (*N*-palmitoyl-*S*-[2,3-bis(palmitoyloxy)-(2RS)-propyl]-[*R*]-cysteinyl-[*S*]-seryl-[*S*]-lysyl-[*S*]-lysyl-[*S*]-lysyl-[*S*]-lysine·3HCl) was purchased from InvivoGen (San Diego, CA, USA). Enzyme-linked immunosorbent assay kits for IL-6, TNF-α, and MCP-1 were obtained from Neobioscience (Shenzhen, China). TurboFect transfection reagent was purchased from Thermo Fisher Scientific (Waltham, MA, USA). Antibodies were purchased from Santa Cruz Biotechnology (CA, USA) or Cell Signaling Tech (Danvers, MA, USA).

Preparation and characterization of SP extract (SPE)

The herbal material of SP was collected from Guiyang (Guizhou province, China) and authenticated by the corresponding author. The voucher specimens (No. SP-002) were deposited at the Institute of Chinese Medical Sciences, University of Macau, Macao, China.

The powdered SP (100 g) was extracted twice with 50% ethanol (1:10, w/v) for 1 h each under reflux. The combined extracts were filtered with filter paper after cooling and then concentrated under reduced pressure to remove the ethanol. The powdered SPE (yield: 27.3%) was obtained by lyophilizing the concentrated sample with a Virtis Freeze Dryer (The Virtis Company, New York, USA).

Quantification of rutin, kirenol and darutoside in SPE was performed using an Agilent HP1100 system (Hewlett Packard, Agilent, USA) coupled with an Elite Hypersil

BDS C-18 analytical column (100 mm × 2.1 mm I.D., 3 μm) (Dalian, China) maintained at 25 °C. Elution was performed with a mobile phase of A (0.2% phosphoric acid in water) and B (0.2% phosphoric acid in ACN) under a gradient program by a linear increase from 10% B to 22% B in the first 30 min, and to 23% B in 10 min, then to 30% in 30 min. The flow rate was 0.35 mL/min, and the injection volume was 10 μL. The analytes were monitored at the UV wavelength of 215 nm. Prior to next injection, the column was washed with 100% B for 5 min and then equilibrated with the initial mobile phase for 10 min.

Cell culture

RAW 264.7 cells were obtained from the American Type Culture Collection (ATCC, Manassa, VA, USA). The cells were maintained in DMEM supplemented with 10% heat-inactivated FBS at 37 °C in humidified 5% CO_2 atmosphere. The Minimum Standards of Reporting Checklist (Additional file 1) contains details of the experimental design, and statistics, and resources used in this study.

Cytotoxicity

The cytotoxicity of SPE on RAW 264.7 cells was detected using the MTT assay combined with lactose dehydrogenase (LDH) assay. In brief, the cells were seeded on a 96-well plate (1×10^4 cells/well) and allowed to adhere overnight. The cells were pretreated with SPE (25–200 μg/mL) for 4 h followed by co-treatment in the presence or absence of Pam_3CSK_4 (200 ng/mL) for 24 h. The cell proliferation was determined using the MTT assay as previous described [33]. The release of LDH in medium was determined using the LDH Cytotoxicity Detection Kit (ThermoFisher Scientific Inc., USA) according to the manufacturer's instructions.

Nitric oxide (NO) production and inflammatory cytokines secretion assays

RAW 264.7 cells were seeded on a 24-well plate (1×10^5 cells/well) and allowed to adhere overnight. The cells were pretreatment with SPE (50, 100 and 200 μg/mL) or CU-CPT22 (4 μM, positive control) for 4 h and then co-treated with addition of Pam_3CSK_4 (200 ng/mL) for another 12 h. NO production was determined by measuring the accumulated nitrite in the culture medium with Griess reagent [33]. Cytokines (TNF-α, IL-6, and MCP-1) secretion in the supernatants of cultured cells was quantified using the enzyme-linked immunosorbent assay kits (Neobioscience, Shenzhen, China) following the manufacturer's instructions.

Capture of intracellular NO generation

RAW 264.7 cells were cultured in glass bottom dish overnight and pretreated with SPE (50, 100 and 200 μg/mL) for 4 h. Subsequently, the cells were co-treated with Pam_3CSK_4 (200 ng/mL) for 12 h and then washed twice with ice-cold PBS. After incubated with 4-amino-5-methylamino-2′,7′-difluorofluorescein diacetate (DAF-FM, 5 μM in PBS) (ThermoFisher Scientific Inc., USA) for 30 min at room temperature, the cells were washed with PBS and then stained with 1 μg/mL Hoechst 33342 for 10 min. The images were obtained by a Leica TCS SP8 laser scanning confocal microscopy (Leica Microsystem, Wetzlar, Germany).

Western blotting analysis

RAW 264.7 cells were treated as described above. The harvested cells were washed thrice with ice-cold PBS and then extracted with RIPA buffer (Beyotime Biotechnology, Shanghai, China) containing protease inhibitor cocktails (ThermoFisher Scientific Inc., USA). The proteins (50 μg for each sample) were separated with SDS-PAGE (8%) and then transferred onto a PVDF membrane. The membranes were blocked with non-fat milk (5% in TBS containing 0.05% Tween-20, w/v) and incubated overnight at 4 °C with antibodies against iNOS, COX-2, p-IκBα, IκBα p-p65, p65 or GAPDH (1:1000). The membranes were then incubated with the corresponding secondary antibody (1:1000) at room temperature for 1 h. The signals were detected using ECL western blotting substrate (ThermoFisher Scientific Inc., USA) and ChemiDoc™ XRS+ system with Image Lab™ software (Bio-Rad Laboratories, Hercules, CA, USA).

Immunofluorescence analysis

RAW 264.7 cells were attached on confocal dish overnight. After pretreatment with SPE (200 μg/mL) for 2 h, the cells were co-treated with Pam_3CSK_4 (200 ng/mL) for another 4 h and then fixed with 4% Paraformaldehyde (PFA) for 10 min at room temperature. The cells were washed thrice with PBS, permeabilized with 0.05% Triton X-100 in PBS for 3 min, and followed by blocking with 3% bovine serum albumin (in PBS, w/v) for 1 h. Thereafter, the cells were incubated with antibody against p65 (1:100) overnight and reacted with Alexa Fluor 488-conjugated secondary antibody (1:1000) for 1 h. The nuclear of the cell was stained with Hoechst 33342. The images were captured with a Leica TCS SP8 laser scanning confocal microscopy.

Luciferase reporter gene assay

RAW 264.7 cells were transiently transfected with NF-κB-luc DNA for 48 h and refreshed with completed DMEM. The transfected cells were seeded in 6 plates overnight and pretreated with SPE (200 μg/mL) or CU-CPT22 (4 μM) for 2 h before Pam_3CSK_4 (200 ng/mL) stimulation for another 4 h. Luciferase activity was determined using a Dual-Glo luciferase assay system kit (Promega, Madison, Wisconsin, USA) following the manufacturer's instructions.

Statistical analysis

Each experiment was performed in triplicate and was repeated for at least thrice. All results were presented as mean ± SD. Variance between two groups was evaluated by one-way ANOVA using the GraphPad Prism software (GraphPad Software, United States). The Newman–Keuls multiple comparison tests were performed for post hoc pairwise comparisons. $P < 0.05$ was considered statistically significant difference.

Results

Characterization of SP extract

The chromatograms of mixed standards and the SP extract were illustrated in Fig. 1. The contents of rutin, kirenol and darutoside in the extract were determined to be 0.27 ± 0.01, 1.81 ± 0.02 and 0.28 ± 0.03%, respectively.

Cytotoxicity

The cytotoxicity of SPE on RAW 264.7 cells were determined using MTT and LDH assays. As illustrated in Fig. 2, SPE did not exert any observable toxicity on RAW 264.7 cells within the concentration ranged from 25 to 200 μg/mL while incubated with or without Pam_3CSK_4 (200 ng/mL) in 24 h. The concentrations of 50, 100 and 200 μg/mL were selected for SPE throughout the study.

SPE suppressed NO release and inflammatory cytokines secretions in Pam_3CSK_4-induced RAW 264.7 cells

Compared to the normal control cells, incubation with Pam_3CSK_4 for 12 h significantly induced the release of NO and secretion of inflammatory cytokines (IL-6, TNF-α, and MCP-1) in RAW 264.7 cells (Fig. 3). However, the stimulations were dose-dependently inhibited by SPE in the concentration ranged from 50 to 200 μg/mL. More than 50% of Pam_3CSK_4-stimulated NO release was observed to be decreased (> 50%) by SPE at the concentration higher than 100 μg/mL (Fig. 3a). The estimated IC_{50} of SPE on NO release was calculated to be 103.6 μg/mL. Moreover, SPE (200 μg/mL) significantly inhibited the Pam_3CSK_4-induced IL-6 (59.98%), TNF-α (42.38%), and MCP-1 (55.10%) (Fig. 3b–d). The inhibitory effects of SPE on Pam_3CSK_4-induced inflammation were comparable to those of the positive control of CU-CPT22 (4 μM).

SPE attenuated Pam_3CSK_4-induced intracellular NO generation

The inhibitory effect of SPE on Pam_3CSK_4-induced intracellular NO generation was determined by confocal microscopy. As illustrated in Fig. 4, Pam_3CSK_4 significantly stimulated the intracellular NO generation in RAW 264.7 cells. This stimulation was attenuated by SPE in a dose-dependent manner (50–200 μg/mL).

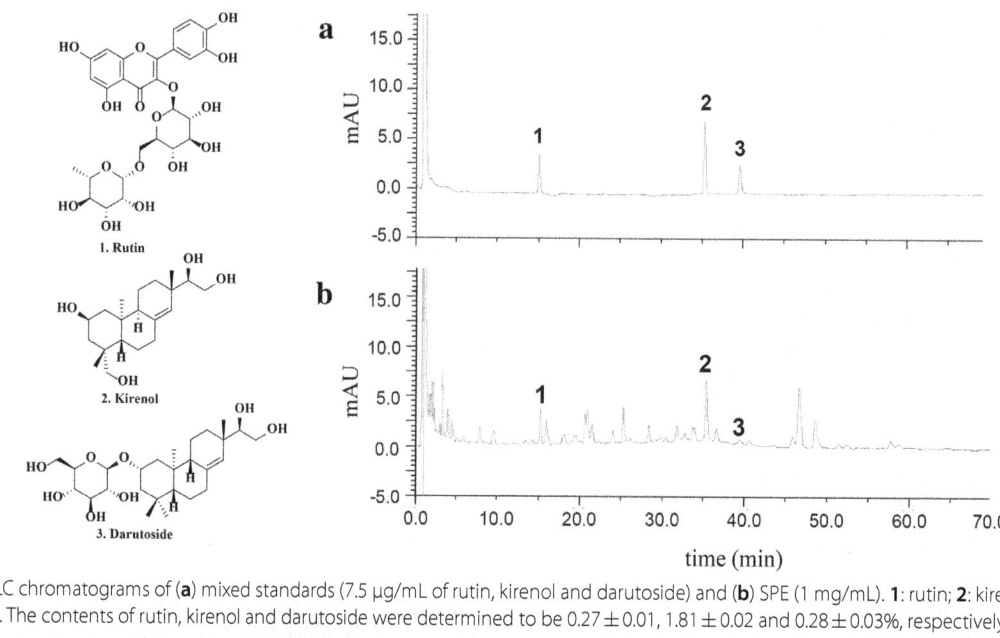

Fig. 1 HPLC chromatograms of (**a**) mixed standards (7.5 μg/mL of rutin, kirenol and darutoside) and (**b**) SPE (1 mg/mL). **1**: rutin; **2**: kirenol; **3**: darutoside. The contents of rutin, kirenol and darutoside were determined to be 0.27 ± 0.01, 1.81 ± 0.02 and 0.28 ± 0.03%, respectively ($n = 3$)

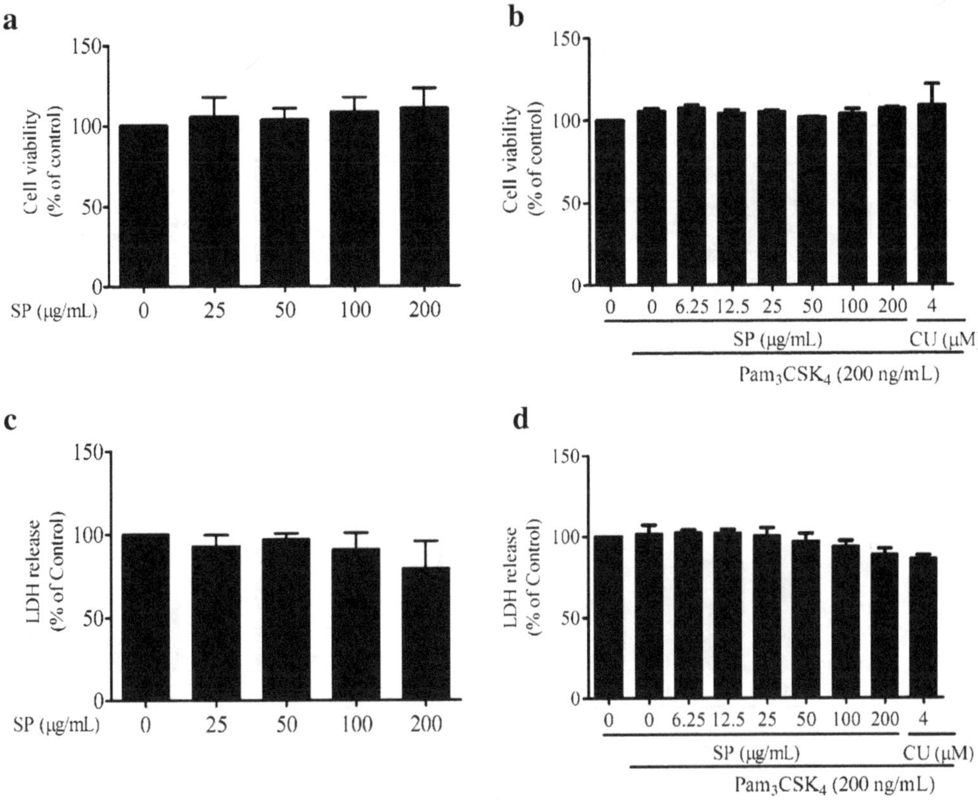

Fig. 2 *Siegesbeckia pubescens* Makino (SP) or SP with Pam_3CSK_4-stimulated did not significantly affect the cell viability and cytotoxicity ($n = 3$). RAW 264.7 cells were treated with SP with different concentrations for 24 h. **a** The cell viability was measured by MTT assay and **c** cell cytotoxicity was measured by LDH assay. RAW 264.7 cells were pretreated with SP for 4 h before Pam_3CSK_4 (200 ng/mL) stimulation for another 12 h. **b** The cell viability was measured by MTT assay and **d** cell cytotoxicity was measured by LDH assay

SPE inhibited Pam_3CSK_4-induced the protein expressions of iNOS and COX-2

The protein expressions of iNOS and COX-2 in SPE-treated RAW 264.7 cells were analyzed by Western blotting assay and illustrated in Fig. 5. SPE was determined to dose-dependently inhibit the Pam_3CSK_4-induced iNOS and COX-2 protein expressions in RAW 264.7 cells. The related amounts of iNOS and COX-2 in SPE-treated cells were determined to be decreased by 61.42 and 74.65% respectively when compared to those in the Pam_3CSK_4-induced cells (Fig. 5b, c). Moreover, the phosphorylation of JNK1/2 and p38, but not ERK1/2, was observed to be increased under Pam_3CSK_4 stimulation; whilst, SPE did not present any influence on the phosphorylation of such proteins.

SPE inactivated Pam_3CSK_4-induced NF-κB signaling

Compared to the untreated cell group, SPE at high concentration (200 μg/mL) was observed to slightly increase the phosphorylation of IκBα but did not influence on the phosphorylation of NF-κB-p65 (Fig. 6a–c). However, under the inflammatory condition, SPE presented dose-dependent inhibition on Pam_3CSK_4-induced phosphorylation of IκBα and NF-κB-p65 in RAW 264.7 cells. The activated p-IκBα and p-NF-κB-p65 were decreased by 26.71 and 34.14%, respectively, while co-treated with SPE at 200 μg/mL for 12 h (Fig. 6a–c). The results suggested the involvement of NF-κB inactivation in Pam_3CSK_4-induced inflammation by SPE. Confirmed by luciferase reporter gene assay, SP significantly attenuated the NF-κB-driven luciferase activity in Pam_3CSK_4-stimulated RAW 264.7 cells (Fig. 6d). Furthermore, the Pam_3CSK_4-induced p65 nuclear translocation was also determined to be attenuated by SPE using the immunofluorescence staining assay (Fig. 7).

Discussion

In this work the anti-inflammatory effect and underlying mechanisms of SP on Pam_3CSK_4-induced inflammation in RAW 264.7 macrophages were investigated and reported.

TLRs have been demonstrated to play critical role in innate immune response in mammals against various infections. Up to date, 10 human TLRs (TLR1-TLR10)

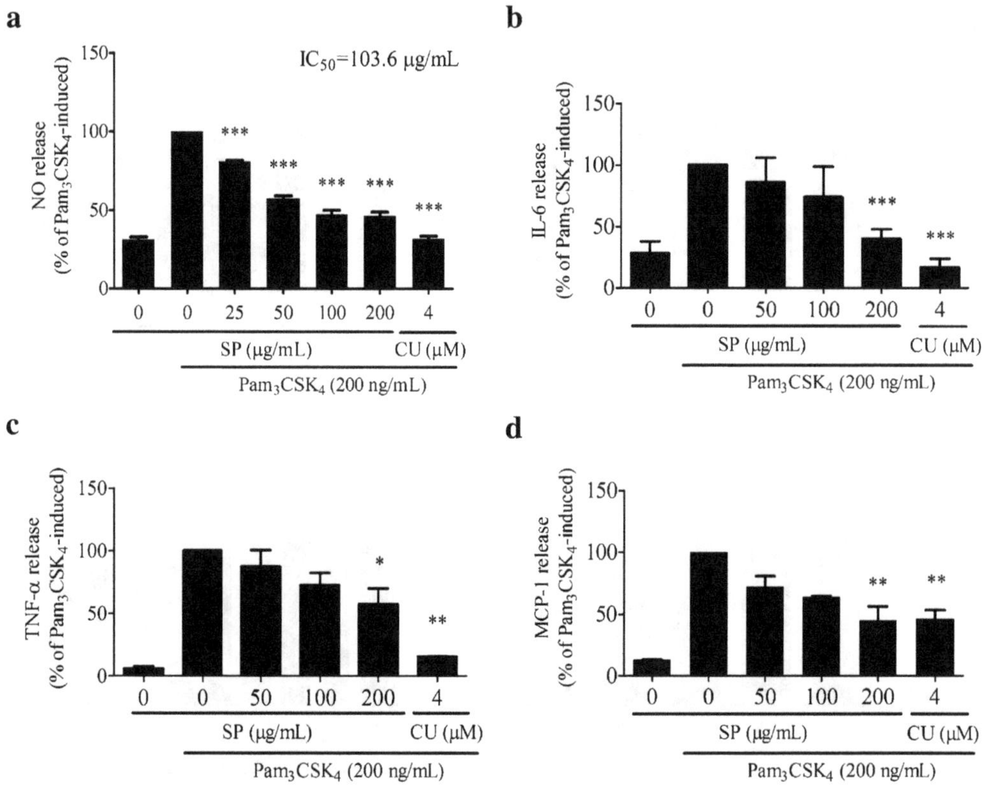

Fig. 3 *Siegesbeckia pubescens* Makino (SP) exhibited anti-inflammatory effects in Pam_3CSK_4-stimulated RAW 264.7 cells ($n = 3$). RAW 264.7 cells were pretreated with SP with different concentrations for 4 h before Pam_3CSK_4 (200 ng/mL) stimulation for another 12 h. **a** Nitric oxide (NO) was determined by Griess assay. TLR1/TLR2 antagonist: CU-CPT22 (CU) was selected as the positive control. We measured the levels of **b** IL-6, **c** TNF-α, and **d** MCP-1 by ELISA assay. *$P < 0.05$ vs. Pam_3CSK_4-induced, **$P < 0.01$ vs. Pam_3CSK_4-induced, ***$P < 0.001$ vs. Pam_3CSK_4-induced

and 12 murine TLRs (TLR1-TLR9 and TLR11-TLR13) have been identified and demonstrated to react to various types of inflammations [13, 14]. Different to TLR4 (mainly response to LPS-induced inflammations), the TLR1–TLR2 heterodimer specifically responses to bacterial tri-acetylated lipopeptides or porins [34]. Activation of TLR1–TLR2 heterodimerization subsequently activates the NF-κB signaling [35] and MAPKs [17] pathways and up-regulates the inflammatory related proteins (such as iNOS and COX-2). Finally, the production of NO and secretion of inflammatory cytokines were increased. Using the specific TLR1–TLR2 heterodimerization stimulator of Pam_3CSK_4 [36], a synthetic tripalmitoylated lipopeptide with the similarity to the bacterial lipoproteins, the inflammatory responses are subsequently induced through activation on NF-κB signaling pathway.

Being a traditional anti-rheumatoid herbal medicine, SP was demonstrated to be beneficial to and has been applied for the management of various chronic inflammatory diseases [26–28]. The inactivation of TLR4-induced NF-κB signaling was identified to be involved in the biological mechanisms of SP on inhibiting the LPS-induced inflammations [32, 37]. However, our preliminary study, we observed that SPE presented more potency on suppressing Pam_3CSK_4-induced than LPS-induced NO release in RAW 264.7 macrophages. The results suggested the inhibition of SP on TLR1-TLR2 activation mediated inflammatory responses might be involved in its potential mechanisms on anti-inflammation. Further investigated in Pam_3CSK_4-stimulated macrophages, SPE improved the inflammatory responses of the cells by decreasing the NO release and cytokines (IL-6, TNF-α, and MCP-1) secretion into the culture medium. The biological mechanisms of such effect were identified to be associated with the suppressions of SPE on Pam_3CSK_4-stimulated NF-κB activation and up-regulation of the protein expressions of iNOS and COX-2. On the other hand, Pam_3CSK_4 stimulated inflammation by activating the MAPKs signaling, but SPE was determined to have no significant influences on the activated p38, ERK and JNK.

Previously, SP has been reported to contain multiple components. Diterpenoids, sesquiterpenoids and flavonoids have been determined to be the major components

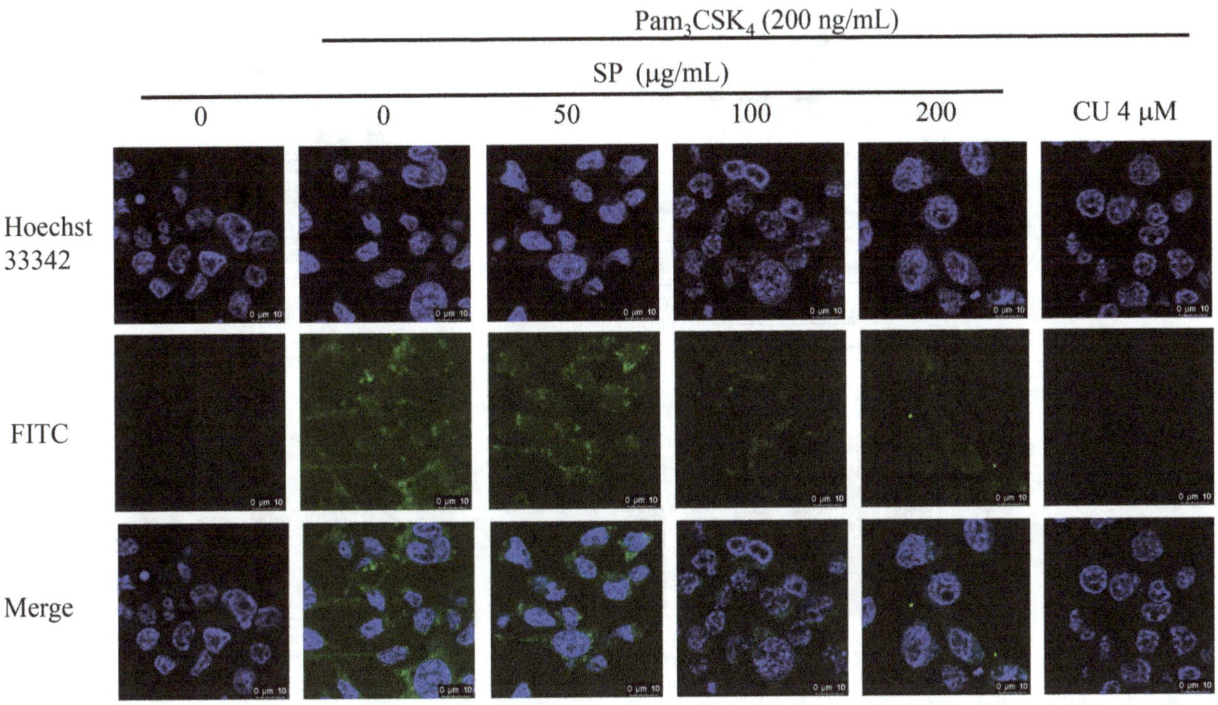

Fig. 4 RAW 264.7 cells were pretreated with *Siegesbeckia pubescens* Makino (SP) ($n = 3$) for 4 h before Pam$_3$CSK$_4$ (200 ng/mL) stimulation for another 12 h. NO was captured by Leica TCS SP8 laser scanning confocal microscope with 5 μM DAF-FM diacetate (4-amino-5-methylamino-2′,7′-difluorofluorescein diacetate). CU-CPT22 (CU) is selected as the positive control

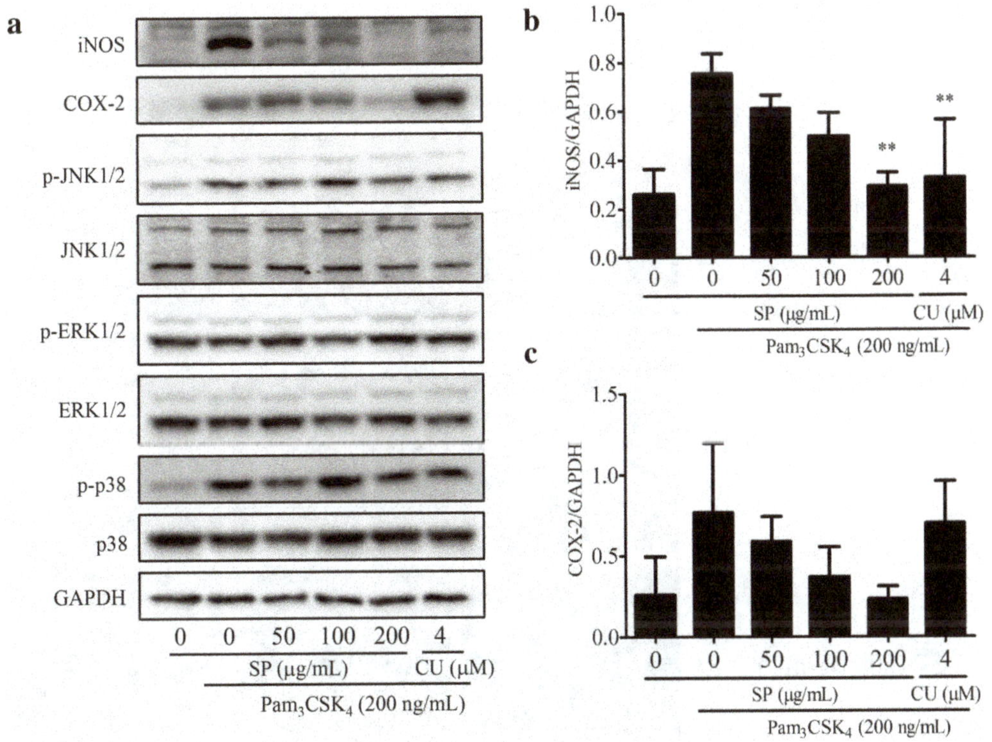

Fig. 5 Effects of *Siegesbeckia pubescens* Makino (SP) on relevant pathways. RAW 264.7 cells were pretreated with SP (0, 50, 100 and 200 μg/mL) for 4 h and followed with Pam$_3$CSK$_4$ (200 ng/mL) addition for 12 h. CU-CPT22 (CU) is selected as the positive control. **a** Proteins was evaluated by Western blotting assay. **b**, **c** Quantification of iNOS and COX-2 protein was detected by densitometric analysis ($n = 3$). $^{**}P < 0.01$ vs. Pam$_3$CSK$_4$-induced

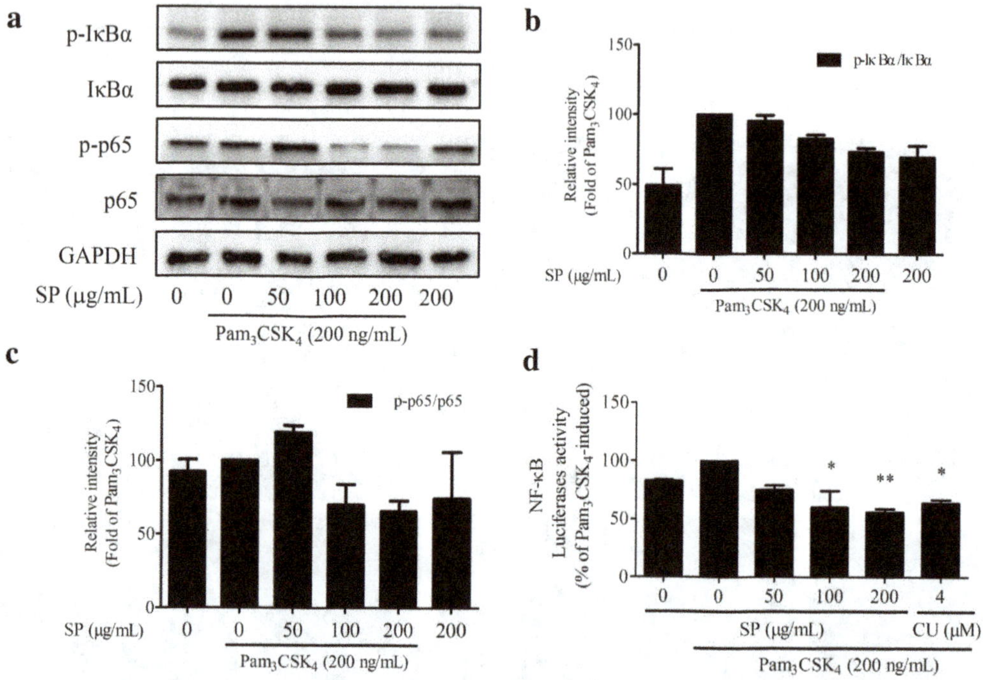

Fig. 6 Effects of *Siegesbeckia pubescens* Makino (SP) on NF-κB pathways ($n = 3$). RAW 264.7 cells were pretreated with SP (0, 50, 100 and 200 μg/mL) for 2 h and followed with Pam_3CSK_4 (200 ng/mL) addition for 4 h. CU-CPT22 (CU) is selected as the positive control. **a** Proteins was evaluated by Western blotting assay. **b**, **c** Quantification was detected by densitometric analysis. **d** RAW 264.7 cells were transfected with NFκB-luc for 48 h. Cells were pretreated with SP 2 h before Pam_3CSK_4 (200 ng/mL) stimulation for another 4 h. Luciferase activity was determined by Dual-Glo Luciferase Assay. *$P < 0.05$ vs. Pam_3CSK_4-induced and **$P < 0.01$ vs. Pam_3CSK_4-induced

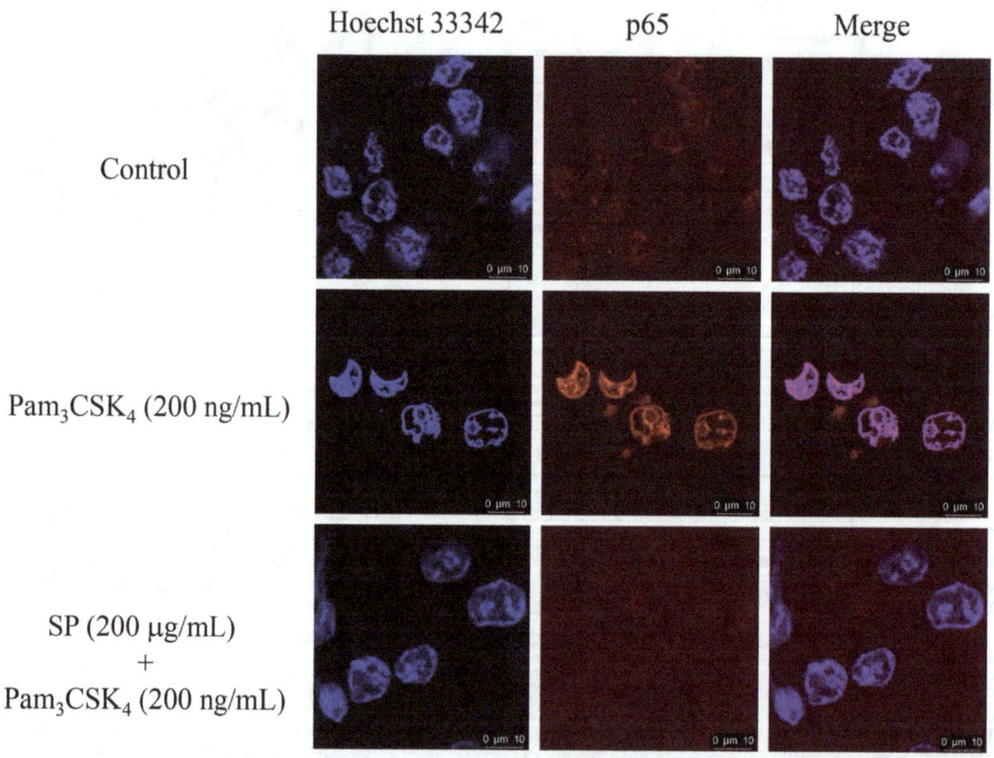

Fig. 7 RAW 264.7 cells were pretreated with 200 μg/mL of *Siegesbeckia pubescens* Makino (SP) ($n = 3$) for 2 h before Pam_3CSK_4 stimulation for another 4 h. NF-κB/p65 nuclear translocation was determined by immunofluorescence assay

in SP [21–24]. Kirenol and darutoside, two *ent*-pimarane-type diterpenoids, were reported to be highly contained in SP [21, 38, 39]. Pharmacologically, the anti-inflammatory effects of SP were partially identified to be related to kirenol and darutoside [40]. Rutin, a widely distributed flavonoid in many plants, has been demonstrated to present various pharmacological activities such as anti-inflammation, anti-oxidant, anti-cancer as well as others [41]. In this study, the chemical compositions of SPE were analyzed using the HPLC method, the contents of the three representative components of kirenol (1.81 ± 0.02%), darutoside (0.28 ± 0.03%) and rutin (0.27 ± 0.01%) in SPE were quantified to be 2.36% in total. Further investigations on other chemical components in SPE as well as their relationship to TLR1-TLR2-activated inflammation are currently under progress in our research team.

Conclusions

In conclusion, the anti-inflammatory activity of SP on Pam_3CSK_4-stimulated RAW 264.7 macrophages was investigated and reported. The results demonstrated that the 50% ethanol extract of SP could effectively decrease Pam_3CSK_4-induced NO release and cytokines secretion in RAW 264.7 cells. The potential biological mechanisms of SP on anti-inflammation were associated with its inactivation on Pam_3CSK_4-stimulated NF-κB signaling.

Abbreviations

SP: *Siegesbeckia pubescens* Makino; SPE: 50% ethanol extract of SP; NF-κB: nuclear factor-κB; MAPK: mitogen-activated protein kinase; TLR: toll-like receptor; Pam_3CSK_4: *N*-palmitoyl-*S*-[2,3-bis(palmitoyloxy)-(2*RS*)-propyl]-[*R*]-cysteinyl-[*S*]-seryl-[*S*]-lysyl-[*S*]-lysyl-[*S*]-lysyl-[*S*]-lysine·3HCl; NO: nitric oxide; COX-2: cyclooxygenase-2; iNOS: inducible nitric oxide synthase; IL-6: interleukin-6; IL-1β: interleukin-1β; TNF-α: tumor necrosis factor-α; MCP-1: monocyte chemoattractant protein-1; LPS: lipopolysaccharide; MTT: 3-(4,5-dimethylthiazol-2-yl)-2,5-diphenyltetrazolium bromide; DMEM: Dulbecco's modified eagle medium; FBS: fetal bovine serum; LDH: lactose dehydrogenase; DAF-FM: 4-amino-5methylamino-2′,7′-difluorofluorescein diacetate.

Authors' contributions

HY and YW organized, conceived, and supervised the study. WS and ZZ designed the study and conducted the experiments. KL, WX and WSC analyzed the data. AKWT edited and revised the manuscript. All authors read and approved the final manuscript.

Author details

[1] Institute of Chinese Medical Sciences, State Key Laboratory of Quality Research in Chinese Medicine, University of Macau, Macao, China. [2] HKBU Shenzhen Research Center, Shenzhen, Guangdong, China. [3] School of Chinese Medicine, Hong Kong Baptist University, Kowloon Tong, Hong Kong, China. [4] Guangdong Key Laboratory for Research and Development of Natural Drugs, Guangdong Medical University, Zhanjiang, China. [5] Academy for Advanced Interdisciplinary Studies, Southern University of Science and Technology, Shenzhen, Guangdong, China. [6] Institute of Chinese Medical Sciences, University of Macau, Room 8008, Building N22, Avenida da Universidade, Taipa, Macao SAR, China. [7] Institute of Chinese Medical Sciences, University of Macau, Room 1050, Building N22, Avenida da Universidade, Taipa, Macao SAR, China.

Acknowledgements

Not applicable.

Competing interests

The authors declare that they have no competing interests.

Consent for publication

Not applicable.

Funding

This study was supported by the National Natural Science Foundation of China (NSFC, No. 81470170), the Research Committee of the University of Macau (SRG2015-00060-ICMS-QRCM, MYRG2017-00178-ICMS, and CPG2014-00012-ICMS), the Guangzhou Science and Technology Innovation funding (EF007/ICMS-YH/2018/GSTIC), the Project funded by China Postdoctoral Science Foundation (No. 2017M622811), and the opening fund of the State Key Laboratory of Quality Research in Chinese Medicine of University of Macau (No. SKL-QRCM-2014-2016).

References

1. Hawiger J. Innate immunity and inflammation: a transcriptional paradigm. Immunol Res. 2001;23(2–3):99–109.
2. Sauaia A, Moore FA, Moore EE. Postinjury inflammation and organ dysfunction. Crit Care Clin. 2017;33(1):167–91.
3. Kunnumakkara AB, Sailo BL, Banik K, Harsha C, Prasad S, Gupta SC, Bharti AC, Aggarwal BB. Chronic diseases, inflammation, and spices: how are they linked? J Transl Med. 2018;16(1):14.
4. Tak PP, Firestein GS. NF-kappaB: a key role in inflammatory diseases. J Clin Invest. 2001;107(1):7–11.
5. Lawrence T. The nuclear factor NF-kappaB pathway in inflammation. Cold Spring Harb Perspect Biol. 2009;1(6):a001651.
6. Shih RH, Wang CY, Yang CM. NF-kappaB signaling pathways in neurological inflammation: a mini review. Front Mol Neurosci. 2015;8:77.
7. Zhang H, Sun SC. NF-κB in inflammation and renal diseases. Cell Biosci. 2015;5:63.
8. Zhang Q, Lenardo MJ, Baltimore D. 30 years of NF-κB: a blossoming of relevance to human pathobiology. Cell. 2017;168(1–2):37–57.
9. Kulms D, Schwarz T. NF-kappaB and cytokines. Vitam Horm. 2006;74:283–300.
10. Hayden MS, Ghosh S. Regulation of NF-κB by TNF family cytokines. Semin Immunol. 2014;26(3):253–66.
11. Lai Y, Dong C. Therapeutic antibodies that target inflammatory cytokines in autoimmune diseases. Int Immunol. 2016;28(4):181–8.
12. Jiménez-Dalmaroni MJ, Gerswhin ME, Adamopoulos IE. The critical role of toll-like receptors–from microbial recognition to autoimmunity: a comprehensive review. Autoimmun Rev. 2016;15(1):1–8.
13. Drexler SK, Foxwell BM. The role of toll-like receptors in chronic inflammation. Int J Biochem Cell Biol. 2010;42(4):506–18.
14. Ospelt C, Gay S. TLRs and chronic inflammation. Int J Biochem Cell Biol. 2010;42(4):495–505.
15. Achek A, Yesudhas D, Choi S. Toll-like receptors: promising therapeutic targets for inflammatory diseases. Arch Pharm Res. 2016;39(8):1032–49.
16. Elshabrawy HA, Essani AE, Szekanecz Z, Fox DA, Shahrara S. TLRs, future potential therapeutic targets for RA. Autoimmun Rev. 2017;16(2):103–13.
17. Lee NY, Lee HY, Lee KH, Han SH, Park SJ. *Vibrio vulnificus* IlpA induces MAPK-mediated cytokine production via TLR1/2 activation in THP-1 cells, a human monocytic cell line. Mol Immunol. 2011;49(1–2):143–54.
18. Funderburg NT, Jadlowsky JK, Lederman MM, Feng Z, Weinberg A, Sieg SF. The toll-like receptor 1/2 agonists Pam(3) CSK(4) and human β-defensin-3 differentially induce interleukin-10 and nuclear factor-κB signalling patterns in human monocytes. Immunology. 2011;134(2):151–60.

19. Khan J, Sharma PK, Mukhopadhaya A. *Vibrio cholerae* porin OmpU mediates M1-polarization of macrophages/monocytes via TLR1/TLR2 activation. Immunobiology. 2015;220(11):1199–209.
20. Broz P, Monack DM. Newly described pattern recognition receptors team up against intracellular pathogens. Nat Rev Immunol. 2013;13(8):551–65.
21. Huo L, Jiang Z, Li H, Wang M, Ye X, Ji B, Guo X. Simultaneous determination of seven major diterpenoids in *Siegesbeckia pubescens* Makino by high-performance liquid chromatography coupled with evaporative light scattering detection. J Sep Sci. 2012;35(19):2585–91.
22. Wang R, Liu YQ, Ha W, Shi YP, Hwang TL, Huang GJ, Wu TS, Lee KH. In vitro anti-inflammatory effects of diterpenoids and sesquiterpenoids from traditional Chinese medicine *Siegesbeckia pubescens*. Bioorg Med Chem Lett. 2014;24(16):3944–7.
23. Yao Y, Liang X, Sun X, Yin L, He H, Guo X, Jiang Z. Rapid extraction and analysis method for the simultaneous determination of 21 bioflavonoids in *Siegesbeckia pubescens* Makino. J Sep Sci. 2015;38(7):1130–6.
24. Wang J, Xie K, Duan H, Wang Y, Ma H, Fu H. Isolation and characterization of diterpene glycosides from *Siegesbeckia pubescens*. Bioorg Med Chem Lett. 2017;27(8):1815–9.
25. Tao HX, Xiong W, Zhao GD, Peng Y, Zhong ZF, Xu L, Duan R, Tsim KWK, Yu H, Wang YT. Discrimination of three Siegesbeckiae Herba species using UPLC-QTOF/MS-based metabolomics approach. Food Chem Toxicol. 2018. https://doi.org/10.1016/j.fct.2017.12.068.
26. Lee M, Kim SH, Lee HK, Cho Y, Kang J, Sung SH. ent-kaurane and ent-pimarane diterpenes from *Siegesbeckia pubescens* inhibit lipopolysaccharide-induced nitric oxide production in BV2 microglia. Biol Pharm Bull. 2014;37(1):152–7.
27. Wang J, Cai Y, Wu Y. Antiinflammatory and analgesic activity of topical administration of *Siegesbeckia pubescens*. Pak J Pharm Sci. 2008;21(2):89–91.
28. Kim HM. Effects of *Siegesbeckia pubescens* on immediate hypersensitivity reaction. Am J Chin Med. 1997;25(2):163–7.
29. Wang J, Duan H, Wang Y, Pan B, Gao C, Gai C, Wu Q, Fu H. ent-Strobane and ent-pimarane diterpenoids from *Siegesbeckia pubescens*. J Nat Prod. 2017;80(1):19–29.
30. Lv D, Guo KW, Xu C, Huang M, Zheng SJ, Ma XH, Pan LH, Wang Q, Yang XZ. Essential oil from *Siegesbeckia pubescens* induces apoptosis through the mitochondrial pathway in human HepG2 cells. J Huazhong Univ Sci Technol Med Sci. 2017;37(1):87–92.
31. Lee SG, Kim M, Kim CE, Kang J, Yoo H, Sung SH, Lee M. Quercetin 3,7-*O*-dimethyl ether from *Siegesbeckia pubescens* suppress the production of inflammatory mediators in lipopolysaccharide-induced macrophages and colon epithelial cells. Biosci Biotechnol Biochem. 2016;80(11):2080–6.
32. Park HJ, Kim IT, Won JH, Jeong SH, Park EY, Nam JH, Choi J, Lee KT. Anti-inflammatory activities of ent-16alpha*H*,17-hydroxy-kauran-19-oic acid isolated from the roots of *Siegesbeckia pubescens* are due to the inhibition of iNOS and COX-2 expression in RAW 264.7 macrophages via NF-kappaB inactivation. Eur J Pharmacol. 2007;558(1–3):185–93.
33. Su T, Yu H, Kwan HY, Ma XQ, Cao HH, Cheng CY, Leung AK, Chan CL, Li WD, Cao H, Fong WF, Yu ZL. Comparisons of the chemical profiles, cytotoxicities and anti-inflammatory effects of raw and rice wine-processed Herba Siegesbeckiae. J Ethnopharmacol. 2014;156:365–9.
34. Jin MS, Kim SE, Heo JY, Lee ME, Kim HM, Paik SG, Lee H, Lee JO. Crystal structure of the TLR1-TLR2 heterodimer induced by binding of a tri-acylated lipopeptide. Cell. 2007;130:1071–82.
35. Cheng K, Gao M, Godfroy JI, Brown PN, Kastelowitz N, Yin H. Specific activation of the TLR1–TLR2 heterodimer by small-molecule agonists. Sci Adv. 2015;1(3):e1400139.
36. Aliprantis AO, Yang RB, Mark MR, Suggett S, Devaux B, Radolf JD, Klimpel GR, Godowski P, Zychlinsky A. Cell activation and apoptosis by bacterial lipoproteins through toll-like receptor-2. Science. 1999;285(5428):736–9.
37. Li H, Kim JY, Hyeon J, Lee HJ, Ryu JH. In vitro antiinflammatory activity of a new sesquiterpene lactone isolated from Siegesbeckia glabrescens. Phytother Res. 2011;25(9):1323–7.
38. Xu FQ, Liu JQ, Wang JT, Huang JP, Zhang J. Simultaneous determination of kirenol and darutoside in Siegesbeckiae Herba by high-performance liquid chromatography. Chin Tradit Pat Med. 2011;33(8):1444–6.
39. Ye XX, Song JX, Ji B, Jiang Z, Guo XJ. Simultaneous determination of five major constituents in *Siegesbeckia pubescens* Makino by HPLC-RID. J Shenyang Pharm Univ. 2014;31(1):36–40.
40. Lu Y, Xiao J, Wu ZW, Wang ZM, Hu J, Fu HZ, Chen YY, Qian RQ. Kirenol exerts a potent anti-arthritic effect in collagen-induced arthritis by modifying the T cells balance. Phytomedicine. 2012;19(10):882–9.
41. Chua LS. A review on plant-based rutin extraction methods and its pharmacological activities. J Ethnopharmacol. 2013;150(3):805–17.

9

A preliminary review of studies on adaptogens: comparison of their bioactivity in TCM with that of ginseng-like herbs used worldwide

Lian-ying Liao[1,2], Yi-fan He[1,2], Li Li[1,2], Hong Meng[1,2], Yin-mao Dong[1,2], Fan Yi[1,2*] and Pei-gen Xiao[3]

Abstract

Modern studies have shown that adaptogens can non-specifically enhance the resistance of human body under a wide range of external stress conditions with a multi-targeted and multi-channel network-like manner, especially by affect the immune-neuro-endocrine system and the hypothalamic–pituitary–adrenal axis. This review article draws the attention to the relationships of adaptogens, tonics from traditional Chinese medicine (TCM) and ginseng-like herbs worldwide, which all have similar plant sources and clinical applications. To clarify the sources and pharmacological mechanisms of these plant-originated adaptogens, which will provide useful information for the utilization of adaptogens to improve the human health. Meanwhile, the TCMs and the world-wide ginseng-like herbs from each region's ethnopharmacology will be beneficial modernization and globalization.

Keywords: Adaptogen, Immune-neuro-endocrine system, HPA axis, Tonics, Ginseng-like herbs worldwide

Introduction

The term of adaptogen was first proposed in 1940 by a scientist from the USSR, namely, N. Lazarev, when he described *Schisandra chinensis* (Turcz.) Bail. and other herbs with the following definition: plant-originated adaptogens that can non-specifically the enhance human body. According to the primary definition of adaptogens, these substances must meet three criteria: first, adaptogens must to be non-specific and must assist the human body in resisting a wide range of adverse conditions, such as physical, chemical or biological stress. These may include environmental pollution, climate change, radiation, infectious diseases, and interpersonal disharmony. Second, adaptogens must maintain homeostasis in humans, that is, these substances can offset or resist physical disorders caused by external stress. Third, adaptogens must not harm the normal functions of the human body.

Then I.Brekhman, a Soviet scientist, studied ginseng in approximately 1950, he extended the concept of adaptogens as follows: medicines that have similar functions as adaptogens can help the body maintain ideal homeostasis under adverse or stressful conditions.

Again, Brekhman and Dardymov further defined plant-originated adaptogens in 1969 [1]. According to this definition, plant-originated adaptogens meet four criteria: first, plant-originated adaptogens must reduce the harm caused by stressed states, such as fatigue, infection, and depression; second, plant-originated adaptogens must have positive excitatory effects on the human body; third, in contrast to traditional stimulants, the excitatory effects produced by plant-originated adaptogens must not cause side effects such as insomnia, low protein synthesis, or excessive energy consumption; fourth, plant-originated adaptogens must not harm the human body.

In the 1990s, a group of scientists, comprised of Hildebert Wagner, George Wikman and Alexander Panossian, performed many studies on adaptogens and proposed the

*Correspondence: fantasyee@btbu.edu.cn
[2] Beijing Key Laboratory of Plant Resources Research and Development, Beijing Technology and Business University, No. 11/33, Fucheng Road, Haidian District, Beijing 100048, People's Republic of China
Full list of author information is available at the end of the article

following definition: adaptogens are natural bioregulators that increase the ability to adapt environmental factors and avoid the damage caused by those factors. In fact, the advantage of adaptogens are they minimized the bodily response to stress, reducing the negative reactions during the alarm phase and eliminating, or at least decreasing, the onset of the exhaustion phase that is part of the so-called general adaptation syndrome [2].

With continuous research for more than half a century, the concept of adaptogens has been continuously modified and perfected. In 1998, the American Food and Drug Administration (FDA) [3] defined an adaptogen as a new kind of metabolic regulator that has been proved to help in environmental adaptation and to prevent external harms. Adaptogen has been generally used as a functional term.

Yance, an American herbal doctor, held a view that adaptogens can improve our ability to recognize, respond, recover, and restore or regenerate. He divided adaptogens into three categories, including primary adaptogens, secondary adaptogens, and adaptogen companions, based on his clinical experience [4]. Primary adaptogens are consistent with the traditional definition of adaptogens and satisfy specific criterias. The criterias contains: abundant scientific research confirmed their adaptogenic characters, guarantee of general resistance and non-specific action in the human body, maintenance or restoration for homeostasis, and adverse- or toxic-effects after prolonged use [5].

Furthermore, some precise scientific experiments demonstrated that adaptogens can enhance the resistance of human body against various external stimuli as non-specific regulators. Adaptogen function mainly by affecting the hypothalamic–pituitary–adrenal (HPA axis) in response to stimulation by external stress. Primary adaptogens can not only maintain or recover homeostasis and allostasis but can also promote anabolic recovery. Primary adaptogens can produce positive stress response and the associated hormone expression. Primary adaptogens strengthen the functioning of each systems, promote optimal response, promote recovery of function, and help regulate energy use by improving the function of neuroendocrine system and enhancing cellular energy transfer, which can make body utilize oxygen, glucose, lipids and proteins very effectively, thus providing us with a steady supply of energy [4].

Another category of adaptogens is secondary adaptogens, which are consistent with most traditional definitions of adaptogens but not all of the criteria of primary adaptogens. Secondary adaptogens cannot influence the HPA axis directly; however, these adaptogens can affect the immune, nervous and endocrine systems. Secondary adaptogens share several common features: first, these adaptogens typically exert influence on the immune, nervous and endocrine systems; second, these adaptogens do not influence the HPA axis, directly; third, these plant-originated adaptogens include fatty acids, sterols and phenols; fourth, these substances can enhance anabolism. While the secondary adaptogens may meet most of the qualifications of primary adaptogens, but they have yet to be studied extensively [5].

Another category is adaptogen companions, which may not satisfy all the traditional standards but can have beneficial effects on the HPA axis and on anabolism to support the functions of adaptogens. Although these kinds of medicinal plants have similar functions as the other two kinds of adaptogens mentioned above, these plants can not formally be called adaptogen. Thus, these plants are classified as adaptogens companions because they can act synergistically with the other two kinds of adaptogens mentioned above, thereby improving the effects of the adaptogens [5].

Currently, studies have confirmed that the following plants are true adaptogens: *Panax ginseng* C.A.Mey, *Schisandra chinensis* (Turcz.) Baill., *Acanthopanax senticosus* (Rupr. et Maxim.) Harms, *Rhodiola crenulata* (Hook. f. et Thoms) S.H.Fu, and *Lepidium meyenii* Walp.

According to web of science database, we searched the key word, adaptogen. Based on the analysis of results, we got a conclusion that more and more researches focus on this field over past 10 years and it showed an increasing tendency from 1999 to 2018, which profiles that it is still a worthwhile direction to explore. Furthermore, we also found out that the many published articles concentrated on the direction of pharmacology pharmacy, biochemistry molecular biology, plant sciences and agriculture. It is still worthy to show its historical development and find out the relationships among adaptogen and tonics and ginseng-like herbs worldwide, which can give a hint to further research in plant-originated adaptogen. Summarized the results of previous studies and our own researches focused on tonics from TCM, we launched out our understanding of adaptogen: Herbs which can non-specific and non-toxicity help human body resist the environmental stress to maintain a homeostasis. The mechanism may multi-targets and multi-channel network to the neuroendocrine system. The adaptogens with tonics from TCM and the world-wide ginseng-like herbs have similar phytochemical and pharmacological properties.

The functions of adaptogens

Adaptogens can affect different tissues and organs, and adjust each of these parts to attain homeostasis.

Adaptogens and adrenal fatigue

Adrenals, the glands of stress, mobilize various stress responses to each stress, including physical, biochemical, hormonal, thermal, internal, external, emotional and mental. Stress rather than pathological damage is the primary cause of adrenal fatigue. Excessive stress may be caused by a single strong stimulatory event or by the accumulation of chronic or repeated stress. When the capacity of the adrenals to secrete enough hormones that can make the necessary physiological, and biochemical compensations for that level of stress cannot meet the requirements of continually excessive pressure, adrenal fatigue occurs. The adrenal gland continues to work under adrenal fatigue but cannot maintain normal homeostasis. On the one hand, if the adrenals can deal well with this circumstance and cortisol levels remain adequately elevated to handle the various stresses, over time, the signs and symptoms of metabolic syndrome, such as muscle wastage, hyperglycemia, and suppresses immune or inflammatory responses [6], begin to appear. On the other hand, if the adrenals are not able to meet the demands, adrenal fatigue appears, usually developing more quickly than metabolic syndrome, and which can become so severe as to disable them [7].

The amount of stress hormone produced by the human body increases under external pressure. Adaptogens can increase the effectiveness of adrenal gland secretion, thereby abolishing excess hormone production [8]. Other studies can prove this statement: In 2001, B.T.Gaffney found that the suggested that Panax ginseng inhibits 11-beta hydroxysteroid dehydrogenase one and *Eleutherococcus senticosus* inhibits catechol-*O*-methyl transferase, both of which reside in close proximity to stress hormone receptors and catalyze the degradation of stress hormones into inactive compounds [9]. In the absence of stress, adaptogens can accelerate the closure of the adrenal gland. Furthermore, adaptogens can increase cellular energy levels and prevent oxidative damages, leading to the maintenance of normal adrenal function. The following plant-originated adaptogens support adrenal function: *Panax quinquefolius* L. [10], *Withania somnifera* [11], *Panax ginseng* C.A.Mey. [9], *Codonopsis pilosula* (Franch.)Nannf. [12], *Eleutherococcus senticosus* (Rupr. & Maxim.) Maxim. [13], *Gynostemma pentaphyllum* (Thunb.) Makino, *Glycyrrhiza uralensis* Fisch.ex DC. [14], *Ganoderma Lucidum* Karst [15], and *Sedum rosea* (L.) Scop [16].

Adaptogens and arthritis

Arthritis is caused by tissue damages and joint diseases, which is typically accompanied by pain and swelling. The most common types of arthritis are osteoarthritis and rheumatoid arthritis. Fibromyalgia maybe an accompanying condition of arthritis; however, it is not considered a form of arthritis because it does not cause inflammation or joint damage.

Adaptogens can reduce arthritis-associated inflammation and pain effectively [17, 18]. The anti-inflammatory effects of the following plant-originated adaptogens can be used to provide relief rheumatoid arthritis: *Withania somnifera* [8, 19], *Panax ginseng* C.A.Mey [20], *Gynostemma pentaphyllum* (Thunb.) Makino [21], *Ganoderma Lucidum Karst* [22], *Sedum rosea* (L.) Scop. [23], and *Glycyrhiza uralensis* Fisch. ex DC. [24].

Adaptogens and sleep

Many people suffer from insomnia and other sleep-related problems. External stress perturbs the normal secretion of circadian cortisol, which is the main cause of sleep-related problems. The secretion of cortisol follows the biological clock and external circadian rhythms. The secretion of cortisol peaks in the morning and then decreases, reaching a minimum value at night. Proper exercise, diet and sleep can help maintain stable cortisol levels in the human body.

Adaptogens help produce cortisol and relieve stress [7, 25]. Studies by Steven Maimes and N. V. Provalova suggest that the following plant-originated adaptogens can act as sleep aids: *Panax quniquefolius* L. [26], *Withania somnifera* (L.) Dunal. [27], *Schisandra chinensis* (Turcz.) Baill. [28], *Gynostemma pentaphyllum* (Thunb.) Makino [29], and *Sedum rosea* (L.) Scop [30].

The following plant-originated adaptogens can alleviate the effects of the time difference syndrome, caused by disruption of physiological rhythm of the human body: *Panax quniquefolius* L., *Panax ginseng* C.A.Mey, *Gynostemma pentaphyllum* (Thunb.) Makino, *Schisandra chinensis* (Turcz.) Baill., and *Sedum rosea* (L.) [31, 32].

Adaptogens and the neuroendocrine system

One of the most important functions of adaptogens is their ability to help stabilize the internal environment of the human body by affecting the neuroendocrine system. The chemicals in plant-originated adaptogens enhance the ability to adapt to external environments and avoid damage [33–35]. A unique feature of adaptogens is that these substances affect the neuroendocrine system and the cellular energy system. Aaptogens can increase the rates of oxygen, protein, fat and sugar utilization. In addition to plant-originated adaptogens, other plants may have some of the functions mentioned above, but plant-originated adaptogens have a broad range of functions and systematically strengthen the stability of the internal environment of the human body [34, 36].

Anti-tumor application of plant-originated adaptogens

Researchers have found that plant-originated adaptogens have a positive influence on all aspects of the health of animals and humans [37]. Cancers studies have shown that plant-originated adaptogen can reduce the risks of cancers [38].

Plant-originated adaptogens play key roles in anti-tumor and multifaceted anticancer mechanisms, such as inhibition of cancer cells production, stabilization of the functions of human body, and promotion of cell repair [39, 40]. The anti-tumor effect of adaptogens is often closely linked to immune mechanisms. In other words, adaptogens can activate macrophages, T-lymphocytes, NK cells and so on to inhibit the growth of tumors and enhance cell-selective apoptosis and intercellular connection [16, 41–43].

The most common chemical anti-tumor medicines currently on the market have side effects such as cytotoxicity and immune suppression. Plant-based immune regulators, for example, plant-originated adaptogens, are generally used as auxiliary treatments to reduce the side effects of these chemical medicines and regain health [44, 45]. Notably, the application of adaptogens improves the tolerance of humans to drug cytotoxicity [46]. Adaptogens can improve the physical conditions of cancer patients in the following ways: first, as modulators of biological responses, adaptogens can the remodel immune mechanism and non-specifically enhance the resistance of the human body [46]; second, adaptogens can promote the production of marrow, increase the amount of blood cells and reduce infection [47]; third, adaptogens affect the entire body, from cells to organs including the liver, kidney, heart and gastrointestinal tract [7]; fourth, adaptogens can strengthen the lethal effects of chemotherapy and radiotherapy on cancer cells [48]; fifth, adaptogens can inhibit the development of multidrug resistance [49]; sixth, adaptogens can inhibit tumor metastasis and cancer cell aggregation [50]; seven, adaptogens can reduce stress hormone levels during immune dysfunction, which is associated with tumor growth [51].

When cancer cells adapt to chemotherapy, the main consequence is the development of multidrug resistance. The most simple mechanism of the development of multidrug resistance is as follows: anti-tumor drug molecules flow out from cancer cells through membrane channel proteins driven by ATP, especially by adjustment of P-glycoprotein pump (Pgp-pump) and due to the effects of breast cancer resistance protein-1 (BCRP/ABCG-2) and multidrug-resistance-associated protein-1 (MRP-1) from thymic cancer cells [52]. Among plant-originated adaptogens, *Panax ginseng* C.A.Mey can substantially reduce multidrug resistance by inhibiting Pgp, and it has been shown that *Panax ginseng* C.A.Mey can prolong the life of the cancer-bearing mice in animal experiments [24, 53]. In addition, epigallocatechin-gallate (EGCG) in *Eurycoma longifolia* can inhibit the expression of Bcl-2 to prevent the development multidrug resistance [54].

Exploration of the mechanism of action of adaptogens

In the case of various stress modes, adaptogens can activate the adjustment of different responses to cope with different forms of stress. Adaptogens are the material basis of the bodily response to the external environment and can act on the immune system and the stress response system, showing in Fig. 1. The non-specific

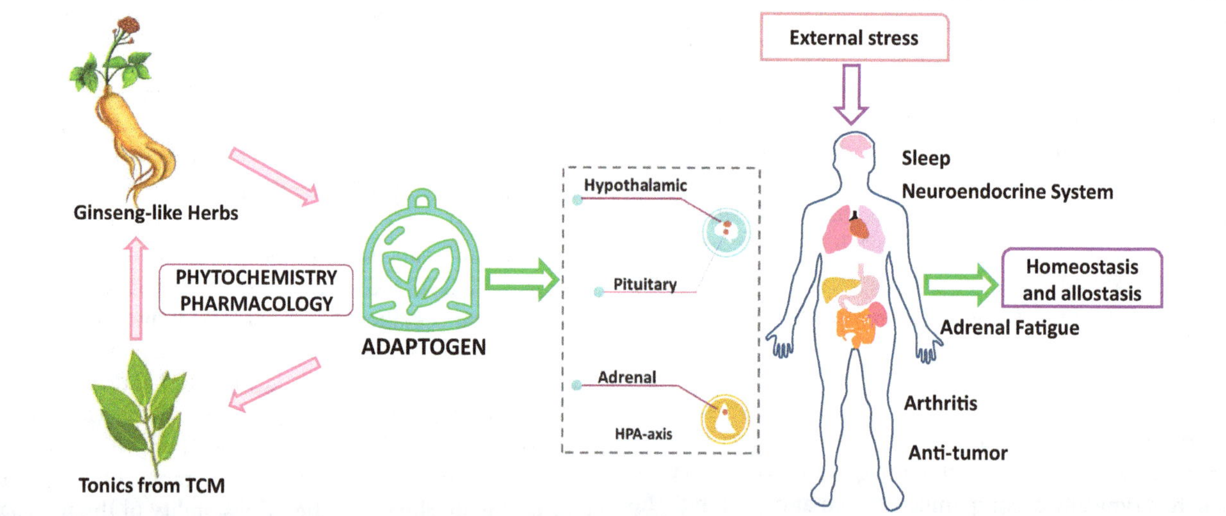

Fig. 1 The mechanism of action of plant-originated adaptogens on human body

response mode, especially the hormone response mode, occurs when homeostasis is not the driving force. When hormone levels exceed the critical level, the complex neurosecretory reactions may have harmful effects [55, 56]. The human stress response system consists of the central nervous system (CNS), which includes neurons of the hypothalamic paraventricular nucleus, and is associated with to corticotropin releasing hormone (CRH), and arginine vasopressin (AVP), and the adrenalin nucleus as well as its distal ends of the brainstem, the HPA axis and the peripheral nervous system [57]. The central coordination system to respond to external pressure consists of CRH neurons, AVP neurons, catecholamine neurons and other cell tissues, and the HPA axis and sympathetic nervous system (SNS) represent the limbs [58]. CRH and catecholamine neurons interact with each other. The SNS and HPA system interact in terms of functions and systematic anatomy. When responding to the external environment, these systems can interact on different levels, for example, catecholamine can stimulate the HPA axis by releasing of CRH, and the hormone produced by the HPA axis can act on the SNS system [33].

Recent studies have shown that the inhibitory effects and long-term overexpression of endogenous glucocorticoids cause stimulatory effects that are adjusted by SNS under stress. The secretion of CRH and AVP increases, which is stimulated by external pressure, thereby promoting the secretion of cortisol and adrenocorticotropic hormone. Furthermore, angiotensin, cytokines and arachidonic acid metabolites participate in the stress response. SNS provides the human body with a fast response mechanism to external stress. In addition to catecholamine, the sympathetic and parasympathetic nervous systems can also secrete a variety of neuropeptides, ATP and nitric oxide (NO) [59]. The following effects are observed upon adjustment the HPA axis: an increase in and regulation of energy circulation; reduction in the feeling of external pressure; enhancement of resistance; improvement of mental concentration; facilitation of deep sleep period after sleep. These functions are all considered the primary function of adaptogens [55, 56, 60].

Adaptogens do not increase the levels of cortisol and NO in the human body under acute physiological loads [6, 31, 61]. Plant-originated adaptogens, for example, *Schisandra chinensis* (Turcz.) Baill, can prevent and resist stress because these substances can activate the secretion of cortisol and NO in the plasms and saliva, allowing the body to adapt to heavier loads. After the consumption of plant-originated adaptogens, physical exercises do not increase the level of cortisol and NO in the human body; in fact, the levels decrease, comparing to those present prior to physical exercise. Thus, adaptogens can increase the level of messenger substances that activate stress (NO) and suppress stress (cortisol).

Adaptogens can improve the stress response system to respond to high levels of external signals in the normal or abnormal states. We should determine the similarities or differences between adaptogens and known classical metabolic regulators. According to the above description, the main difference may be that adaptogen can stimulate the CNS. It is now possible to obtain additional information at the biochemical level and identify analogues adrenal cortex hormone analogue, catecholamine analogue and so indicating that the active ingredients have similar structures.

Adaptogens and Chinese tonics

There is much overlap between these medicines and many tonics are internationally recognized as plant-originated adaptogens [2].

In traditional Chinese medicine, it is believed that harmony and balance are indispensable for health and the concepts of yin and yang are used to diagnose and cure disease [62]. Medicines that can supplement deficiency and weakness, correct the pathological bias caused by deficiency in both qi and blood, and treat the syndrome of qi deficiency are called tonics in traditional Chinese medicine (Qì, in the context of Chinese medicine, can be defined as the physiological processes of the body.). According to the differences in the properties, functions and indications of tonics, these medicines can be divided into qi-supplementing medicines, yang-supplementing medicines, blood-supplementing medicines, and yin-supplementing medicines. The common species of tonics and their functions are listed in Table 1.

Tonics have wide range of applications in traditional Chinese medicine and can be used under the conditions of low body resistance and weak constitution or when the human body is finding it difficult to fight severe diseases, this function of tonics is similar to that of plant-originated adaptogens [78]. Tonics typically are adaptogens, but not always. They are similar in the following aspects: First, the clinical application and mechanisms of action of these substances are similar. Based on their current applications, tonics and plant-originated adaptogens can be described as substances that regulate human bodily functions in order to attain homeostasis. The primary effects exhibited by these substances are regulation of the immune system, improving the disorders of the nervous system, anti-fatigue effects and overall nourishment. In terms of specific mechanisms, both medicines can affect the HPA axis in the immune-neuro-endocrine system, thereby achieving the above pharmacological effects [79]. Second, the plants of origin of these substances are similar [2]. Chinese herbs considered to be both adaptogens

Table 1 Various tonics and their features

Classification	Scientific name	Immunity	Neuroendocrine	Anti-stress	Anti-inflammatory	Anti-age	Hypolipidemic	Hypoglycemic	Anti-tumor	References
Qi-supplementing medicines	*Panax ginseng* C.A.Mey	√	√	√	√	√	√	√	√	[42]
	Codonopsis pilosula (Franch.) Nannf.	√	√	√	√	√		√	√	[63]
	Pannax quinquefolius L.	√	√	√			√			[42]
	Rhodiola crenulata (Hook.f. et Thoms) S.H.Fu	√	√	√	√	√				[48]
	Astragalus membranaceus (Fisch.) Bunge.	√	√	√	√	√				[64]
	Glycyrrhiza uralensis Fisch.	√	√		√		√			[65]
	Acanthopan-ax senticosus (Rupr. et Maxim.) Harms	√	√	√	√			√	√	[13]
	Atractylodes macrocephala Koidz.	√	√	√					√	[64]
Blood-supplementing medicines	*Angelica sinensis* (Oliv.) Diels	√			√	√	√			[64]
	Fallopia multiflora (Thunb.) Harald.	√				√	√			[66]
	Cynanchum otophyllum Schneid.	√	√		√					[67]
Yang-supplementing medicines	*Cuscuta chinensis* Lam.	√	√							[68]
	Epimedium brevicornu Maxim.	√	√	√	√					[69]
	Psoralea corylifolia Linn.	√	√						√	[70]
	Stachys geobombycis C.Y.Wu	√	√	√		√			√	[68]
	Cynomorium songaricum *Rupr.*	√	√							[71]
Yin-supplementing medicines	*Asparagus cochinchinensis* (Lour.) Merr.	√		√	√				√	[72]
	Ophiopogon japonicus (Linn. f.) Ker-Gawl	√	√		√	√		√		[73]
	Polygonatum odoratum	√	√		√					[74]
	Fructus Ligustri Lucidi.	√		√						[75]
	Cornus officinalis Sieb.et Zucc.	√				√				[76]
	Lycium chinense Mill.	√		√		√	√	√	√	[77]

and tonics include the following: *Panax ginseng* C.A.Mey, *Panax quniquefolius* L., *Panax notoginseng* (Burkill) F.H.Chen, *Eleutherococcus senticosus* (Rupr. & Maxim.) Maxim, *Sedum rosea* (L.) Scop., and *Schisandra chinensis* (Turcz.) Baill. According to the terminology used in traditional Chinese medicine, the mechanism of action of plant-originated adaptogens is to achieve equilibrium in both yin and yang, showing great vitality [80].

Based on the chemical composition, common tonics can be divided into following several categories in Table 2.

According to Panossian's conclusion, the main active chemical components can be divided into the following two categories. The first category includes terpenoids with four-ring skeletons that are similar to cortisol: sitoindosides (*Withania somnifera*), cucurbitacin-R-saponin (*Bryonia dioica*). The second category includes aromatic compounds with structures similar to that of catecholamine: (a) lignans: eleuteroside E (*Acanthopanax senticosus* (Rupr. et Maxim) Harms), schisandrin b (*Schisandra chinensis* (Turcz.)); (b) phenylpropane derivatives: syringin (*Acanthopanax senticosus* (Rupr. et Maxim) Harms), cinnamyl glycoside (*Rhodiola crenulata* (Hook.f. et Thoms) S.H.Fu); (c) phenylethane derivatives: salidroside.

Tonics have the following functions: enriching and activating blood (promoting the secretion of erythropoietin and inducing the production of stimulatory factors, for example, macrophage colonies, to activate blood), regulating cellular and humoral immunity, and affecting cytokine activity. These functions are similar with those of the plant-originated adaptogens mentioned above. Plant-originated adaptogens are generally considered to be the "elite of herbs" [5], and in Chinese medicine, tonics are considered the highest grade of medicine [81]. In traditional Chinese medicine theory, tonics are also considered to be top grades in traditional Chinese medicine. It is helpful to expand the range of plant-originated adaptogen species and to have an in-depth analysis about the mechanism of tonic traditional Chinese medicine.

Adaptogens and ginseng species worldwide

Many regions, ethnic groups and countries, they have their own medical histories and habits. Continuous development and transfer of knowledge through generations leads to the formation of unique medicinal systems such as traditional Chinese medicine and Indian ayurvedic medicine. Coincidentally, in different regions and medical systems, there are several medicinal plants that are considered to be national treasures or that are called ginseng locally. There is much overlap between plant-originated adaptogens and ginseng species worldwide. Furthermore, most ginseng species worldwide are internationally recognized as plant-originated adaptogens. Both ginseng-like herbs worldwide and plant-originated adaptogens have very similar clinical applications. Ginseng species are widely used by local communities world-wide because these plants can enhance the resistance of the human body and can have various beneficial effects, such as anti-fatigue, anti-ageing, anti-stress, anti-anxiety, anti-inflammatory, and anti-depression. Furthermore, ginseng species may improve the circulatory system and immune system [34], which correlates precisely to the function of adaptogens.

Most medicinal plants called ginseng belong to Araliaceous, but there are also other medicinal plants that belong to other families. For example, *Withania somnifera*, which belongs to Slanaceae, is called Indian ginseng; this plant has nourishing and strengthening effects and can delay ageing [47]. *Panax japonicus*, which belongs to Solanaceae is called Japanese ginseng; this plants have tonifying, strengthening and anti-fatigue effects [82]. *Eurycoma longifolia*, which belongs to Simaroubaceae is called Malaysian ginseng; this plant can be used as a postpartum tonic or aphrodisiac [83]. *Lepidium meyerii*, which belongs to Brassicaceae, is called Peruvian ginseng; this plant can be used for natural nutrient, can enhance fertility effectively, and has anti-fatigue effects. The common ginsengs species from different countries and their functions are listed in The results of modern pharmacological studies show that these medicinal plants called ginseng have effects on the neuroendocrine and immune systems, which is similar to the mechanism of action of plant-originated adaptogens, the elite of herbs. However, there have been few studies on the chemical compositions, mechanisms of action, traditional curative effects and similarities of these types of medicinal plants. Comparisons with ginseng species from around the world are helpful for widening the spectrum of plant-originated adaptogen species and for in-depth analysis of the mechanism of action of ginseng species worldwide. The functions and the main functional ingredients of common ginseng-like herbs worldwide were showed in Table 3.

Current difficulties and prospects of adaptogens

Plant-originated adaptogens have been demonstrated to regulate stress-related changes, at least in animal experiments. However, even after more than 40-years of herbal research, there are very few drugs that have been successfully introduced as adaptogens in modern medicine. Most of these kinds of plant-based medicines are considered to be plant-originated adaptogens and the remaining few are immune enhancers, anabolic agents and antioxidants, which are the same as plant-originated adaptogens. Therefore, there are many difficulties associated

Table 2 Based on the chemical composition, common tonics can be divided into following several categories

Category	Specific tonics
Saponin	*Panax ginseng* C.A.Mey.
	Panax japonicus C.A.Mey.
	Codonopsis pilosula (Franch.) Nannf.
	Codonopsis lanceolata (Siebold & Zucc.) Benth. & Hook.f. ex Trautv.
	Glycyrrhiza uralensis Fisch. ex DC.
	Eleutherococcus senticosus (Rupr. & Maxim.) Maxim.
	Ophiopogon japonicus (Thunb.) Ker Gawl.
	Asparagus cochinchinensis (Lour.) Merr.
	Cornus officinalis Siebold & Zucc.
	Trigonella foenum-graecum L.
	Ipomoea batatas (L.) Lam.
	Ziziphus jujuba Mill.
	Broussonetia papyrifera (L.) L'Hér. ex Vent.
	Cynomorium songaricum Rupr.
	Ligustrum lucidum W.T.Aiton
Coumarin	*Psoralea corylifolia* L.
	Clinopodium megalanthum (Diels) C.Y.Wu & S.J.Hsuan ex H.W.Li
	Lycium chinense Mill.
	Glycyrrhiza uralensis Fisch. ex DC.
	Eleutherococcus senticosus (Rupr. & Maxim.) Maxim.
	Panax ginseng C.A.Mey.
	Astragalus membranaceus Fisch. ex Bunge
Flavonoids	*Epimedium brevicornu* Maxim.
	Astragalus membranaceus Fisch. ex Bunge
	Panax ginseng C.A.Mey.
	Eucommia ulmoides Oliver
	Psoralea corylifolia L.
	Glycyrrhiza uralensis Fisch. ex DC.
	Cuscuta chinensis Lam.
	Trigonella foenum-graecum L.
	Taxillus sutchuenensis (Lecomte) Danser
	Dendrobium nobile Lindl.
Alkaloids	*Trigonella foenum-graecum* L.
	Epimedium brevicornu Maxim.
	Cistanche deserticola Ma
	Polygonatum odoratum (Mill.) Druce
	Phlomis umbrosa Turczaninow
	Ilex cornuta Lindl. & Paxton
	Allium tuberosum Rottler ex Spreng.
	Cuscuta chinensis Lam.
	Dendrobium nobile Lindl.
	Aconitum carmichaeli Debeaux
	Lilium brownii var.viridulum Baker
Volatile oils	*Atractylodes macrocephala* Koidz.
	Alpinia oxyphylla Miq.
	Angelica sinensis (Oliv.) Diels

Table 2 (continued)

Category	Specific tonics
	Clinopodium megalanthum (Diels) C.Y. Wu & Hsuan ex H.W.
	Psoralea corylifolia L.
	Epimedium brevicornu Maxim.
	Trigonella foenum-graecum L.
Amino acids	*Rehmannia glutinosa* (Gaertn.) DC.
	Stachys geobombycis C.Y.Wu
	Asparagus cochinchinensis (Lour.) Merr.
	Glycyrrhiza uralensis Fisch. ex DC.
	Panax ginseng C.A.Mey
	Trigonella foenum-graecum L.
	Lycium chinense Mill.
Polysaccharides	*Astragalus membranaceus* Fisch. ex Bunge
	Eleutherococcus senticosus (Rupr. & Maxim.) Maxim.
	Polygonatum sibiricum Redouté
	Panax ginseng C.A.Mey.
Other	*Fallopia multiflora* (Thunb.) Haraldson
	Cynanchum otophyllum C.K.Schneid.
	Rehmannia glutinosa (Gaertn.) DC.
	Epimedium brevicornu Maxim.
	Eucommia ulmoides Oliver

with judging whether a plant is a plant-originated adaptogen or not [94].

Adaptogens are stress response modifiers that non-specifically increase resistance to various stressors, thereby promoting adaptation and survival. Adapting to environmental challenges are multistep processes that involve diverse mechanisms and interactions. Multiple molecular networks are involved that coordinate both intracellular and extracellular stress signaling. The metabolic regulation of homeostasis by adaptogens at the cellular and systems levels is associated with multiple targets [95]. To date, the main problem in the research of mechanism of adaptogens, is the lack of suitable stress-response animal models. The stress responses system can be divided into three parts: stressor, stress response and stress performance [96]. The stressor is the object that induces physical strain; therefore, a stressor may be biological (infection), physical (external force, extreme environment), chemical (medicine, ethanol), or psychological (sadness, argument). When an organism is exposed to a stressor, the neuroendocrine system of the body changes. It is easy to study stress performances because these effects are visible [97].

Therefore, stress is known to lead to high blood pressure, myocardial ischemia, depression and even cancer. Briefly, stress performance is the manifestation of the final effect of the stress response on the target organ.

Table 3 Ginseng-like herbs worldwide with similar functions as those of plant-originated adaptogens

Scientific name	Common name	Family	Common function	Main functional ingredient
Panax ginseng C.A.Mey	Asian ginseng	Araliaceae	Used for strengthening, nourishing, adjusting blood pressure and restoring heart function, neurasthenia and physical weakness [42]	Ginsenoside [84]
Pannax quinquefolius L.	American ginseng	Araliaceae	Used to treat qi and yin deficiency, endogenous heat, kechuan, sputum, asthenic fever, dysphoria, thirst, and dry mouth and throat [42]	Ginsenoside, etc. [84]
Panax notoginseng (Burk.) F.H.Chen	Notoginseng	Araliaceae	Used for dispersing blood stasis and haemostasis and relieving swelling and pain [85]	Notoginseng saponins, Dencichine, etc. [84]
Panax japonicus	Japanese ginseng	Araliaceae	Used for dispersing blood stasis and haemostasis, relieving swelling and pain, eliminating phlegm and arresting coughing and for tonifying deficiency and strengthening [86]	Chikusetsusaponin, pseudo ginsenoside F11, Panax japonicus polysaccharide, etc. [86]
Panax pseudoginseng Wall. var. major (Burkill) H. L. Li	Himalayan ginseng	Araliaceae	Used to treat qi and yin deficiency, dysphoria, thirst, asthenia coughing, injuries from falling down, joint pain, haemoptysis, haematemesis and bleeding wounds [86]	Majoroside, etc. [86]
Eleutherococcus senticosus	Siberian ginseng	Araliaceae	Used for regulating body disorders, improving the circulatory system, to treat fatigue, for promoting blood circulation for removing blood stasis, invigorating the stomach and for diuresis and so on [13, 87]	Eleutheroside, acanthopanax senticosus polysaccharide, etc. [13, 87]
Withania somnifera	Indian ginseng	Solanaceae	Used for strengthening; nourishing;its anti-ageing, anti-stress, antioxidation, anti-tumor, anti-anxiety, anti-inflammatory, anti-depression properties; immune regulation; improving cognitive function and so on [19]	Withanolides and other steroid esters and withanine and other alkaloids [88]
Pfaffia paniculata	Brazilian ginseng	Amaranthaceae	Often used as a tonic, to relieve fatigue effectively, improve sexual function, and lower blood pressure, blood sugar and blood lipid levels [89]	Pfaffic acid and its glycoside, for example, pfaffosides A–F, and nortiperpene and its glycoside, etc. [86]
Eurycoma longifolia	Malaysian ginseng	Simaroubaceae	Used for its anticancer, anti-malaria properties, improving male sexual dysfunction, sterilizing, lowering blood pressure and treating diabetes [54]	Diterpenes with quassinoid skeletons and alkaloids such as canthin-6-one, mainly, biphenyl lignin and squalene derivatives [54]
Lepidium meyerii	Peruvian ginseng	Brassicaceae	Used as s natural nutrient, for enhancing fertility effectively and for its anti-fatigue properties [90]	Marca amide, marca alkaloids, etc. [91]
Talinum paniculatum	Folk ginseng	Talinaceae	Used as a medicinal tonic and for strengthening, nourishing, improving qi, replenishing blood, aiding digestion, promoting fluid production, quenching thirst and treating cough and phlegm containing blood [92]	Terpenoids, coumarins, volatile oils, and polysaccharides, etc. [93]

However, it remains challenging to study various steps of this stress response [98]. First, this difficulty is associated with the stressor because it is difficult to quantify external stressors, especially psychological stressors, for example, sadness. In addition, we know little about the interactions between stressors and the body. The specific response of mechanisms induced by stressors affect broad-spectrum stress response. Second, this difficulty is associated with the stress response. In the terms of development, hormones, neurotransmitters, neuro-regulators and cytokines, which are involved in the response have been identified, but the specific functions of these proteins divisions remain unknown. The identity of the first substance to regulate the stress response remains unclear, and it has not been determined whether there are different mechanisms for different stressors. There are no definitive results regarding the specific mechanisms and pathway changes of that lead to conversion of the status from unsuitable to suitable. As a result, it is impossible to differentiate and characterize the different stages of stress response (including adaptation), making the response difficult to quantify [97]. Therefore, scientists use "prevention of stress manifestation" as a guideline to evaluate the anti-stress properties of a drug [99]. Third, the difficulty is associated with stress expression. According to the strength and severity of the stressor, different changes are observed. Genetic or other external factors (species, day–night cycles, gender, age and physiological state of tissues or organs) also affect the extent of overall stress expression. The difficulties mentioned above will appear in the process of the mechanism of action of adaptogens; therefore, it is necessary to further discuss the mechanisms, targets, similarities and differences associated with the pharmacological functions.

To date, various studies and practical applications have shown that plant-originated adaptogens are a kind of elite herbal medicine, playing an important role in human health and helping the human body resist various stress factors. However, the clinical application of plant-originated adaptogens and their use in health care products remains in the preliminary stage. Categorization of plant-originated adaptogens, clarification of their pharmacological functions, and the determination of the similarities and differences between adaptogens, tonics and ginseng species worldwide, will help in effective utilization of plant-originated adaptogens, and provide a new way to guarantee human health.

Authors' contributions

Conceptualization, P-GX and FY; Methodology, LL, HM, and Y-MD; Writing—original draft preparation, L-YY; Writing—review and editing, Y-FH. All authors read and approved the final manuscript.

Author details

[1] Key Laboratory of Cosmetics, China National Light Industry, Beijing Technology and Business University, No. 11/33, Fucheng Road, Haidian District, Beijing 100048, People's Republic of China. [2] Beijing Key Laboratory of Plant Resources Research and Development, Beijing Technology and Business University, No. 11/33, Fucheng Road, Haidian District, Beijing 100048, People's Republic of China. [3] Institute of Medicinal Plant Development, Chinese Academy of Medical Sciences, Peking Union Medical College, Beijing, 151 Malianwa North Road, Haidian District, Beijing 100193, People's Republic of China.

Acknowledgements

We are very grateful to Pr. Yong PENG (Institute of Medicinal Plant Development, Chinese Academy of Medical Sciences, Peking Union Medical College, Beijing) for his valuable suggestions.

Competing interests

The authors declare that they have no competing interests.

Consent for publication

I, the corresponding author give my consent for my article to be publish in Chinese Medicine.

Funding

This study was supported by the Beijing Technology and Business University Youth Scholars Fund (PXM2018_014213_000033) and the Key Laboratory of Cosmetics, China National Light Industry, Beijing Technology and Business University Innovation Fund (KLC 2017 YB2).

References

1. Brekhman II, Dardymov IV. New substances of plant origin which increase nonspecific resistance. Ann Rev Pharmacol Toxicol. 1969;9(1):419–30.
2. Mendes FR. Tonic, fortifier and aphrodisiac: adaptogens in the Brazilian folk medicine. Revista Brasileira de Farmacognosia. 2011;21(4):754–63.
3. Winslow LC, Kroll DJ. Herbs as medicines. Arch Intern Med. 1998;158(20):2192–9.
4. Yance DR, Tabachnik B. Breakthrough solutions in herbal medicine adaptogenic formulas: the way to vitality. Townsend Lett. 2007;282:86–90.
5. Yance DR. Adaptogens in medical herbalism: elite herbs and natural compounds for mastering stress, aging, and chronic disease. New York: Simon and Schuster; 2013. p. 103–7.
6. Panossian A, Wikman G. Evidence-based efficacy of adaptogens in fatigue, and molecular mechanisms related to their stress-protective activity. Curr Clin Pharmacol. 2009;4(3):198–219.
7. Winston D, Maimes S. Adaptogens: herbs for strength, stamina, and stress relief. Rochester: Inner Traditions/Bear & Co; 2007. p. 48–53.
8. Bhatia N, Jaggi AS, Singh N, Anand P, Dhawan R. Adaptogenic potential of curcumin in experimental chronic stress and chronic unpredictable stress-induced memory deficits and alterations in functional homeostasis. J Nat Med. 2011;65(3–4):532–43.
9. Gaffney B, Hügel H, Rich P. *Panax ginseng* and *Eleutherococcus senticosus* may exaggerate an already existing biphasic response to stress via inhibition of enzymes which limit the binding of stress hormones to their receptors. Med Hypotheses. 2001;56(5):567–72.
10. Awang D. The anti-stress potential of North American ginseng (*Panax quinquefolius* L.). J Herbs Spices Med Plants. 1998;6(2):87–91.
11. Sengupta P, Agarwal A, Pogrebetskaya M, Roychoudhury S, Durairajanayagam D, Henkel R. Role of *Withania somnifera* (Ashwagandha) in the management of male infertility. Reprod Biomed Online. 2017;36:311–26.
12. Liu K, Wang Z, Rong P. Puerarin decoction with cassia twig combined with auricular acupoint plaster and acupuncture in the treatment of 38 tension headache patients. Int J Clin Acupuncture. 2017;26(1):871.
13. Huang L, Zhao H, Huang B, Zheng C, Peng W, Qin L. *Acanthopanax senticosus*: review of botany, chemistry and pharmacology. Int J Pharm Sci. 2011;66(2):83–97.
14. Wang J, Gao W, Zhang L, Huang L. Establishment and quality assessment of tissue cultures in *Glycyrrhiza uralensis* Fisch. Appl Biochem Biotechnol. 2013;169(2):588–94.
15. Lu H, Kyo E, Uesaka T, Katoh O, Watanabe H. A water-soluble extract from cultured medium of *Ganoderma lucidum* (Rei-shi) mycelia suppresses azoxymethane-induction of colon cancers in male F344 rats. Oncol Rep. 2003;10(2):375–9.

16. Chen SP, Huang Liu R, Lu TM, Wei JCC, Wu TC, Tsai WY, et al. Complementary usage of *Rhodiola crenulata* (L.) in chronic obstructive pulmonary disease patients: the effects on cytokines and T cells. Phytother Res. 2015;29(4):518–25.
17. Bhattacharya A, Ghosal S, Bhattacharya S. Anti-oxidant effect of *Withania somnifera* glycowithanolides in chronic footshock stress-induced perturbations of oxidative free radical scavenging enzymes and lipid peroxidation in rat frontal cortex and striatum. J Ethnopharmacol. 2001;74(1):1–6.
18. Kropotov A, Kolodnyak O, Koldaev V. Effects of Siberian ginseng extract and ipriflavone on the development of glucocorticoid-induced osteoporosis. Bull Exp Biol Med. 2002;133(3):252–4.
19. Singh N, Bhalla M, de Jager P, Gilca M. An overview on ashwagandha: a Rasayana (Rejuvenator) of ayurveda. Afr J Tradit Complement Altern Med. 2011;8:5S.
20. Choi YS, Kang EH, Lee EY, Gong HS, Kang HS, Shin K, et al. Joint-protective effects of compound K, a major ginsenoside metabolite, in rheumatoid arthritis: in vitro evidence. Rheumatol Int. 2013;33(8):1981–90.
21. Razmovski-Naumovski V, Huang TH-W, Tran VH, Li GQ, Duke CC, Roufogalis BD. Chemistry and pharmacology of *Gynostemma pentaphyllum*. Phytochem Rev. 2005;4(2–3):197–219.
22. Ho YW, Yeung JS, Chiu PK, Tang WM, Lin ZB, Man RY, et al. Ganoderma lucidum polysaccharide peptide reduced the production of proinflammatory cytokines in activated rheumatoid synovial fibroblast. Mol Cell Biochem. 2007;301(1–2):173–9.
23. Perfumi M, Mattioli L. Adaptogenic and central nervous system effects of single doses of 3% rosavin and 1% salidroside *Rhodiola rosea* L. extract in mice. Phytother Res. 2007;21(1):37–43.
24. Zhu L, Wei H, Wu Y, Yang S, Xiao L, Zhang J, et al. Licorice isoliquiritigenin suppresses RANKL-induced osteoclastogenesis in vitro and prevents inflammatory bone loss in vivo. Int J Biochem Cell Biol. 2012;44(7):1139–52.
25. Provalova N, Skurikhin E, Pershina O, Suslov N, Minakova MY, Dygai A, et al. Mechanisms underling the effects of adaptogens on erythropoiesis during paradoxical sleep deprivation. Bull Exp Biol Med. 2002;133(5):428–32.
26. Chanana P, Kumar A. GABA-BZD receptor modulating mechanism of *Panax quinquefolius* against 72-h sleep deprivation induced anxiety like behavior: possible roles of oxidative stress, mitochondrial dysfunction and neuroinflammation. Front Neurosci. 2016;10:84.
27. Deshpande A, Irani N, Balakrishnan R. Study protocol and rationale for a prospective, randomized, double-blind, placebo-controlled study to evaluate the effects of Ashwagandha (*Withania somnifera*) extract on nonrestorative sleep. Medicine. 2018;97:26.
28. Zhang C, Zhao X, Mao X, Liu A, Liu Z, Li X, et al. Pharmacological evaluation of sedative and hypnotic effects of schizandrin through the modification of pentobarbital-induced sleep behaviors in mice. Eur J Pharmacol. 2014;744:157–63.
29. Takemoto T, Arihara S, Nakajima T, Okuhira M. Studies on the constituents of gynostemma-pentaphyllum makino. 1. structures of gypenoside-I-XIV. yakugaku zasshi. J Pharm Soc Japan. 1983;103(2):173–85.
30. Darbinyan V, Aslanyan G, Amroyan E, Gabrielyan E, Malmström C, Panossian A. Clinical trial of *Rhodiola rosea* L. extract SHR-5 in the treatment of mild to moderate depression. Nordic J Psychiatry. 2007;61(5):343–8.
31. Panossian A, Wikman G, Kaur P, Asea A. Adaptogens exert a stress-protective effect by modulation of expression of molecular chaperones. Phytomedicine. 2009;16(6–7):617–22.
32. Provino R. The role of adaptogens in stress management. Aus J Med Herbalism. 2010;22(2):41.
33. Panossian A, Wagner H. Stimulating effect of adaptogens: an overview with particular reference to their efficacy following single dose administration. Phytother Res. 2010;19(10):819–38.
34. Panossian A, Wikman G. Effects of adaptogens on the central nervous system and the molecular mechanisms associated with their stress—protective activity. Pharmaceuticals. 2010;3(1):188–224.
35. Carlini E. Plants and the central nervous system. Pharmacol Biochem Behav. 2003;75(3):501–12.
36. Mendes FR, Carlini EA. Brazilian plants as possible adaptogens: an ethnopharmacological survey of books edited in Brazil. J Ethnopharmacol. 2007;109(3):493–500.
37. de Oliveira DR, Leitão SG. Fortifier, tonic, and rejuvenating plants and the adaptogen concept. Berlin: Introduction to Ethnobiology: Springer; 2016. p. 151–61.
38. Arushanyan E. Systemic and cellular mechanisms of anti-tumor activity of plant adaptogens. Vopr Onkol. 2009;55(1):15–23.
39. Wiegant F, Surinova S, Ytsma E, Langelaar-Makkinje M, Wikman G, Post J. Plant adaptogens increase lifespan and stress resistance in *C. elegans*. Biogerontology. 2009;10(1):27–42.
40. Iaremenko K. Adaptogens as means of the prevention of malignant tumors. Vopr Onkol. 1989;35(8):912–9.
41. Winters M. Ancient medicine, modern use: *Withania somnifera* and its potential role in integrative oncology. Altern Med Rev. 2006;11:4.
42. Patel S, Rauf A. Adaptogenic herb ginseng (Panax) as medical food: status quo and future prospects. Biomed Pharmacother. 2017;85:120–7.
43. Kaur P, Makanjuola VO, Arora R, Singh B, Arora S. Immunopotentiating significance of conventionally used plant adaptogens as modulators in biochemical and molecular signalling pathways in cell mediated processes. Biomed Pharmacother. 2017;95:1815–29.
44. Loo WT, Jin L, Chow LW, Cheung MN, Wang M. *Rhodiola algida* improves chemotherapy-induced oral mucositis in breast cancer patients. Expert Opin Invest Drugs. 2010;19(sup1):S91–100.
45. Barton DL, Soori GS, Bauer BA, Sloan JA, Johnson PA, Figueras C, et al. Pilot study of *Panax quinquefolius* (American ginseng) to improve cancer-related fatigue: a randomized, double-blind, dose-finding evaluation: NCCTG trial N03CA. Supportive Care Cancer. 2010;18(2):179.
46. Barton DL, Liu H, Dakhil SR, Linquist B, Sloan JA, Nichols CR, et al. Wisconsin Ginseng (*Panax quinquefolius*) to improve cancer-related fatigue: a randomized, double-blind trial, N07C2. J Natl Cancer Instit. 2013;105(16):1230–8.
47. Mishra L-C, Singh BB, Dagenais S. Scientific basis for the therapeutic use of *Withania somnifera* (ashwagandha): a review. Altern Med Rev. 2000;5(4):334–46.
48. Chiang H-M, Chen H-C, Wu C-S, Wu P-Y, Wen KC. Rhodiola plants: chemistry and biological activity. J Food Drug Anal. 2015;23(3):359–69.
49. Treasure J, editor. Herbal medicine and cancer: an introductory overview. Seminars in oncology nursing. New York: Elsevier; 2005.
50. Tavakoli J, Miar S, Zadehzare MM, Akbari H. Evaluation of effectiveness of herbal medication in cancer care: a review study. Iranian J Cancer Prev. 2012;5(3):144.
51. Meissner HO, Mscisz A, ReichBilinska H, Mrozikiewicz P, BobkiewiczKozlowska T, Kedzia B, et al. Hormone-Balancing effect of Pre-Gelatinized organic maca (*Lepidium peruvianum* Chacon): (III) clinical responses of early-postmenopausal women to Maca in double blind, randomized, placebo-controlled, crossover configuration, outpatient study. Int J Biomed Sci. 2006;2(4):375–94.
52. Chai S, To KK, Lin G. Circumvention of multi-drug resistance of cancer cells by Chinese herbal medicines. Chin Med. 2010;5(1):26.
53. Yang Z, Wang J-R, Niu T, Gao S, Yin T, You M, et al. Inhibition of *P*-glycoprotein leads to improved oral bioavailability of compound K, an anticancer metabolite of red ginseng extract produced by gut microflora. Drug Metabol Disposit. 2012;40(8):1538–44.
54. Rehman SU, Choe K, Yoo HH. Review on a traditional herbal medicine, *Eurycoma longifolia* Jack (Tongkat Ali): its traditional uses, chemistry, evidence-based pharmacology and toxicology. Molecules. 2016;21(3):331.
55. Panossian A, Oganessian A, Ambartsumian M, Gabrielian E, Wagner H, Wikman G. Effects of heavy physical exercise and adaptogens on nitric oxide content in human saliva. Phytomedicine. 1999;6(1):17–26.
56. Panossian A, Wikman G, Wagner H. Plant adaptogens III. Earlier and more recent aspects and concepts on their mode of action. Phytomedicine. 1999;6(4):287–300.
57. Chrousos GP, Gold PW. The concepts of stress and stress system disorders: overview of physical and behavioral homeostasis. JAMA. 1992;267(9):1244–52.
58. Chrousos GP. Stress and disorders of the stress system. Nat Rev Endocrinol. 2009;5(7):374.
59. Wardle J, Sarris J. Clinical naturopathy: an evidence-based guide to practice. New York: Elsevier Health Sciences; 2014.
60. Panossian A, Hambardzumyan M, Hovhanissyan A, Wikman G. The adaptogens Rhodiola and Schizandra modify the response to immobilization stress in rabbits by suppressing the increase of phosphorylated stress-

activated protein kinase, nitric oxide and cortisol. Drug Target Insights. 2007;2:117739280700200011.
61. Darbinyan V, Kteyan A, Panossian A, Gabrielian E, Wikman G, Wagner H. Rhodiola rosea in stress induced fatigue—a double blind cross-over study of a standardized extract SHR-5 with a repeated low-dose regimen on the mental performance of healthy physicians during night duty. Phytomedicine. 2000;7(5):365–71.
62. Unschuld PU. Huang Di Nei Jing Su Wen Nature, Knowledge, Imagery in an Ancient Chinese Medical Text: With an Appendix: The Doctrine of the Five Periods and Six Qi in the Huang Di Nei Jing Su Wen. California: Univ of California Press; 2003.
63. Gao S-M, Liu J-S, Wang M, Cao T-T, Qi Y-D, Zhang B-G, et al. Traditional uses, phytochemistry, pharmacology and toxicology of Codonopsis: a review. J Ethnopharmacol. 2018;219:50–70.
64. Xie J-H, Jin M-L, Morris GA, Zha X-Q, Chen H-Q, Yi Y, et al. Advances on bioactive polysaccharides from medicinal plants. Crit Rev Food Sci Nutr. 2016;56(sup1):S60–84.
65. Asl MN, Hosseinzadeh HJP, Derivatives TEoNP. Review of pharmacological effects of *Glycyrrhiza* sp. and its bioactive compounds. Phytother Res. 2008;22(6):709–24.
66. Lin L, Ni B, Lin H, Zhang M, Li X, Yin X, et al. Traditional usages, botany, phytochemistry, pharmacology and toxicology of *Polygonum multiflorum* Thunb.: a review. J Ethnopharmacol. 2015;159:158–83.
67. Parker S, May B, Zhang C, Zhang AL, Lu C, Xue CC. A pharmacological review of bioactive constituents of *Paeonia lactiflora* Pallas and *Paeonia veitchii* Lynch. Phytother Res. 2016;30(9):1445–73.
68. Donnapee S, Li J, Yang X, A-h Ge, Donkor PO, X-m Gao, et al. *Cuscuta chinensis* Lam.: a systematic review on ethnopharmacology, phytochemistry and pharmacology of an important traditional herbal medicine. J Ethnopharmacol. 2014;157:292–308.
69. Chen X-J, Tang Z-H, Li X-W, Xie C-X, Lu J-J, Wang Y-T. Chemical constituents, quality control, and bioactivity of Epimedii Folium (Yinyanghuo). Am J Chin Med. 2015;43(05):783–834.
70. Chopra B, Dhingra AK, Dhar KLJF. *Psoralea corylifolia* L. (Buguchi)—folklore to modern evidence. Fitoterapia. 2013;90:44–56.
71. Cui Z, Guo Z, Miao J, Wang Z, Li Q, Chai X, et al. The genus Cynomorium in China: an ethnopharmacological and phytochemical review. J Ethnopharmacol. 2013;147(1):1–15.
72. Negi J, Singh P, Joshi G, Rawat M, Bisht V. Chemical constituents of Asparagus. Pharmacognosy Rev. 2010;4(8):215.
73. Chen M-H, Chen X-J, Wang M, Lin L-G, Wang Y-TJJ. *Ophiopogon japonicus*—a phytochemical, ethnomedicinal and pharmacological review. J Ethnopharmacol. 2016;181:193–213.
74. Zhao P, Zhao C, Li X, Gao Q, Huang L, Xiao P, et al. The genus Polygonatum: a review of ethnopharmacology, phytochemistry and pharmacology. J Ethnopharmacol. 2017;214:274–91.
75. Gao L, Li C, Wang Z, Liu X, You Y, Wei H, et al. Ligustri Lucidi Fructus as a traditional Chinese medicine: a review of its phytochemistry and pharmacology. Nat Product Res. 2015;29(6):493–510.
76. Huang J, Zhang Y, Dong L, Gao Q, Yin L, Quan H, et al. Ethnopharmacology, phytochemistry, and pharmacology of *Cornus officinalis* Sieb. et Zucc. J Ethnopharmacol. 2017;213:280–301.
77. Yao X, Peng Y, Xu LJ, Li L, Wu QL, Xiao PG. Phytochemical and biological studies of Lycium medicinal plants. Chem Biodiver. 2011;8(6):976–1010.
78. Panossian AG. Adaptogens: tonic herbs for fatigue and stress. Altern Complement Ther. 2003;9(6):327–31.
79. Li H, Liu S-Y, Wang B. Progress of the regulation effect of ginsenosides on HPA axis. Yao xue xue bao = Acta Pharmaceutica Sinica. 2014;49(5):569–75.
80. You J, Roh KB, Li Z, Liu G, Tang J, Shin S, et al. The antiaging properties of *Andrographis paniculata* by activation epidermal cell stemness. Molecules. 2015;20(9):17557–69.
81. Zhu Y-P. Chinese materia medica: chemistry, pharmacology and applications. New York: CRC Press; 1998. p. 24–8.
82. Ng T. Pharmacological activity of sanchi ginseng (*Panax notoginseng*). J Pharm Pharmacol. 2006;58(8):1007–19.
83. Yeng C, Wai-Mei P, Alan K-WM, Choon-Keat C, Bin-Seng L, Sreenivasan S, et al. Decreased expression of alpha-2-HS glycoprotein in the sera of rats treated with *Eurycoma longifolia* extract. Front Pharmacol. 2015;6(211):1–6.
84. Yang W-z HuY, W-y Wu, Ye M, Guo D-A. Saponins in the genus Panax L. (Araliaceae): a systematic review of their chemical diversity. Phytochemistry. 2014;106:7–24.
85. Wang T, Guo R, Zhou G, Zhou X, Kou Z, Sui F, et al. Traditional uses, botany, phytochemistry, pharmacology and toxicology of Panax notoginseng (Burk.) FH Chen: a review. J Ethnopharmacol. 2016;188:234–58.
86. Zabelinskaja-Mackova AA. Ginseng as panacea: its chemical composition and physiological influence.
87. Huang L-Z, Huang B-K, Ye Q, Qin L-P. Bioactivity-guided fractionation for anti-fatigue property of *Acanthopanax senticosus*. J Ethnopharmacol. 2011;133(1):213–9.
88. Özdemir Z, Bildziukevich U, Wimmerová M, Macůrková A, Lovecká P, Wimmer Z. Plant adaptogens: natural medicaments for 21st century? ChemistrySelect. 2018;3(7):2196–214.
89. Costa C, Quaglio A, Di Stasi LJJ. *Pfaffia paniculata* (Brazilian ginseng) extract modulates Mapk and mucin pathways in intestinal inflammation. J Ethnopharmacol. 2018;213:21–5.
90. Gonzales GF. Ethnobiology and ethnopharmacology of *Lepidium meyenii* (Maca), a plant from the Peruvian highlands. Evid Based Complement Altern Med. 2012;2012:193496.
91. Xia C, Chen J, Deng J-L, Zhu Y-Q, Li W-Y, Jie B, et al. Novel macamides from maca (*Lepidium meyenii* Walpers) root and their cytotoxicity. Phytochem Lett. 2018;25:65–9.
92. Ramos MPO, Silva GDDF, Duarte LP, Peres V, Miranda RRS, Souza GHBD, et al. Antinociceptive and edematogenic activity and chemical constituents of *Talinum paniculatum* Willd. J Chem Pharm Res. 2010;2(6):265–74.
93. Reis LFD, Cerdeira CD, Paula BF, Silva JJD, Coelho LF, Silva MA, et al. Chemical characterization and evaluation of antibacterial, antifungal, antimycobacterial, and cytotoxic activities of *Talinum paniculatum*. Revista do Instituto de Medicina Tropical de São Paulo. 2015;57(5):397–405.
94. Singh N, Nath R, Lata A, Singh S, Kohli R, Bhargava K. *Withania somnifera* (ashwagandha), a rejuvenating herbal drug which enhances survival during stress (an adaptogen). Int J Crude Drug Res. 1982;20(1):29–35.
95. Panossian A. Understanding adaptogenic activity: specificity of the pharmacological action of adaptogens and other phytochemicals. Ann N Y Acad Sci. 2017;1401(1):49–64.
96. Maslova L, Kondrat'ev B, Maslov L, Lishmanov I. The cardioprotective and antiadrenergic activity of an extract of *Rhodiola rosea* in stress. Eksperimental'naia i klinicheskaia farmakologiia. 1994;57(6):61–3.
97. Spasov AA, Wikman GK, Mandrikov VB, Mironova IA, Neumoin VV. A double-blind, placebo-controlled pilot study of the stimulating and adaptogenic effect of *Rhodiola rosea* SHR-5 extract on the fatigue of students caused by stress during an examination period with a repeated low-dose regimen. Phytomedicine. 2000;7(2):85–9.
98. Verma S, Rajeevan V, Bordia A, Jain V. Greater cardamom (*Amomum subulatum* Roxb.)—a cardio-adaptogen against physical stress. J Herb Med Toxicol. 2010;4(2):55–8.
99. Bhattacharya S, Muruganandam A. Adaptogenic activity of *Withania somnifera*: an experimental study using a rat model of chronic stress. Pharmacol Biochem Behav. 2003;75(3):547–55.

10

Global ecological regionalization of 15 *Illicium* species: nature sources of shikimic acid

Xiang Zhang[1†], Xiangxiao Meng[2†], Jie Wu[2†], Linfang Huang[1*] and Shilin Chen[2*]

Abstract

Background: *Illicium* plants are relevant officinal and ornamental species that are native in Eastern Asia, and they are the main sources of shikimic acid. Shikimic acid is an important component of Tamiflu, which is recognized for its ability to resist avian influenza by the World Health Organization. To determine areas where 15 *Illicium* species can be grown and to understand the importance of species diversity, we should enhance the prediction of suitable areas.

Methods: In this study, the global potential distribution of 15 *Illicium* species was predicted using a geographic information system for global medicinal plants.

Results: Results showed that the possible suitable areas for these plants in China covered 1357.68 × 10^4 km^2 (56%), and the second-largest area spanning 527.42 × 10^4 km^2 was found in the United States. *Illicium verum* Hook, an edible species with the highest shikimic acid content among them, grew in areas of 59.92 × 10^4 (48%), 64.04 × 10^4 (19%), and 60.53 × 10^4 km^2(18%) in China, the United States, and Brazil, respectively. *Illicium.difengpi* B. N. Chamg, an endangered species, was distributed in an area of 19.03 × 10^4 km^2 or 95% of the total area in China.

Conclusions: This research provided a guarantee for the demand of Tamiflu, presented strategies that helped protect endangered species, and provided a reference for species cultivation and introduction.

Keywords: Shikimic acid, *Illicium* plants, Geographic information system for global medicinal plants, Ecological suitable areas

Background

Shikimic acid (3,4,5-trihydroxy-1-cyclohexene-1-carboxylic acid) is commonly known as the main natural raw material of Tamiflu, which is recognized as the first drug to treat avian influenza in clinical settings [1–3]. The main sources of shikimic acid are *Illicium* plants, which are naturally distributed in Southeast China, the United States, Burma, and Vietnam [4] (Table 1). A total of 34 kinds of *Illicium* plants exist, and 15 of them (*I. verum* Hook. f., *I. henryi* Diels, *I. majus* Hook. f. & Thoms., *I. simonsii* Maxim., *I. micranthum* Dunn, *I. dunnianum* Tutch., *I. lanceolatum* A. C. Smith, *I. fargesii* Finet & Gagnep, *I. jiadifengpi* B. N. Chang, *I. difengpi* B. N. Chamg, *I. ternstroemioides* A. C. Smith, *I. macranthum* A. C. Smit, *I. oligandrum* Merr, et al. Chun, *I. brevistylum* A. C. Smith, and *I. pachyphyllum* A. C. Smith) can be used as Chinese herbal medicines for the treatment of rheumatoid arthritis, injuries, abdominal distention, and vomiting [5, 6]. Currently, they are mainly distributed in South and Southeast China, such as Hunan, Fujian and Guangxi. Among these species, *I. verum* Hook. f., an edible plant which is listed in the Pharmacopoeia of China (2015 edition) and European Pharmacopoeia (7th edition). *I. difengpi* B. N. Chamg is listed in the Pharmacopoeia of China (2015 edition) and recorded in the Information System of Chinese Rare and Endangered Plants (http://rep.iplant.cn/protlist).

As traditional herbal medicines, *Illicium* plants have been technically investigated on active ingredient synthesis. Here are two ways for shikimic acid synthesis including biosynthetic pathways and chemical pathways. Figure 1a shows the shikimate pathway, which serves as

*Correspondence: lfhuang@implad.ac.cn; slchen@icmm.ac.cn
†Xiang Zhang, Xiangxiao Meng and Jie Wu are co-first authors
[1] Institute of Medicinal Plant Development, Chinese Academy of Medical Sciences and Peking Union Medical College, Beijing 100193, China
[2] Institute of Chinese Materia Medica, China Academy of Chinese Medical Sciences, Beijing 100700, China

Table 1 Distribution points of 15 kinds of *Illicium* plants

Latin names of species	Distribution	Sampling points
I. verum	In China, western and southern of Guangxi, southern of Zhejiang, Jiangxi, Hunan and Chongqing, south-central Fujian, southwest of Guangdong and Guizhou, southeast of Hainan, Yunnan, etc.	61
I. henryi	In China, Anhui, Jiangxi, Fujian, Henan, Guangdong, Guangxi, Chongqing, Yunnan, southern of Shanxi and Gansu, northern of Hubei, from west to northwest of Hubei, from east to southeast of Sichuan, from eastern to northern of Guizhou, etc.	171
I. majus	Guangxi, Guizhou, Chongqing, Yunnan, Hunan, southwest of Hubei, from western to northern of Guangdong, from central to south central of Sichuan in China, southern of Burma, northern of Vietnam, etc.	128
I. simonsii	Southwest of Sichuan (Xichang, Huili, Puge),from northwest to southeast of Guizhou, northwest, northeast and central Yunnan in China, northern of Burma, northeast of India, etc.	95
I. micranthum	In China, Hunan, Guangdong, Hongkong, Sichuan, Guizhou, Chongqing, Yunnan, western of Hubei, from central to northern of Guangxi, etc.	93
I. dunnianum	In China, Guangdong, Hongkong, Guangxi, southern of Fujian, southwest of Hunan, southern and southwest of Guizhou, southeast of Sichuan, etc.	80
I. lanceolatum	In China, Anhui, Zhejiang, Jiangxi, Fujian, Hubei, Hunan, Guizhou, southern of Jiangsu, southeast of Henan, etc.	76
I. fargesii	In China, Chongqing, western of Hubei, northeast of Yunnan, from northwest to southwest of Hunan, from northern to northeast of Guangxi, from eastern to northeast of Guizhou, from eastern to central of Sichuan, etc.	72
I. jiadifengpi	In China, Jiangxi, Fujian, Hongkong, southern of Anhui, southwest of Zhejiang, northeast of Guangxin, northern of Guangdong, southeast of Hubei, from southern to eastern of Hunan, etc.	69
I. difengpi	In China, Guangxin, southeast of Yunnan, etc.	61
I. ternstroemioides	In China, Fujian, Guangdong, Hongkong, Guangxi, southern of Hunan, southeast of Yunnan, etc.	58
I. macranthum	In China, southeast and western of Yunnan, southeast of Tibet, etc.	42
I. oligandrum	South of Guangxi, Hainan in China, Vietnam, etc.	37
I. brevistylum	In China, Guangdong, Guangxi, southern of Hunan, southeast of Yunnan, Fujian, Hongkong, etc.	29
I. pachyphyllum	In China, southwest of Guangdong and Hunan, southeast and northeast of Guizhou, etc.	22

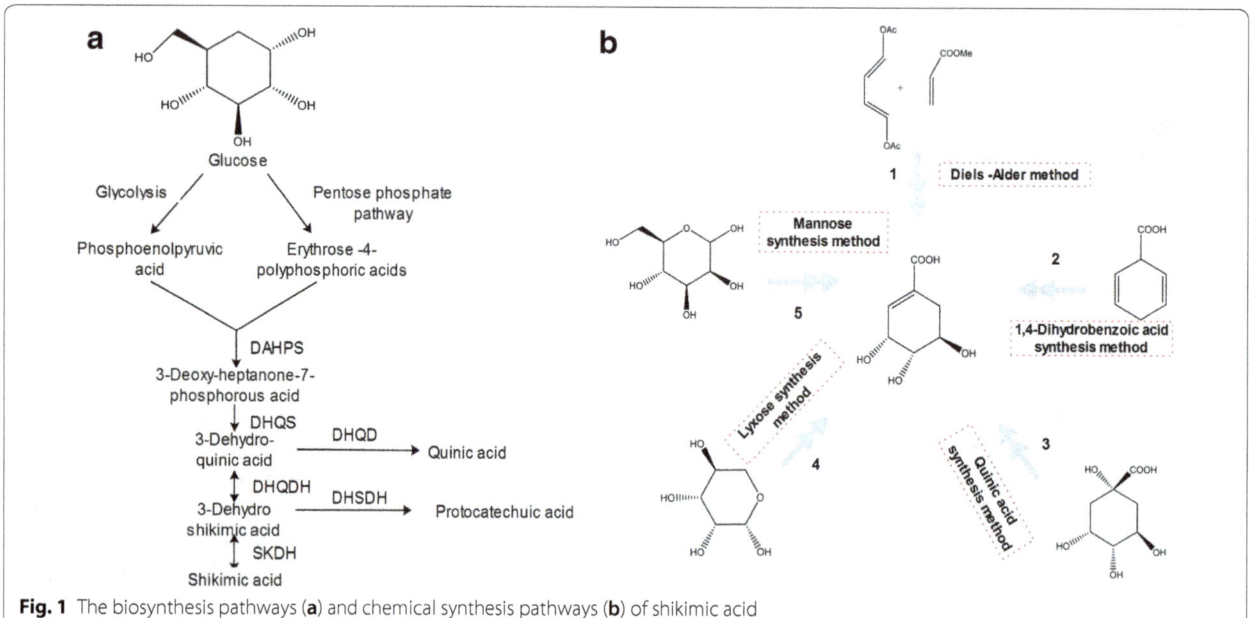

Fig. 1 The biosynthesis pathways (**a**) and chemical synthesis pathways (**b**) of shikimic acid

an intermediate product in this pathway to form essential aromatic amino acids [7–11]. The whole biosynthetic pathway of shikimic acid involves six steps with uncontrollable conditions and a low product yield of 36%. Besides, five routes of shikimic acid synthesis (Fig. 1b) have been reported [12–14]. Diels–Alder method [1, 9] possess a low product yield (15%). Quinic acid is used to produce shikimic acid with more than 7 days [8]. The route with the raw material of mannose which is a novel and simplified strategy has five steps and a low product yield of 25% [9]. Tamiflu plays a key role in resisting avian influenza [10, 15]. Tamiflu synthesis has been widely examined which need shikimic acid as raw material, and research on the suitable distribution areas of the 15 *Illicium* species has revealed that these plants as natural sources of shikimic acid can be efficient materials to obtain Tamiflu. Nevertheless, the product yield of shikimic acid is low and synthetic procedure is complex, and the possible ecologically suitable areas for *Illicium* plants are largely unknown [16, 17].

We collated high-quality ground-point data to analyze favorable growing areas for future applications, and we used seven environmental factors to understand the current climate conditions for *Illicium* plant farming. According to ecological niche, we can assess the habitats which are conducive for the growth of the 15 *Illicium* species by using a geographic information system for global medicinal plants (GMPGIS), a software could predict the potential distribution of species based on the climate factors analysis and has been applied in many species such as *Panax ginseng* [18]. Our analyses primarily focused on identifying their suitable habitats of *Illicium* species at a global scale and determining appropriate areas where they could be introduced and cultivated worldwide. This study could enhance our understanding of the distribution range of *Illicium* plants, address problems related to shikimic acid supply, and provide strategies to help protect *I. difengpi* B. N. Chamg, which is an endangered species.

Methods

Data sources of target species

Illicium plants are evergreen trees or shrubs, and they are suited to mountain climate. In this research, the occurrence data points of modeling species distribution were carefully screened to reduce sampling bias and sampling errors from four resources [7, 19]: (1) Chinese Virtual Herbarium (CVH) (http://www.cvh.ac.cn/); (2) National Specimen Information Infrastructure (NSII) (http://www.nsii.org.cn/2017/home.php); (3) literatures; and (4) field work. The number of sampling points is listed in Table 1. Using the website http://www.gpsspg.com/maps.htm, we can obtain the latitude and longitude of each point, and the range of the latitude and longitude of the sampling points is shown in Additional file 1: Table S1.

Environmental variables for modeling

Environmental variables play important roles in determining the potential species' distribution at a global scale. Hence, these variables are widely used to predict the possible suitable habitats of species. In the present study, the environmental characteristics of 15 *Illicium* species were characterized by determining seven environmental variables (annual mean temperature, mean temperature of the coldest quarter, annual precipitation, mean temperature of the warmest quarter, humidity, annual radiation, and soil), which were examined according to statistics, ecology, and botany, as well as their close relationship with plant growth.

GMPGIS modeling

We modeled the potential regions of the 15 *Illicium* species by using the GMPGIS. This system has been verified successfully and has been used to predict potential distributions of many plant species, such as *Panax ginseng* C.A. Mey and *Panax notoginseng* (Burk.) F. H. et al. in China [18, 20, 21]. The following equations were utilized during the prediction of suitable distribution of the 15 *Illicium* species.

Data were standardized as follows:

$$\chi' = \frac{\chi - \min}{\max - \min}$$

Similarity clustering analysis was conducted using the following equation:

$$d_{ij} = \sqrt{(\chi_{11} - \chi_{12})^2 + (\chi_{12} - \chi_{22})^2 + L + (\chi_{p1} - \chi_{p2})^2}$$
$$= \left[\sum \frac{p}{k=1} (\chi_{ki} - \chi_{kj})^2\right]^{\frac{1}{2}}$$

According to the results of distance calculation [$Mind_{ij}$, $Maxd_{ij}$], we reclassified the distance raster, and the areas at 99.9% similarity were considered the suitable distribution with maximum similarities. Besides, after the intersection between the distance layer which is reclassified and the soil layer, the coincident suitable areas for climate and soil conditions could be obtained.

The Minimum Standards of Reporting Checklist contains details of the experimental design, and statistics, and resources used in this study (Additional file 2).

Results

Analysis of seven environmental variables

The specific ranges of the seven environmental variables of the 15 *Illicium* species are shown in Table 2. Different species exist in various soil types. The boxplots containing six environmental variables of the 15 *Illicium* species are illustrated in Fig. 2. Most of the variables showed large ranges in group 1 followed by

Table 2 Range values of the environmental variables for 15 kinds of *Illicium* plants

Chinese name of species	Annual mean temperature/°C	Mean temperature of coldest quarter/°C	Mean temperature of warmest quarter/°C	Annual precipitation/mm	Annual humidity/%	Annual radiation /W m^{-2}
I. verum	11.7–24.0	1.9–18.4	18.9–28.7	909–2266	58.2–77.1	121.9–156.0
	Soil types lixisols, acrisols, fluvisols, etc.					
I. henryi	4.5–22.3	−4.9–14.7	13.7–28.5	697–2107	53.9–76.2	121.5–146.5
	Soil types lixisols, chernozems, plinthosols, arenosols, acrisols, ferralsols, leptosols, etc.					
I. majus	8.9–22.6	−0.8–16.2	17.3–28.5	915–1933	56.2–76.1	120.7–150.6
	Soil types arenosols, lixisols, acrisols, rock debris, chernozems, inland waterways, etc.					
I. simonsii	4.9–20.7	−1.3–14.9	9.8–27.5	782–1675	53.3–73.1	121.9–150.8
	Soil types chernozems, arenosols, acrisols, leptosols, lixisols, luvisols, etc.					
I. micranthum	7.8–23.4	−1.3–18.5	16.1–29.1	865–2077	57.8–77.1	118.5–156.1
	Soil types acrisols, lixisols, arenosols, rhogosols, chernozems, fluvisols, etc.					
I. dunnianum	11.2–23.0	−0.1–16.2	19.9–28.8	553–2203	59.9–76.0	122.1–148.6
	Soil types acrisols, lixisols, arenosols, chernozems, luvisols, rhogosols, etc.					
I. lanceolatum	9.3–21.2	0.1–14.0	17.2–28.5	1092–2305	71.4–76.3	121.8–145.1
	Soil types acrisols, lixisols, anthrosols, arenosols, chernozems, luvisols, etc.					
I. fargesii	6.9–21.5	−2.4–13.3	15.3–28.0	793–1988	60.9–73.2	122.2–137.7
	Soil types acrisols, lixisols, arenosols, rhogosols, chernozems, etc.					
I. jiadifengpi	9.8–22.0	0.6–13.7	18.2–28.7	1457–2104	70.8–73.9	126–142.7
	Soil types acrisols, lixisols, arenosols, rhogosols, etc.					
I. difengpi	16.6–23.0	9.6–15.7	21.6–29.2	1216–1680	72.4–75.2	126.4–137.7
	Soil types acrisols, lixisols, arenosols, rhogosols, chernozems, leptosols, etc.					
I. ternstroemioides	15.1–25.3	5.2–20.9	21.8–28.6	1143–1941	71.8–76.9	123.9–147.6
	Soil types acrisols, fluvisols, chernozems, chernozems, etc.					
I. macranthum	9.5–23.3	4.1–18.5	13.9–28.4	977–1719	63.5–72.7	127.0–153.8
	Soil types acrisols, lixisols leptosols, etc.					
I. oligandrum	20.0–25.2	12.8–20.9	23.5–28.4	1408–1722	72.9–76.9	130.6–147.6
	Soil types acrisols, fluvisols, lixisols, arenosols, etc.					
I. brevistylum	13.3–21.0	3.5–12.5	22.2–28.6	1247–2077	71.1–72.9	123.9–139.4
	Soil types acrisols, chernozems, etc.					
I. pachyphyllum	16.4–17.8	6.1–7.9	25.8–26.6	1190–1505	71.9–72.1	124.1–126.5
	Soil types acrisols, etc.					

15, especially annual mean temperature, mean temperature of the coldest quarter, and annual precipitation. These significant differences could be attributed to different growth environments required by various species.

Ecological niche

Each environmental variable' range was divided into six segments on average, and the area (km^2) of each segment for the 15 *Illicium* species is shown in Fig. 3. These plants were widely distributed at annual mean temperature of 11.5 –22.0 °C, mean temperature of −0.7–16.9 °C in the coldest quarter, and annual precipitation of 551–2016 mm. Furthermore, the potential suitable areas were larger at a mean temperature of 19.6–29.4 °C in the warmest quarter, humidity of 61.2–75.2%, and annual radiation of 124.7–156.2 W m^2.

Analysis of the suitable distribution of the 15 *Illicium* species

The suitable habitat maps based on the occurrence points of the 15 *Illicium* species in CVH, NSII databases, and field work are shown in Figs. 4 and 5 and in Additional file 3: Figure S1. The 15 *Illicium* species are mainly located in the latitude range of 45°S–45°N, which is south and southeast of China, east of the USA, and south of Brazil. The core area in China where these plants are mainly distributed is 1357.68 × 10^4 km^2, which ranks first and accounts for 56% of the total area worldwide. This ranking is followed by the USA with suitable areas of 527.42 × 10^4 km^2. Figure 5 demonstrates that most of the areas in China are climatically suitable for *I. difengpi*, and only a small area spanning approximately 5% exists outside of China. Additional file 3: Figure S1 shows that *I. pachyphyllum*is located only in China.

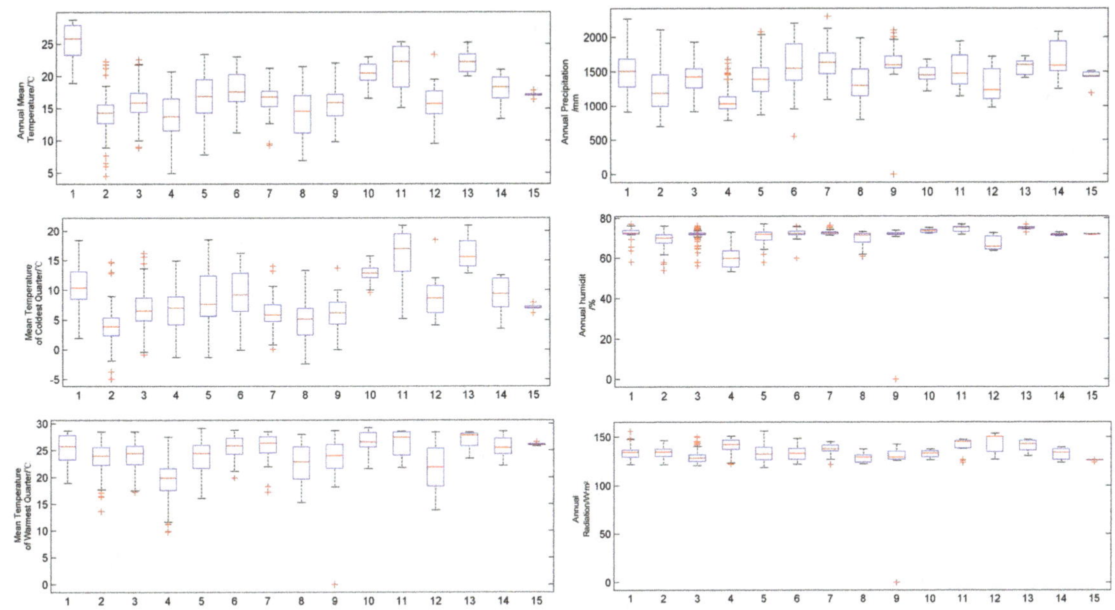

Fig. 2 Boxplot chart of the environmental variables. (1, *I. verum*; 2, *I. henryi*; 3, *I. majus*; 4, *I. simonsii*; 5, *I. micranthum*; 6, *I. dunnianum*; 7, *I. lanceolatum*; 8, *I. fargesii*; 9, *I. jiadifengpi*; 10, *I. difengpi*; 11, *I. ternstroemioides*; 12, *I. macranthum*; 13, *I. oligandrum*; 14, *I. brevistylum*; 15, *I. pachyphyllum*)

According to the map, the potential suitable habitats of the 15 *Illicium* species are found in six provinces in China (Fig. 6): Guangxi, Yunnan, Hunan, Guizhou, Sichuan, and Hubei. The specific suitable areas of each *Illicium* plant in China and other countries are shown in Additional file 1: Tables S2, S3.

a. *I. verum* Hook. f, an edible plant whose main producing area is Guangxi from China, which is recognized by National Health and Family Planning Commission, has a potential habitat with a total area of 377.9×10^4 km^2 (19%) worldwide. It also covers approximately 64.04×10^4 km^2 (18%) in the USA and 60.5×10^4 km^2 (48%) in Brazil. The core areas are approximately 158.8×10^4 km^2, which are mainly located in Yunnan, Guangxi, Hunan, and other places in China.
b. *I. henryi* Diels is a Chinese endemic species and its main producing areas are Shannxi and Gansu. Its favorable area measured approximately 407.4×10^4 km^2 worldwide. It is distributed at 100.3×10^4 km^2 (25%) in the USA, which has the second-largest coverage. This species also thrives at 23.3×10^4 (6%) and 16.4×10^4 km^2 (4%) in France and Italy, respectively. The core areas cover 176.3×10^4 km^2 (43%) in Yunnan, Guangxi, Guangdong, and Hunan in China.
c. *I. majus* Hook. f is mainly produced in Hunan which has a suitable habitat with an area of 275.9×10^4 km^2 worldwide. Its favorable habitats in the USA, Brazil, and Japan cover 70.1×10^4 (25%), 13.1×10^4 (5%), and 6.5×10^4 km^2 (6%), respectively. The core areas account for 59%, or approximately 62.0×10^4 km^2, of the land area in Guangxi, Yunnan, Hunan, and Sichuan in China.
d. *I. simonsii* Maxim is prevailingly occurred in Guizhou and Sichuan. It has a globally potential suitable area of 272.6×10^4 km^2. It covers 78.9×10^4 (29%), 14.5×10^4 (5%), 14.0×10^4 (5%), and 5.7×10^4 km^2 (3%) suitable areas in the USA, Spain, Italy, and France, respectively. The core areas spanning 113.5×10^4 km^2 (42%) are mainly distributed in Yunnan, Hunan, and Guizhou provinces in China.
e. *I. micranthum* Dunn, is a native species chiefly in Fujian and Hubei, in China. The area of its suitable habitat is approximately 435.37×10^4 km^2. Its distribution areas in the USA, Brazil, and Japan are 107.86×10^4 (24%), 56.38×10^4 (13%), and 9.04×10^4 km^2 (13%), respectively. The core areas spanning 190.7×10^4 km^2 (44%) are mainly located in Hunan, Guangxi, and Yunnan in China.
f. *I. dunnianum* Tutch, is a species endemic to China mainly in Fujian and Hunan. Its suitable habitat worldwide has a land area of 263.1×10^4 km^2. This species also covers an area of 47.2×10^4 km^2 (18%) in the USA. The core areas spanning 62% are mainly distributed in China, especially in Guangxi, Hunan, and Jiangxi provinces.

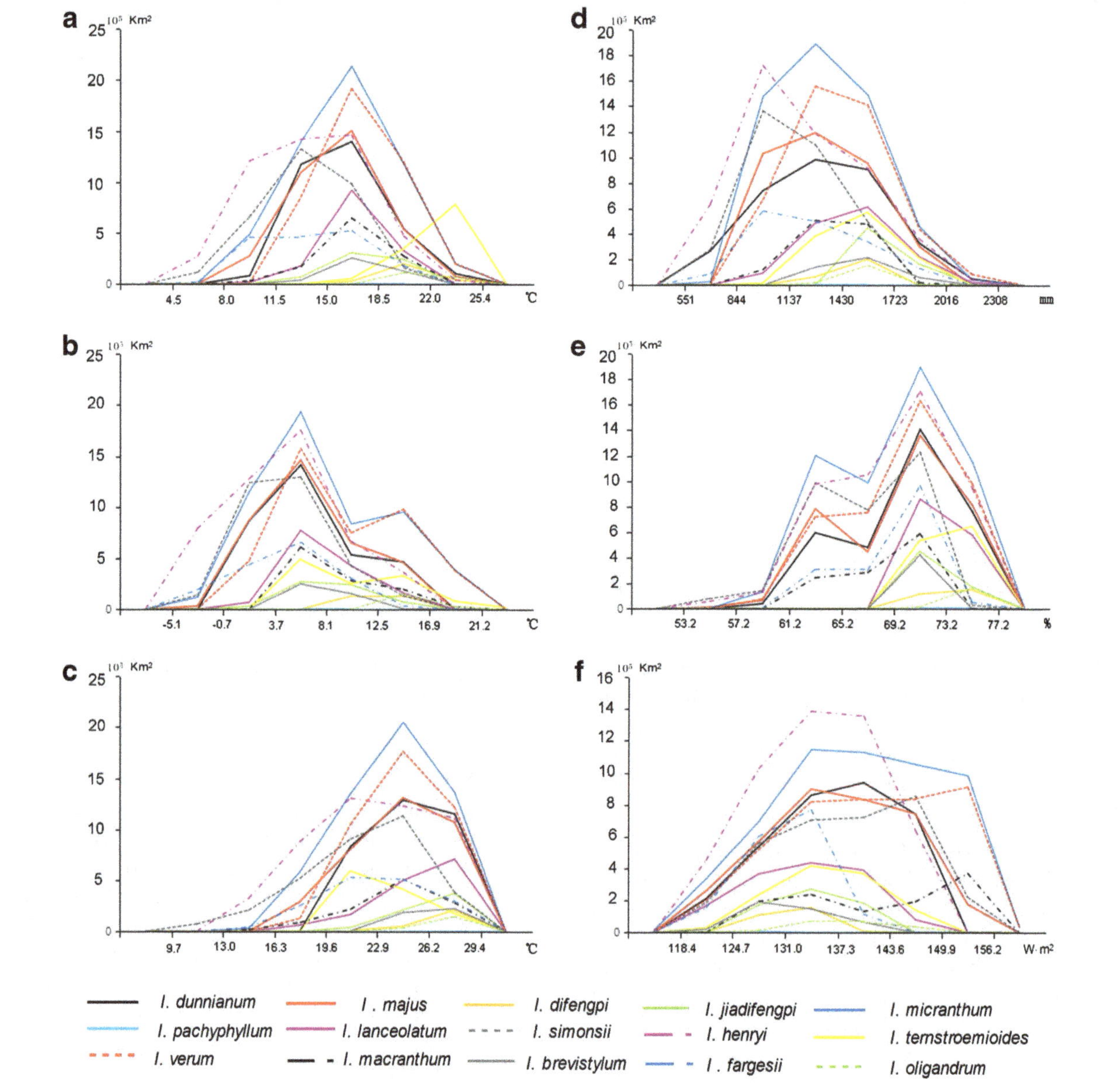

Fig. 3 The ecological niche of every environmental variables. **a** Annual mean temperature; **b** mean temperature of coldest quarter; **c** mean temperature of warmest quarter; **d** annual precipitation; **e** annual humidity and annual radiation

g. *I. lanceolatum* A. C. Smith is a native species in China and mostly in Jiangsu and Anhui. It possess a potential suitable area of 109.1×10^4 km^2 worldwide. This species covers an area of approximately 8% of the total distribution area in Brazil. It is also distributed in Vietnam, Japan, and the USA with respective areas of 1.4×10^4, 1.6×10^4, and 0.2×10^4 km^2, which account for 1%. Its potential suitable habitat with an area of 95.1×10^4 km^2 (87%) is located in China, particularly in Hunan, Jiangxi, and Guangxi provinces.

h. *I. fargesii* Finet & Gagnep is a species endemic to China, its main producing areas are Guizhou and Hunan. It has a suitable area of 135.2×10^4 km^2. This species covers 31.8×10^4 (24%) and 5.8×10^4 km^2 (4%) in the USA and Japan. Its potential distribution area in China is 71.7×10^4 km^2 (53%) spanning Guizhou, Hunan, and Guangxi provinces.

i. *I. jiadifengpi* B. N. Chang principally grows in Anhui and Zhejiang, which has a suitable habitat with an area of 45.4×10^4 km^2 worldwide. This species respectively covers 0.6×10^4 and 0.5×10^4

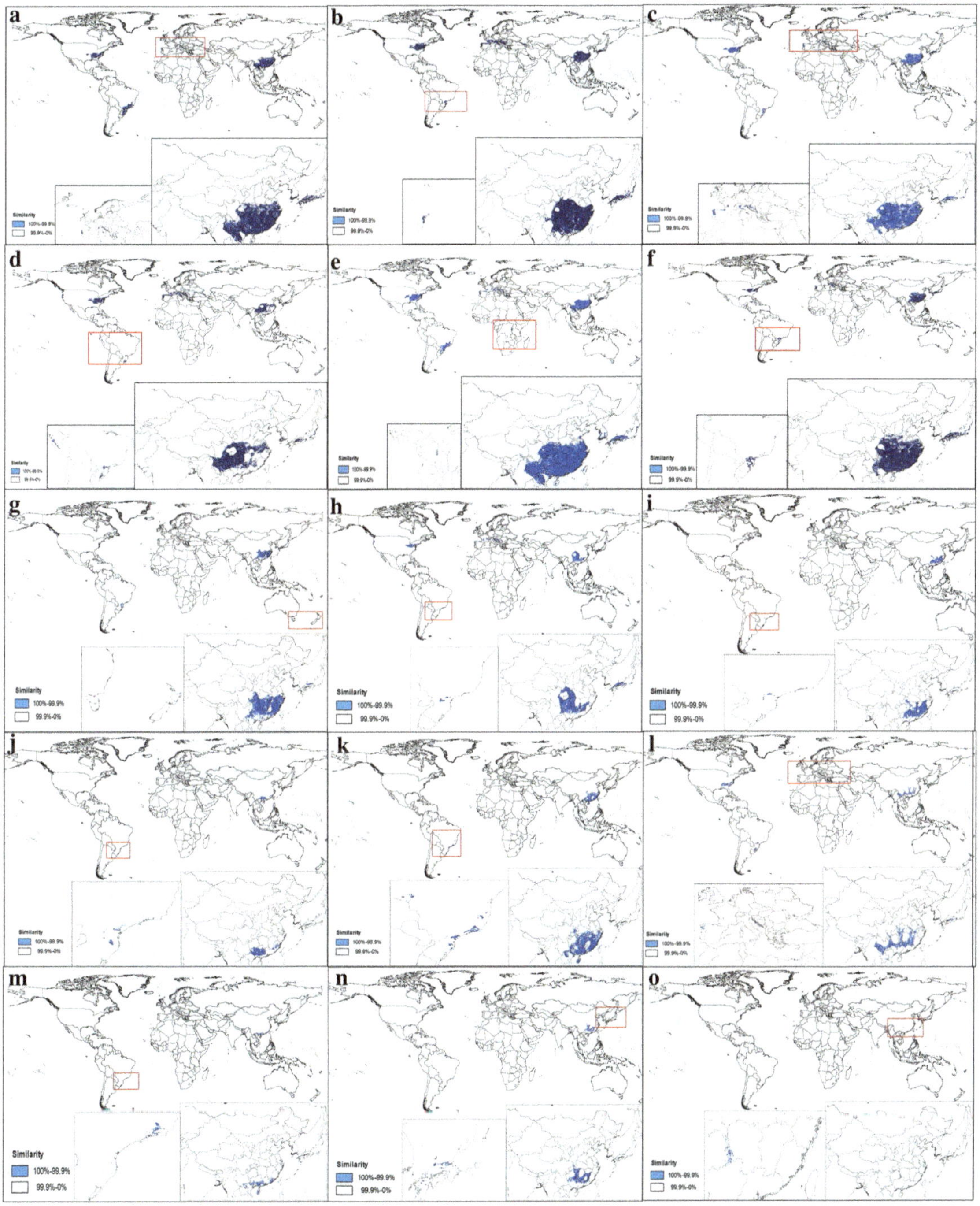

Fig. 4 Suitable areas in China and in the world of 15 *illicium* plants. (**a** *I. verum*; **b** *I. henryi*; **c** *I. majus*; **d** *I. simonsii*; **e** *I. micranthum*; **f** *I. dunnianum*; **g** *I. lanceolatum*; **h** *I. fargesii*; **i** *I. jiadifengpi*; **j** *I. difengpi*; **k** *I. ternstroemioides*; **l** *I. macranthum*; **m** *I. oligandrum*; **n** *I. brevistylum*; **o** *I. pachyphyllum*)

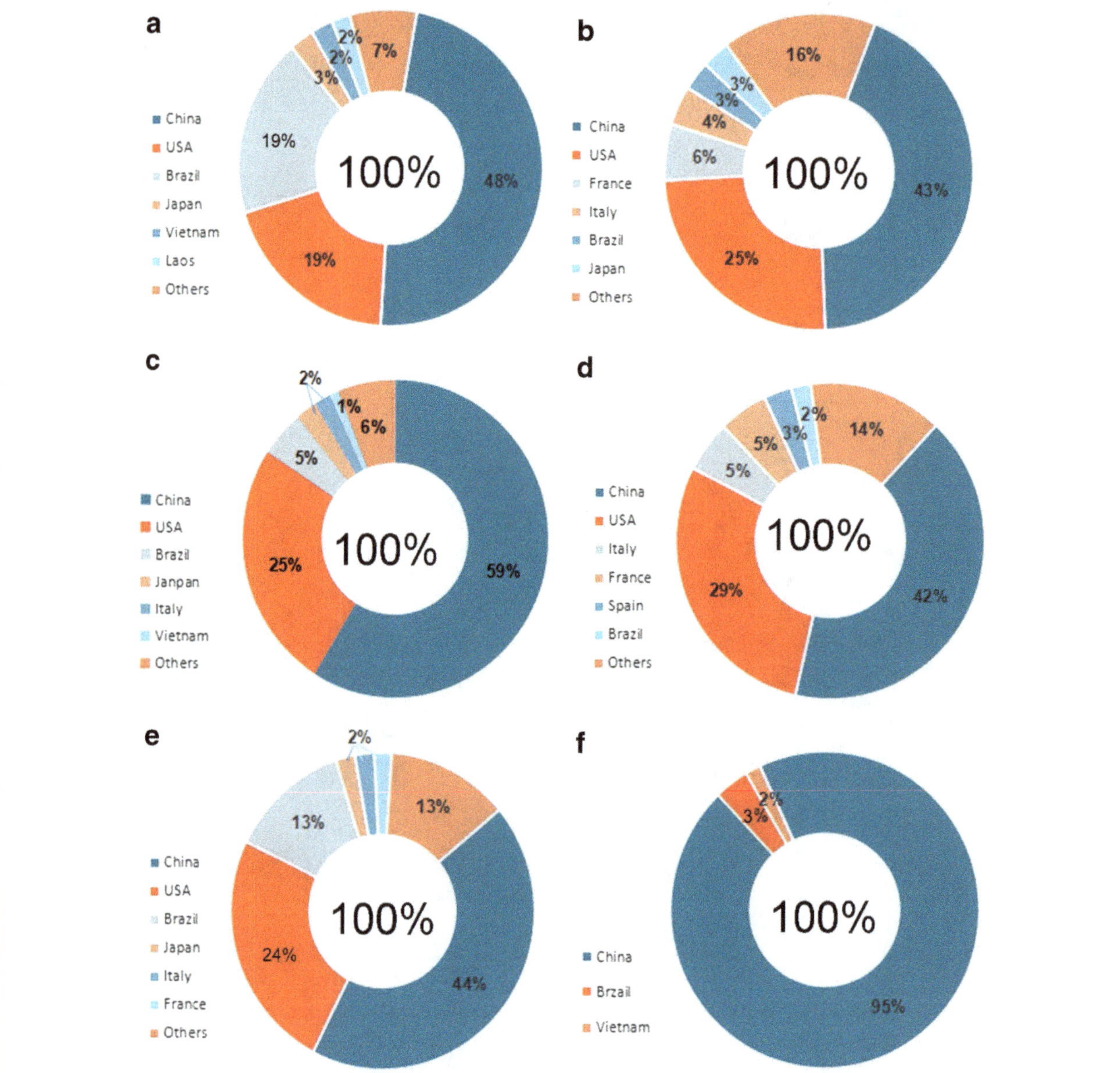

Fig. 5 The ratio of suitable areas in the world of six typical *Illicium* plants. (**a** *I. verum;* **b** *I. henryi;* **c** *I. majus;* **d** *I. simonsii;* **e** *I. micranthum,* **f** *I. difengpi*)

km^2, or equivalent to 1% of the total area worldwide, in Japan and Brazil. A large proportion of the area corresponding to 45.4×10^4 km^2 (98%) is mainly distributed in Anhui, Zhejiang, Guangxi, and Guangdong provinces in China.

j. *I. difengpi* B. N. Chamg prevailingly grows in Guangxi and Yunnan, China and is recorded as endangered in the Endangered Species Act, it covers a potential suitable area of 20.1×10^4 km^2. This species is distributed in 0.7×10^4 (3%) and 0.3×10^4 km^2 (2%) in Vietnam and Brazil, respectively. Its largest suitable area is 19.0×10^4 km^2 (95%), which is mainly located in Guangxi and southeast of Yunnan in China.

k. *I. ternstroemioides* A. C. Smith, a native species in China, mainly in Hainan, has a total potential suitable area of 88.7×10^4 km^2. This species covers 6.8×10^4 (8%) and 4.3×10^4 km^2 (5%) in Brazil and Vietnam, respectively. The core areas measuring 76.7×10^4 km^2 (85%) are mainly located in Hainan, Fujian, Hunan, and Guangdong provinces in China.

l. *I. macranthum* A. C. Smith primarily occurred in Yunnan, China, has a total potential suitable area of 89.9×10^4 km^2. This species is distributed in

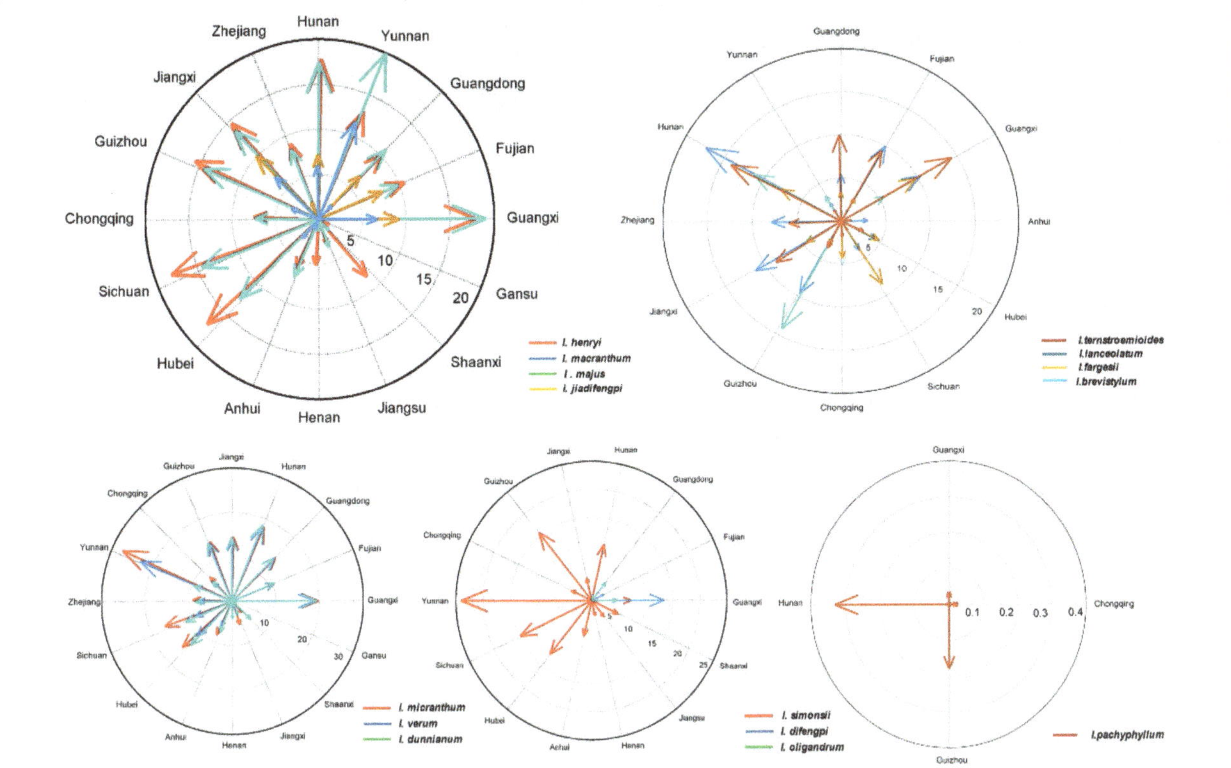

Fig. 6 Suitable areas in every provinces in China of 15 *illicium* plants

areas of 27.3×10^4 (30%) and 9.6×10^4 km^2 (12%) in the USA and Brazil, respectively. This species also occupies the largest suitable habitat area of 44.6×10^4 km^2 (49%) found in Yunnan and Jiangxi provinces in China.

m. *I. oligandrum* Merr.et Chun, chiefly grows in Guangxi and Hainan from China, has a total potential suitable area of 13.6×10^4 km^2. This species respectively covers 2.53×10^4 (18%) and 9.9×10^4 km^2 in Vietnam and China (Guangdong and Guangxi provinces), and this coverage accounts for 73% of the total area worldwide.

n. *I. brevistylum* A. C. Smith, a species endemic to China, mainly in Fujian and Hunan, has a globally potential distribution area of 31.8×10^4 km^2. It covers 0.6×10^4 km^2 (2%) in Japan and 31.2×10^4 km^2 (98%) in other regions, such as Fujian, Guangdong, Guangxi, and Hunan provinces in China.

o. *I. pachyphyllum* A. C. Smith, another species endemic to China, principally in Hunan and Guangdong, has a potential suitable habitat with an area of 0.5×10^4 km^2 in Hunan, Guizhou, and Guangxi provinces in China. This observation is consistent with our current findings.

Discussion

In this study, spatial analysis was conducted using GMPGIS to define the spatial distribution of habitat suitability and the range of each variable for two classes of habitats of 15 *Illicium* species. According to the analysis of environmental variables, it is easy to be concluded that different *Illicium* species exist in different requirement on a growing environment. In addition, Our GMPGIS models successfully showed that the most suitable climate condition for these plants are annual mean temperature of 11.5–22.0 °C, mean temperature of − 0.7–16.9 °C in the coldest quarter, and annual precipitation of 551–2016 mm, in which are roughly consistent with the known regions where the 15 *Illicium* species exist and mostly located in a large range from S 45° to N 45°. On the basis of the climatic suitable maps of these plants, we can conclude that they covered an area of 1356.75×10^4 km^2 in China, which ranked first, followed by the USA with an area of 527.42×10^4 km^2. We speculated that the reason for China topped the rankings is not only China has vast areas could grow *Illicium* plants, but also there are many endemic species in China such as *I. fargesii*, *I. brevistylum* and *I. pachyphyllum*. *I. verum* with a high shikimic acid content is mainly distributed in China (48%) and in the USA (19%). The suitable habitats of *I. difengpi* cover 95, 3, and 2% in China, Brazil, and Vietnam, respectively.

Conclusion

According to the data on suitable habitats, we recommended that *I. verum* can be expanded to suitable regions, such as southeast of China and south of Brazil, to solve problems on shikimic acid shortage. *I. difengpi* can be introduced to Vietnam and Brazil and can thus mitigate its risk of becoming endangered. Some species, such as *I. henryi, I. micranthum,* and *I. dunnianum,* which are endemic to China, can be introduced and cultivated in the USA or other favorable regions. This approach possibly addresses the high demands for shikimic acid, protects the diversity of rare or endangered species, and helps governments establish various protection strategies for future ecological conservation.

Abbreviations

GMPGIS: geographic information system for global medicinal plants; CVH: Chinese Virtual Herbarium; NSII: National Specimen Information Infrastructure.

Authors' contributions

LFH and SLC conceived the ideas and designed methodology; XZ collected and analyzed the data of 15 *Illicium* species together with XXM and JW; XZ was a major contributor in writing the manuscript. All authors read and approved the final manuscript.

Acknowledgements

This study is supported and sponsored by the National Natural Science Foundation of China (No. 81473315) and the CAMS Innovation Fund for Medical Sciences, Grant CIFMS (No. 2016-I2M-3-015).

Competing interests

The authors declare that they have no competing interests.

Consent for publication

All of authors consent to publication of this study in Journal of Chinese Medicine.

Funding

This study was supported by the National Natural Science Foundation of China (No. 81473315) and the CAMS Innovation Fund for Medical Sciences, Grant CIFMS (No. 2016-I2M-3-015).

References

1. Rawat G, Tripathi P, Saxena RK. Expanding horizons of shikimic acid. Appl Microbiol Biotechnol. 2013;97:4277–87.
2. Bochkov DV, Sysolyatin SV, Kalashnikov AI, Surmacheva IA. Shikimic acid: review of its analytical, isolation, and purification techniques from plant and microbial sources. J Chem Biol. 2012;5:5–17.
3. Farina V, Brown JD. Tamiflu: the supply problem. Angew Chem. 2006;45(44):7330–4. https://doi.org/10.1002/anie.200602623.
4. Pang X. Research progress in shikimic acid. Heilongjiang Med J. 2011;24(5):700–2.
5. Li G, Du S, Wen Z. Mapping the climatic suitable habitat of oriental arborvitae (*Platycladus orientalis*) for introduction and cultivation at a global scale. Sci Rep. 2016;6:30009.
6. Lin Q. Medicinal plant resources of Illicium L. Chin Tradit Herbal Drugs. 2002;2002(7):81–4.
7. Yi YJ, Cheng X, Yang ZF, Zhang SH. Maxent modeling for predicting the potential distribution of endangered medicinal plant (*H. riparia* Lour) in Yunnan, China. Ecol Eng. 2016;92:260–9.
8. Box JM, Harwood LM, Humphreys JL, Morris GA, Redon PM, Whitehead RC. Dehydration of quinate derivatives: synthesis of a difluoromethylene homologue of shikimic acid. Synlett. 2002;2002:0358–60.
9. Ghosh S, Chisti Y, Banerjee UC. Production of shikimic acid. Biotechnol Adv. 2012;30:1425.
10. Nie LD, Shi XX, Ko KH, Lu WD. A short and practical synthesis of oseltamivir phosphate (Tamiflu) from (−)-shikimic acid. J Org Chem. 2009;74:3970.
11. Huang LF, Wang ZH, Chen SL. Hypericin: chemical synthesis and biosynthesis. Chin J Nat Med. 2014;12:81–8.
12. Zhang, Lu T, Zhang H, Cheng FM, Liu J. Recent progress in the synthesis of tamiflu. Chin J Org Chem. 2013;33:1235.
13. Kou YH, Lei Y. Synthesis of shikimic acid. J Shaanxi Univ Sci Technol. 2011;29(3):53–9.
14. Zhan Y, Ouyang H. The study on the process of application and preparation of Shikimic acid. Chem Intermed. 2012;9(5):1–5.
15. Liu Y. Research advance in Shikimic acid. Chem Ind Times. 2007;2007(3):54–7.
16. Guo Y, Li X, Zhao Z, Wei H, Gao B, Gu W. Prediction of the potential geographic distribution of the ectomycorrhizal mushroom *Tricholoma matsutake* under multiple climate change scenarios. Sci Rep. 2017;7:46221.
17. Manyangadze T, Chimbari MJ, Gebreslasie M, Ceccato P, Mukaratirwa S. Modelling the spatial and seasonal distribution of suitable habitats of schistosomiasis intermediate host snails using Maxent in Ndumo area, KwaZulu-Natal Province, South Africa. Parasites Vectors. 2016;9:572.
18. Liang S, Jie WU, Xi-Wen LI, Jiang XU, Dong LL, Sang MC, Sun CZ, Fujihara N, Chen SL. A study of global ecological adaptability and field selection practices of *Panax ginseng*. China J Chin Mater Med. 2016;41(18):3314–22.
19. Liu D, Wang R, Gordon DR, Sun X, Chen L, Wang Y. Predicting plant invasions following China's Water Diversion Project. Environ Sci Technol. 2017;51:1450.
20. Meng XX, Huang LF, Dong LL, Xi-Wen LI, Wei FG, Chen ZJ, Jie WU, Sun CZ, Yu-Qi YU, Chen SL. Analysis of global ecology of *Panax notoginseng* in suitability and quality. Acta Pharm Sin. 2016;51(9):1483–93.
21. Huang L, Xie C, Duan B, Chen S. Mapping the potential distribution of high artemisinin-yielding *Artemisia annua* L. (Qinghao) in China with a geographic information system. Chin Med. 2010;5:18.

11

Bioactive polysaccharides from natural resources including Chinese medicinal herbs on tissue repair

Qiu Li, Yiming Niu, Panfei Xing and Chunming Wang*

Abstract

Background: Functional polysaccharides can be derived from plants (including herbs), animals and microorganisms. They have been widely used in a broad of biomedical applications, such as immunoregulatory agents or drug delivery vehicles. In the past few years, increasing studies have started to develop natural polysaccharides-based biomaterials for various applications in tissue engineering and regenerative medicine.

Main body: We discuss in this article the emerging applications of natural polysaccharides—particularly those derived from Chinese medicine—for wound healing. First, we introduce natural polysaccharides of three natural sources and their biological activities. Then, we focus on certain natural polysaccharides with growth factor-binding affinities and their inspired polymeric tools, with an emphasis on how these polysaccharides could possibly benefit wound healing. Finally, we report the latest progress in the discovery of polysaccharides from Chinese medicinal herbs with identified activities favouring tissue repair.

Conclusion: Natural polysaccharides with clearly elucidated compositions/structures, identified cellular activities, as well as desirable physical properties have shown the potential to serve as therapeutic tools for tissue regeneration.

Keywords: Polysaccharides, Chinese medicinal herbs, Biomedical applications

Background

The carbohydrates, along with proteins, lipids and nucleic acids, are regarded as the major biomacromolecules. Most carbohydrates found in nature existing as polysaccharides are composed of monosaccharides [1], which can be found in almost all kingdoms of life, such as the algae [2] (e.g. alginate), plants [3] (e.g. starch and cellulose), microbes [4] (e.g. zymosan and dextran) and animals [5] (e.g. hyaluronic acid and heparin). Polysaccharides can be classified according to their electric charge: cationic polysaccharide [6] (chitin, chitosan), anionic polysaccharide [7, 8] (heparin, hyaluronic acid, alginic acid and chondroitin sulfate) and nonionic polysaccharide [9] (dextran, starch, and cellulose). In terms of chemical composition, polysaccharides can also be classified as the homo-polysaccharide [10] containing a single type of monosaccharide and hetero-polysaccharide [11] containing two or more different types of monosaccharides. For example, cellulose consists of unique glucose and heparin consists of the α-L-idopyranosyluronic acid 2-sulfate and 2-deoxy-2-sulfoamino-α-D-glucopyranose 6-sulfate [12]. Based on the different glycosides linked with glycan, polysaccharides also exist in the forms of proteoglycans, glycolipids and glycoconjugates. The rapid development of bioanalytical technology has enabled to understand the structure of polysaccharides and utilise their functions. Polysaccharides, together with oligosaccharides, not only serve as the building blocks of the life but also mediate many biological signals, including cell–cell communication [13], immune recognition [14], and mitogenesis [15].

These findings motivate the development of polysaccharides for biomedical applications—as therapeutic

*Correspondence: cmwang@umac.mo
State Key Laboratory of Quality Research in Chinese Medicine, Institute of Chinese Medical Sciences, University of Macau, Avenida da Universidade, Macau SAR, China

agents, drug carriers and tissue scaffolds. For instance, starch and glycogen have long been used as biofuels [16], adjuvants and food additives [17]. More applications of polysaccharides are also inspired by their native functions in constructing the extracellular matrix and supporting cell adhesion and proliferation [18]. However, unlike proteins that can be more accurately characterised and 'bottom-up' synthesised, polysaccharides are generally very difficult to characterise for a precise structure, based on the current technical conditions. Polysaccharides have diverse chemical structure, composition, molecular weight, potential and linking sequence, all of which result in different functionality and biological activity [19]. Therefore, it is both interesting and challenging to obtain novel, functional polysaccharides and elucidate the relationship between its structure and activity. Successful understanding of the mechanism of biological effects requires multidisciplinary knowledge and various technologies. Here, we concisely review the previous research into naturally derived functional polysaccharides in biomedical science, and discuss the potential of those derived from Chinese medicine in tissue regeneration, which may represent a promising direction in this field of research [20–28] (Table 1).

Table 1 Various polysaccharides in nature

Polysaccharides	Source	Functions
Starch	Plants	Storage, drug adjuvant
Cellulose	Plants	Cell structure, food additives
Pectin	Plants	Food additives
Alginate	Microorganism	Drug adjuvant
Carrageenan	Microorganism	Food additives
Heparin	Animals	Animal tissue structure, therapeutic agents
Hyaluronan	Animals	Animal tissue structure, therapeutic agents
Chondroitin sulfate	Animals	Animal tissue structure
Heparin sulfate	Animals	Animal tissue structure
Chitin and chitosan	Animals	Tissue scaffolds

Plant polysaccharides: biological activities and biomedical applications

In the past decades, the polysaccharides derived from herbs, such as various Chinese medicines, have attracted much attention in a multiple of fields. Numerous researches indicate that polysaccharides can be used in many fields and have a diverse of therapeutic properties, such as antioxidant activity [29], antitumor activity [30], the effect of promoting wound healing [31] and immunostimulatory activity [32].

Firstly, plant polysaccharides have been used for industrial applications, e.g. pharmaceuticals, biomaterials, food stuff and nutrition, and biofuels. For example, a variety of indigestible plant polysaccharides including cellulose, hemicelluloses, pectins, oligosaccharides, gums, was defined as the dietary fiber by the Food and Agriculture Organization (FAO). Among these, cellulose and hemicellulose can directly stimulate the bowel movement, which is the most widely spreading polymeric material in nature, is a fibrous, tough, water-insoluble material. The cellulose commonly found in the cell walls of plants-stalks, stems or trunks, is a linear polysaccharide consisting of β-D-glucan units linked by (1 → 4) glycosidic bonds [33]. The materials based on the cellulose have been extensively used in biomedical field [34], such as the adsorbent beads, filter, artificial tissue, and protective clothing. Among these applications, the cellulose due to the mechanical strength and biocompatibility, can be applied for tissue engineering [35], including engineering vascular tissue, and a series of other tissues, such as bone, cartilage, skeletal muscle, cardiac muscle, and heart valves. Additionally, cellulose has also been used to establish nano-fibrous carrier for liver cells and create tubes for regeneration of damaged peripheral nerves. Gu performed the research of creating carriers for delivery and differentiation of mesenchymal stem cells [36]. However, the applications of the cellulose are limited by the solubility in common organic solvents. It is difficult to melt due to the strong intermolecular and intramolecular hydrogen bonds.

Secondly, herbs have been used to treat kinds of illnesses and modern pharmacological experiments have identified that the main or key components of herbal medicines generally include much ingredients. Of these fractions in herbal medicines, polysaccharides have been identified as major active ingredients, responsible for various pharmacological activities. Although the detailed mechanism of these effects is under exploration, the immunostimulatory activities of many polysaccharides are confirmed. It appears that immune cells, especially macrophages [3], involve this regulating process. Macrophages play a vital role in kinds of complex microbicidal functions, including the surveillance [37], chemotaxis [38], phagocytosis [39], and degradation of the target organisms. And polysaccharides can modulate the function of macrophages. The studies about the effects of plant polysaccharides on macrophage functions have demonstrated that glycan can enhance macrophage functions, which include activating phagocytic ability [40], increasing the cytotoxic activity against the tumour cells, reactive oxygen species (ROS) and nitric oxide (NO) production, and secretion of cytokines and chemokines, such as tumour necrosis factor (TNF-α), interleukin-1β (IL-1β), IL-6, IL-12 and so on [41]. For example, Schepetkin and Quinn extracted a polysaccharide from the cones of *Juniperus scopulorum*, which composed of arabinogalactan, and showed significant immunomodulatory effect to the murine macrophages [42]. It was certified that the polysaccharide caused the increasing expression of macrophage iNOS and NO, enhanced secretion of cytokines like IL-1, IL-6, IL-12, IL-10 and TNF-α. Popov and Ovodov isolated and obtained a pectic polysaccharide from *Silene vulgaris*, which can enhance the myeloperoxidase activity of macrophage via extracellular Ca^{2+}, whereas, the polysaccharide obtained from the same species can show the same effect without the extracellular Ca^{2+}. We can conclude that the polysaccharides from the same plant may induce different signal transductions. Luk found that polysaccharides extracted from the *Tripterygium wilfordii* exhibited the effect of suppressing the secretion of TNF-α and expression of some proteins (CD11c, CD18, CD14 and CD54) in human monocytic THP-1 cells [43, 44]. Additionally, polysaccharides derived from herbs can also induce macrophage hematopoiesis [3]. Song found that polysaccharides from *Chelidonium majus* could increase the amount of granulocyte–macrophage colony-forming cells in experimental animals [45]. Meanwhile, a polysaccharide from *Aloe barbadensis* also showed significant hematopoietic effect and induced production of monocytes [46].

We found that polysaccharides from plants activate macrophages mainly via the interaction with specific receptors on cells, which are usually known as pattern recognition receptors. Macrophages could bind and interact with the polysaccharides through toll-like receptor 4 (TLR4) [47], CD14 [48], dectin-1 [49] and mannose receptor [50], among others. After the activation of the receptors, it can lead to downstream signal and production of pro-inflammatory factors. Ando and Kataoka found that polysaccharides extracted from *Carthamus tinctorius* could active the macrophage through TLR4, inducing downstream signals and expression of TNF-α and NO [51]. Further, the test in vitro was performed in peritoneal macrophage from the C3H/HeJ mice which have a point mutation in the TLR4 gene and the activating effect disappeared. Moreover, regarding the polysaccharides from the roots of *Astragalus membranaceus*, the results also showed that the relative response disappeared in the peritoneal macrophage from the C3H/HeJ mice [52]. It suggested that the TLR4 receptor involved the signal transaction of macrophage activation.

In summary, carbohydrates may interact with macrophages and regulate these cells in diverse mechanisms, some of which are shown in Fig. 1. For example, carbohydrates interact with the TLR4/MD-2 complex resulting in

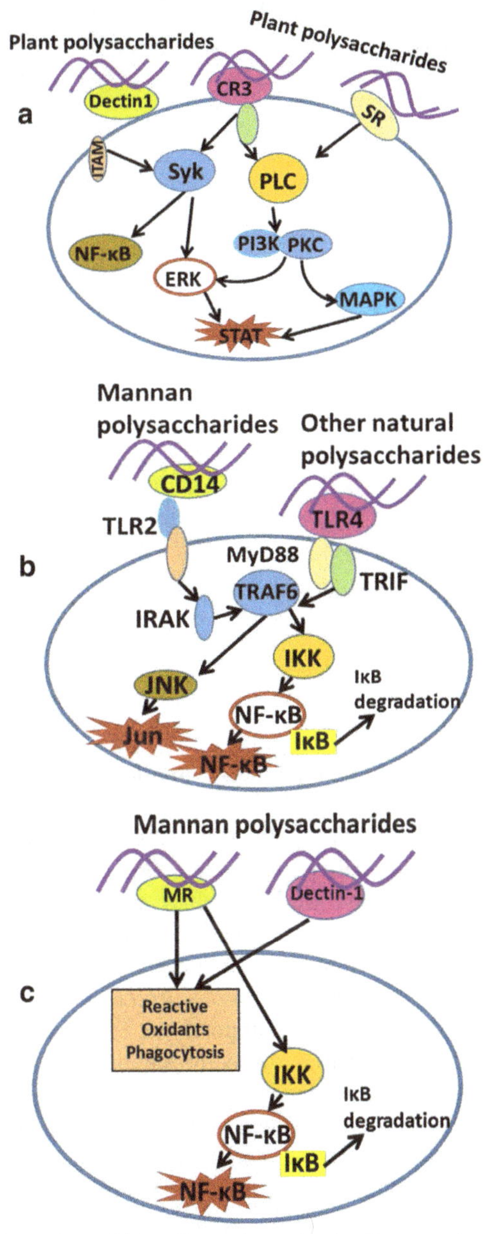

Fig. 1 **a–c** Potential signalling pathways involved in macrophage activation by plant polysaccharides [3, 53]

dimerisation of two TLR4/MD-2 complexes, recruitment of two adaptor molecules, MyD88 and TRIF, and activation of intracellular signalling pathways (NF-κB) [53]. The mannose receptor is also a potential receptor inducing macrophage phagocytosis, endocytosis and NF-κB signalling pathways. Additionally, CR3 is involved in the activation of phosphoinositide-3-kinase (PI3K), the mitogen-activated protein kinase (MAPK) and NF-κB signalling pathways (Table 2; [54–60]).

Table 2 The polysaccharides derived from herbs in nature

Polysaccharides	Composition	Source	Physiological effects
Cellulose	β-(1-4)-Linked-glucopyranose	Grains, fruit, vegetables	Cell structure, food additives, regulate bowel movement
Juniperus scopolorum polysaccharide	β-Galactopyranose, and α-arabinofuranose	*Juniperus scopulorum*	Immunomodulatory effect to the murine macrophages
Konjac glucomannan polysaccharide	β-(1-4)-Linked-glucose, β-(1-4)-linked-mannose	*Amorphophallus konjac* plant	Cholesterol lowering and immunoregulation
Chelidonium majus polysaccharide	Galactose, mannose, glucose in the molar ratio of 5:4:1	*Chelidonium majus*	An effective antitumor immunostimulator
Reishi polysaccharide	Arabinose, rhamnose, xylose, mannose, glucose at the different ratios	*Ganoderma lucidum*	Stimulating the expression of inflammatory cytokines
Ginseng polysaccharide	(1-4)-Linked homogalacturonan backbone	*Ginseng*, the root of *Panax ginseng*	Anti-rotavirus activity
Bletilla striata polysaccharide	α-Mannose, β-mannose and β-glucose at the ratio of 2.4:1	*Bletilla striata*	Modulating the function of macrophages
Eucommia ulmoides polysaccharide	Mannose, galactose, glucose, arabinose, rhamnose, and galacturonic acid	*Eucommia ulmoides*	Binding PDGF-BB growth factor and anti-inflammatory effect
Astragalus polysaccharides	Rhamnose, arabinose and glucose in a molar ratio of 1:6.25:17.86	The roots of *Astragalus*	The effect of immunomodulatory
Pectin	α-(1-4)-D-Galacturonic acid and rhamnose	Plant primary cell wall	Food additives

Animal-derived polysaccharides: potential biomedical functions

Except for functional polysaccharides from herbs, the polysaccharides derived from animals also play a vital role as tissue composition and exhibit significant effect in biomedical science. Among these, extracellular matrix in animal tissues, composed of an interlocking meshwork of heteropolysaccharides and fibrous proteins, is filled with a gel-like material, which supports cell adhesion, growth and provides a porous pathway for the diffusion of nutrients and oxygen to individual cells [61]. For instance, the heteropolysaccharides, called glycosaminoglycans, are a family of linear polymers composed of repeating disaccharide units [62]. Glycosaminoglycans (GAGs) include hyaluronic acid, heparin and heparan sulfate, chondroitin sulfate (CS), dermatan sulfate, keratin sulfate. In addition to GAGs, the chitosan and chitin also belong to animal derived polysaccharides, which are widely used in biomedical science.

Heparin and heparan sulfate

Heparin possessing highly sulfated, linear structure is an important member of glycosaminoglycans (GAGs), which consists in repeated units of sulfonated hexuronic acid ($1 \rightarrow 4$) D-glucosamine. The residue of uronic acid in heparin consisting of α-L-iduronic acid (IdoA) or β-D-glucuronic acid (GlcA) can be sulfated at 2-*O* position. The residue of glucosamine can present unmodified (GlcN), *N*-sulfonated (GlcNS), or *N*-acetylated (GlcNAc), with various *O*-sulfations at the 3-*O* and 6-*O* positions [63]. And heparan sulfate has a higher ratio of IdoA residues and sulfate groups.

Heparin can be biosynthesized and stored in mast cells, whereas heparan sulfate as a proteoglycan, mainly exists on the surface of cells and in extracellular matrix of tissue. Heparin widely used as one of the oldest drug in clinic plays part in many physiological and pathophysiological processes, such as angiogenesis, cell adhesion, cell growth, inflammation and anticoagulation [64, 65]. Numerous researches indicated that heparin could modulate the relative biological processes via binding with the basic amino acid groups of proteins, such as binding with growth factors [66], forming the complex to stabilize growth factors and prolong the function of growth factors. For example, Shah and Revzin prepared bioactive heparin-based hydrogel systems, which showed sustained release of hepatocyte growth factor [67]. The common function of heparin is the anticoagulation activity which induce the effect by interacting with the serine protease inhibitor antithrombin III [68]. With regard to heparan sulfate, it is reported that heparan sulfate on the cell surface serves as the receptors of adhesion for many bacterial pathogens [69].

Although heparin as clinical drug has been used for treating venous thrombosis, pulmonary embolism, and acute coronary syndrome [70], there are still some limitations including having the risks of potential bleeding and heparin-induced thrombocytopenia [71]. Thus, the low molecular weight heparin obtained from the unfractionated heparin were developed into therapeutic agent to alleviating side effects in clinic [72]. Certainly, more understanding of the structure–activity relationship is required in the relative biological processes. We can further explore the drugs derived from heparin and heparan sulfate to improve therapeutic effect in clinic.

Hyaluronic acid

The hyaluronic acid owning high molecular weight [73], which is an anionic and non-sulfate polysaccharide and consists of alternating units of D-glucuronic acid, and *N*-acetyl-D-glucosamine, is the component of ECM. It was discovered by Karl Meyer and his assistant, John Palmer in 1934. The hyaluronic acid is a naturally substance which is naturally existing in our body, and has crucial biological functions in our body [74, 75]. In human body, it is found in most connective tissues, especially in the eyes and joints. The use of hyaluronic acid in some eye surgeries including the cataract removal, corneal transplantation, and repair of a detached retina and other eye injuries, has been approved by FDA. It can be injected into the eye during the process to aid instead natural fluids [76].

According to numerous studies, hyaluronic acid (HA) owns various biological activities. It has chondroprotective effects in vivo and can evidently influence on the articular cartilage [77]. It was reported that exogenous HA could promote the synthesis of proteoglycan, modulate the functions of immune cells, and reduce the activity of proinflammatory cytokines [78]. Additionally, HA has the prominent ability of water retention and play a vital role in regulating tissue hydration and osmotic balance [79]. Because of the highly hygroscopicity, HA can significantly regulate the physical properties of ECM. Hyaluronic acid with special structure is usually considered as a prominent signalling molecule, which can interact with cell surface receptors and thereby modulate cell adhesion, migration, and proliferation [80, 81]. Among these signals, CD44 can bind with HA and the relative signal pathways were confirmed in hematopoietic cells from CD44-deficient mice [82]. The results suggested that there are CD44-independent mechanisms for the guidance of gene expression by HA. Above all, HA has been widely used for more than 20 years over the world due to the biocompatibility and biodegradability. Scientists have made great progress of HA applications in biomedical science. However, the mechanism of HA interacting with the cells need to be explored more clearly and the clinical application of the material derived from HA still has a long way to go.

Chitosan and chitin

Chitosan, the deacetylated derivative of chitin obtained from arthropods usually exists in the form of granules, sheets, or powders. Chitosan and chitin are both linear polysaccharides, composed of the repeated units of N-acetyl-2-amino-2-deoxy-D-glucose (N-acetylated groups) and 2-amino-2-deoxy-D-glucose residues (N-deacetylated groups, amino groups). Chitosan as a heteropolysaccharide also includes linear β-1,4-linked units [83]. Numerous studies suggest that chitosan and chitin can be used for various applications in tissue engineering [84], like wound healing, and drug delivery [85]. They can be engineered versatile formations such as the gels [86], membranes [87], nanofibers, nanoparticles [88], and sponges [89]. At present, many studies trying to develop the chitinous scaffolds in tissue engineering were reported and have made great progress [90]. These chitosan scaffolds exhibited the significant effect on supporting and aiding the generation of extracellular matrix containing abundant proteoglycan in vivo. Additionally, the chitosan and chitin are also widely used as the skin substitutes in tissue engineering [91]. It attributes to the excellent properties of chitin including hemostasis and biocompatible [92], which can facilitate tissue regeneration and generation of the extracellular matrix. And the chitosan was also demonstrated that it could promote wound healing via accelerating the infiltration of polymorphonuclear (PMN) cells at the wound site [93].

Polysaccharides derived from microorganism: functions and applications

Polysaccharides derived from the microorganism are also one class of the major polysaccharides existed in nature. Microbial polysaccharides may be neutral (e.g. dextran, scleroglucan) or acidic (xanthan, gellan) in nature. Some of these polysaccharides such as the glycogen serve as storage compound. Moreover, microbial polysaccharides present a great potential for medical, pharmaceutical and biomedical applications, such as wound dressings, biomaterials, and tissue regeneration.

Alginate

Alginate is a class of naturally existing anionic polymer, which can be extracted from brown algae cell walls, including *Macrocystis pyrifera, Laminaria hyperborea, Ascophyllum nodosum.* Alginate is a linear polysaccharide composing of the repeated units of 1,4-linked β-D-mannuronate (M) and 1,4-α-L-guluronate residues (G). The common alginate usually derived from algal owns highly different physical–chemical heterogeneity which can affect their quality and induce different applications [94]. The alginate possessing kinds of outstanding properties has been extensively studied for biomedical applications [95], including their biocompatibility, low toxicity, low cost, and moderate gelation induced by divalent cations such as Ca^{2+}.

The alginate gel formed by the inducing of divalent cations can be used for wound healing [96], therapeutic agents, proteins delivery [97], and cell transplantation [98]. The wound dressing made by alginate can stimulate the extracellular matrix and establish a moist environment, which could decrease the risk of bacterial infection at the injured site, and accelerate the wound healing rate. Drug and protein systems which can deliver bioactive agents and biomacromolecules, were fabricated by alginate, and could release bioactive molecules in a controlled manner. The alginate gels are also applied for cell transplantation in tissue engineering [99]. It can deliver cells to the designated site, providing artificial matrix for neovascularization. Additionally, the alginate gels can also be orally administrated or injected into body, which can be used in pharmaceutical filed [100].

Dextran

Dextran, a high molecular-weight polysaccharide, composed of α-1,6 linking glucose of the backbone, α-1,4 linking glucose of side chain. The dextran extracted from different microbial strain possesses different structures [101]. After the crosslinking of the dextran, it usually can be used for the separation and purification of biomacromolecules. Due to its biocompatibility, it also can be applied as the plasma expander for biomedical application (Table 3; [102, 103]).

Polysaccharides to enrich growth factors for wound healing

Traumatic injury is a leading cause of mortality in many countries. Accelerating the healing, while minimising the aesthetic impact on patients and restoring full functions the tissue, remains an unmet clinical goal. Although minor injuries in healthy bodies generally heal, the healing of large injuries is often hampered by many factors, such as the age of the patient, infection at the wound site and chronic diseases. The detailed mechanisms are poorly understood.

To most organs and tissues, wound healing has three overlapping stages: inflammation, proliferation and remodelling. In all stages—in particular the second and third, multiple families of growth factors play essential, diverse and co-ordinated roles. For example, several members in the vascular endothelial growth factor (VEGF) and fibroblast growth factor (FGF) families are primary mediators of angiogenesis, while several FGFs also direct fibroblast proliferation and migrations. The platelet-derived growth factor family (PDGF), in particular the PDGF-BB variant, is required for vascular maturation; while transforming growth factors (TGFs) regulate the collagen synthesis. Importantly, many growth factors are bound and protected by glycosaminoglycans (GAGs)—which are anionic, sulphated polysaccharides—in mammalian tissues. In the absence of GAGs, the growth factors cannot be enriched and may easily be degraded or diffused.

This feature provides an exciting opportunity for the design of growth factor-binding polysaccharides for

Table 3 The different kinds of non-plant-origin polysaccharides in nature

Polysaccharides	Composition	Source	Physiological effects
Alginate	Repeated units of 1,4-linked β-mannuronate and 1,4-α-guluronate residues	Brown algae (Phaeophyceae)	Wound healing, therapeutic agents and proteins delivery, and cell transplantation
Carrageenan	Repeating galactose units and 3,6 anhydrogalactose	Red edible seaweeds	Food additives and immunoregulatory effect
Mushroom polysaccharides	β-Glucans and heteropolysaccharides	Mushrooms	Antiobesity, antidiabetes, anticancer, and antibiotic properties
Heparin	Repeated units of sulfonated hexuronic acid (1 → 4)-glucosamine	Porcine intestinal mucosa	Animal tissue structure, binding affinity for growth factors, and anticoagulation
Hyaluronan	Alternating units of D-glucuronic acid, and *N*-acetyl-D-glucosamine	Synovial fluid, the vitreous fluid of the eye, umbilical cords and chicken combs	Natural fluids, wound dressing, chondroprotective effects
Chondroitin sulfate	Alternating sugars (*N*-acetylgalactosamine and glucuronic acid)	Cartilage of animals	Animal tissue structure, dietary supplement for treatment of osteoarthritis
Heparin sulfate	A glucuronic acid (GlcA) linked to *N*-acetylglucosamine	Animals	Animal tissue structure
Chitin and chitosan	Repeated units of *N*-acetyl-2-amino-2-deoxyd-glucose and 2-amino-2-deoxy-dglucose residues	Crab or shrimp shells and fungal mycelia	Wound healing, and drug delivery

wound healing, which, compared with conventional polysaccharides scaffolds as dressing, possess clearer and more specific bioactivities. Numerous attempts have been performed for engineering polysaccharide scaffolds to bind and enrich growth factors, which showed better effect on wound repair than free growth factors. For example, researchers fabricated a heparin-based hydrogel consisting of thiolated heparin and diacrylated poly (ethylene glycol) using photo polymerisation, which was loaded with human epidermal growth factor (hEGF) for skin repair in mice. It showed a sustained release profile of hEGF in vitro and an accelerated healing of skin incision in vivo, in comparison with using free hEGF alone [104]. In another study, Wu and Xiao explored a heparin-based coacervate composed of poly (ethylene argininylaspartate digylceride) (PEAD) as a reservoir, heparin as a bridge, and fibroblast growth factor-2 (FGF-2) as a cargo. The regenerative effect of this scaffold was evaluated in mice with full-thickness excisional skin wounds. The results indicated that this coacervate exhibited faster wound closure, compared with the control and free FGF-2 groups [105]. Additionally, numerous synthetic polymers are devised to mimic the action of GAGs. For instance, a supramolecular polyelectrolyte complexation with sulfonated polyrotaxanes (PRXs) loaded with bone morphogenetic protein 2 (BMP-2) was fabricated, which enhanced the osteogenetic differentiation of BMP-2 in vitro and improved the healing of a calvarial defect in mice [106]. A more direct approach, as demonstrated by Wang and colleagues, was to isolate a fraction from heparan sulfate, named HS^{7+}, which had a higher binding affinity for VEGF-A than the crude sugars. The results in vitro and in vivo demonstrated the potential for vascular therapy of HS^{7+} targeted at enhancing the bioactivity of VEGF-A [107].

Polysaccharides from Chinese medicinal herbs—new prospects in tissue engineering

In the past decades, lots of polysaccharides were obtained from Chinese medicinal herbs; there are many polysaccharides that have received massive attention as promising biomaterials for various applications because of their biocompatible, safe and biodegradable properties. As summarized by above, polysaccharides from Chinese medicinal herbs have comprehensive physiological activity in human body. Meanwhile, much studied indicated that polysaccharides play a vital role in regulating the immune system. However, few attentions focus on the development of polysaccharides from Chinese medicinal herbs as functional biomaterials in tissue engineering.

As mentioned above, macrophages can be activated by many polysaccharides in the nature through relatively specific membrane receptors. The interactions between certain saccharide units (e.g. mannose, β-glucan) and receptors induce multiple cellular responses. According to this property, the polysaccharides can be developed into biomaterial matrices for tissue engineering. For example, as a traditional Chinese medicine, *Bletilla striata* has long been applied for stop bleeding and wound healing. The *B. striata* polysaccharide is obtained from *B. striata*, which composed of α-mannose, β-mannose and β-glucose at the mole ratio of 2.4:1. It can be widely used in tissue regeneration. Luo found that after the wound treated with BSP gel, it was proved to control the inflammatory responses and accelerate the wound closure [108]. In another study, the cotton gauze coated with aqueous extract of *B. striata* polysaccharide showed better healing effect [109].

Further, *B. striata* polysaccharide (BSP), as a typical glucomannan, derived from a Chinese medicinal herb was studied for its bioactivity in modulating macrophages. It was demonstrated that BSP could modulate the function of macrophages via binding mannose receptor and regulating downstream signals [110]. This polysaccharide also could active macrophages and regulates the secretion of cytokines for regeneration of engineered tissues. Accordingly, Niu found a polysaccharide from *B. striata*, which can be used for modulating the phenotype of host macrophage after the acetylation of this polysaccharide. The results suggested that the polysaccharide can stimulate macrophages into a pro-osteogenic phenotype; further, the scaffold manufactured by the polysaccharide had a competent ability as an innovative and efficacious platform to harness the power of host immunity for enhancing the regenerative performance of engineered tissue constructs. This research innovatively modulates the function of macrophages in tissue engineering.

Except for BSP, another polysaccharide, derived from *Konjac*, also is a glucomannan, which can be used for wound healing due to its excellent physical and chemical properties. Fan fabricated a film of a blend of *Konjac* glucomannan (KGM) and chitosan. It was indicated that this film showed a strong antibiotic effect and haemostatic efficiency compared with conventional materials [111]. Meanwhile, Feng found that the natural polysaccharide form *Konjac* glucomannan had affinitive for macrophages, and stimulate them to release growth factors and cytokines [112]. They further modified this polysaccharide with heparin, and then designed an injectable hydrogel scaffold composed of KGM polysaccharide and heparin. They evaluated the efficacy of this scaffold in promoting angiogenesis in situ. The results demonstrated that this scaffold based on polysaccharides had a prominent potential in regenerative medicine.

It is concluded that the glucomannan can interact with mannose receptor. As mentioned in the last section, it is an interesting direction to discover carbohydrates of non-animal source with growth factor-binding ability. Accordingly, Li obtained a polysaccharide from *Eucommia ulmoides*, named EUP3, containing a proportion of galacturonic acid [58]. Unlike animal derived polysaccharides—glycosaminoglycans binding various growth factors, EUP3 polysaccharide had no significant affinity for VEGF-A and FGF-2, but had a clear affinity for PDGF-BB. Further, Li developed EUP3 into a growth factor-affinitive scaffold using electrospinning technology [113]. The results indicated that this scaffold based on EUP3 polysaccharide could accelerate angiogenesis and promote wound healing via sequestering PDGF-BB growth factor.

As we concluded above, polysaccharides from the Chinese medicinal herbs have a promising potential for the applications in tissue engineering. Numerous researches have been performed for engineering suitable polysaccharide scaffolds via interdisciplinary biotechnologies. Above all, compared with polysaccharides from animals, which are often amorphous and have weakly mechanical properties, the polysaccharides from Chinese medicinal herbs have better mechanical properties. Moreover, the polysaccharides from animals often have the risk of immune response and other side effects. Therefore, because of the limitations of animal-derived polysaccharides, it has a promising prospect that screening the polysaccharides from the Chinese medicinal herbs, which have specific properties, can be applied in tissue engineering.

Conclusions

Polysaccharides are natural biomaterials which are inexpensive, and most of them are easily obtained. The special structure diversities and physiochemical properties of polysaccharides can be exerted successfully, and lots of polysaccharides have been developed into functional biomaterial matrices. In sum, they have been applied in tissue engineering by mainly three approaches: (1) compatible materials for tissue regeneration, (2) drug delivery materials, and (3) immunoregulatory agents.

However, although lots of polysaccharides were obtained and various bioactivities of polysaccharides were applied in tissue engineering, the mechanism of polysaccharides interacting with bodies was still unclear due to the complicated structures. The detailed mechanisms and structure–activity relationship should be studied further. Moreover, it is a challenge that obtains the functional polysaccharides with high purity and characterizes the structure of polysaccharides. Additionally, in terms of the application of functional polysaccharides in tissue regeneration, although numerous researches have been carried out for developing the functional scaffolds, there is still a long way to transform from research to clinic. At present, there are still many limitations which include the immunogenicity of scaffolds, high cost and high failure rate. Developing the ideal polysaccharide scaffolds, which can be used in clinic, must satisfy these requirements: the clear structure of polysaccharides; definite bioactivities, security and biocompatibility, and appropriately physico-chemical properties. We suppose that the Chinese medicinal herbs could be a potential and abundant natural source for developing promising biomaterials in future.

Abbreviations

ROS: reactive oxygen species; NO: nitric oxide; TNF-α: tumour necrosis factor; IL-1β: interleukin-1β; HA: hyaluronic acid; GAGs: glycosaminoglycans; ECM: extracellular matrix.

Authors' contributions

QL wrote the manuscript; YN and PX helped in analysing the references; CW revised the manuscript. All authors read and approved the final manuscript.

Acknowledgements

Not applicable.

Competing interests

The authors declare that they have no competing interests.

Consent for publication

Not applicable.

Funding

This study was financially supported by the funding grants from Fundo para o Desenvolvimento das Ciências e da Tecnologia, Macau (FDCT 126/2016/A3, 080/2016/A2), the University of Macau (MYRG2016-00031-ICMS-QRCM, and MYRG2015-00160-ICMS-QRCM), the open fund of the State Key Laboratory of Quality Research in Chinese Medicine, University of Macau (No. 005), and National Science Foundation of China (51503232).

References

1. Aachary AA, Prapulla SG. Xylooligosaccharides (XOS) as an emerging prebiotic: microbial synthesis, utilization, structural characterization, bioactive properties, and applications. Compr Rev Food Sci Food Saf. 2011;10(1):2–16.
2. Rinaudo M. Biomaterials based on a natural polysaccharide: alginate. TIP. 2014;17(1):92–6.
3. Schepetkin IA, Quinn MT. Botanical polysaccharides: macrophage immunomodulation and therapeutic potential. Int Immunopharmacol. 2006;6(3):317–33.

4. Yang L, Zhang L-M. Chemical structural and chain conformational characterization of some bioactive polysaccharides isolated from natural sources. Carbohydr Polym. 2009;76(3):349–61.
5. Zhao W, Liu W, Li J, Lin X, Wang Y. Preparation of animal polysaccharides nanofibers by electrospinning and their potential biomedical applications. J Biomed Mater Res Part A. 2015;103(2):807–18.
6. Yudovin-Farber I, Azzam T, Metzer E, Taraboulos A, Domb AJ. Cationic polysaccharides as antiprion agents. J Med Chem. 2005;48(5):1414–20.
7. Xiao Z, Tappen BR, Ly M, Zhao W, Canova LP, Guan H, et al. Heparin mapping using heparin lyases and the generation of a novel low molecular weight heparin. J Med Chem. 2011;54(2):603–10.
8. Funami T, Nakauma M, Noda S, Ishihara S, Asai I, Inouchi N, et al. Effects of some anionic polysaccharides on the gelatinization and retrogradation behaviors of wheat starch: soybean-soluble polysaccharide and gum arabic. Food Hydrocolloids. 2008;22(8):1528–40.
9. Dalheim MØ, Arnfinnsdottir NB, Widmalm G, Christensen BE. The size and shape of three water-soluble, non-ionic polysaccharides produced by lactic acid bacteria: a comparative study. Carbohydr Polym. 2016;142:91–7.
10. Korakli M, Vogel RF. Structure/function relationship of homopolysaccharide producing glycansucrases and therapeutic potential of their synthesised glycans. Appl Microbiol Biotechnol. 2006;71(6):790–803.
11. Amid B, Mirhosseini H. Influence of chemical extraction on rheological behavior, viscoelastic properties and functional characteristics of natural heteropolysaccharide/protein polymer from *Durio zibethinus* Seed. Int J Mol Sci. 2012;13(11):14871–88.
12. Hurst RE, Poon MC, Griffith MJ. Structure–activity relationships of heparin. Independence of heparin charge density and antithrombin-binding domains in thrombin inhibition by antithrombin and heparin cofactor II. J Clin Invest. 1983;72(3):1042–5.
13. Powderly WG, Schreiber JR, Pier GB, Markham RB. T cells recognizing polysaccharide-specific B cells function as contrasuppressor cells in the generation of T cell immunity to *Pseudomonas aeruginosa*. J Immunol. 1988;140(8):2746.
14. González-Fernández Á, Faro J, Fernández C. Immune responses to polysaccharides: lessons from humans and mice. Vaccine. 2008;26(3):292–300.
15. Kumbar SG, Toti US, Deng M, James R, Laurencin CT, Aravamudhan A, et al. Novel mechanically competent polysaccharide scaffolds for bone tissue engineering. Biomed Mater. 2011;6(6):065005.
16. Mascal M, Nikitin EB. Direct, high-yield conversion of cellulose into biofuel. Angew Chem. 2008;120(41):8042–4.
17. Englyst HN, Anderson V, Cummings JH. Starch and non-starch polysaccharides in some cereal foods. J Sci Food Agric. 1983;34(12):1434–40.
18. Frantz C, Stewart KM, Weaver VM. The extracellular matrix at a glance. J Cell Sci. 2010;123(24):4195–200.
19. Bohn JA, BeMiller JN. (1 → 3)-β-D-glucans as biological response modifiers: a review of structure-functional activity relationships. Carbohydr Polym. 1995;28(1):3–14.
20. Pinkert A, Goeke DF, Marsh KN, Pang S. Extracting wood lignin without dissolving or degrading cellulose: investigations on the use of food additive-derived ionic liquids. Green Chem. 2011;13(11):3124–36.
21. May CD. Industrial pectins: sources, production and applications. Carbohydr Polym. 1990;12(1):79–99.
22. Sarei F, Dounighi NM, Zolfagharian H, Khaki P, Bidhendi SM. Alginate nanoparticles as a promising adjuvant and vaccine delivery system. Indian J Pharm Sci. 2013;75(4):442.
23. Aliste AJ, Vieira FF, Del Mastro NL. Radiation effects on agar, alginates and carrageenan to be used as food additives. Radiat Phys Chem. 2000;57(3):305–8.
24. DiGabriele AD, Lax I, Chen DI, Svahn CM. Structure of a heparin-linked biologically active dimer of fibroblast growth factor. Nature. 1998;393(6687):812.
25. Liao Y-H, Jones SA, Forbes B, Martin GP, Brown MB. Hyaluronan: pharmaceutical characterization and drug delivery. Drug Deliv. 2005;12(6):327–42.
26. Dong-An W, Varghese S, Sharma B, Strehin I, Fermanian S, Gorham J, et al. Multifunctional chondroitin sulphate for cartilage tissue-biomaterial integration. Nat Mater. 2007;6(5):385.
27. Dietrich CP, Nader HB, Straus AH. Structural differences of heparan sulfates according to the tissue and species of origin. Biochem Biophys Res Commun. 1983;111(3):865–71.
28. Berger J, Reist M, Mayer JM, Felt O, Peppas N, Gurny R. Structure and interactions in covalently and ionically crosslinked chitosan hydrogels for biomedical applications. Eur J Pharm Biopharm. 2004;57(1):19–34.
29. Wang J, Zhang Q, Zhang Z, Li Z. Antioxidant activity of sulfated polysaccharide fractions extracted from *Laminaria japonica*. Int J Biol Macromol. 2008;42(2):127–32.
30. Chen Y, Xie M-Y, Nie S-P, Li C, Wang Y-X. Purification, composition analysis and antioxidant activity of a polysaccharide from the fruiting bodies of *Ganoderma atrum*. Food Chem. 2008;107(1):231–41.
31. Ueno H, Mori T, Fujinaga T. Topical formulations and wound healing applications of chitosan. Adv Drug Del Rev. 2001;52(2):105–15.
32. Ramberg JE, Nelson ED, Sinnott RA. Immunomodulatory dietary polysaccharides: a systematic review of the literature. Nutr J. 2010;9(1):54.
33. Poletto M, Ornaghi H, Zattera A. Native cellulose: structure, characterization and thermal properties. Materials. 2014;7(9):6105.
34. Onofrei M, Filimon A. Cellulose-based hydrogels: designing concepts, properties, and perspectives for biomedical and environmental applications. Polymer science: research advances, practical applications and educational aspects. 2016;108–20.
35. Domingues RMA, Gomes ME, Reis RL. The potential of cellulose nanocrystals in tissue engineering strategies. Biomacromolecules. 2014;15(7):2327–46.
36. Gu H, Yue Z, Leong WS, Nugraha B, Tan LP. Control of in vitro neural differentiation of mesenchymal stem cells in 3D macroporous, cellulosic hydrogels. Regen Med. 2010;5(2):245–53.
37. O'Riordan M, Yi CH, Gonzales R, Lee K-D, Portnoy DA. Innate recognition of bacteria by a macrophage cytosolic surveillance pathway. Proc Natl Acad Sci. 2002;99(21):13861–6.
38. Truman LA, Ford CA, Pasikowska M, Pound JD, Wilkinson SJ, Dumitriu IE, et al. CX3CL1/fractalkine is released from apoptotic lymphocytes to stimulate macrophage chemotaxis. Blood. 2008;112(13):5026–36.
39. Bratosin D, Mazurier J, Tissier JP, Estaquier J, Huart JJ, Ameisen JC, et al. Cellular and molecular mechanisms of senescent erythrocyte phagocytosis by macrophages. A review. Biochimie. 1998;80(2):173–95.
40. Wang W-S, Hung S-W, Lin Y-H, Tu C-Y, Wong M-L, Chiou S-H, et al. The effects of five different glycans on innate immune responses by phagocytes of hybrid tilapia and Japanese eels *Anguilla japonica*. J Aquat Anim Health. 2007;19(1):49–59.
41. Rabinovich GA, Toscano MA. Turning 'sweet' on immunity: galectin–glycan interactions in immune tolerance and inflammation. Nat Rev Immunol. 2009;9(5):338–52.
42. Schepetkin IA, Faulkner CL, Nelson-Overton LK, Wiley JA, Quinn MT. Macrophage immunomodulatory activity of polysaccharides isolated from *Juniperus scopolorum*. Int Immunopharmacol. 2005;5(13):1783–99.
43. Wong K-F, Yuan Y, Luk JM. *Tripterygium wilfordii* bioactive compounds as anticancer and anti-inflammatory agents. Clin Exp Pharmacol Physiol. 2012;39(3):311–20.
44. Luk JM, Lai W, Tam P, Koo MWL. Suppression of cytokine production and cell adhesion molecule expression in human monocytic cell line THP-1 by *Tripterygium wilfordii* polysaccharide moiety. Life Sci. 2000;67(2):155–63.
45. Song J-Y, Yang H-O, Pyo S-N, Jung I-S, Yi S-Y, Yun Y-S. Immunomodulatory activity of protein-bound polysaccharide extracted from *Chelidonium majus*. Arch Pharmacal Res. 2002;25(2):158–64.
46. Hamman J. Composition and applications of aloe vera leaf gel. Molecules. 2008;13(8):1599.
47. Hsu H-Y, Hua K-F, Lin C-C, Lin C-H, Hsu J, Wong C-H. Extract of Reishi polysaccharides induces cytokine expression via TLR4-modulated protein kinase signaling pathways. J Immunol. 2004;173(10):5989.
48. Hua K-F, Hsu H-Y, Chao LK, Chen S-T, Yang W-B, Hsu J, et al. Ganoderma lucidum polysaccharides enhance CD14 endocytosis of LPS and promote TLR4 signal transduction of cytokine expression. J Cell Physiol. 2007;212(2):537–50.
49. Hollmig ST, Ariizumi K, Cruz JPD. Recognition of non-self-polysaccharides by C-type lectin receptors dectin-1 and dectin-2. Glycobiology. 2009;19(6):568–75.

50. Zamze S, Martinez-Pomares L, Jones H, Taylor PR, Stillion RJ, Gordon S, et al. Recognition of bacterial capsular polysaccharides and lipopolysaccharides by the macrophage mannose receptor. J Biol Chem. 2002;277(44):41613–23.
51. Ando I, Tsukumo Y, Wakabayashi T, Akashi S, Miyake K, Kataoka T, et al. Safflower polysaccharides activate the transcription factor NF-κB via Toll-like receptor 4 and induce cytokine production by macrophages. Int Immunopharmacol. 2002;2(8):1155–62.
52. Zhao KS, Mancini C, Doria G. Enhancement of the immune response in mice by *Astragalus membranaceus* extracts. Immunopharmacology. 1990;20(3):225–33.
53. Kim SJ, Kim HM. Dynamic lipopolysaccharide transfer cascade to TLR4/MD2 complex via LBP and CD14. BMB Rep. 2017;50(2):55.
54. Liao W, Luo Z, Liu D, Ning Z, Yang J, Ren J. Structure characterization of a novel polysaccharide from *Dictyophora indusiata* and its macrophage immunomodulatory activities. J Agric Food Chem. 2015;63(2):535–44.
55. Wang Y, Liu J, Li Q, Wang Y, Wang C. Two natural glucomannan polymers, from Konjac and Bletilla, as bioactive materials for pharmaceutical applications. Biotechnol Lett. 2015;37(1):1–8.
56. Baek S-H, Lee JG, Park SY, Bae ON, Kim D-H, Park JH. Pectic polysaccharides from *Panax ginseng* as the antirotavirus principals in ginseng. Biomacromolecules. 2010;11(8):2044–52.
57. Niu Y, Li Q, Xie R, Liu S, Wang R, Xing P, et al. Modulating the phenotype of host macrophages to enhance osteogenesis in MSC-laden hydrogels: design of a glucomannan coating material. Biomaterials. 2017;139:39–55.
58. Li Q, Guo G, Meng F, Wang HH, Niu Y, Zhang Q, et al. A naturally derived, growth factor-binding polysaccharide for therapeutic angiogenesis. ACS Macro Lett. 2016;5(5):617–21.
59. Li Q, Feng Y, He W, Wang L, Wang R, Dong L, et al. Post-screening characterisation and in vivo evaluation of an anti-inflammatory polysaccharide fraction from *Eucommia ulmoides*. Carbohydr Polym. 2017;169:304–14.
60. Xu DJ, Xia Q, Wang JJ, Wang PP. Molecular weight and monosaccharide composition of Astragalus polysaccharides. Molecules. 2008;13(10):2408.
61. Rusnati M, Presta M. Interaction of angiogenic basic fibroblast growth factor with endothelial cell heparan sulfate proteoglycans. Int J Clin Lab Res. 1996;26(1):15–23.
62. DeAngelis PL. Glycosaminoglycan polysaccharide biosynthesis and production: today and tomorrow. Appl Microbiol Biotechnol. 2012;94(2):295–305.
63. Casu B, Naggi A, Torri G. Re-visiting the structure of heparin. Carbohydr Res. 2015;403:60–8.
64. Nikitovic D, Mytilinaiou M, Berdiaki A, Karamanos NK, Tzanakakis GN. Heparan sulfate proteoglycans and heparin regulate melanoma cell functions. Biochimica et Biophysica Acta (BBA) General Subjects. 2014;1840(8):2471–81.
65. Peysselon F, Ricard-Blum S. Heparin–protein interactions: from affinity and kinetics to biological roles. Application to an interaction network regulating angiogenesis. Matrix Biol. 2014;35:73–81.
66. Kadomatsu K, Kishida S, Tsubota S. The heparin-binding growth factor midkine: the biological activities and candidate receptors. J Biochem. 2013;153(6):511–21.
67. You J, Park S-A, Shin D-S, Patel D, Raghunathan VK, Kim M, et al. Characterizing the effects of heparin gel stiffness on function of primary hepatocytes. Tissue Eng Part A. 2013;19(23–24):2655–63.
68. Chen Y, Lin L, Agyekum I, Zhang X, St. Ange K, Yu Y, et al. Structural analysis of heparin-derived 3-*O*-sulfated tetrasaccharides: antithrombin binding site variants. J Pharm Sci. 2017;106(4):973–81.
69. Feizi T, Haltiwanger RS. Editorial overview: carbohydrate–protein interactions and glycosylation: glycan synthesis and recognition: finding the perfect partner in a sugar-coated life. Curr Opin Struct Biol. 2015;34:vii–ix.
70. Mulloy B, Hogwood J, Gray E, Lever R, Page CP. Pharmacology of heparin and related drugs. Pharmacol Rev. 2016;68(1):76–141.
71. Greinacher A. Heparin-induced thrombocytopenia. N Engl J Med. 2015;373(3):252–61.
72. Xu Y, Cai C, Chandarajoti K, Hsieh P-H, Li L, Pham TQ, et al. Homogeneous low-molecular-weight heparins with reversible anticoagulant activity. Nat Chem Biol. 2014;10(4):248–50.
73. Cyphert JM, Trempus CS, Garantziotis S. Size matters: molecular weight specificity of hyaluronan effects in cell biology. Int J Cell Biol. 2015;2015:8.
74. Papakonstantinou E, Roth M, Karakiulakis G. Hyaluronic acid: a key molecule in skin aging. Dermatoendocrinology. 2012;4(3):253–8.
75. Jordan AR, Racine RR, Hennig MJP, Lokeshwar VB. The role of CD44 in disease pathophysiology and targeted treatment. Front Immunol. 2015;6:182.
76. Collins MN, Birkinshaw C. Hyaluronic acid based scaffolds for tissue engineering—a review. Carbohydr Polym. 2013;92(2):1262–79.
77. Elmorsy S, Funakoshi T, Sasazawa F, Todoh M, Tadano S, Iwasaki N. Chondroprotective effects of high-molecular-weight cross-linked hyaluronic acid in a rabbit knee osteoarthritis model. Osteoarthritis Cartilage. 2014;22(1):121–7.
78. Menzel EJ, Farr C. Hyaluronidase and its substrate hyaluronan: biochemistry, biological activities and therapeutic uses. Cancer Lett. 1998;131(1):3–11.
79. Chan RW, Tayama N. Biomechanical effects of hydration in vocal fold tissues. Otolaryngol Head Neck Surg. 2002;126(5):528–37.
80. Lokeshwar VB, Iida N, Bourguignon LYW. The cell adhesion molecule, GP116, is a new CD44 variant (ex14/v10) involved in hyaluronic acid binding and endothelial cell proliferation. J Biol Chem. 1996;271(39):23853–64.
81. Lam J, Truong NF, Segura T. Design of cell–matrix interactions in hyaluronic acid hydrogel scaffolds. Acta Biomater. 2014;10(4):1571–80.
82. Naor D. Editorial: interaction between hyaluronic acid and its receptors (CD44, RHAMM) regulates the activity of inflammation and cancer. Front Immunol. 2016;7:39.
83. Younes I, Rinaudo M. Chitin and chitosan preparation from marine sources. Structure, properties and applications. Mar Drugs. 2015;13(3):1133.
84. Croisier F, Jérôme C. Chitosan-based biomaterials for tissue engineering. Eur Polym J. 2013;49(4):780–92.
85. Anitha A, Sowmya S, Kumar PTS, Deepthi S, Chennazhi KP, Ehrlich H, et al. Chitin and chitosan in selected biomedical applications. Prog Polym Sci. 2014;39(9):1644–67.
86. Mukhopadhyay P, Sarkar K, Bhattacharya S, Bhattacharyya A, Mishra R, Kundu PP. pH sensitive *N*-succinyl chitosan grafted polyacrylamide hydrogel for oral insulin delivery. Carbohydr Polym. 2014;112:627–37.
87. Lin W-C, Lien C-C, Yeh H-J, Yu C-M, Hsu S-H. Bacterial cellulose and bacterial cellulose–chitosan membranes for wound dressing applications. Carbohydr Polym. 2013;94(1):603–11.
88. Ragelle H, Riva R, Vandermeulen G, Naeye B, Pourcelle V, Le Duff CS, et al. Chitosan nanoparticles for siRNA delivery: optimizing formulation to increase stability and efficiency. J Control Release. 2014;176:54–63.
89. Huang X, Sun Y, Nie J, Lu W, Yang L, Zhang Z, et al. Using absorbable chitosan hemostatic sponges as a promising surgical dressing. Int J Biol Macromol. 2015;75:322–9.
90. Mutsenko VV, Gryshkov O, Lauterboeck L, Rogulska O, Tarusin DN, Bazhenov VV, et al. Novel chitin scaffolds derived from marine sponge *Ianthella basta* for tissue engineering approaches based on human mesenchymal stromal cells: biocompatibility and cryopreservation. Int J Biol Macromol. 2017;104:1955–65.
91. Mohd Hilmi AB, Halim AS, Jaafar H, Asiah AB, Hassan A. Chitosan dermal substitute and chitosan skin substitute contribute to accelerated full-thickness wound healing in irradiated rats. Biomed Res Int. 2013;2013:13.
92. Zhang W, Sun Y-L, Chen D-H. Effects of chitin and sepia ink hybrid hemostatic sponge on the blood parameters of mice. Mar Drugs. 2014;12(4):2269.
93. Mendoza G, Zavala J, Garza-Madrid M, Tamez A, Zavala-Pompa A, Brito G, et al. Biosafety of chitosan and collagen vitrigel membranes in the corneal endothelium of young New Zealand Rabbits. Invest Ophthalmol Vis Sci. 2013;54(15):1666.
94. Lee KY, Mooney DJ. Alginate: properties and biomedical applications. Prog Polym Sci. 2012;37(1):106–26.
95. Martins M, Barros AA, Quraishi S, Gurikov P, Raman SP, Smirnova I, et al. Preparation of macroporous alginate-based aerogels for biomedical applications. J Supercrit Fluids. 2015;106:152–9.
96. De Leon-Peralta EJ, Brudno Y, Kwee BJ, Mooney DJ. Improving wound healing through the use of tetrazine-modified alginate. FASEB J. 2016;30(1 Supplement):1177.1110.

97. Jain D, Bar-Shalom D. Alginate drug delivery systems: application in context of pharmaceutical and biomedical research. Drug Dev Ind Pharm. 2014;40(12):1576–84.
98. Pipeleers D, Keymeulen B. Boost for alginate encapsulation in beta cell transplantation. Trends Endocrinol Metab. 2016;27(5):247–8.
99. Venkatesan J, Bhatnagar I, Manivasagan P, Kang K-H, Kim S-K. Alginate composites for bone tissue engineering: a review. Int J Biol Macromol. 2015;72:269–81.
100. Choudhary S, Reck JM, Carr AJ, Bhatia SR. Hydrophobically modified alginate for extended release of pharmaceuticals. Polym Adv Technol. 2018;29(1):198–204.
101. Siddiqui NN, Aman A, Silipo A, Qader SAU, Molinaro A. Structural analysis and characterization of dextran produced by wild and mutant strains of *Leuconostoc mesenteroides*. Carbohydr Polym. 2014;99:331–8.
102. Howard JM, Ebert RV, Bloom WL, Sloan MH. The present status of dextran as a plasma expander. Am J Surg. 1959;97(5):593–6.
103. Friedman M. Mushroom polysaccharides: chemistry and antiobesity, antidiabetes, anticancer, and antibiotic properties in cells, rodents, and humans. Foods. 2016;5(4):80.
104. Goh M, Hwang Y, Tae G. Epidermal growth factor loaded heparin-based hydrogel sheet for skin wound healing. Carbohydr Polym. 2016;147:251–60.
105. Wu J, Ye J, Zhu J, Xiao Z, He C, Shi H, et al. Heparin-based coacervate of FGF2 improves dermal regeneration by asserting a synergistic role with cell proliferation and endogenous facilitated VEGF for cutaneous wound healing. Biomacromolecules. 2016;17(6):2168–77.
106. Terauchi M, Inada T, Kanemaru T, Ikeda G, Tonegawa A, Nishida K, et al. Potentiating bioactivity of BMP-2 by polyelectrolyte complexation with sulfonated polyrotaxanes to induce rapid bone regeneration in a mouse calvarial defect. J Biomed Mater Res A. 2017;105(5):1355–63.
107. Wang C, Poon S, Murali S, Koo C-Y, Bell TJ, Hinkley SF, et al. Engineering a vascular endothelial growth factor 165-binding heparan sulfate for vascular therapy. Biomaterials. 2014;35(25):6776–86.
108. Luo Y, Diao H, Xia S, Dong L, Chen J, Zhang J. A physiologically active polysaccharide hydrogel promotes wound healing. J Biomed Mater Res A. 2010;94A(1):193–204.
109. Venkatrajah B, Malathy VV, Elayarajah B, Rajendran R, Rammohan R. Biopolymer and *Bletilla striata* herbal extract coated cotton gauze preparation for wound healing. J Med Sci. 2012;12(6):148.
110. Zhan X, Jia L, Niu Y, Qi H, Chen X, Zhang Q, et al. Targeted depletion of tumour-associated macrophages by an alendronate–glucomannan conjugate for cancer immunotherapy. Biomaterials. 2014;35(38):10046–57.
111. Fan L, Cheng C, Qiao Y, Li F, Li W, Wu H, et al. GNPs-CS/KGM as hemostatic first aid wound dressing with antibiotic effect. In vitro and in vivo study. PLoS ONE. 2013;8(7):e66890.
112. Feng Y, Li Q, Wu D, Niu Y, Yang C, Dong L, et al. A macrophage-activating, injectable hydrogel to sequester endogenous growth factors for in situ angiogenesis. Biomaterials. 2017;134:128–42.
113. Li Q, Niu Y, Diao H, Wang L, Chen X, Wang Y, et al. In situ sequestration of endogenous PDGF-BB with an ECM-mimetic sponge for accelerated wound healing. Biomaterials. 2017;148:54–68.

12

Pharmacological effects of medicinal components of *Atractylodes lancea* (Thunb.) DC.

Xie Jun[1†], Peng Fu[2†], Yu Lei[1] and Peng Cheng[1*]

Abstract

Atractylodes lancea Thunb. DC. (AL) has a long history as one of the important herbs used in East Asia. This review is on the purpose of providing a comprehensive summary of the pharmacological effects of AL and its extractions. The potential application of AL on the disease could be attributed to its pharmacological properties such as anti-cancer, anti-inflam-matory and other essential effects. Hence, this review aims at providing evidence of the pharmacological activities of AL as one of natural products used in clinical trial.

Keywords: Natural product, AL, Pharmacological activities

Background

Atractylodes lancea Thunb. DC. (AL) has a long history as one of the important herbs used in East Asia. AL is grown mainly in Hubei and Jiangsu. In traditional Chinese medicine (TCM), the rhizome of AL tastes pungent and bitter, and belongs to spleen, stomach and liver meridian. AL could eliminate dampness, strengthen the spleen, eliminating wind and dispersing cold. According to TCM theory, AL was traditionally used to treat rheumatic diseases, digestive disorders, night blindness, and influenza [1]. AL was generally applied into traditional decoction, such as Ermiao Powder, Simiao Powder, Yueju-Wan and several other famous decoctions. Recently, it was interesting to find the extract from AL could also exert anti-cancer, anti-obesity and anti-inflammatory effects [2]. AL contains sesquiterpenes, sesquiterpenoids, polyethylene alkynes, phytosterols and etc., such as elemol, β-selinene and atractylone [3, 4]. Sesquiterpenes are a class of natural products composed of three isoprene units, derived from the 15-carbon farnesyl pyrophosphate. Sesquiterpenoids are extensively distributed in nature with 15-carbon after biochemical modifications of sesquiterpenes. Alkynes are a class of organic compounds composed of at least one carbon–carbon triple bond, easily undergoing oxidative cleavage. Phytosterols are a subgroup of the steroids. Steroids are a class of organic molecules composed of seventeen carbon atoms, with four rings arranged in a specific molecular configuration. Especially, this review article will concentrate on the major constituents identified in AL with multi-pharmacological activities [5, 6]. The names are shown in Table 1 and structures are shown in Fig. 1.

Pharmacological effects

Atractylodes lancea Thunb. DC.

Opisthorchis viverrini (OV)-induced cholangiocarcinoma (CCA) is the common cancer between male and female, especially in Thailand. Recent study exhibited that the ethanol extract of AL exerted an inhibitory effect on OV-induced CCA animal model without obvious toxicity through oral administration for 30 days according to the results from positron emission tomography-computed tomography and male Syrian hamsters [7]. In order to explore the effect of AL rhizome on gastrointestinal motility, the atropine-, dopamine-, and 5-hydroxytryptamine (5-HT)-treated mice were adopted in the study. The results exerted that 1 mg/kg extract could vitally suppress dopamine-induced gastric emptying and gastrointestinal motility decrease through intraperitoneal injection. The extract at the concentration of 1000 mg/kg could restrict

*Correspondence: pengchengchengdu@126.com
†Xie Jun and Peng Fu contributed equally to this work
1 Chengdu University of Traditional Chinese Medicine, Chengdu, China
Full list of author information is available at the end of the article

Table 1 The chemical information of major components of AL

Chemical name	Formula	Type of compound	Molecular weight (g/mol)
Atractylenolide I	$C_{15}H_{18}O_2$	Sesquiterpene	230.30
AtractylenolideII	$C_{15}H_{20}O_2$	Sesquiterpene	232.32
Atractylenolide III	$C_{15}H_{20}O_3$	Sesquiterpene	248.32
Atractylone	$C_{15}H_{20}O$	Sesquiterpenoid	216.32
Hinesol	$C_{15}H_{26}O$	Sesquiterpenoid	216.3
β-Eudesmol	$C_{15}H_{26}O$	Sesquiterpenoid	222.37
Atractylodin	$C_{13}H_{10}O$	Polyethylene alkyne	182.22
Stigmasterol	$C_{29}H_{48}O$	Phytosterol	412.69
β-Sitosterol	$C_{29}H_{50}O$	Phytosterol	414.71

atropine-induced small intestinal motility decrease, and the extract of 500 mg/kg dose could block 5-HT-induced gastric emptying and small intestinal motility decrease [8]. Additionally, AL exerted anti-gastric ulcer effect in the rat model through decreasing inflammatory mediators (i.e. tumor necrosis factor-α (TNF-α), interleukin-8 (IL-8), IL-6), and prostaglandin E_2 (PGE_2) and increasing epidermal growth factor (EGF) and trefoil factor2 (TFF2) [9]. Soil-borne fungal pathogens reduced 30% yields of peanuts [10]. Recently, it was reported that intercropping with the peanuts, AL could also suppress soil-borne fungal diseases through the inhibition of *Fusarium oxysporum* growth [11]. Petroleum ether (PE) extraction from AL showed an inhibitory effect on BGC-823 and SGC-7901 human gastric cancer cells. PE fraction could induce apoptosis, cell cycle arrest, and mitochondrial transmembrane potential changes [12]. A recent report exerted that MeOH extract of AL could inhibit nitric oxide (NO) production in lipopolysaccharide-stimulated murine macrophage-like RAW264.7 cells and induce granulocyte-colony stimulating factor (G-CSF) secretion in murine normal colonic epithelial MCE301 cells. NO is a free radical [13]. The ethanol extract of AL exerted an essential inhibitory effect on lipase with the IC_{50} 9.06 μg/mL in a human pancreatic lipase assay, and exhibited anti-obesity effect on a high-fat diet-induced obesity mice model at the high concentration of 500 mg/kg [14]. The water extracts from AL showed the antagonistic activity against serotonin receptors and an inhibitory effect on the selective 5-HT2A/2C agonist 1-(2,5-dimethoxy-4-iodophenyl)-2-aminopropane-induced head-twitch response in mice [15]. Water extracts from AL reduced triptolide-induced toxicity through the down-regulation of the hepatic expression of CYP3A. In the meantime, AL could improve anti-inflammatory effects of triptolide. These findings suggested that AL could inhibit toxicity and increase therapeutic activity of triptolide through combination [16].

Atractylenolide I

Atractylenolide I (ATL-I), a sesquiterpene, can be extracted from *Rhizoma Atractylodis Macrocephalae* (RAM) and AL [17]. ATL-I is soluble in Ethanol and Methanol, and is stable without exposure to light or moisture. ATL-I exerted multiple therapeutic activities, such as anti-cancer, anti-inflammatory and anti-atopic effects [18–20]. ATL-I was identified in AL as one of the main components in 2009 [21]. Bladder cancer ranks the second most common urological worldwide [22]. ATL-I recently was demonstrated to have the anti-tumor effect on bladder cancer in vivo and in vitro. It was found that ATL-I increased the p21 level and decreased the level of cyclin B1, CDK1 and Cdc25c, resulting in the inhibition of bladder cancer cell proliferation. Further study showed that ATL-I could induce cell cycle arrest in G2/M phase. Additionally, ATL-I had a stimulatory effect on apoptosis through the suppression of PI3 K/Akt/mTOR signaling pathway. The animal study showed that ATL-I could inhibit tumor growth without the obvious toxicity [17]. Leukemia refers to a type of cancers generally starting from the bone marrow and resulting in abnormal white blood cells. Recent studies showed that ATL-I could inhibit AML and CML leukemia cell proliferation and growth. MTT assay showed that ATL-I could inhibit K562 CML and U937 AML. ELISA and IF assay exhibited that ATL-I could induce apoptosis. Additionally, ATL-I also promoted caspase-3 and caspase-9 activation through the cleavage of pro-caspase-3 and pro-caspase-9. Caspase-3 and caspase-9 are an enzymes initiating apoptotic pathway. Also, ATL-I could increase the CD14 and CD68 markers, leading to the cell differentiation of ATL-I-treated leukemia cells [23]. Melanoma belongs to the skin cancer [24]. Recent researches showed that ATL-I could inhibit human melanoma cells growth through the induction of apoptosis. Further study exerted that ATL-I could suppress melanoma cell migration through the inhibition on p-JAK2, p-STAT3, MMP-2 and MMP-9. MMP-2 and MMP-9 are matrix metallopeptidases involved in invasion and metastasis in multiple cancers. Interestingly, the overexpression of STAT3 would at least partly reverse the anti-cancer effect of ATL-I on melanoma cells [25]. The clinical study about the evaluation of therapeutic effect of ATL-I on gastric cancer cachexia patients has been conducted in recent years. According to the results about appetite, body weight, mid-arm muscle circumference, Karnofsky performance status (KPS) status, ATL-I could improve appetite and KPS

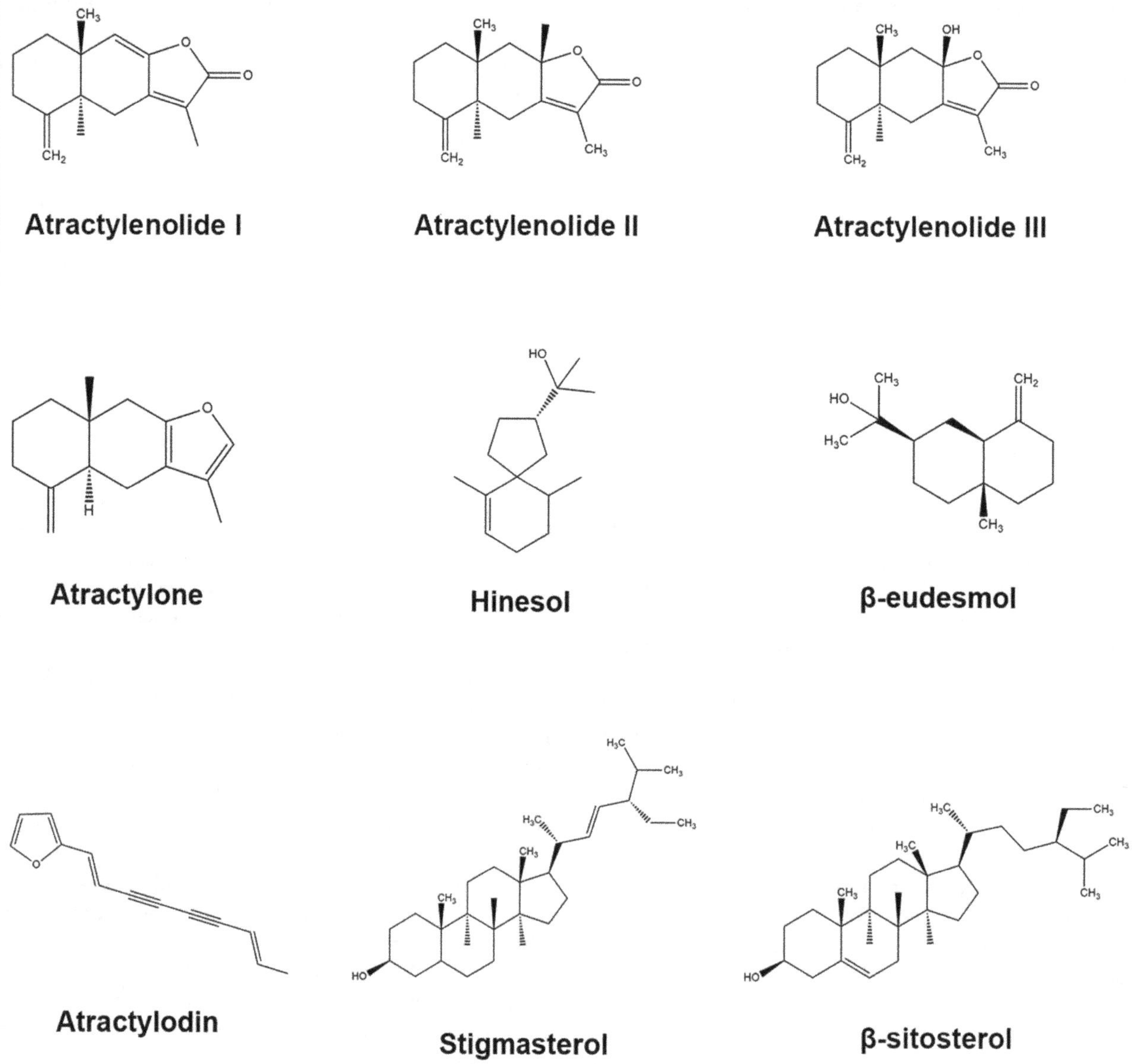

Fig. 1 The chemical structures of pure compounds extracted from AL (drawing via ChemDraw)

status. Meanwhile, the IHC staining results showed that ATL-I could increase TNF-α expression and reduce IL-1 and proteolysis-inducing factor (PIF) production [26]. Intestinal epithelial (IEC-6) cells showed an important role in gastrointestinal disease with the ability to promote and accelerate the healing of mucosal ulcers and wounds. Recent study found that ATL-I could promote IEC-6 cell migration and proliferation, with an increase of cytosolic free Ca^{2+} concentration (Ca^{2+}). Further study exerted that ATL-I could increase TRPC1 and PLC-$_{\gamma 1}$ in IEC-6 cells [27]. Moreover, ATL-I suppressed vascular smooth muscle cell proliferation, migration, lipid peroxidation and inflammatory responses induced by oxidized modified low-density lipoprotein [28]. A present research indicated that ATL-I had a protective effect on the acute lung injury in the lipopolysaccharide (LPS)-induced mice. The detailed mechanism was associated with suppression of toll like receptor 4 (TLR4) expression and NF-κB activation. NF-κB could promote the transcription of oncogenic genes, cytokine production and cell survival after inducers stimulation, such as ROS, TNFα and IL-1β. It was found that ATL-I powerfully suppressed lung wet-to-dry weight ratio. Simultaneously, attenuating the LPS-induced pathological changes in lung tissues included inflammatory cells infiltration, interalveolar septal thickening, and edema. The further study showed that treatment with ATL-I considerably down-regulated the release of TNF-α, IL-6, IL-1β, and IL-13, which were detected by ELISA. However, ATL-I could enhance the expression of IL-10 in BALF. LPS could induce conformational changes in the TLR4 receptors to activate TLR4. TLR4 activation would promote NF-κB expression and inflammatory cytokine production. Additionally, ATL-I also had an inhibitory effect on the LPS-induced TLR4 expression and NF-κB activation, which were measured by western blot analysis [29]. It was interesting that recent study showed that ATL-I could inhibit uridine 5′-iphospho-glucuronosyltransferases (UGTs) isoforms, especially UGT2B7 [30]. Additionally, ATL-I could inhibit 5-LOX production to decrease allergic response [31].

Atractylenolide II

Atractylenolide II (ATL-II), a sesquiterpene, can be extracted from RAM and AL, exerting anti-cancer and anti-inflammatory activities. The melting point of ATL-II is 383 °C. ATL-II was identified in AL in 1998 [32]. Recent study showed that suppression of STAT3 signaling had a promoting effect on the anti-melanoma action of AT-II in B16 and A375 cells. 48 h AT-II treatment showed a dose-dependent manner inhibitory effect on p-STAT3, p-Src, and Mcl-1 and Bcl-xL in B16 and A375 cells. However, the suppressive effect of AT-II would be mostly reversed after the restoration of active variant of STAT3. The animal studies showed that 14-day administration of AT-II could obviously suppress tumor growth and inhibit STAT3 activation [33]. A present study manifested that AT-II could significantly inhibit human gastric carcinoma cell HGC-27 and AGS growth and migration in a dose-dependent manner. Further study showed that AT-II could suppress Bcl-2, p-Akt and p-ERK expression, and increase Bax expression [34].

Atractylenolide III

Atractylenolide III (ATL-III), a sesquiterpene, is the major component in RAM, and could be extracted from AL. The melting point of ATL-III is 200–201 °C, and the freezing point of ATL-III is 392–394 °F. ATL-III showed the cytotoxic effect on cancer cells and the anti-inflammatory effect on macrophages [35, 36]. ATL-III was identified in AL in 2008 [37]. Mast cells could promote atopic dermatitis [38]. It was demonstrated that ATL-III possessed anti-tumor activity on TSLP-stimulated human mast cell, HMC-1 cells. The detailed mechanism was that ATL-III could inhibit the murine double minute 2 levels, mast cell proliferation, IL-13 and phosphorylated signal transducer and activator of transcription. In the mean time, ATL-III could promote p53 expression. Additionally, the release of pro-inflammatory cytokines stimulated by TSLP (IL-6, TNF-α, and IL-8) was reduced by ATL-III. Furthermore, the Bcl2 and pro-caspase-3 levels could be down regulated by ATL-III, whereas the caspase-3 activation and cleaved PARP levels could be up regulated by ATL-III [39]. Recent study showed that ATL-III exhibited anti-inflammatory effect on LPS-triggered RAW264.7 mouse macrophages. The detailed mechanism was associated with the inhibitory effect of ATL-III on the production of NO, PGE2, TNF-α and IL-6, and the suppressive effect of ATL-III on NF-κB and mitogen-activated protein kinase (MAPK) signaling pathways. ATL-III could dose-dependently inhibit NO, TNF-α, PGE2 and IL-6 release, and high concentration of ATL-III (100 μM) could suppress cytokines cyclooxygenase-2 (COX-2) expression via the inhibition on the activation of NF-κB and ERK1/2 [40]. Additionally, ATL-III exerted a neuroprotective effect in rats with learning and memory impairment through the inhibition of ROS production and protein kinase C levels [41].

Atractylone

Atractylone was one of the main sesquiterpenic constituents of AL, displaying the anti-inflammatory action and anti-hepatotoxic effect [42–44]. The boiling point is 285.00–286.00 °C. Atractylone was identified in AL in 2006, reaching 9.35% [45]. Atractylone showed an inhibitory effect on allergic inflammation in an ovalbumin (OVA)-induced AR animal model. Further study exerted that Atractylone could also suppress caspase-1/NF-κB/MAPKs activation phorbol 12-myristate 13-acetate and calcium ionophore A23187 (PMACI)-induced human mast cell line (HMC-1) cells. In the animal model, Atractylone decreased rub scores, and reduced IL-1, IL-4, IL-5, IL-6, IL-13, COX-2, intercellular adhesion molecule-1, and macrophage inflammatory protein-2 expression [46]. Recently, atractylone could decrease influenza A virus (IAV)-induced pulmonary injury at the concentration of 40 mg/kg for 5 days in mice model. Further study showed that atractylone could inhibit IL-6, TNF-α and IL-1β, but promote Toll-like receptor 7 (TLR7), MyD88, tumor necrosis factor receptor-associated factor 6 interferon-β (IFN-β) expression [47]. It was reported that atractylone exerted a salutary effect on the mast cell-mediated allergic reactions. The results exhibited that atractylone could suppress compound 48/80-induced rat peritoneal mast cells (RPMCs) degranulation intracellular Ca^{2+} level ($[Ca^{2+}]$), tryptase release, and histamine release. Additionally, atractylone could inhibit compound 48/80-induced p56lck tyrosine kinase activity in RPMCs. Also, atractylone showed an inhibitory effect on histidine decarboxylase activity and expression in PMACI-induced HMC-1 cells. Further study showed that atractylone could also inhibit tryptase and histamine releases in

PMACI-induced HMC-1 cells. Atractylone could inhibit morphological alteration and filamentous actin formation in stem cell factor-stimulated RPMCs animal model [48].

Hinesol

Hinesol is a sesquiterpenoid, which was 5–9% in AL. Hinesol exhibited the cytotoxic effect on cancer cells and a strong anti-inflammatory effect. Hinesol was clarified in AL in 2003 [49]. Hinesol could reduce nuclear fragmentation and DNA fragmentation, indicating that hinesol had an inhibitory effect on human leukemia HL-60 cells through apoptosis. The further study showed that hinesol could modulate c-Jun signaling pathway through the activation of c-Jun N-terminal kinase (JNK) [50]. A recent study indicated that hinesol could show the anti-gastric ulcer effect through a significant inhibitory effect on H^+, K^+-ATPase activity. The concentration of ATP and K^+ could not modulate the inhibitory effect of hinesol, but the increase of Mg^{2+} concentration could promote the inhibitory effect of hinesol. Also, hinesol displayed a moderate inhibitory effect on Mg^{2+}-ATPase and Ca^{2+}-ATPase activity [51].

β-Eudesmol

β-Eudesmol, a sesquiterpenoid alcohol, is the main constituent of AL. β-Eudesmol can be also extracted from *Teucrium ramosissimum* [52]. The melting point of β-eudesmol is 72–74 °C. Particularly, β-eudesmol demonstrated a strong inhibitory effect on cancer, and β-eudesmol could protect neuron from inflammatory damage. CCA, or bile duct cancer, which was an uncommon adenocarcinoma that originated from the epithelial cells of bile ducts, is becoming a vital public health problem worldwide. Recent study exerted that β-eudesmol could improve the anti-cancer effect of 5-fluorouracil and doxorubicin in human CCA KKU-100 cells with the high expression of NAD (P) H-quinone oxidoreductase 1 (NQO1). Also, β-eudesmol could inhibit cell growth, migration, NQO1 expression and activity in CCA [53]. β-Eudesmol showed an inhibitory effect on CCA growth and metastasis in CCA-xenografted nude mouse model according to the results from positron emission tomography-computed tomography (PET-CT). Also, β-eudesmol could prolong the survival time of CCA mice model [54]. Another study exerted that β-eudesmol could also induce apoptosis, cell cycle arrest at G1 phase, and the cleavage of caspase 3 and caspase 7 in CCA [55]. Primary liver cancer is the third-leading cause of cancer death all over the world [56]. Recent studies showed that β-eudesmol isomers could inhibit proliferation of human hepatocellular carcinoma Hep-G2 cells through the induction of apoptosis, according to haematoxylin–eosin and acridine orange ethidium bromide staining results. Further study showed that β-eudesmol could decrease mitochondrial membrane potential and activate caspases [57]. Recently, β-eudesmol showed the anti-tumor activities in human lung and colon cancer cells. Further study exerted that β-eudesmol (200 μM) significantly decreased A549 cells migration towards type IV collagen (54% inhibition) and fibronectin (60% inhibition). Meanwhile, β-eudesmol (200 μM) also inhibited HT29 cell migration toward type IV collagen and fibronectinline with inhibition of 76% and 63%, respectively [52]. Abnormal angiogenesis was involved in diverse diseases, such as tumor and diabetic retinopathy. Recently, β-eudesmol showed an inhibitory effect on angiogenesis partly via the arrest of the ERK signaling pathway, suggesting that β-eudesmol could be considered as the drug candidate for treatment of angiogenic diseases. In detail, β-eudesmol had an inhibitory effect on the multiplication of porcine brain microvascular endothelial cells and human umbilical vein endothelial cells (HUVEC). Additionally, β-eudesmol could inhibit the migration of HUVEC, and at the high concentration β-eudesmol could inhibit the ERK1/2 phosphorylation and suppress angiogenesis in subcutaneously implanted Matrigel plugs in mice and in adjuvant-induced granuloma in mice [58]. Another study showed that β-eudesmol had an inhibitory effect on angiogenesis via inhibiting CREB activation in growth factor signaling pathway, herein demonstrating β-eudesmol as an inhibitory compound of tumor growth. β-Eudesmol at the concentration ranging from 50 to 100 μM had an inhibitory effect on the proliferation of HUVEC stimulated with vascular endothelial growth factor (VEGF, 30 ng/ml) and basic fibroblast growth factor (bFGF, 30 ng/ml). In addition, β-eudesmol at the concentration of 100 μM also had a blocking effect on the phosphorylation of cAMP response element binding protein (CREB) triggered by VEGF 30 ng/ml in HUVEC. β-Eudesmol at the concentration ranging from 10 to 100 μM suppressed proliferation of HeLa, SGC-7901, and BEL-7402 tumor cells in a time-and dose-dependent manner. Moreover, treatment with β-eudesmol (2.5–5 mg/kg) markedly suppressed the growth of H22 and S180 mouse tumor growth in vivo [59]. Pheochromocytoma mainly refers to a neuroendocrine tumor of the adrenal glands. β-Eudesmol could induce neurite extension in rat pheochromocytoma cells (PC-12), accompanying with inhibition of $[^3H]$ thymidine incorporation. Meanwhile, β-eudesmol also stimulated the improvement of $[Ca^{2+}]$. Moreover, β-eudesmol concentration-dependently led to an accumulation of inositol phosphates, and β-eudesmol could increase the p-MAPK time-dependently [60]. Recently, β-eudesmol was reported to modify the sensitivity of diabetic mice to depolarizing blockers so as to increase the susceptibility to these compounds. By investigating phrenic nerve-diaphragm muscles in normal and alloxan-diabetic mice, β-eudesmol exhibited the potentiating/promoting effect on neuromuscular blockade. Pretreatment with β-eudesmol enhanced the blocking action of succinylcholine to a greater degree in diabetic muscles than in normal ones. 30-min pretreatment in normal muscles could make the effect saturated,while 60-min pretreatment in diabetic muscles could make further potentiation [61]. It was reported that β-eudesmol could block the nicotinic acetylcholine receptor (nAChR) channel in both open and closed conformations, resulting in potentiating the neuromuscular blockade induced by succinylcholine (SuCh). The blocking effect of SuCh (0.1–10 μM) with β-eudesmol on nAChR channel activity was investigated by using the cell-attached patch clamp technique. Pretreatment with β-eudesmol (20 μM) had no effect on resting membrane potential and ACh-activated channel activities. β-Eudesmol decreased SuCh (above 0.3 μM)-induced prolongation of channel open time and reduced the frequency of channel opening in the presence of SuCh (above 3 μM) in ACh-activated channel currents regulated by SuCh [62]. β-Eudesmol could potentiate the effect of phenylene-polymethylene-bis-ammonium (PMBA) derivatives on neuromuscular blockades in alloxan-diabetic mice [63]. Current study manifested that the intragastric injection of β-eudesmol to rats could inhibit efferent adrenal sympathetic nerve activity (ASNA). The knock-out of TRPA1 could block the inhibitory effect of β-eudesmol on ASNA, and subdiaphragmatic vagotomy could promote the suppression of β-eudesmol on ASNA, suggesting that β-eudesmol could modulate ASNA through TRPA1 and afferent vagus nerve [7]. It was reported that β-eudesmol had the ability of modifying the chemical composition of the workers cuticle, to impair nestmate recognition, initiate alarm behavior and result in nestmate aggression [64]. Recent study showed that β-eudesmol pre-treatment on mouse diaphragm muscles for 30–60 min could promote $[Ca^{2+}]$ and twitch tension induced by succinylcholine as nicotinic acetylcholine receptor channel [65].

Atractylodin

Atractylodin (Atr), a polyethylene alkyne, could be extracted from AL, exerting the anti-inflammatory activities. The melting point of Atr is 52 °C. A present study showed that atractylodin (Atr) could inhibit LPS-induced inflammatory responses. Namely, Atr could suppress myeloperoxidase (MPO) activity, the wet-to-dry weight ratio of the lungs, protein leakage, infiltration of inflammatory cells, TNF-α, IL-6, IL-1β and monocyte chemoattractant protein (MCP)-1 secretion. The mechanism was that Atr could down-regulate nucleotide-binding domain- (NOD-) like receptor protein 3 (NLRP3) inflammasome and TLR4 activation [66]. Another study reported that Atr exhibited anti-inflammatory effects and ameliorated concurring dysmotility in constipation-prominent (CP) and diarrheaprominent (DP) rats. The detailed mechanism was associated with the reduction of the plasma pro-inflammatory cytokines such as TNF-α, IL-1β, and IL-6 [67].

Stigmasterol

Stigmasterol is an unsaturated phytosterol, and could extracted from soybean, calabar bean, rape seed, American Ginseng, AL and etc. The melting point of stigmasterol is 160–164 °C. Stigmasterol showed diverse pharmacological effects, such as anti-inflammotory, anti-nociceptive and anti-diabetic activities. Recent study exerted that stigmasterol could inhibit OVA-induced airway inflammatory damage in guinea pigs through intraperitoneal injection. More precisely, stigmasterol could suppress eosinophils, lymphocytes, and monocytes proliferation and inhibit peribronchiolar, perivascular, and alveolar infiltration of inflammatory cells. Stigmasterol could also inhibit vascular cell adhesion molecule-1 (VCAM-1) and OVA-specific immunoglobulin E (OVA sIgE) expression. VCAM-1 could medicate the adhesion of lymphocytes, monocytes, eosinophils, and basophils to vascular endothelium after the endothelial cells are stimulated by cytokines [68]. Recent study showed stigmasterol could improve memory and behavioral impairments in vanadium-induced neurotoxicity. More precisely, stigmasterol could reduce escape latency and prolong swimming time in Morris water maze. Also, stigmasterol could promote activities of antioxidant enzymes, and inhibit oxidative stress markers as well as lipid peroxidation in mice hippocampal homogenates [69]. A recent study showed that stigmasterol could protect mice from LPS-induced fever response. Further study exerted that stigmasterol relived organ damage and dearth rate [70]. Recently, stigmasterol exerted the synergistic antibiotic effect as adjuvant of ampicillin against both Gram positive and Gram-negative bacteria from clinical isolates. The inhibitory effect of ampicillin and stigmasterol alone is extremely ineffective, but the combination of stigmasterol-ampicillin significantly suppress colony counts, yielding 98.7% [71]. *Trypanosoma congolense* could induce the disease nagan in diverse animals. Stigmasterol showed antitrypanosomal activity against *Trypanosoma congolense* infection through reducing sialidase [72]. Moreover, a present study exhibited that stigmasterol displayed a mosquito larvicidal activity through neurotoxicity [73]. A present study displayed that stigmasterol showed anti-nociceptive effect on male albino Swiss mice model according to the results from

Table 2 The anti-cancer effects of major components of AL

Chemical name	Tumor suppressive effect	Potential targets	Function study	References
Atractylenolide I	Anti-bladder cancer effect	↓PI3K/Akt/mTOR	In vitro and In vivo	[17]
	Anti-leukemia effect	↑CD14/CD68	In vitro	[23]
	Anti-melanoma effect	↓p-JAK2/p-STAT3	In vitro	[25]
Atractylenolide II	Anti-melanoma effect	↓p-STAT3/p-Src	In vitro and in vivo	[33]
	Anti-gastric cancer effect	↓p-Akt/p-ERK	In vitro	[34]
Hinesol	Anti-leukemia effect	↓c-Jun	In vitro	[50]
β-Eudesmol	Anti-bile duct cancer effect	↓NQO1	In vitro and in vivo	[53, 54]
β-Sitosterol	Anti-melanoma effect	↓JNK	In vitro	[77]
	Anti-gastric cancer effect	↑PTEN/p-AMPK	In vitro and in vivo	[78]

acetic-acid writhing test, surgical incision, partial sciatic nerve ligation and complete Freund's adjuvant. Further study exerted that naloxone could not block the anti-nociceptive effect of stigmasterol [74]. Recent study indicated that stigmasterol exhibited anti-diabetic activity in vitro and in vivo. Stigmasterol could increase GLUT4 translocation and expression. In the animal model, stigmasterol could reduce insulin resistance and oral glucose tolerance with the decrease of fasting blood-glucose levels and blood lipid indexes [75]. Recently, stigmasterol and β-sitosterol could suppress colitis in dextran sulfate sodium (DSS)-induced colitis in C57BL/6J male mice fed a high fat Western-style diet. β-Sitosterol and stigmasterol critically suppressed colon shortening, decreased fecal hemoglobin content, and inhibited the severity of colitis in the middle as well as distal colon through the inactivation of NF-κB. Particularly, stigmasterol could reduce COX-2 and CSF-1 [76].

β-Sitosterol

β-Sitosterol is a phytosterol, and could be extracted from *Nigella sativa, Serenoa repens, Cucurbita pepo, Pygeum africanum*, AL and etc. The melting point of β-sitosterol is 136–140 °C. β-Sitosterol displayed cytotoxic effect on cancer cells and an anti-inflammatory activity. Multiple myeloma refers to a cancer of plasma cells. Recently, it was reported that β-sitosterol could display cytotoxicity on multiple myeloma U266 cells through apoptosis. Further study showed that β-sitosterol could increase production, activate AMP-activated protein kinase (AMPK) acetyl-CoA carboxylase (ACC) and JNK pathways, with a decrease of p-AKT, S6K and vascular VEGF [77]. Gastric cancer refers to the cancer starting from stomach. Recently, β-sitosterol exerted the anti-cancer effect on AGS human gastric adenocarcinoma cells through apoptosis. Further study showed that β-sitosterol could increase phosphatase and tensin homolog (PTEN) and p-AMPK expression, and decrease Hsp90 protein. Moreover, β-sitosterol could inhibit tumor weight and volume according in AGS xenograft animal study [78]. Recent study showed that β-sitosterol exerted the anti-inflammatory activity on rat model according to the rat paw edema test and the rat pleurisy assay [79]. A recent study manifested that β-sitosterol could ameliorate high fat diet induced dyslipidemia and hepatotoxicity in Swiss albino mice [80].

Conclusion

In recent time, herbs and extractions from TCM have been widely considered as the complementary and alternative medicine (CAM) for various diseases treatment [81, 82]. AL has been used as TCM for thousands of years, and current studies found that AL and some of its pure compounds exerted diverse biological activities. It is interesting to find that most of major components could exert cytotoxic effects on cancer cells, especially melanoma (Table 2). However, the animal studies are insufficient. Also, the effects of these drugs on normal cells and healthy animals are lacking. Meanwhile, it is worthwhile to explore the pharmacological activities of minor components identified in AL. Nevertheless, further studies to identify other pure compounds for drug development and novel pharmacological activities of AL are still necessary to facilitate research and development.

Abbreviations

ACC: acetyl-CoA carboxylase; AL: *Atractylodes lancea* Thunb. DC; AMPK: AMP-activated protein kinase; ASNA: adrenal sympathetic nerve activity; ATL-I: atractylenolide I; ATL-II: atractylenolide II; ATL-III: atractylenolide III; Atr: atractylodin; bFGF: basic fibroblast growth factor; [Ca^{2+}]: Ca^{2+} concentration; CAM: complementary and alternative medicine; CCA: cholangiocarcinoma; CP: constipation-prominent; CREB: cAMP response element binding protein; COX-2: cyclooxygenase-2; DP: diarrheaprominent; DSS: dextran sulfate sodium; EGF: epidermal growth factor; G-CSF: granulocyte-colony stimulating factor; HUVEC: human umbilical vein endothelial cells; 5-HT: 5-hydroxytryptamine; IAV: influenza A virus; IFN-β: tumor necrosis factor receptor-associated factor 6 interferon-β; IL-8: interleukin-8; JNK: c-Jun N-terminal kinase; KPS: Karnofsky performance status; LPS: lipopolysaccharide; MAPK: mitogen-activated protein kinase; MCP: monocyte chemoattractant protein; MPO: myeloperoxidase;

nAChR: nicotinic acetylcholine receptor; NO: nitric oxide; NOD: nucleotide-binding domain; NQO1: NAD(P)H-quinone oxidoreductase 1; OV: opisthorchis viverrini; OVA: ovalbumin; OVA sIgE: OVA-specific immunoglobulin E; PE: petroleum ether; PET-CT: positron emission tomography-computed tomography; PGE2: prostaglandin E2; PIF: proteolysis-inducing factor; PMACI: phorbol 12-myristate 13-acetate and calcium ionophore A23187; PMBA: phenylene-polymethylene-bis-ammonium; PTEN: phosphatase and tensin homolog; SuCh: succinylcholine; TFF2: trefoil factor2; TLR4: toll like receptor 4; TNF-α: tumor necrosis factor-α; UGT: uridine 5′-iphospho-glucuronosyltransferases; VCAM-1: vascular cell adhesion molecule-1; VEGF: vascular endothelial growth factor.

Authors' contributions
XJ and PF drafted the manuscript. YL drew Fig. 1. PC designed and revised the manuscript. All authors read and approved the final manuscript.

Author details
[1] Chengdu University of Traditional Chinese Medicine, Chengdu, China. [2] West China School of Pharmacy, Sichuan University, Chengdu, China.

Acknowledgements
Not applicable.

Competing interests
The authors declare that they have no competing interests.

Consent for publication
All of authors consent to publication of this work in Chinese Medicine.

Funding
National Natural Science Foundation of China No. 81630101 supported this work.

References

1. Qian S, Wang L, Duan J, Feng H. The research progress in chemical constituents and biological activities of *Atractylodes lancea* DC. Chin Tradit Herbal Drugs. 2006;18:8–11.
2. Koonrungsesomboon N, Nabangchang K, Karbwang J. Therapeutic potential and pharmacological activities of *Atractylodes lancea* (Thunb.) DC. Asian Pac. J Trop Med. 2014;7:421.
3. Zhang Y, Wang Z, Zhu J, Chen B, Li Y. Determination of atractylodin in rat plasma by HPLC-UV method and its application to a Pharmacokinetic study. J Liq Chromatogr R T. 2012;35:778–87.
4. Huo Y, Liu YQ, Bai ZX, Cai Q. Determination of (4E, 6E, 12E)-tetradecatriene-8,10-diyne-1,3-diyl diacetate in rat plasma and tissues by HPLC-UV method and their application to a pharmacokinetic and tissue distribution study. J Anal Methods Chem Biol. 2014;2014:1–7.
5. Liu Q, Kong D, Luo J, Kong W, Guo W, Yang M. Quantitative and fingerprinting analysis of Atractylodes rhizome based on gas chromatography with flame ionization detection combined with chemometrics. J Sep Sci. 2016;39:2517.
6. Duan JA, Wang L, Qian S, Su S. A new cytotoxic prenylated dihydrobenzofuran derivative and other chemical constituents from the rhizomes of *Atractylodes lancea* DC. Arch Pharm Res. 2008;31:965–9.
7. Ohara K, Katayama M, Nagai K. β-eudesmol, an oxygenized sesquiterpene, affects efferent adrenal sympathetic nerve activity via transient receptor potential ankyrin 1 in rats. Neurosci Lett. 2018;684:18–24.
8. Kimura Y, Sumiyoshi M. Effects of an *Atractylodes lancea* rhizome extract and a volatile component β-eudesmol on gastrointestinal motility in mice. J Ethnopharmacol. 2012;141:530–6.
9. Yu Y, Jia TZ, Cai Q, Jiang N, Ma MY, Min DY, Yuan Y. Comparison of the anti-ulcer activity between the crude and bran-processed *Atractylodes lancea* in the rat model of gastric ulcer induced by acetic acid. J Ethnopharmacol. 2015;160:211–8.
10. Wang M, Chen X. Obstacle and countermeasure of sustainable high yield for peanut in low-hilly red soil region. J Peanut Sci. 2005;34:17–22.
11. Mitsuboshi M, Kioka Y, Noguchi K, Asakawa S. Evaluation of suppressiveness of soils exhibiting soil-borne disease suppression after long-term application of organic amendments by the co-cultivation method of pathogenic fusarium oxysporum and indigenous soil microorganisms. Microbes Environ. 2018;33:58–65.
12. Zhao M, Wang Q, Ouyang Z, Han B, Wang W, Wei Y, Wu Y, Yang B. Selective fraction of *Atractylodes lancea* (Thunb.) DC. and its growth inhibitory effect on human gastric cancer cells. Cytotechnology. 2014;66:201–8.
13. Shimato Y, Ota M, Asai K, Atsumi T, Tabuchi Y, Makino T. Comparison of byakujutsu (Atractylodes rhizome) and sojutsu (*Atractylodes lancea* rhizome) on anti-inflammatory and immunostimulative effects in vitro. J Nat Med. 2018;72:192–201.
14. Jiao P, Tseng-Crank J, Corneliusen B, Yimam M, Hodges M, Hong M, Maurseth C, Oh M, Kim H, Chu M, Jia Q. Lipase inhibition and antiobesity effect of *Atractylodes lancea*. Planta Med. 2014;80:577–82.
15. Murayama C, Wang CC, Michihara S, Norimoto H. Pharmacological effects of "jutsu" (Atractylodis rhizome and Atractylodis lanceae rhizome) on 1-(2,5-dimethoxy-4-iodophenyl)-2-aminopropane (DOI)-induced head twitch response in mice (I). Molecules. 2014;19:14979–86.
16. Wei Y, Sui DJ, Xu HM, Ouyang Z, Wu N, Wang DJ, Zhang XY, Qian DW. *Atractylodes lancea* rhizome water extract reduces triptolide-induced toxicity and enhances anti-inflammatory effects. Chin J Nat Med. 2017;15:905–11.
17. Yu R, Yu BX, Chen JF, Lv XY, Yan ZJ, Cheng Y, Ma Q. Anti-tumor effects of Atractylenolide I on bladder cancer cells. J Exp Clin Cana Res. 2016;35:40.
18. Wang CC, Lin SY, Cheng CH, Hou WC. Pro-oxidant and cytotoxic activities of atractylenolide I in human promyeloleukemic HL-60 cells. Food Chem Toxicol. 2006;44:1308–15.
19. Wang CH, Duan HJ, He LC. Inhibitory effect of atractylenolide I on angiogenesis in chronic inflammation in vivo and in vitro. Eur J Pharmacol. 2002;612:143–52.
20. Lim H, Lee JH, Kim J, Kim YS, Kim HP. Effects of the rhizomes of *Atractylodes japonica* and atractylenolide I on allergic response and experimental atopic dermatitis. Arch Pharm Res. 2004;35:2007–12.
21. Wang C, He L, Wang N, Liu F. Screening anti-inflammatory components from chinese traditional medicines using a peritoneal macrophage/cell membrane chromatography-offline-gc/ms method. J Chromatogr B Analyt Technol Biomed Life Sci. 2009;877:3019–24.
22. Carneiro BA, Meeks JJ, Kuzel TM, Scaranti M, Abdulkadir SA, Giles FJ. Emerging therapeutic targets in bladder cancer. Cancer Treat Rev. 2015;41:170–8.
23. Huang HL, Lin TW, Huang YL, Huang RL. Induction of apoptosis and differentiation by atractylenolide-1 isolated from *Atractylodes macrocephala* in human leukemia cells. Bioorg Med Chem Lett. 2016;26:1905–9.
24. Tentori L, Lacal PM, Graziani G. Challenging resistance mechanisms to therapies for metastatic melanoma. Trends Pharmacol Sci Rep. 2013;34:656–66.
25. Fu XQ, Chou JY, Li T, Zhu PL, Li JK, Yin CL, Su T, Guo H, Lee KW, Hossen MJ, Chou GX, Yu ZL. The JAK2/STAT3 pathway is involved in the anti-melanoma effects of atractylenolide I. Exp Dermatol. 2018;27:201–4.
26. Liu Y, Jia Z, Dong L, Wang R, Qiu G. A randomized pilot study of atractylenolide I on gastric cancer cachexia patients. Evid-Based Comp Alt. 2008;5:337–44.
27. Song HP, Hou XQ, Li RY, Yu R, Li X, Zhou SN, Huang HY, Cai X, Zhou C. Atractylenolide I stimulates intestinal epithelial repair through polyamine-mediated Ca(2+) signaling pathway. Phytomedicine. 2017;28:27–35.
28. Li W, Zhi W, Liu F, He Z, Wang X, Niu X. Atractylenolide I restores HO-1 expression and inhibits Ox-LDL-induced VSMCs proliferation, migration and inflammatory responses in vitro. Exp Cell Res. 2017;353:26–34.
29. Zhang JL, Huang WM, Zeng QY. Atractylenolide I protects mice from lipopolysaccharide-induced acute lung injury. Eur J Pharmacol. 2015;765:94–9.
30. Zhang Q, Cao YF, Ran RX, Li RS, Wu X, Dong PP, Zhang YY, Hu CM, Wang WM. Strong specific inhibition of UDP-glucuronosyltransferase 2B7 by atractylenolide I and III. Phytother Res. 2016;30:25–30.

31. Lim H, Lee JH, Kim J, Kim YS, Kim HP. Effects of the rhizomes of *Atractylodes japonica* and atractylenolide I on allergic response and experimental atopic dermatitis. Arch Pharm Res. 2012;35:2007–12.
32. Resch M, Steigel A, Chen ZL, Bauer R. 5-Lipoxygenase and cyclooxygenase-1 inhibitory active compounds from *Atractylodes lancea*. J Nat Prod. 1998;61:347–50.
33. Fu XQ, Chou GX, Kwan HY, Tse AK, Zhao LH, Yuen TK, Cao HH, Yu H, Chao XJ, Su T, Cheng BC, Sun XG, Yu ZL. Inhibition of STAT3 signalling contributes to the antimelanoma action of atractylenolide II. Exp Dermatol. 2014;23:855–7.
34. Tian S, Yu H. Atractylenolide II inhibits proliferation, motility and induces apoptosis in human gastric carcinoma cell lines HGC-27 and AGS. Molecules. 2017;22:1886.
35. Wang CC, Chen LG, Yang LL. Cytotoxic activity of sesquiterpenoids from *Atractylodes ovata* on leukemia cell lines. Planta Med. 2002;68:204–8.
36. Li CQ, He LC, Jin JQ. Atractylenolide I and atractylenolide III inhibit lipopolysaccharide-induced TNF-a and NO production in macrophages. Phytother Res. 2007;21:347–53.
37. Wang HX, Liu CM, Liu Q, Gao K. Three types of sesquiterpenes from rhizomes of *Atractylodes lancea*. Phytochemistry. 2008;69:2088–94.
38. Theoharides TC, Cochrane DE. Critical role of mast cells in inflammatory diseases and the effect of acute stress. J Neuroimmunol. 2004;146:1–12.
39. Yoou MS, Nam SY, Jin MH, Lee SY, Kim MS, Roh SS, Choi IH, Woo N, Lim S, Kim DH, Jang JB, Kim HM, Jeong HJ. Ameliorative effect of atractylenolide III in the mast cell proliferation induced by TSLP. Food Chem Toxicol. 2017;106:78–85.
40. Ji GQ, Chen RQ, Wang L. Anti-inflammatory activity of atractylenolide III through inhibition of nuclear factor-kappaB and mitogen-activated protein kinase pathways in mouse macrophages. Immunopharm Immunot. 2016;38:98–102.
41. Zhao H, Ji ZH, Liu C, Yu XY. Neuroprotection and mechanisms of atractylenolide III in preventing learning and memory impairment induced by chronic high-dose homocysteine administration in rats. Neuroscience. 2015;290:485–91.
42. Hwang JM, Tseng TH, Hsieh YS, Chou FP, Wang CJ, Chu CY. Inhibitory effect of atractylon on tert-butyl hydroperoxide induced DNA damage and hepatic toxicity in rat hepatocytes. Arch Toxicol. 2013;70:660–4.
43. Sin KS, Kim HP, Lee WC, Pachaly P. Pharmacological activities of the constituents of Atractylodes rhizomes. Arch Pharm Res. 1989;12:236–8.
44. Kiso Y, Tohkin M, Hikino H. Mechanism of antihepatotoxic activity of atractylon, I: effect on free radical generation and lipid peroxidation. Planta Med. 2015;51:97–100.
45. Guo FQ, Huang LF, Zhou SY, Zhang TM, Liang YZ. Comparison of the volatile compounds of Atractylodes, medicinal plants by headspace solid-phase microextraction-gas chromatography–mass spectrometry. Anal Chim Acta. 2006;570:73–8.
46. Kim HY, Nam SY, Hwang SY, Kim HM, Jeong HJ. Atractylone, an active constituent of KMP6, attenuates allergic inflammation on allergic rhinitis in vitro and in vivo models. Mol Immunol. 2016;78:121–32.
47. Cheng Y, Mai JY, Hou TL, Ping J, Chen JJ. Antiviral activities of atractylon from Atractylodis Rhizoma. Mol Med Rep. 2016;14:3704–10.
48. Han NR, Moon PD, Nam SY, Ryu KJ, Yoou MS, Choi JH, Hwang SY, Kim HM, Jeong HJ. Inhibitory effects of atractylone on mast cell-mediated allergic reactions. Chem-biol Interact. 2016;258:59–68.
49. Nakai Y, Kido T, Hashimoto K, Kase Y, Sakakibara I, Higuchi M, Sasaki H. Effect of the rhizomes of *Atractylodes lancea* and its constituents on the delay of gastric emptying. J Ethnopharmacol. 2003;84:51–5.
50. Masuda Y, Kadokura T, Ishii M, Takada K, Kitajima J. Hinesol, a compound isolated from the essential oils of *Atractylodes lancea* rhizome, inhibits cell growth and induces apoptosis in human leukemia HL-60 cells. J Nat Med. 2015;69:332–9.
51. Satoh K, Nagai F, Kano I. Inhibition of H+, K+-ATPase by hinesol, a major component of So-jutsu, by interaction with enzyme in the E1 state. Biochem Pharmacol. 2000;59:881–6.
52. Ben Sghaier M, Mousslim M, Pagano A, Ammari Y, Luis J, Kovacic H. beta-eudesmol, a sesquiterpene from *Teucrium ramosissimum*, inhibits superoxide production, proliferation, adhesion and migration of human tumor cell. Environ Toxicol Pharm. 2016;46:227–33.
53. Srijiwangsa P, Ponnikorn S, Na-Bangchang K. Effect of of vacic H. beta-eusuppression-enhanced sensitivity of cholangiocarcinoma cells to chemotherapeutic agents. BMC. Pharmacol Toxicol. 2018;19:32.
54. Plengsuriyakarn T, Karbwang J, Na-Bangchang K. Anticancer activity using positron emission tomography-computed tomography and pharmacokinetics of beta-eudesmol in human cholangiocarcinoma xenografted nude mouse model. Clin Exp Pharmacol. 2015;42:293–304.
55. Kotawong K, Chaijaroenkul W, Muhamad P, Na-Bangchang K. Cytotoxic activities and effects of atractylodin and β-eudesmol on the cell cycle arrest and apoptosis on cholangiocarcinoma cell line. J Pharmacol Sci. 2018;136:51–6.
56. Ferlay J, Soerjomataram I, Dikshit R, Eser S, Mathers C, Rebelo M, Parkin DM, Forman D, Bray F. Cancer incidence and mortality worldwide: sources, methods and major patterns in GLOBOCAN 2012. Int J Cancer. 2015;136:E359–86.
57. Bomfim DS, Ferraz RP, Carvalho NC, Soares MB, Pinheiro ML, Costa EV, Bezerra DP. Eudesmol isomers induce caspase-mediated apoptosis in human hepatocellular carcinoma HepG2 cells. Basic Clin Pharmacol. 2013;113:300–6.
58. Tsuneki H, Ma EL, Kobayashi S, Sekizaki N, Maekawa K, Sasaoka T, Wang MW, Kimura I. Antiangiogenic activity of beta-eudesmol *in vitro* and *in vivo*. Eur J Pharmacol. 2005;512:105–15.
59. Ma EL, Li YC, Tsuneki H, Xiao JF, Xia MY, Wang MW, Kimura I. Beta-eudesmol suppresses tumour growth through inhibition of tumour neovascularisation and tumour cell proliferation. J Asian Nat Prod Res. 2008;10:159–67.
60. Obara Y, Aoki T, Kusano M, Ohizumi Y. Beta-eudesmol induces neurite outgrowth in rat pheochromocytoma cells accompanied by an activation of mitogen-activated protein kinase. J Pharmacol Exp Ther. 2002;301:803–11.
61. Muroi M, Tanaka K, Kimura I, Kimura M. Beta-eudesmol (a main component of *Atractylodes lancea*)-induced potentiation of depolarizing neuromuscular blockade in diaphragm muscles of normal and diabetic mice. Jpn J Pharmacol. 1989;50:69–71.
62. Nojima H, Kimura I, Kimura M. Blocking action of succinylcholine with beta-eudesmol on acetylcholine-activated channel activity at end-plates of single muscle cells of adult mice. Brain Res. 1992;575:337–40.
63. Kimura M, Kimura I, Muroi M, Tanaka K, Nojima H, Uwano T. Different modes of potentiation by beta-eudesmol, a main compound from *Atractylodes lancea*, depending on neuromuscular blocking actions of p-phenylene-polymethylene bis-ammonium derivatives in isolated phrenic nerve-diaphragm muscles of normal and alloxan-diabetic mice. Jpn J Pharmacol. 1992;60:19–24.
64. Marinho CG, Della Lucia TM, Ribeiro MM, Magalhaes ST, Guedes RN, Jham GN. Interference of beta-eudesmol in nestmate recognition in Atta sexdens rubropilosa (Hymenoptera: Formicidae). B Entomol Res. 2008;98:467–73.
65. Kimura I, Tsuneki H, Kondoh T, Kimura M. Enhancing effect by nicotinic acetylcholine receptor channel blockers, including beta-eudesmol, on succinylcholine-induced inhibition of twitch tension and intracellular Ca^{2+} in mouse diaphragm muscle. J Pharmacol Exp Ther. 1991;256:24–8.
66. Tang F, Fan K, Wang K, Bian C. Atractylodin attenuates lipopolysaccharide-induced acute lung injury by inhibiting NLRP3 inflammasome and TLR4 pathways. J Pharmacol Sci. 2018;136:203–11.
67. Yu C, Xiong Y, Chen D, Li Y, Xu B, Lin Y, Tang Z, Jiang C, Wang L. Ameliorative effects of atractylodin on intestinal inflammation and co-occurring dysmotility in both constipation and diarrhea prominent rats. Korean J Physiol Pha. 2017;21:1–9.
68. Antwi AO, Obiri DD, Osafo N. Stigmasterol modulates allergic airway inflammation in guinea pig model of ovalbumin-induced asthma. Mediat Inflamm. 2017;1:1. https://doi.org/10.1155/2017/2953930.
69. Adebiyi OE, Olopade JO, Olayemi FO. Sodium metavanadate induced cognitive decline, behavioral impairments, oxidative stress and down regulation of myelin basic protein in mice hippocampus: ameliorative roles of β-spinasterol, and stigmasterol. Brain Behav. 2018;8:e01014.
70. Antwi AO, Obiri DD, Osafo N, Forkuo AD, Essel LB. Stigmasterol inhibits lipopolysaccharide-induced innate immune responses in murine models. Int Immunopharmacol. 2017;53:105–13.

71. Yenn TW, Arslan Khan M, Amiera Syuhada N, Chean Ring L, Ibrahim D, Tan WN. Stigmasterol: an adjuvant for beta lactam antibiotics against beta-lactamase positive clinical isolates. Steroids. 2017;128:68–71.
72. Aminu R, Umar IA, Rahman MA, Ibrahim MA. Stigmasterol retards the proliferation and pathological features of *Trypanosoma congolense* infection in rats and inhibits trypanosomal sialidase in vitro and in silico. Biomed Pharmacother. 2017;89:482–9.
73. Gade S, Rajamanikyam M, Vadlapudi V, Nukala KM, Aluvala R, Giddigari C, Karanam NJ, Barua NC, Pandey R, Upadhyayula VSV, Sripadi P, Amanchy R, Upadhyayula SM. Acetylcholinesterase inhibitory activity of stigmasterol & hexacosanol is responsible for larvicidal and repellent properties of *Chromolaena odorata*. BBA-Gen Subjects. 2017;1861:541–50.
74. Walker CIB, Oliveira SM, Tonello R, Rossato MF, da Silva Brum E, Ferreira J, Trevisan G. Anti-nociceptive effect of stigmasterol in mouse models of acute and chronic pain. N-S Arch Pharmacol. 2017;390:1163–72.
75. Wang J, Huang M, Yang J, Ma X, Zheng S, Deng S, Huang Y, Yang X, Zhao P. Anti-diabetic activity of stigmasterol from soybean oil by targeting the GLUT4 glucose transporter. Food Nutr Res. 2017;61:1364117.
76. Feng S, Dai Z, Liu A, Wang H, Chen J, Luo Z, Yang CS. β-Sitosterol and stigmasterol ameliorate dextran sulfate sodium-induced colitis in mice fed a high fat Western-style diet. Food Funct. 2017;8:4179–86.
77. Sook SH, Lee HJ, Kim JH, Sohn EJ, Jung JH, Kim B, Kim JH, Jeong SJ, Kim SH. Reactive oxygen species-mediated activation of AMP-activated protein kinase and c-Jun N-terminal kinase plays a critical role in beta-sitosterol-induced apoptosis in multiple myeloma U266 cells. Phytother Res. 2014;28:387–94.
78. Shin EJ, Choi HK, Sung MJ, Park JH, Chung MY, Chung S, Hwang JT. Anti-tumour effects of beta-sitosterol are mediated by AMPK/PTEN/HSP90 axis in AGS human gastric adenocarcinoma cells and xenograft mouse models. Biochem Pharmacol. 2018;152:60–70.
79. Paniagua-Pérez R, Flores-Mondragón G, Reyes-Legorreta C, Herrera-López B, Cervantes-Hernández I, Madrigal-Santillán O, Morales-González JA, Álvarez-González I, Madrigal-Bujaidar E. Evaluation of the anti-inflammatory capacity of beta-sitosterol in rodent assays. Afr J Tradit Complement Altern Med. 2017;14:123–30.
80. Sikder K, Das N, Kesh SB, Dey S. Quercetin and beta-sitosterol prevent high fat diet induced dyslipidemia and hepatotoxicity in Swiss albino mice. Indian J Exp Biol. 2014;52:60–6.
81. Lewith G, Britten N, Paterson C. Complementary and alternative medicine (CAM) and cancer: the kind face of complementary medicine. Int J Surg. 2010;8:81.
82. Hsiao WL, Liu L. The role of traditional Chinese herbal medicines in cancer therapy-from TCM theory to mechanistic insights. Planta Med. 2010;76:1118–31.

13

Corni Fructus: a review of chemical constituents and pharmacological activities

Yu Dong[1], Zhe-Ling Feng[1], Hu-Biao Chen[2], Fu-Sheng Wang[3] and Jia-Hong Lu[1*]

Abstract

Cornus officinalis Sieb. et Zucc. is part of the genus *Cornus* of the family *Cornaceae*. Ripening and dry fruits (*Corni Fructus*) are recognized as an essential herb medicine in the traditional Chinese medicine (TCM) and have been widely used for over 2000 years. This review provides a comprehensive summary of *Corni Fructus* (CF), including the botany, phytochemistry, traditional use, and current pharmacological activities. According to the basic theory of TCM, CF usually participates in various Chinese medicinal formulae to exert the essential roles in replenishing liver and kidney, arresting seminal emission and sweat. Based on modern pharmacological studies, about 90 compounds have been isolated and identified from CF. In vivo and in vitro experimental studies indicate that CF exhibits extensive pharmacological activities including hypoglycemic, antioxidant, anti-inflammatory, anticancer, neuroprotective, hepatoprotective, and nephroprotective activities. However, only about 18% of chemical constituents in CF were tested. It means the potential pharmacological activities and clinical values of CF need to be further investigated.

Keywords: *Cornus officinalis* Sieb. et Zucc., *Corni Fructus*, Shan Zhu Yu, Phytochemistry, Pharmacological activity

Background

Cornus officinalis Sieb. et Zucc., commonly known as Shan Zhu Yu/山茱萸 (in Chinese), Asiatic Dogwood, and Japanese Cornel Dogwood, is a deciduous shrub or dungarunga in the genus *Cornus* (family *Cornaceae*). It is a heliophilous plant that grows in the warm-temperate zone. The most suitable growth temperature is between 20 and 30 °C, it also has a specific cold resistance that can temporarily grow in −18 °C low-temperature zone. *Cornus officinalis* Sieb. et Zucc. can be found in Anhui, Gansu, Jiangsu, Jiangxi, Shandong, Shanxi in China, Korea, and Japan. It usually grows in 400–1500 m high mountain slope, forest or forest edge. Ripening fruits are picked during September and October and dried in the air for medical uses [1, 2].

About 2200 years ago, *Cornus officinalis* Sieb. et Zucc. fructus (usually known as *Corni Fructus*) was first recorded in *Shen Nong's Materia Medica* (Fig. 1). According to the basic theory of TCM, CF is characterized as replenishing liver and kidney, arresting seminal emission and sweat for its sour, astringent, and tepid properties [1]. It is used to treat four series of clinical symptoms. The first part of symptoms contains vertigo, tinnitus, weakness of the waist and knees which are caused by liver and kidney deficiency. CF is usually combined with *Radix Rehmanniae Praeparata, Dioscoreae Rhizoma, Alismatis Rhizoma, Moutan Cortex, Poria* to make Liuwei Dihuang Wan (六味地黄丸) replenish liver and kidney Yin [3]. For patients with kidney Yang deficiency, CF helps *Cinnamomi Cortex, Aconiti Lateralis Radix Praeparata* to reinforce Yang from Yin, e.g., Jingui Shenqi Wan (金匮肾气丸) [4]. The second part of symptoms contains spermatorrhoea and polydipsia. For patients with kidney deficiency, CF is frequently used with *Radix Rehmanniae Praeparata, Dioscoreae Rhizoma, Cervi Cornu Pantotrichum, Psoraleae Fructus.* For patients with dysfunction of the urinary bladder, CF is often applied with *Mantidis Oötheca, Rubi Fructus, Rosae Laevigatae Fructus.* The third part of symptom contains hypermenorrhea. CF is usually combined with *Radix Rehmanniae Praeparata, Angelica Sinensis, Radix Paeoniae Alba* to make Guchong Tang (固冲汤) preserve

*Correspondence: jiahonglu@umac.mo
[1] State Key Laboratory of Quality Research in Chinese Medicine, Institute of Chinese Medical Sciences, University of Macau, Room 7015, N22, Avenida da Universidade, Taipa, Macau SAR, People's Republic of China
Full list of author information is available at the end of the article

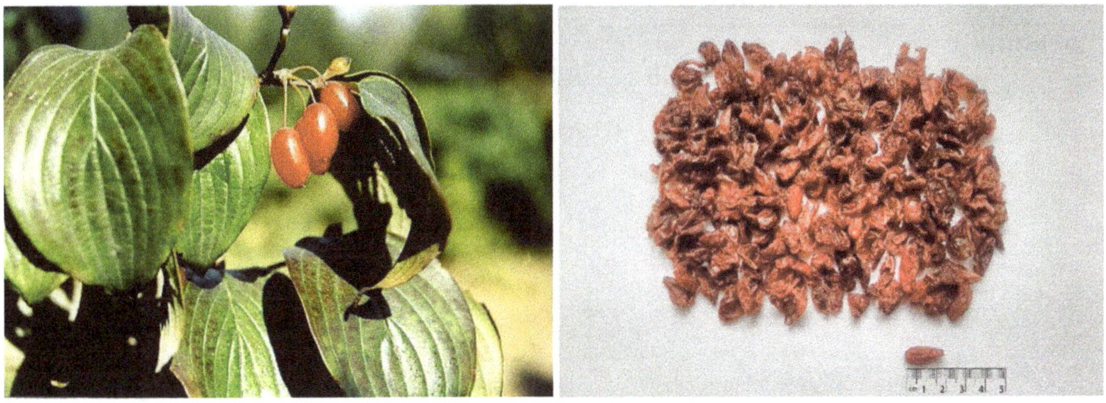

Fig. 1 *Corni Fructus*: **a** crude fruits, **b** processed fruits

Primordial Qi and stop Blood [5]. The fourth part of symptoms contains profuse cold sweating, pale complexion, cold limbs, and a feeble pulse. For patients with the Yang depletion syndrome, *Ginseng Radix et Rhizoma*, *Aconiti Lateralis Radix Praeparata*, and CF are applied in Laifu Tang (来复汤) to restore Yang from collapse. Medical practices indicate that CF can be combined with either Yin-tonifying or Yang-invigorating herbs to act as the sovereign drug or adjuvant drug in Chinese medicinal formulae and treat different types of TCM syndromes. Besides, CF is primarily made into the honey bolus to treat chronic diseases while is usually made into the decoction to treat acute conditions.

Chemical constituents

About 90 compounds have been isolated and identified from CF, including terpenoids, flavonoids, tannins, polysaccharides, phenylpropanoids, sterols, carboxylic acids, furans, and mineral substances. Chemical constituents are listed in Table 1. Among them, iridoids, tannins, and flavonoids are the major components. Their chemical structures are shown in Figs. 2, 3, 4 and 5.

Terpenoids (1–26) and flavonoids (27–39)

Most terpenoids and flavonoids in CF shared two similar isolation processes. Firstly, CF was percolated with ethanol to acquire the solvent which was then evaporated under reduced pressure. The resulting extract was suspended in water and then partitioned with ethyl acetate for several times. Finally, the extract was subjected to column chromatography over silica gel to yield compounds. Secondly, CF was grounded into powder and then subjected to supercritical carbon dioxide to yield extract. The resulting extract was subjected to GC–MS to identify the chemical components. So far, 26 terpenoids and 13 flavonoids have been isolated and identified from CF. Among terpenoids, the pharmacological activities of sweroside (**1**), loganin (**5**), cornuside (**23**), ursolic acid (**24**), and oleanolic acid (**25**) have been further assayed, and a wide range of pharmacological activities has been revealed. Furthermore, two types of flavonoids namely kaempferol (**28**), quercetin (**33**), and their derivatives are the essential flavonoids.

Tannins (40–69)

During the isolation process, CF was firstly homogenized in acetone and then filtered to acquire an aqueous solution which was sequentially extracted with diethyl ether and ethyl acetate. The extract was subjected to column chromatography to give compounds. Finally, the chemical structure and molecular weight were determined using nuclear magnetic resonance (NMR) spectroscopy. To date, 30 tannic acids have been isolated from CF. Tsutomu HATANO identified 28 of them. Many tannic acids in this Chinese herb have the large molecular weight, e.g., the molecular weight of Cornusiins A–F and Camptothins A–B are even larger than 1000 Da [6, 7], because dimers and trimers exist in these types of tannic acids.

Polysaccharides (70–79)

Wu and Yin identified most polysaccharides in CF [8, 9]. In their isolation process, hot water or petroleum ether was initially used for combining with assistant ultrasonic and microwave to break the cell wall to isolate polysaccharides. Further separation and purification were achieved by the combination of several techniques, e.g., fractional precipitation, ethanol precipitation, ion-exchange chromatography and affinity chromatography. Finally, infrared spectroscopy analysis and morphological analysis were used to determine the physiochemical and structural features of the polysaccharide.

Table 1 Chemical constituents identified from CF

No.	Chemical class	Compound name	Chemical formula	Exact mass	References
	Terpenoids				
1	Iridoids	Sweroside	$C_{16}H_{22}O_9$	358.1264	[73]
2		Loganic acid	$C_{16}H_{24}O_{10}$	376.1369	[19]
3		Cornin	$C_{17}H_{24}O_{10}$	388.1369	[73]
4		7-Dehydrologanin	$C_{17}H_{24}O_{10}$	388.1369	[74]
5		Loganin	$C_{17}H_{26}O_{10}$	390.1526	[74]
6		7-α-Morroniside	$C_{17}H_{26}O_{11}$	406.1475	[75]
7		7-β-Morroniside	$C_{17}H_{26}O_{11}$	406.1475	[75]
8		7-α-*O*-Methyl-morroniside	$C_{18}H_{28}O_{11}$	420.1632	[75]
9		7-β-*O*-Methyl-morroniside	$C_{18}H_{28}O_{11}$	420.1632	[75]
10		7-α-*O*-Ethyl-morroniside	$C_{18}H_{29}O_{11}$	421.1710	[75]
11		7-β-*O*-Ethyl-morroniside	$C_{18}H_{29}O_{11}$	421.1710	[75]
12		7-α-*O*-Butyl-morroniside	$C_{21}H_{34}O_{11}$	462.2101	[43]
13		7-β-*O*-Dimethyl-butanedioate morroniside	$C_{23}H_{34}O_{15}$	550.1898	[76]
14		Logmalicids A	$C_{21}H_{29}O_{14}$	505.1557	[24]
15		Logmalicids B	$C_{21}H_{29}O_{14}$	505.1557	[24]
16		Cornusfuroside A	$C_{25}H_{34}O_{13}$	542.1999	[77]
17		Cornusfuroside B	$C_{25}H_{34}O_{13}$	542.1999	[77]
18		Cornusfuroside C	$C_{25}H_{34}O_{13}$	542.1999	[77]
19		Cornusfuroside D	$C_{29}H_{34}O_{15}$	622.1898	[77]
20	Secoiridoids	Linalool	$C_{10}H_{18}O$	154.1358	[78]
21		Linalool oxide	$C_{10}H_{18}O_2$	170.1307	[79]
22		Secoxyloganin	$C_{17}H_{24}O_{11}$	404.1319	[24]
23		Cornuside	$C_{24}H_{30}O_{14}$	542.1636	[74]
24	Triterpenoids	Ursolic acid	$C_{30}H_{48}O_3$	456.3603	[74]
25		Oleanolic acid	$C_{30}H_{48}O_3$	456.3603	[15]
26		Arjunglucoside II	$C_{36}H_{58}O_{10}$	650.4030	[74]
	Flavonoids				
27		Naringenin	$C_{15}H_{12}O_5$	272.0685	[74]
28		Kaempferol	$C_{15}H_{10}O_6$	286.0477	[79]
29		Kaempferide	$C_{16}H_{12}O_6$	300.0634	[80]
30		Kaempferol-3-*O*-β-D-galactopyranoside	$C_{21}H_{20}O_{11}$	448.1006	[24]
31		Kaempferol-3-*O*-β-D-glucoside	$C_{21}H_{20}O_{11}$	448.1006	[74]
32		Kaempferol-3-*O*-β-D-rutinoside	$C_{27}H_{30}O_{15}$	594.1585	[24]
33		Quercetin	$C_{15}H_{10}O_7$	302.0427	[79]
34		Quercetin-3-*O*-β-D-galactopyranoside	$C_{21}H_{20}O_{12}$	464.0955	[24]
35		Quercetin-3-*O*-β-D-glucuronide	$C_{21}H_{18}O_{13}$	478.0747	[24]
36		Quercetin-3-*O*-β-D-glucuronide methyl ester	$C_{22}H_{20}O_{13}$	492.0904	[24]
37		Quercetin-3-*O*-β-D-(6-n-butyl glucuronide)	$C_{25}H_{25}O_{13}$	533.1295	[15]
38		(−)-Epicatechin-3-*O*-gallate	$C_{22}H_{18}O_{10}$	442.0900	[15]
39		Isoquercitrin	$C_{21}H_{20}O_{12}$	464.0955	[80]

Table 1 (continued)

No.	Chemical class	Compound name	Chemical formula	Exact mass	References
	Tannins				
40		Gallic acid	$C_7H_6O_5$	170.0215	[74]
41		7-*O*-Galloyl-D-sedoheptulose	$C_{14}H_{18}O_{11}$	362.0849	[19]
42		Gemin D	$C_{27}H_{22}O_{18}$	634.0806	[6, 7]
43		Oenothein C	$C_{34}H_{24}O_{22}$	784.0759	[6, 7]
44		3-*O*-Galloyl-D-glucose	$C_{13}H_{16}O_{10}$	332.0743	[6, 7]
45		2,3-Di-*O*-galloyl-D-glucose	$C_{20}H_{20}O_{14}$	484.0853	[6, 7]
46		1,2,3-Tri-*O*-galloyl-β-D-glucose	$C_{27}H_{24}O_{18}$	636.0963	[6, 7]
47		1,2,6-Tri-*O*-galloyl-β-D-glucose	$C_{27}H_{24}O_{18}$	636.0963	[6, 7]
48		1,2,3,6-Tetra-*O*-galloyl-β-D-glucose	$C_{34}H_{28}O_{22}$	788.1072	[6, 7]
49		Tellimagrandin I	$C_{34}H_{26}O_{22}$	786.0916	[6, 7]
50		Tellimagrandin II	$C_{41}H_{30}O_{26}$	938.1025	[6, 7]
51		Isocoriariin F	$C_{34}H_{26}O_{23}$	802.0865	[6, 7]
52		Coriariin F	$C_{34}H_{26}O_{23}$	802.0865	[6, 7]
53		Rugosin B	$C_{41}H_{30}O_{27}$	954.0974	[6, 7]
54		Isorugosin B	$C_{41}H_{30}O_{27}$	954.0974	[6, 7]
55		Isoterchebin	$C_{41}H_{30}O_{27}$	954.0974	[6, 7]
56		Isorugosin A	$C_{48}H_{34}O_{31}$	1106.1084	[6, 7]
57		Rugosin D	$C_{82}H_{58}O_{52}$	1874.1894	[6, 7]
58		Isorugosin D	$C_{82}H_{58}O_{52}$	1874.1894	[6, 7]
59		Camptothin A	$C_{61}H_{46}O_{40}$	1418.1565	[6, 7]
60		Camptothin B	$C_{75}H_{54}O_{48}$	1722.1785	[6, 7]
61		Cornusiin B	$C_{48}H_{30}O_{30}$	1086.0822	[6, 7]
62		Cornusiin A	$C_{68}H_{50}O_{44}$	1570.1675	[6, 7]
63		Cornusiin D	$C_{75}H_{54}O_{48}$	1722.1785	[6, 7]
64		Cornusiin E	$C_{82}H_{58}O_{52}$	1874.1894	[6, 7]
65		Cornusiin F	$C_{95}H_{70}O_{62}$	2202.2325	[6, 7]
66		Cornusiin C	$C_{102}H_{74}O_{66}$	2354.2434	[6, 7]
67		Methyl tri-*O*-methylgallate	$C_{11}H_{14}O_5$	226.0841	[6, 7]
68		Dimethyl hexamethoxydiphenate	$C_{22}H_{26}O_{10}$	450.1526	[6, 7]
69		Trimethyl-octa-*O*-methylvaloneate	$C_{32}H_{36}O_{15}$	660.2054	[6, 7]
	Polysaccharides				
70		Co-4			[8]
71		COP-1			[9]
72		COP-2			[9]
73		COP-3			[9]
74		COP-4			[9]
75		FCAP1			[81]
76		FCP5-A			[8]
77		PFCA-III			[8]
78		PFCC-I			[8]
79		SZYP-2			[8]
	Other compounds				
80	Phenylpropanoids	*p*-Hydroxycinnamic acid	$C_9H_8O_3$	164.0473	[74]
81		Caffeic acid	$C_9H_8O_4$	180.0423	[15]
82		Caftaric acid monomethyl ester	$C_{14}H_{14}O_9$	326.2556	[15]
83		Caffeoyltartaric acid dimethyl ester	$C_{15}H_{16}O_9$	340.0794	[76]
84	Sterols	β-Sitosterol	$C_{29}H_{50}O$	414.7067	[15]
85		Daucosterol-6′-malate	$C_{39}H_{64}O_{10}$	692.4499	[80]

Table 1 (continued)

No.	Chemical class	Compound name	Chemical formula	Exact mass	References
86	Carboxylic acids	Succinic acid	$C_4H_6O_4$	118.0266	[85]
87		Malic acid	$C_4H_6O_5$	134.0215	[85]
88		Methylmalic acid	$C_5H_8O_5$	148.0372	[74]
89		Citric acid	$C_6H_8O_7$	192.0270	[85]
90		Butoxysuccinic acid	$C_8H_{14}O_5$	190.1938	[15]
91	Furans	5-Hydroxymethylfurfural	$C_6H_6O_3$	126.0317	[73]
92		Dimethyltetrahydrofuran cis-2,5-dicarboxylate	$C_8H_{12}O_5$	188.0685	[79]
93	Mineral substances	Ca, Fe, K, Mg, Mn, Zn			[82]

Other compounds (80–93)

Four phenylpropanoids, two sterols, five carboxylic acids, two furans, and several mineral substances have also been determined. Among them, 5-hydroxymethylfurfural exhibits diverse biological activities. Besides, Chen, Li, and Wen identified 32, 16, and 48 volatile compounds by GC–MS, respectively [10–12].

Pharmacological activities

Although just a few chemical constituents from CF are assayed for their biological activities, these components displayed diverse pharmacological activities. Detailed biological activities are summarized in Table 2.

Hypoglycemic activity and diabetic target organs protective activity

Diabetes mellitus (DM) is a group of long-term and chronic metabolic disorders which are associated with high serum glucose levels. Compared with the no treatment diabetic animal model group, CF extract (at 300 mg kg^{-1} 2 day^{-1} and 400 mg kg^{-1} day^{-1} p.o.), loganin, morroniside, and ursolic acid (each at 200 mg kg^{-1} day^{-1} p.o.) for 4 weeks can significantly decrease fasting blood glucose and alleviate polyphagia, polydipsia, polyuria, and weight loss [13, 14]. In He's study, metformin (at 200 mg kg^{-1} day^{-1} p.o.) demonstrated better effect [14]. Besides, loganin, morroniside, ursolic acid, and butyl morroniside (each at 100 μmol L^{-1}) can protect the pancreatic β-cells from high glucose-induced excessive oxidative stress and apoptosis [14, 15], may further increase the insulin release. Compared with the insulin treatment, CF extract, (−)-epicatechin-3-*O*-gallate, and caftaric acid monomethyl ester (each at 50 μmol L^{-1}) can also significantly inhibit α-glucosidase activity to slow down the elevation of serum glucose levels [14, 16, 17] and suppress the hepatic gluconeogenesis by decreasing the protein and mRNA levels of PEPCK in vitro [15, 18].

Also, CF extract, iridoid glycosides, and the single compound can decrease 24 h urine protein and serum levels of urea nitrogen and creatinine. To be specific, loganin, morroniside, and 7-*O*-galloyl-D-sedoheptulose (each at 20–100 mg kg^{-1} day^{-1} p.o.) for 10 days and 8 weeks can significantly inhibit both AGE/RAGE formation [19–22] and CTGF production [23] in db/db mice or STZ-induced diabetic nephropathy model. They can also significantly alleviate diabetic organ injury by decreasing the production of NF-κB and its downstream synthetases and cytokines [19–25], increasing antioxidant enzyme production [19, 26, 27], and suppressing apoptotic cell death [27, 28].

Antioxidant activity

Long-term oxidative stress will generate excessive ROS to oxidize protein, lipids, DNA and then cause cell death, tissue damage, and organ dysfunction. Ideal antioxidant drugs are required to regulate the defense system and scavenge excessive ROS. Studies indicated that morroniside (at 1, 10, 100 μmol L^{-1}) for 24 h and total saponins (at 60 and 120 mg kg^{-1} day^{-1} p.o.) for 4 weeks regulated Ca^{2+} and NO release [29, 30], the aqueous extract (at 0.25–2.0 mg mL^{-1}) for 20 h modulated GSH redox cycle [31], the aqueous extract, the ethanol extract (at 0.01–0.1 mg mL^{-1}), morroniside (at 0.05–2 μg mL^{-1}), and ursolic acid (at 0.05–2 μg mL^{-1}) for 24 h promoted antioxidant enzymes syntheses [31–33] to inhibit lipid peroxidation [29], 5-hydroxymethylfurfural (at 100–400 μmol L^{-1}) for 3 days decreased ROS release [34], morroniside (at 100 μmol L^{-1}) for 2 days recovered cell cycle to normal state [35]. Mentioned effects significantly together reduced the oxidative stress-induced damages compared with the no treatment group.

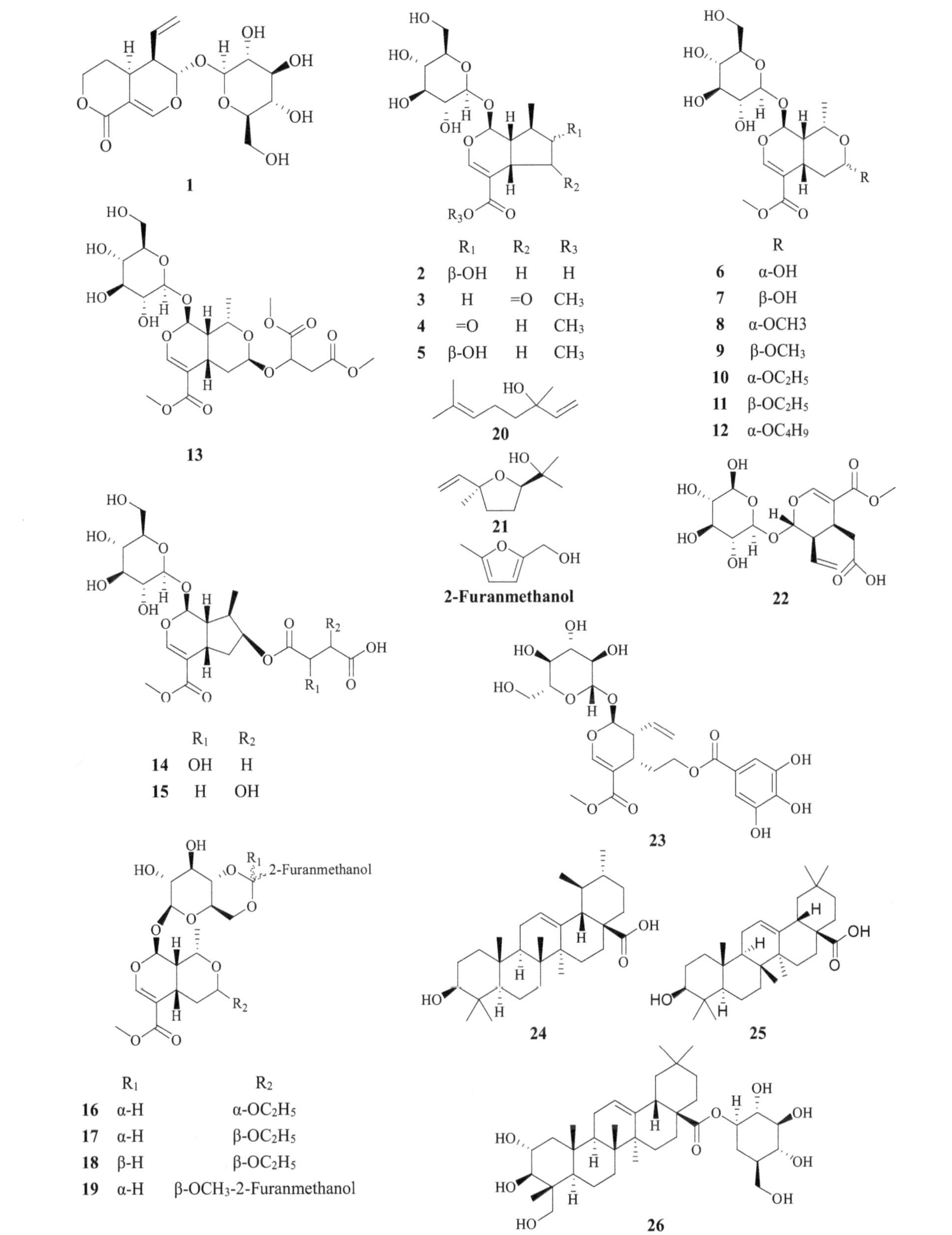

Fig. 2 Structures of chemical constituents from *Corni Fructus*

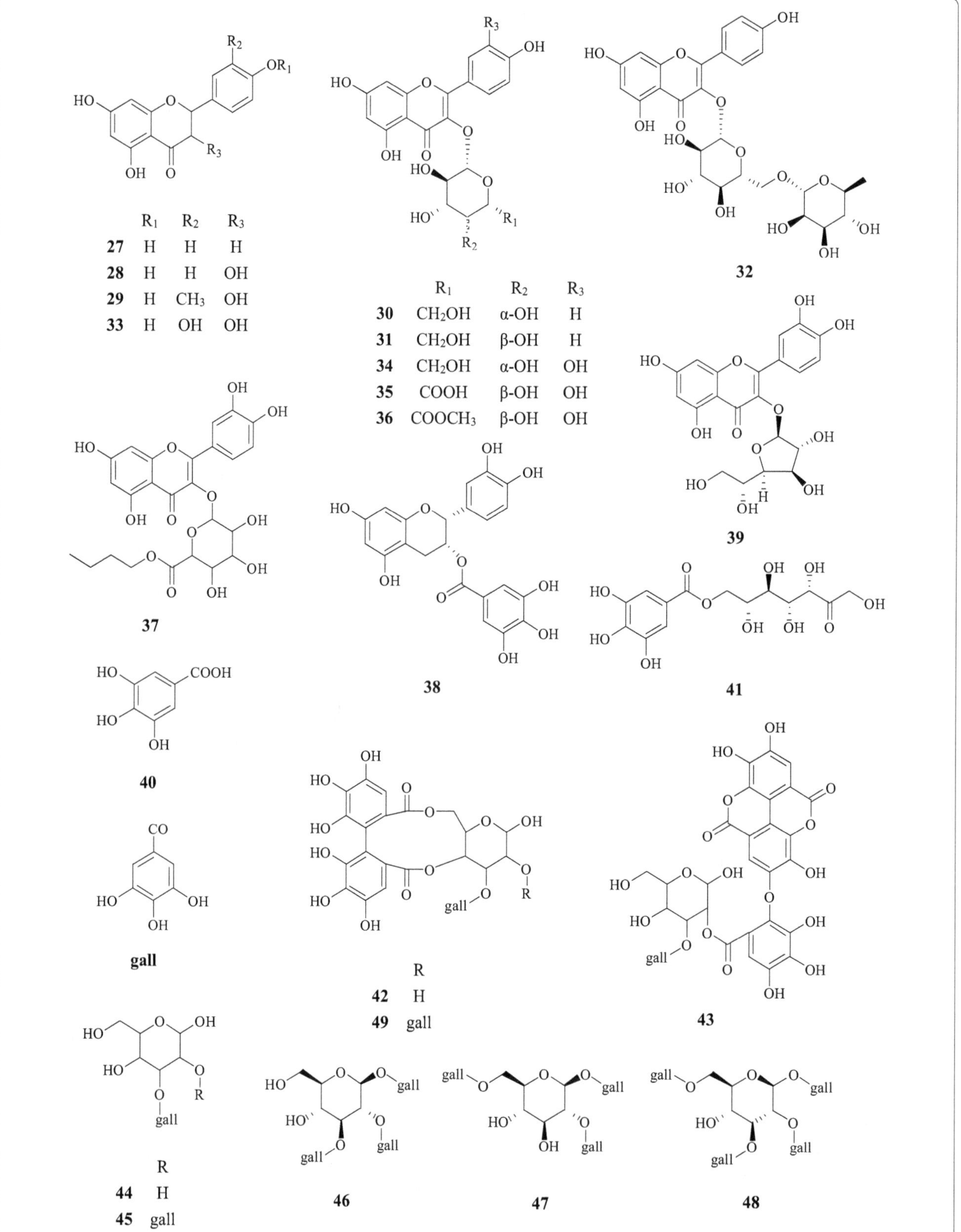

Fig. 3 Structures of chemical constituents from *Corni Fructus*

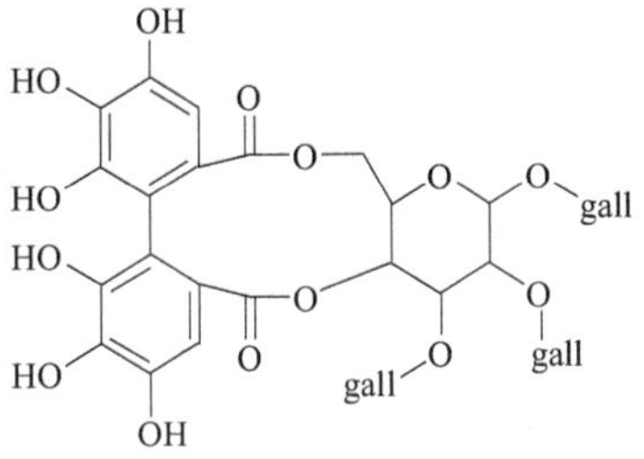

50

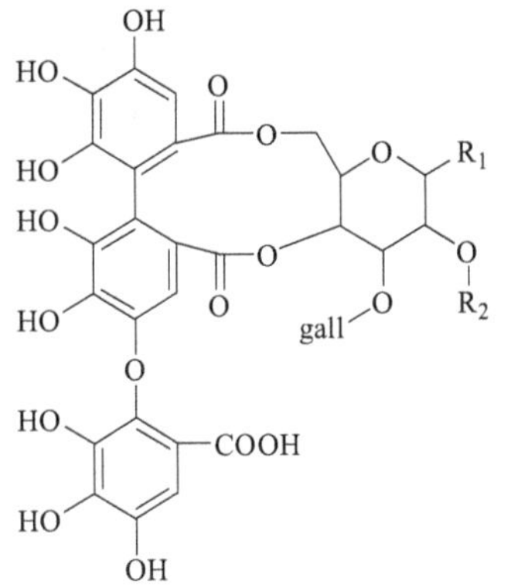

	R_1	R_2
51	OH	H
54	OH	gall
56	O-gall	gall

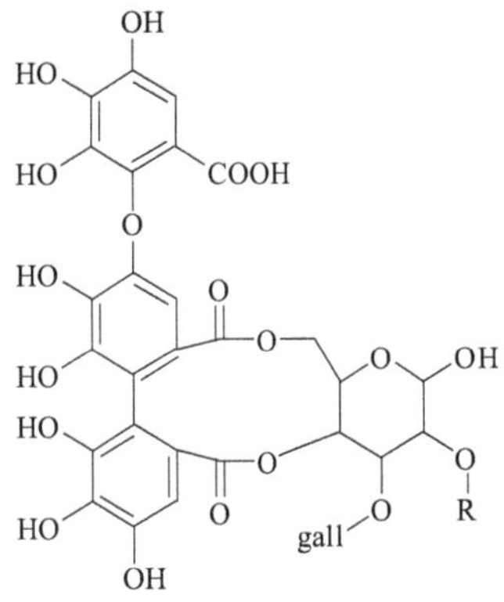

	R
52	H
53	gall

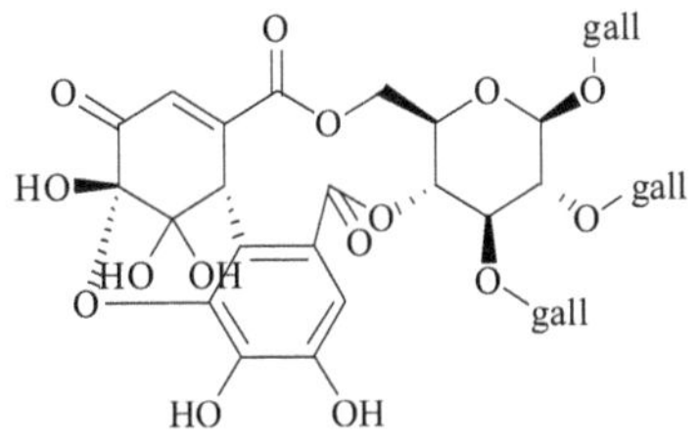

55

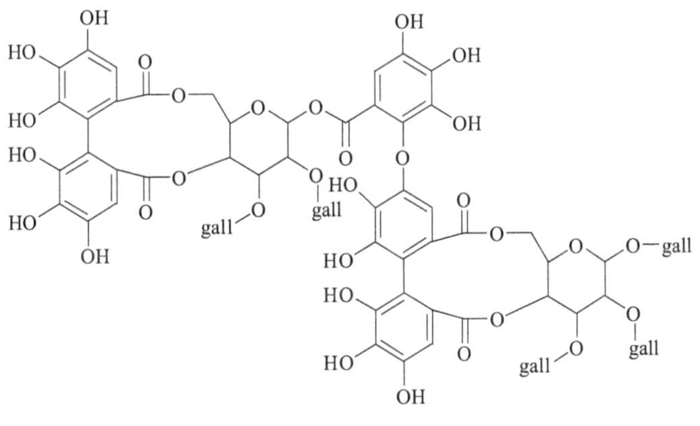

57

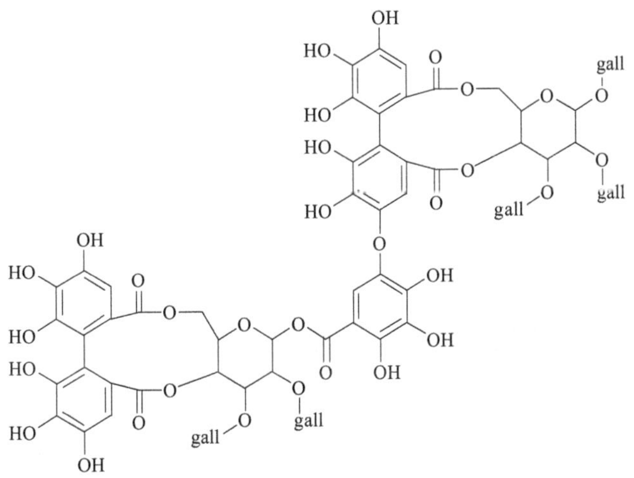

58

Fig. 4 Structures of chemical constituents from *Corni Fructus*

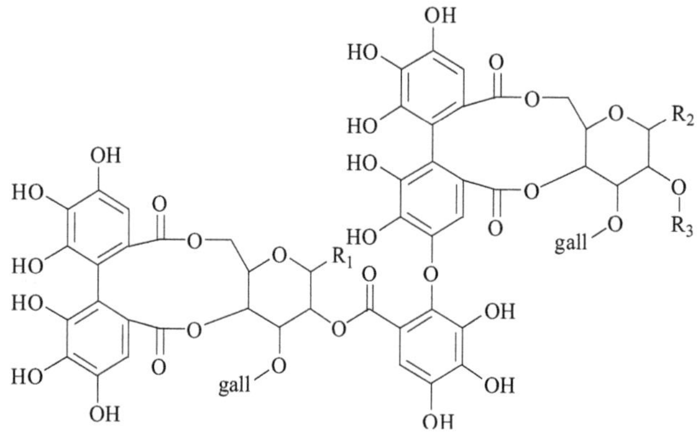

	R1	R2	R3
59	OH	OH	H
60	OH	O-gall	gall
62	OH	OH	gall
63	O-gall	OH	gall
64	O-gall	O-gall	gall

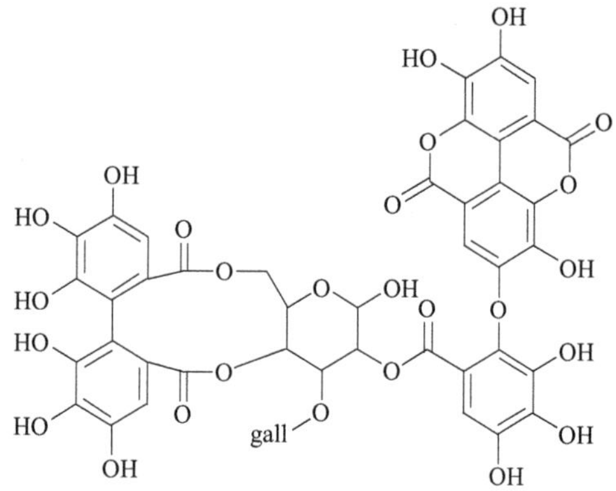

61

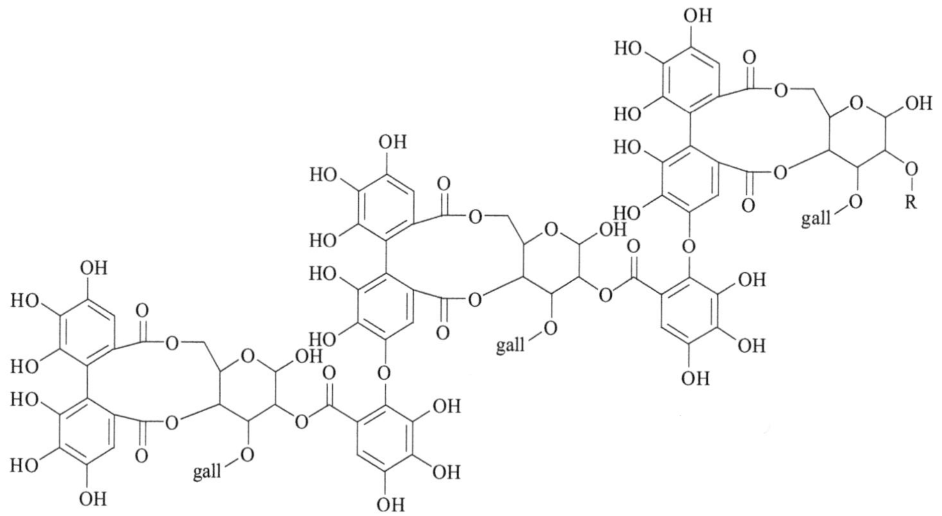

	R
65	H
66	gall

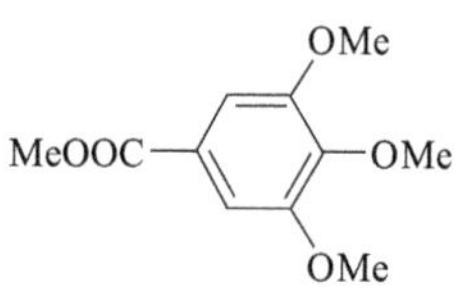

67

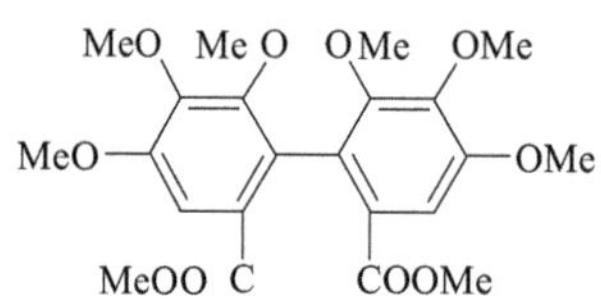

68

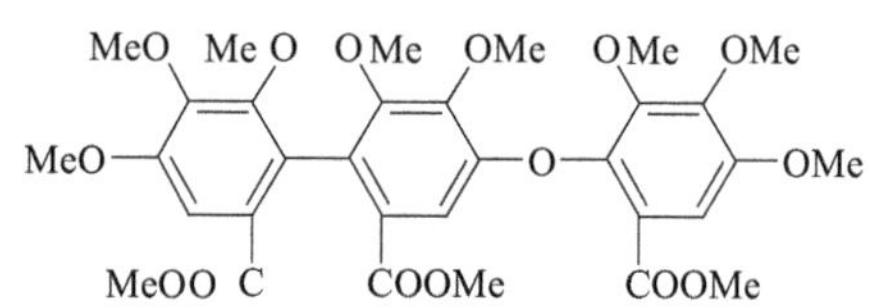

69

Fig. 5 Structures of chemical constituents from *Corni Fructus*

Table 2 Summary of pharmacological activities of CF

Extracts or compounds	Disease models	Specific effects	References
Hypoglycemic activity			
Oleanolic acid	Fasting rat	Decrease plasma glucose levels. Regulate ACh release from nerve terminals to activate muscarinic M3 receptors in the pancreatic cells and increase C-peptide and insulin release	[83]
Iridoid glycosides	STZ-induced rat as DM model	Show α-glucosidase inhibition activity in vitro and decrease serum glucose levels in vivo	[16]
Loganin Morroniside Ursolic acid	STZ-induced mice as DM model, HepG2 cell lines	Show α-glucosidase inhibition activity in vitro. Decrease fasting blood glucose and alleviate weight loss, polydipsia, and polyphagia. Increase SOD activity and ROS scavenging activity. Attenuate aldose reductase activity and decrease MDA plasma level and renal somatic indices in mice	[14]
Butyl morroniside (−)-Epicatechin-3-*O*-gallate Caftaric acid monomethyl ester	High glucose-induced BRIN-BD11 and H4IIE cell lines as in vitro DM model	Increase glucose uptake efficiency. Reduce PEPCK mRNA level and NO production. Inhibit pancreatic β-cell death	[15]
Aqueous extract	STZ-induced rat as diabetic organs injury model	Decrease levels of glucose and TC in serum, and α-SMA expression in kidney. Improve the pathohistological injury of pancreas, kidney, lung, and liver	[13]
Aqueous extract	Normal rat	Show α-glucosidase inhibition activity in vitro, and exhibit hypoglycemic effect via oral sucrose tolerance test in vivo	[17]
Aqueous extract	Dexamethasone and 8-bromo-cAMP-induced BRIN-BD11 and H4IIE cell lines as in vitro DM model	Increase insulin release. Decrease PEPCK mRNA level	[18]
Nephroprotective activity			
Loganin	STZ-induced rat and high glucose-induced HK-2 as in vivo and in vitro diabetic nephropathy model	Improve renal function. Decrease CTGF level in kidney and serum via ERK signaling pathway	[23]
Morroniside Loganin 7-*O*-Galloyl-D-sedoheptulose	Db/db mice as obesity-associated type 2 diabetic nephropathy model	Suppress formation of AGEs and TBARS in the kidney. Reduce the production of SREBP-1&2, NF-κB p65, COX-2, and iNOS. Decrease GSH/GSSG ratio and levels of serum glucose, TC, and TG	[19]
7-*O*-Galloyl-D-sedoheptulose	STZ-induced rat as diabetic nephropathy model	Decrease serum creatinine, renal glucose, and urinary protein. Reduce the production of AGE, RAGE, HO-1, intracellular glycation, CML, GA-pyridine, and TBARS	[21]
Iridoid glycosides	STZ-induced rat as diabetic nephropathy model	Suppress over-deposition of fibronectin and laminin in the kidney. Reduce protein and mRNA levels of TGF-β1 in serum and glomeruli	[25]
Iridoid glycosides Triterpene acids	Db/db mice as obesity-associated type 2 diabetic nephropathy model	Improve the histological injury of kidney and pancreas. Ameliorate the structural alterations in mesangial cells and the podocytes in the renal cortex. Inhibit ECM accumulation in the kidney. Decrease 24 h urine protein and serum levels of urea nitrogen and creatinine. Increase insulin release, and decrease fasting blood glucose and levels of TC, TG, and GSP. Attenuate food consumption, water intake, and urine volume. Reduce the production of RAGE, NF-κB, SphK1, and TGF-β	[22]
CF extract	STZ-induced rat as diabetic nephropathy model	Inhibit AGE formation in the kidney. Attenuate hyperglycemia and proteinuria. Reduce the production of RAGE, NF-κB, TGF-β1, and CML	[20]

Table 2 (continued)

Extracts or compounds	Disease models	Specific effects	References
Ethanol extract	High glucose-induced mesangial cells as in vitro diabetic nephropathy model	Decrease the production of Col V, FN, and IL-6	[24]
Myocardial protection activity			
Morroniside	High glucose-induced rat as diabetic cardiomyopathy model	Inhibit myocardial cell apoptosis. Elevate Bcl-2 production and decrease expressions of Bax and caspase-3	[28]
Triterpene acids	STZ-induced rat as diabetic cardiomyopathy model	Inhibit the ventricular remodeling and regulate the systolic and diastolic function of the left ventricle. Increase insulin release and reduce serum glucose levels. Enhance GSX and SOD activity. Increase the production of calstabin 2, PLB, and SERCA2a. Decrease protein and mRNA levels of ECE, iNOS, MDA, ET-1, and propreET-1	[26]
Testis-protective activity			
Iridoid glycosides	STZ-induced rat as diabetic testicular damage model	Improve the pathohistological injury of testes and pancreas. Increase serum insulin release and decrease blood glucose levels. Alleviate weight loss, polydipsia, polyphagia, and polyuria. Increase CAT and SOD activity. Reduce the production of AGEs, RAGE, ROS, MDA, and p-p38 MAPK. Down-regulate Bax/Bcl-2 ratio and spermatogenic cell apoptosis	[27]
Antioxidant activity			
Morroniside	Hydrogen peroxide-induced SH-SY5Y cell line as in vitro neurodegenerative disorder model	Suppress intracellular accumulation of Ca^{2+}. Increase SOD activity and reduce the loss of MMP. Inhibit cytotoxicity	[29]
Morroniside	High ambient glucose-induced endothelial cell injury model	Attenuate cellular morphological damage. Repair cell cycle progression and improve cell viability	[35]
Ursolic acid	Hydrogen peroxide-induced HEI-OC1 cell line as in vitro inner ear diseases model	Increase antioxidant enzymes expressions, e.g., CAT and GPX. Suppress lipid peroxidation	[32]
5-Hydroxymethylfurfural	High glucose-induced HUVECs as in vitro oxidative stress model	Decrease levels of ROS, IL-8, JNK1, and JNK2/3. Increase P-Akt production	[34]
Total saponins	STZ-induced rat as a diabetic oxidative stress model	Regulate NO release and endothelium-dependent relaxation on the mesenteric artery. Reduce blood glucose levels	[30]
Aqueous extract	Hypoxanthine and xanthine oxidase-induced bovine PAECs as in vitro oxidative stress model	Regulate GSH redox cycle. Increase the intracellular GSH production and the activity of GSH peroxidase and GSH disulfide reductase. Reduce the intracellular level of GSH disulfide. Increase CAT and SOD activity and inhibit the production of hydrogen peroxide and superoxide anion	[31]
Ethanol extract	LPS-induced RAW 264.7 macrophage cells as in vitro oxidative stress model	Attenuate xanthine oxidase activity and ROS production. Induce the production of antioxidant enzymes, e.g., CAT, GSX, Cu/Zn-SOD, and Mn-SOD	[33]
Anti-inflammatory activity			
Cornuside	TNF-α-induced HUVECs as in vitro inflammation model	Decrease the production of ICAM-1, VCAM-1, MCP-1, and NF-κB. Inhibit NF-κB p65 translocation	[36]
Cornuside	LPS-induced RAW 264.7 macrophage cells as in vitro inflammation model	Decrease the production of COX-2, iNOS, PGE_2, NO, IL-1β, IL-6, and TNF-α. Suppress the translocation of NF-κB p65, the phosphorylation and degradation of IκB-α, and the phosphorylation of ERK1/2, JNK1/2, and p38	[38]

Table 2 (continued)

Extracts or compounds	Disease models	Specific effects	References
Aqueous extract	LPS-induced RAW 264.7 macrophage cells as in vitro inflammation model	Decrease protein and mRNA levels of COX-2 and iNOS. Reduce PGE_2 and NO production	[37]
Anticancer activity			
Aqueous extract	HSC-2, HSC-3, HSC-4, Ca9-22, NA cell lines as in vitro oral squamous cell carcinoma model	Produce broad radical peak under alkaline condition and increase the cytotoxicity and superoxide anion scavenging activity of vitamin C	[39]
Aqueous extract	E2-induced MCF-7 cell line as in vitro ER^+ human mammary carcinoma model	Inhibit cell line anchorage-independent growth and reduce the mitogenically inert metabolite E3 formation	[40]
Aqueous extract	Parental ER^+ MCF-7 cell line as in vitro human mammary carcinoma model	Suppress cell line anchorage-independent growth and induce G1 or G2/M arrest and apoptosis. Increase anti-proliferative E2 metabolites production	[41]
Aqueous extract	HepG2, SKHep1 and PLC/PRF/5 cell lines as in vitro hepatocellular carcinoma model	Inhibit cell proliferation. Exhibit free radicals scavenging activity and suppress lipid peroxidation and xanthine oxidase production	[42]
Neuroprotective activity			
Cornuside 1,2,3-Tri-*O*-galloyl-β-D-glucose 1,2,3,6-Tetra-*O*-galloyl-β-D-glucose Tellimagrandin I Tellimagrandin II Isoterchebin	In vitro enzyme activities assay	Exhibit synergetic inhibitory activities against BACE1 and ChE	[45]
Morroniside	MCAO-induced rat as focal cerebral ischemia model	Decrease the infarction volume and improve neurological function. Increase GSH expression and SOD activity. Decrease the production and activity of MDA and caspase-3 in ischemic cortex tissues	[47]
5-Hydroxymethylfurfural	Hydrogen peroxide-induced rat hippocampal neurons as in vitro neurodegenerative disorder model	Enhance Bcl-2 production and suppress expressions of Bax, caspase-3, and p53	[84]
Iridoid glycosides	MCAO-induced rat as focal cerebral ischemia model	Improve neurological function. Increase the number of BrdU-positive cells and nestin-positive cells in the subventricular zone, and the number of new mature neurons and blood vessels in the striatum. Increase protein and mRNA levels of VEGF and Flk-1	[46]
Iridoid glycosides	Fimbria-fornix transected rat as cerebral ischemia model	Decrease neuron loss in the hippocampus and improve memory deficits. Increase the production of BDNF, NGF, Bcl-2, SYP, Trk A, and GAP-43, and decrease the production of Bax and Cyt c	[49]
7*R*-*O*-Methyl-morroniside 7*S*-*O*-Methyl-morroniside 7-*O*-Butyl-morroniside Loganin Morroniside	Glutamate-induced HT22 cell lines as in vitro hippocampal cell injury	Improve cell viability	[43]

Table 2 (continued)

Extracts or compounds	Disease models	Specific effects	References
Iridoid glycosides	*Mycobacterium tuberculosis* and guinea-pig myelin basic protein-induced experimental autoimmune encephalomyelitis rat as multiple sclerosis model	Increase the number of mature oligodendrocytes and reduce the number of oligodendrocyte progenitor cells. Inhibit the process of T cell entry to the central nervous system and attenuate microglia activation. Increase BDNF expression and decrease phosphorylation of JAK/STAT1/3 and inflammatory cytokines production, e.g., IL-1β, IFN-γ, TNF-α	[48]
Iridoid glycosides	*Mycobacterium tuberculosis* and myelin oligodendrocyte glycoprotein-induced experimental autoimmune encephalomyelitis mouse as multiple sclerosis model	Decrease BDNF and NGF loss in the spinal cord	[50]
Aqueous extract	PC 12 cell lines	Increase cell neurite outgrowth. Inhibit extracellular Ca^{2+} influx, and protein and mRNA levels of STIM1	[44]
Hepatoprotective activity			
5-Hydroxymethylfurfural	Hydrogen peroxide-induced L02 cell lines as in vitro hepatitis model	Promote S phase into G2/M phase and recover cell cycle to normal. Reduce NO production and caspase-4 activity and inhibit hepatocyte apoptosis	[51]
5-Hydroxymethylfurfural	Hydrogen peroxide-induced L02 cell lines as in vitro hepatitis model	Improve hepatocyte morphology and reduce caspase-3&9 expressions	[52]
5-Hydroxymethylfurfural	D-Galactosamine/TNF-α-induced L02 cell lines as in vitro acute liver injury model	Inhibit hepatocyte apoptosis. Increase Bcl-2 production and decrease intracellular Ca^{2+} level and production of ATF4, Bax, CHOP, PERK, and p-eIF2α	[53]
7-*O*-Galloyl-D-sedoheptulose	Db/db mice as obesity-associated type 2 diabetic liver injury model	Improve hepatic histological damage and decrease serum levels of ALT, AST, and blood glucose. Attenuate water intake, food consumption, and body weight gain. Decrease the production of AP-1, NF-κB p65, IL-6, TNF-α, ICAM-1, MCP-1, AGEs, RAGE, GA-pyridine, pentosidine, CEL, CMA, CML, leptin, resistin, p-ERK1/2, and p-JNK	[54]
Ethanol extract	Acetaminophen-induced mice as liver injury model	Increase levels of CAT, HO-1, and SOD. Suppress lipid peroxidation	[55]
Improving osteoporosis activity			
Sweroside	Rat osteoblasts and human MG-63 cell lines	Stimulate the osteocalcin secretion. Increase cell proliferation and inhibit apoptotic cell death. Increase ALP activity	[56]
CF extract	RANKL-induced mice BMDM as in vitro osteoclast differentiation model	Suppress osteoclast differentiation. Reduce protein and mRNA levels of c-Fos, NFATc1, OSCAR, and TRAP. Inhibit phosphorylation of p-38 and c-JNK and degradation of I-κB	[57]
Promoting melanogenesis activity			
Methanol extract	Melan-a cell lines	Increase the production and activity of tyrosinase. Increase MITF-M mRNA level and TRP-1&2 production	[58]
Immunomodulatory activity			
Aqueous extract	C57BL/6 mice are transplanted with a skin graft from Balb/C donors	Prolong skin allograft survival. Reduce the number of graft-infiltrating T cells and inhibit their proliferation. Decrease intracellular IL-12 expression by intragraft DCs and IFN-γ expression by graft-infiltrating T cells. Reduce intragraft IL-12 mRNA level	[59]

Table 2 (continued)

Extracts or compounds	Disease models	Specific effects	References
Lung-protective activity			
Oleanolic acid Ursolic acid	Epidermal growth factor—and phorbol ester-induced NCI-H292 cell lines as in vitro airway diseases model	Decrease protein and mRNA levels of MUC5AC mucin	[60]
Aqueous extract	Ovalbumin-induced BALB/c mice as allergic asthma model	Inhibit eosinophil infiltration and ameliorate allergic airway inflammation and airway hyperresponsiveness. Decrease the production of IL-5&13 and OVA-specific IgE	[61]
Vasorelaxation activity			
Cornuside	Phenylephrine-contracted rat aorta and HUVEC	Dilate vascular smooth muscle in the rat and increase cGMP production in vitro	[62]
Antiviral activity			
Aqueous extract	CVA16 infected Vero cells as in vitro HFMD model	Inhibit CVA16 replication	[63]

Anti-inflammatory activity

Prolonged and incurable inflammation may cause many diseases, e.g., atherosclerosis, cancer, ulcerative colitis. In LPS and TNF-α-induced cell inflammation models, compared with the no treatment group, CF aqueous extract (at 0.2, 1, 5 mg mL^{-1}) and cornuside (at 1, 10, 50 μmol L^{-1}) for 24 h significantly inhibited NF-κB p65 translocation, down-regulated COX-2 and iNOS production, finally decreased PGE_2 and NO levels to control excessive inflammatory responses [36–38].

Anticancer activity

CF aqueous extract significantly enhanced both the cytotoxicity and superoxide anion scavenging activity of vitamin C at 0.5 and 36 μg mL^{-1}, respectively. Together with CF aqueous extract, vitamin C further inhibited proliferation and induced apoptosis in several human oral squamous cell carcinoma cell lines. Compared with no treatment, the proliferation inhibition rate was at 1.3–71.0% [39]. Furthermore, the aqueous extract (at 1.0 mg mL^{-1}) for 2 days significantly exhibited anti-ER^+ human mammary carcinoma activity by inhibiting cell anchorage-independent growth, regulating the metabolism of E2 and E3 [40], and influencing cell cycle progression and cellular apoptosis [41]. Finally, the aqueous extract has been tested for its cancer inhibitory effect in several hepatocellular carcinomas and leukemic cell lines. The study indicated that the aqueous extract inhibited the tumor cell proliferation in a dose-dependent manner at 0.11–0.337 mg mL^{-1}, exhibited oxygen free radicals scavenging activity (at 50 μg mL^{-1}), attenuated xanthine oxidase production (at 2.62 mg mL^{-1}) and lipid peroxidation (at 0.892 mg mL^{-1}) [42]. In this study, CF aqueous extract exhibited the similar effects compared with 5-fluorouracil (at 0.5, 1, 5 μg mL^{-1}).

Neuroprotective activity

Many compounds in CF were further tested for the neuroprotective effects. 7*R*-*O*-Methyl-morroniside, 7*S*-*O*-methyl-morroniside, 7-*O*-butyl-morroniside, loganin, and morroniside (each at 10 and 50 μmol L^{-1}) for 1 h significantly protected the neurons against glutamate-induced neurotoxicity up to about 78% compared with the no treatment group [43]. CF aqueous extract (at 60 μg mL^{-1}) significantly inhibited the extracellular Ca^{2+} influx to increase cell neurite outgrowth [44]. Also, cornuside, isoterchebin, and tellimagrandin II (each at 25–100 μmol L^{-1}) displayed anti-Alzheimer's disease potential due to their synergetic inhibitory activities against BACE1 and ChE [45].

Cerebral ischemia, multiple sclerosis, and neurodegenerative disorder models are applied in animal experiments. Iridoid glycosides (at 60 and 180 mg kg^{-1} day^{-1} p.o.) for 1–4 weeks and morroniside (at 90 and 270 mg kg^{-1} day^{-1} p.o.) for 3 days significantly decreased the infarction volume, increased the number of new mature neurons and blood vessels, and improved nervous system function [46, 47]. Also, iridoid glycosides (at 50–180 mg kg^{-1} day^{-1} p.o.) for 3–4 weeks can significantly promote NGF and BDNF production [48–50], and repair the abnormal functions of microglia, oligodendrocyte, and T cell to maintain the central nervous system homeostasis [48].

Hepatoprotective activity

In hepatitis cell models, 5-hydroxymethylfurfural (at 0.2–1 and 0.79 μmol L^{-1}) for 24 h has been shown to protect hepatocytes from H_2O_2 induced-cytotoxicity by significantly decreasing NO and intracellular Ca^{2+} levels, inhibiting abnormal production of apoptosis-related proteins and recovering back to regular cell cycle [51–53]. In hepatitis animal models, 7-*O*-galloyl-D-sedoheptulose (at 20 and 100 mg kg^{-1} day^{-1} p.o.) for 6 weeks and CF ethanol extract (at 100–500 mg kg^{-1} day^{-1} p.o.) for 1 week significantly decreased the serum marker enzymes of hepatic damage, weakened the oxidative stress by promoting antioxidant enzymes production and inhibiting lipid peroxidation, finally improved hepatic histological injury [54, 55].

Other pharmacological activities

In addition to the mentioned pharmacological activities, CF has also been reported to exert multiple bioactivities. Firstly, sweroside (at 7.5 μg mL^{-1}) for 1 week significantly promoted the proliferation and differentiation of osteoblasts via the regulation of osteocalcin [56]. Also, CF extract (at 0–100 μg mL^{-1}) for 4 days significantly inhibited osteoclast differentiation in a dose-dependent manner via the inhibition of the signaling cascades NF-κB/c-Fos/NFATc1 to improve osteoporosis [57]. Secondly, CF methanol extract (at 3.125–12.5 μg mL^{-1}) for 3 days significantly up-regulated synthesis and activity of tyrosinase, raised TRP-1&2 translation associating with increasing transcription of MITF-M, finally promoted melanogenesis by 36.1% [58]. Thirdly, CF aqueous extract possesses immunomodulatory activity. In C57BL/6 mice that were transplanted with a skin graft from Balb/C donors, CF extract significantly prolonged skin allograft survival synergistically by suppressing Th1 response, promoting regulatory T cell generation, and enhancing its suppressive function [59]. Fourthly, CF shows lung-protective activity via two studies. In the cellular test, oleanolic acid (at 10 and 100 μmol L^{-1}) and ursolic acid (at 100 μmol L^{-1}) for 30 min' pretreatment significantly down-regulated MUC5AC mucin whose excessive level would impair airway defenses to cause serious airway diseases [60]. In an animal experiment, CF aqueous extract (at 50 and 200 mg kg^{-1} 3 day^{-1} p.o.) for 5 weeks significantly decreased the production of inflammatory mediators and reduced eosinophil infiltration, finally attenuated allergic airway inflammation and airway hyperresponsiveness [61]. Fifthly, cornuside significantly dilated vascular smooth muscle in phenylephrine-contracted rat aorta via the up-regulation of cGMP level to show its vasorelaxation activity [62]. Finally, among in vitro screening of antiviral drugs for treating hand, foot, and mouth disease (HFMD) infection, CF aqueous extract (at 0.4 μg mL^{-1}) for 2 days significantly inhibited CVA16 replication in cellular level [63].

Conclusion

CF is recognized as a fundamental constituent part of tonifying Yin and Yang prescription because of its harmonious and complementary features according to the basic theory of TCM. It possesses the properties of sour and astringent. Firstly, sour and sweet herbs can be combined to nourish Yin, it can act as the sovereign and ministerial drug among *Radix Rehmanniae Praeparata, Dioscoreae Rhizoma, Lycii Fructus, Ligustri Lucidi Fructus, Schisandrae Chinensis Fructus.* Also, sour and astringent properties exhibit their function of astringing and storing. It also behaves as the sovereign and the ministerial drug that combines with *Euryales Semen, Sepiae Endoconcha, Mantidis Oötheca, Rubi Fructus, Paeoniae Radix Alba* to treat spermatorrhea, urorrhagia, metrorrhagia and metrostaxis, and excessive perspiration. Finally, CF can be as the adjuvant and conductant drug to alleviate warm and dry features of Yang-reinforcing drugs.

Chemical constituents from terpenoids, flavonoids, tannins, and furans exhibited diverse biological activities, including hypoglycemic, neuroprotective, heart-protective, hepatoprotective, nephroprotective, testis-protective activities. Pharmacological activities are outlined in Fig. 6. In these studies, bioactive components from CF mainly alleviated the damage of target organs by antioxidant activity, anti-inflammatory activity, and anti-apoptosis activity, i.e., up-regulating the expressions and activities of antioxidant enzymes, down-regulating the levels of cytokines and chemokines, and modulating the abnormal expressions of apoptotic death associated proteins.

Hypoglycemic activity and alleviating diabetic target organs damage are critical pharmacological activities among the broad spectrum of pharmacological activities of CF. Morroniside, loganin, oleanolic acid, ursolic acid, and 7-*O*-galloyl-D-sedoheptulose exhibited the similar efficacy compared with the conventional oral hypoglycemic drugs (acarbose and metformin). In vivo studies, they reduced serum glucose levels and alleviated unusual symptoms caused by diabetes. In cellular assays, they protected pancreatic β cell from oxidative damage, increased insulin release, improved insulin resistance, displayed α-glucosidase inhibition activity, and

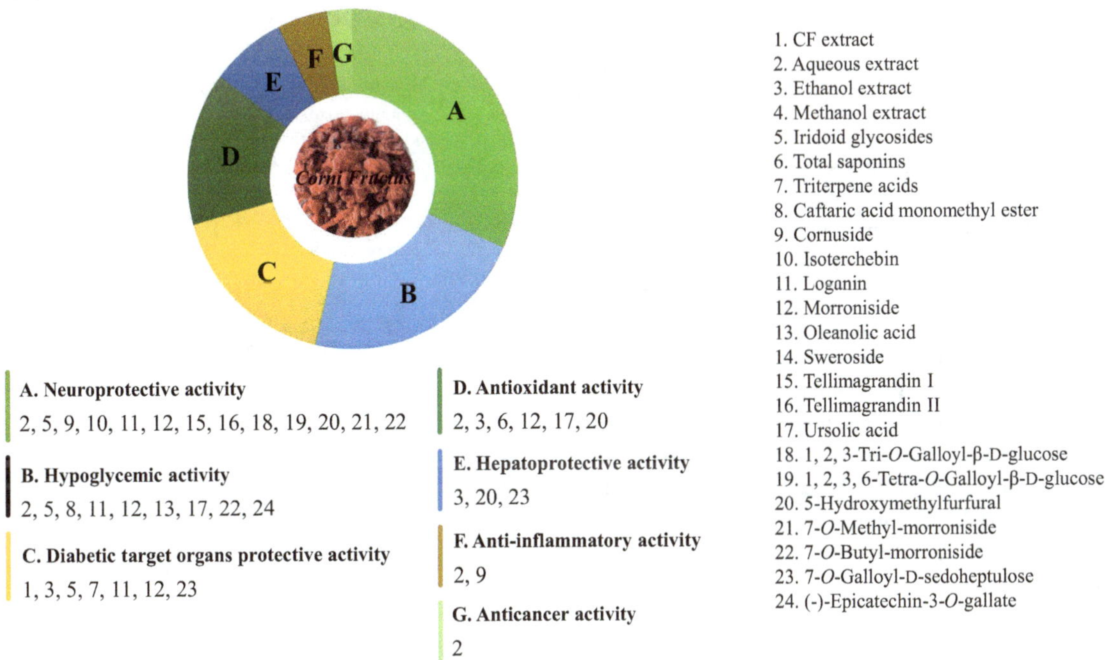

Fig. 6 The various pharmacological activities of the extract and chemical compounds identified from *Corni Fructus*

suppressed liver gluconeogenesis. Also, compounds alleviated the high-glucose triggered target organs damage by attenuating oxidative stress, inflammation, and apoptosis, finally kept the essential function of target organs stable. CF has also been widely used to treat DM in clinical work. For example, Jingui Shenqi Wan and Liuwei Dihuang Wan are two classic Chinese medicinal formulae which contain CF. Clinical trials indicated that Jingui Shenqi Wan and Liuwei Dihuang Wan could decrease serum glucose levels, alleviate typical DM symptoms and repair target organs injury [64–67]. Diverse anti-diabetes and anti-diabetic complication pharmacological activities make CF a potential herb to become the complementary drug for treating DM.

Another significant biological activity is the neuroprotection. In cerebral ischemia rat model and neurodegenerative disorder cellular model, iridoid glycosides (e.g., morroniside) and 5-hydroxymethylfurfural increased the number of new mature neurons and blood vessels and exerted anti-oxidative stress, anti-inflammation, and anti-apoptosis properties. In cerebral ischemia rat model and multiple sclerosis rats and mice models, iridoid glycosides also enhanced the levels of brain-derived neurotrophic factor and nerve growth factor. Current studies showed that the pathogenic mechanisms of neurodegenerative diseases have the close relationship with autophagy deficiency and abnormal proteins aggregate clearance dysfunction [68, 69]. In addition to the anti-apoptotic activity, pharmacological activities of CF on the regulation of autophagy can be further explored. Furthermore, many classic Chinese medicinal formulae have been used to treat neurological disorders belonging to liver and kidney deficiency [70–72]. For example, Liuwei Dihuang Wan treats insomnia, Zuogui Wan (左归丸) treats epilepsy and vertigo, Dabu Yinjian (大补阴煎) treats a headache, Zuogui Wan and Dihuang Yinzi (地黄饮子) treats stroke, and Huanshao Dan (还少丹) treats dementia. CF plays a vital role in nourishing liver and kidney Yin in these Chinese medicinal formulae.

However, about 90 compounds have been isolated and identified from CF, only 18% compounds are further assayed for their pharmacological activities in vivo and in vitro. It indicates that pharmacological activities of the remaining 90% chemical components are still unknown yet. Moreover, current studies do not provide enough evidence to verify the drug binding sites of active ingredients of CF. For example, it is difficult to judge whether these active ingredients bind the G protein coupled receptor, ion channels, transmembrane receptor kinases, or nuclear receptors to work. Therefore, more systematic and detailed pharmacological studies on CF need to be fulfilled in the future.

Abbreviations

ACh: acetyl choline; AGEs: advances glycation endproducts; ALP: alkaline phosphatase; ALT: alanine aminotransferase; AST: aspartate aminotransferase; ATF4: activating transcription factor 4; BACE1: b-site amyloid precursor protein cleaving enzyme 1; Bax: bcl-2-associated X; Bcl-2: B-cell lymphoma-2; BDNF: brain-derived neurotrophic factor; BMDM: bone marrow-derived macrophages; BrdU: bromodeoxyuridine; CAT: catalase; CEL: Ne-(carboxyethyl) lysine; ChE: cholinesterase; CHOP: C/EBP homologous protein; CMA: Ne-(carboxymethyl)arginine; CML: Ne-(carboxymethyl)lysine; Col V: collagen V; COX-2: cyclooxygenase-2; CTGF: connective tissue growth factor; CVA16: Coxsackie virus A group 16 strain; Cyt c: cytochrome C; DCs: dendritic cells; E2: 17β-estradiol; E3: estrone; ECE: endothelin converting enzyme; ECM: extracellular matrix; ER^+: estrogen receptor-positive; ERK1/2: extracellular-signal-related kinase 1/2; ET-1: endothelin-1; FN: fibronectin; GAP-43: growth-associated protein-43; GC–MS: gas chromatography–mass spectrometry; GPX: glutathione peroxidase; GSH: glutathione; GSP: glycated serum protein; GSSG: glutathione disulfide; HK-2: human renal proximal tubular epithelial cells; HO-1: heme oxygenase-1; HUVECs: human umbilical vein endothelial cells; ICAM-1: intercellular adhesion molecule-1; iNOS: inducible nitric oxide synthase; IFN: interferon; IL: interleukin; JNK: c-Jun N-terminal kinase; LPS: lipopolysaccharide; MAPK: mitogen-activated protein kinase; MCAO: middle cerebral artery occlusion; MCP-1: monocyte chemoattractant protein 1; MDA: malondialdehyde; MITF-M: microphthalmia-associated transcription factor-M; MMP: mitochondrial membrane potential; NF-kB: nuclear factor-kappa B; NFATc1: nuclear factor of activated T cells cytoplasmic 1; NGF: nerve growth factor; NO: nitric oxide; OSCAR: osteoclast-associated receptor; OVA: ovalbumin; *p*-eIF2α: *p*-eukaryotic initiation factor 2 alpha; PAECs: pulmonary artery endothelial cells; PEPCK: phosphoenolpyruvate carboxykinase; PERK: protein kinase R (PKR)-like endoplasmic reticulum kinase; PGE_2: prostaglandin E_2; PLB: phospholamban; p.o.: per os; RAGE: receptor of AGE; RANKL: receptor activator of nuclear factor kappa-B ligand; ROS: reactive oxygen species; SERCA2a: sarcoplasmic reticulum Ca^{2+}-ATPase 2a; SOD: superoxide dismutase; SPHK1: sphingosine kinase 1; SREBP-1&2: sterol regulatory element binding protein-1&2; STIM1: sensor protein stromal interaction molecule 1; STZ: streptozotocin; SYP: synaptophysin; TBARS: thiobarbituric acid-reactive substance; TC: triglyceride; TG: total cholesterol; TGF: transforming growth factor; TNF-α: tumor necrosis factor-α; TRAP: tartrate-resistant acid phosphatase; Trk A: tyrosine receptor kinase A; TRP-1&2: tyrosinase-related protein-1&2; VCAM-1: vascular cell adhesion molecule-1; VEGF: vascular endothelial growth factor.

Authors' contributions

YD conducted literature searches, extracted and analyzed data and drafted the manuscript and prepared tables and figures. ZLF contributed to the proofreading of chemical constituents and structures. FSW contributed to the draft of the fundamental theories of traditional Chinese medicine of the review. HBC contributed to the revisions of the manuscript. JHL designed the study, developed and revised the manuscript and is the corresponding author. All authors read and approved the final manuscript.

Author details

[1] State Key Laboratory of Quality Research in Chinese Medicine, Institute of Chinese Medical Sciences, University of Macau, Room 7015, N22, Avenida da Universidade, Taipa, Macau SAR, People's Republic of China. [2] School of Chinese Medicine, Hong Kong Baptist University, Hong Kong, SAR, People's Republic of China. [3] Ulcerous Vascular Surgical Department, Beijing Traditional Chinese Medicine Hospital Affiliated to Capital Medical University, Beijing, People's Republic of China.

Acknowledgements

Not applicable.

Competing interests

The authors declare that they have no competing interests.

Consent for publication

Not applicable.

Funding
This work was supported by Macau government Grants FDCT-022/2015/A1 and FDCT-092-2015-A3, the University of Macau Grants MYRG2016-0019-ICMS-QRCM and MYRG2017-00147-ICMS awarded to Jia-Hong Lu.

References

1. Chinese Pharmacopoeia Commission. People's Republic of China pharmacopoeia 2015 edition, 1st part. Beijing: China Medical Science Press; 2015. p. 27–8.
2. Xiang CK. Research progress on resources and active components of *Cornus officinalis*. Hebei Med J. 2016;38:1886–9.
3. Song XY, Chen Q, Qi XY. Effect of Liuwei Dihuang pill on erythrocyte aldose reductase activity in early diabetic nephropathy patients. Chin J Integr Tradit West Med. 2004;24:1087–90.
4. Liu XD, Fu J, Feng MZ, Zhang ZH. Effect of Jinggui Shenqi pill combined with nifedipine for the treatment of elderly hypertensive patients with spleen–kidney Yang deficiency syndrome. China J Chin Mater Med. 2015;40:4908–12.
5. Wang Y, Wang C. Three cases of clinical application of Guchong Decoction. China J Tradit Chin Med Pharm. 2010;25:2041–3.
6. Hatano T, Ogawa N, Kira R, Yasuhara T, Okuda T. Tannins of cornaceous plants. I. Cornusiins A, B and C, dimeric monomeric and trimeric hydrolyzable tannins from *Cornus officinalis*, and orientation of valoneoyl group in related tannins. Chem Pharm Bull. 1989;37:2083–90.
7. Hatano T, Ogawa N, Kira R, Yasuhara T, Okuda T. Tannins of cornaceous plants. II. Cornusiins D, E and F, new dimeric and trimeric hydrolyzable Tannins from *Cornus officinalis*. Chem Pharm Bull. 1989;37:2665–9.
8. Wu Y, Wang X, Shen B, Kang L, Fan E. Extraction, structure, and bioactivities of the polysaccharides from *Fructus corni*. Recent Pat Food Nutr Agric. 2013;5:57–61.
9. Yin X, You Q, Jiang Z, Zhou X. Optimization for ultrasonic-microwave synergistic extraction of polysaccharides from *Cornus officinalis* and characterization of polysaccharides. Int J Biol Macromol. 2016;83:226–32.
10. Chen H, Zhang HJ, Zhang MJ, Xiao ZH. Orthogonal test for optimization of extraction condition for volatile components of *Cornus officinalis* and extract analysis by GC–MS. J Third Mil Med Univ. 2007;29:1079–82.
11. Li GY, Yao YX, Ding X. Studies on chemistry component and the biological activity of petroleum ether extraction from pre- and post-processed of *Cornus officinalis*. Zhong Yao Cai. 2010;33:192–5.
12. Wen YY, Ren Q, Zhang GM, Li AN, Ding ZE. Analysis of the essential oils from *Cornus officinalis* by simultaneous distillation extraction coupled with gas chromatography–mass spectrometry. Food Ferment Ind. 2010;36:166–70.
13. Han Y, Jung HW, Park YK. Selective therapeutic effect of *Cornus officinalis* fruits on the damage of different organs in STZ-induced diabetic rats. Am J Chin Med. 2014;42:1169–82.
14. He K, Song S, Zou Z, Feng M, Wang D, Wang Y, Li X, Ye X. The hypoglycemic and synergistic effect of loganin, morroniside, and ursolic acid isolated from the fruits of *Cornus officinalis*. Phytother Res. 2015;30:283–91.
15. Lin MH, Liu HK, Huang WJ, Huang CC, Wu TH, Hsu FL. Evaluation of the potential hypoglycemic and beta-cell protective constituents isolated from *Corni Fructus* to tackle insulin-dependent diabetes mellitus. J Agric Food Chem. 2011;59:7743–51.
16. He LH. Comparative study on alpha-glucosidase inhibitory effects of total iridoid glycosides in the crude products and the wine-processed products from *Cornus officinalis*. Yakugaku Zasshi. 2011;131:1801–5.
17. Park CH, Noh JS, Tanaka T, Uebaba K, Cho EJ, Yokozawa T. The effects of *Corni Fructus* extract and its fractions against α-glucosidase inhibitory activities in vitro and sucrose tolerance in normal rats. Am J Chin Med. 2011;39:367–80.
18. Chen CC, Hsu CY, Chen CY, Liu HK. *Fructus Corni* suppresses hepatic gluconeogenesis related gene transcription, enhances glucose responsiveness of pancreatic beta-cells, and prevents toxin induced beta-cell death. J Ethnopharmacol. 2008;117:483–90.
19. Yokozawa T, Kang KS, Park CH, Noh JS, Yamabe N, Shibahara N, Tanaka T. Bioactive constituents of *Corni Fructus*: the therapeutic use of morroniside, loganin, and 7-*O*-galloyl-D-sedoheptulose as renoprotective agents in type 2 diabetes. Drug Discov Ther. 2010;4:223–34.
20. Yamabe N, Kang KS, Goto E, Tanaka T, Yokozawa T. Beneficial effect of *Corni Fructus*, a constituent of Hachimi-jio-gan, on advanced glycation end-product-mediated renal injury in streptozotocin-treated diabetic rats. Biol Pharm Bull. 2007;30:520–6.
21. Yamabe N, Kang KS, Park CH, Tanaka T, Yokozawa T. 7-*O*-galloyl-D-sedoheptulose is a novel therapeutic agent against oxidative stress and advanced glycation endproducts in the diabetic kidney. Biol Pharm Bull. 2009;32:657–64.
22. Lv X, Dai G, Lv G, Chen Y, Wu Y, Shen H, Xu H. Synergistic interaction of effective parts in *Rehmanniae Radix* and *Cornus officinalis* ameliorates renal injury in C57BL/KsJ-db/db diabetic mice: involvement of suppression of AGEs/RAGE/SphK1 signaling pathway. J Ethnopharmacol. 2016;185:110–9.
23. Jiang WL, Zhang SP, Hou J, Zhu HB. Effect of loganin on experimental diabetic nephropathy. Phytomedicine. 2012;19:217–22.
24. Ma W, Wang KJ, Cheng CS, Yan GQ, Lu WL, Ge JF, Cheng YX, Li N. Bioactive compounds from *Cornus officinalis* fruits and their effects on diabetic nephropathy. J Ethnopharmacol. 2014;153:840–5.
25. Xu HQ, Hao HP. Effects of iridoid total glycoside from *Cornus officinalis* on prevention of glomerular overexpression of transforming growth factor beta 1 and matrixes in an experimental diabetes model. Biol Pharm Bull. 2004;27:1014–8.
26. Qi MY, Liu HR, Dai DZ, Li N, Dai Y. Total triterpene acids, active ingredients from *Fructus Corni*, attenuate diabetic cardiomyopathy by normalizing ET pathway and expression of FKBP12.6 and SERCA2a in streptozotocin-rats. J Pharm Pharmacol. 2008;60:1687–94.
27. Chen Y, Wu Y, Gan X, Liu K, Lv X, Shen H, Dai G, Xu H. Iridoid glycoside from *Cornus officinalis* ameliorated diabetes mellitus-induced testicular damage in male rats: involvement of suppression of the AGEs/RAGE/p38 MAPK signaling pathway. J Ethnopharmacol. 2016;194:850–60.
28. Pi WX, Feng XP, Ye LH, Cai BC. Combination of morroniside and diosgenin prevents high glucose-induced cardiomyocytes apoptosis. Molecules. 2017;22:163.
29. Wang W, Sun F, An Y, Ai H, Zhang L, Huang W, Li L. Morroniside protects human neuroblastoma SH-SY5Y cells against hydrogen peroxide-induced cytotoxicity. Eur J Pharmacol. 2009;613:19–23.
30. Liu Y, Liu H, Zhang J. Total saponins of *Cornus officinalis* Sieb. ameliorates the endothelium dependent relaxation of mesenteric artery by regulating nitric oxide release in streptozotocin-induced diabetic rats. Zhong Nan Da Xue Xue Bao Yi Xue Ban. 2012;37:757–64.
31. Peng Q, Wei Z, Lau BH. *Fructus corni* enhances endothelial cell antioxidant defenses. Gen Pharmacol. 1998;31:221–5.
32. Yu HH, Hur JM, Seo SJ, Moon HD, Kim HJ, Park RK, You YO. Protective effect of ursolic acid from *Cornus officinalis* on the hydrogen peroxide-induced damage of HEI-OC1 auditory cells. Am J Chin Med. 2009;37:735–46.
33. Hwang KA, Hwang YJ, Song J. Antioxidant activities and oxidative stress inhibitory effects of ethanol extracts from *Cornus officinalis* on raw 264.7 cells. BMC Complement Altern Med. 2016;16:196.
34. Cao G, Cai H, Cai B, Tu S. Effect of 5-hydroxymethylfurfural derived from processed *Cornus officinalis* on the prevention of high glucose-induced oxidative stress in human umbilical vein endothelial cells and its mechanism. Food Chem. 2013;140:273–9.
35. Xu HQ, Hao HP, Zhang X, Pan Y. Morroniside protects cultured human umbilical vein endothelial cells from damage by high ambient glucose. Acta Pharmacol Sin. 2004;25:412–5.
36. Kang DG, Moon MK, Lee AS, Kwon TO, Kim JS, Lee HS. Cornuside suppresses cytokine-induced proinflammatory and adhesion molecules in the human umbilical vein endothelial cells. Biol Pharm Bull. 2007;30:1796–9.
37. Chu Q, Hashimoto K, Satoh K, Wang Q, Sakagami H. Effect of three herbal extracts on NO and PGE2 production by activated mouse macrophage-like cells. In Vivo. 2009;544:537–44.
38. Choi YH, Jin GY, Li GZ, Yan GH. Cornuside suppresses lipopolysaccharide-induced inflammatory mediators by inhibiting nuclear factor-kappa B activation in RAW 264.7 macrophages. Biol Pharm Bull. 2011;34:959–66.

39. Chu Q, Satoh K, Kanamoto T, Terakubo S, Nakashima H, Wang Q, Sakagami H. Antitumor potential of three herbal extracts against human oral squamous cell lines. Anticancer Res. 2009;29:3211–9.
40. Telang NT, Li G, Sepkovic DW, Bradlow HL, Wong GY. Anti-proliferative effects of Chinese herb *Cornus officinalis* in a cell culture model for estrogen receptor-positive clinical breast cancer. Mol Med Rep. 2012;5:22–8.
41. Telang N, Li G, Katdare M, Sepkovic D, Bradlow L, Wong G. Inhibitory effects of Chinese nutritional herbs in isogenic breast carcinoma cells with modulated estrogen receptor function. Oncol Lett. 2016;12:3949–57.
42. Chang JS, Chiang LC, Hsu FF, Lin CC. Chemoprevention against hepatocellular carcinoma of *Cornus officinalis* in vitro. Am J Chin Med. 2004;32:717–25.
43. Jeong EJ, Kim TB, Yang H, Kang SY, Kim SY, Sung SH, Kim YC. Neuroprotective iridoid glycosides from *Cornus officinalis* fruits against glutamate-induced toxicity in HT22 hippocampal cells. Phytomedicine. 2012;19:317–21.
44. Wang X, Liu J, Jin N, Xu D, Wang J, Han Y, Yin N. *Fructus corni* extract-induced neuritogenesis in PC12 cells is associated with the suppression of stromal interaction molecule 1 expression and inhibition of Ca^{2+} influx. Exp Ther Med. 2015;9:1773–9.
45. Bhakta HK, Park CH, Yokozawa T, Tanaka T, Jung HA, Choi JS. Potential anticholinesterase and β-site amyloid precursor protein cleaving enzyme 1 inhibitory activities of cornuside and gallotannins from *Cornus officinalis* fruits. Arch Pharm Res. 2017;40:836–53.
46. Yao RQ, Zhang L, Wang W, Li L. Cornel iridoid glycoside promotes neurogenesis and angiogenesis and improves neurological function after focal cerebral ischemia in rats. Brain Res Bull. 2009;79:69–76.
47. Wang W, Xu J, Li L, Wang P, Ji X, Ai H, Zhang L, Li L. Neuroprotective effect of morroniside on focal cerebral ischemia in rats. Brain Res Bull. 2010;83:196–201.
48. Yin L, Chen Y, Qu Z, Zhang L, Wang Q, Zhang Q, Li L. Involvement of JAK/STAT signaling in the effect of cornel iridoid glycoside on experimental autoimmune encephalomyelitis amelioration in rats. J Neuroimmunol. 2014;274:28–37.
49. Zhao L, Ding Y, Zhang L, Li L. Cornel iridoid glycoside improves memory ability and promotes neuronal survival in fimbria–fornix transected rats. Eur J Pharmacol. 2010;647:68–74.
50. Qu Z, Zheng N, Zhang Y, Zhang L, Liu J, Wang Q, Yin L. Preventing the BDNF and NGF loss involved in the effects of cornel iridoid glycoside on attenuation of experimental autoimmune encephalomyelitis in mice. Neurol Res. 2016;38:831–7.
51. Ding X, Wang MY, Yao YX, Li GY, Cai BC. Protective effect of 5-hydroxymethylfurfural derived from processed *Fructus Corni* on human hepatocyte L02 injured by hydrogen peroxide and its mechanism. J Ethnopharmacol. 2010;128:373–6.
52. Wang MY, Zhao FM, Peng HY, Lou CH, Li Y, Ding X, Yu XY, Yang GM, Xu DQ, Jiang LH, Zhang X, Ye LH, Cai BC. Investigation on the morphological protective effect of 5-hydroxymethylfurfural extracted from wine-processed *Fructus corni* on human L02 hepatocytes. J Ethnopharmacol. 2010;130:424–8.
53. Jiang ZQ, Ma YX, Li MH, Zhan XQ, Zhang X, Wang MY. 5-Hydroxymethylfurfural protects against ER stress-induced apoptosis in GalN/TNF-α-injured L02 hepatocytes through regulating the PERK-eIF2α signaling pathway. Chin J Nat Med. 2015;13:896–905.
54. Park CH, Noh JS, Tanaka T, Roh SS, Lee JC, Yokozawa T. Polyphenol isolated from *Corni Fructus*, 7-*O*-galloyl-D-sedoheptulose, modulates advanced glycation endproduct-related pathway in type 2 diabetic db/db mice. Arch Pharmacal Res. 2015;38:1270–80.
55. Lee NH, Seo CS, Lee HY, Jung DY, Lee JK, Lee JA, Song KY, Shin HK, Lee MY, Seo YB, Kim H, Ha H. Hepatoprotective and antioxidative activities of *Cornus officinalis* against acetaminophen-induced hepatotoxicity in mice. Evid Based Complement Altern Med. 2012;2012:1–8.
56. Sun H, Li L, Zhang A, Zhang N, Lv H, Sun W, Wang X. Protective effects of sweroside on human MG-63 cells and rat osteoblasts. Fitoterapia. 2013;84:174–9.
57. Kim JY, Kim YK, Choi MK, Oh J, Kwak HB, Kim JJ. Effect of *Cornus Officinalis* on receptor activator of nuclear factor-kappaB ligand (RANKL)-induced osteoclast differentiation. J Bone Metab. 2012;19:121.
58. An YA, Hwang JY, Lee JS, Kim YC. *Cornus officinalis* methanol extract upregulates melanogenesis in melan-a cells. Toxicol Res. 2015;31:165–72.
59. Liu X, Zeng YQ, Liang YZ, Zou C, Liu H, Qiu F, Liang CL, Jin XW, Su ZR, Dai Z. Medicinal herbs *Fructus corni* and *Semen cuscutae* suppress allograft rejection via distinct immune mechanisms. Oncotarget. 2016;7:35680.
60. Cho K, Lee HJ, Lee SY, Woo H, Lee MN, Seok JH, et al. Oleanolic acid and ursolic acid derived from *Cornus officinalis* Sieb. et Zucc. suppress epidermal growth factor- and phorbol ester-induced MUC5AC mucin production and gene expression from human airway epithelial cells. Phytother Res. 2011;25:760–4.
61. Kim SH, Kim BK, Lee YC. Effects of *Corni fructus* on ovalbumin-induced airway inflammation and airway hyper-responsiveness in a mouse model of allergic asthma. J Inflamm. 2012;9:9.
62. Kang DG, Choi DH, Lee JK, Lee YJ, Moon MK, Yang SN, Kwon TO, Kwon JW, Kim JS, Lee HS. Endothelial NO/cGMP-dependent vascular relaxation of cornuside isolated from the fruit of *Cornus officinalis*. Planta Med. 2007;73:1436–40.
63. Song JH, Park K, Shim A, Kwon BE, Ahn JH, Choi YJ, Kim JK, Yeo SG, Yoon K, Ko HJ. Complete sequence analysis and antiviral screening of medicinal plants for human Coxsackievirus A16 isolated in Korea. Osong Public Health Res Perspect. 2015;6:52–8.
64. Wu HZ. The clinical effect of Jinkui Shenqi pill on type 2 diabetes. Pharmacol Clin Chin Mater Med. 2013;29:191–3.
65. Liu ZW. Curative effect valuation on Jingui Senqi pill in the treatment of diabetic nephropathy. Chin J Basic Med Tradit Chin Med. 2014;20(821–2):31.
66. Li X, Li Y. Clinical study on Liuwei Dihuang pills combined with liraglutide and metformin in treatment of type 2 diabetes mellitus. Drugs Clin. 2016;31:1146–50.
67. He K, Zhu LH, Lu XW. Clinical observation of Liuwei Dihuang pills combined with metformin in the treatment of type 2 diabetes. Chin Tradit Pat Med. 2016;38:50–2.
68. Menzies FM, Fleming A, Rubinsztein DC. Compromised autophagy and neurodegenerative diseases. Nat Rev Neurosci. 2015;16:345–57.
69. Nah J, Yuan J, Jung YK. Autophagy in neurodegenerative diseases: from mechanism to therapeutic approach. Mol Cells. 2015;38:381–9.
70. Zhou ZY. Chinese internal medicine. Beijing: China Press of Traditional Chinese Medicine; 2003. p. 157, 176, 183, 308, 316, 327.
71. Lin SK, Yan SH, Lai JN, Tsai TH. Patterns of Chinese medicine use in prescriptions for treating Alzheimer's disease in Taiwan. Chin Med. 2016;11:12.
72. Yeung WF, Chung KF, Zhang NL, Zhang SP, Yung KP, Chen PX, Ho YY. Identification of Chinese medicine syndromes in persistent insomnia associated with major depressive disorder: a latent tree analysis. Chin Med. 2016;11:4.
73. Cai H, Cao G, Cai B. Rapid simultaneous identification and determination of the multiple compounds in crude *Fructus Corni* and its processed products by HPLC–MS/MS with multiple reaction monitoring mode. Pharm Biol. 2013;51:273–8.
74. Zhang YE, Liu EH, Li HJ, Li P. Chemical constituents from the fruit of *Cornus officinalis*. Chin J Nat Med. 2009;7:365–7.
75. Han SY, Pan Y, Ding G, Cai BC. Application of 1H-NMR and 13C-NMR spectra in the structure identification of iridoids from *Cornus officinalis*. Chin Arch Tradit Chin Med. 2004;22:56–9.
76. Park JY, Han AR, Kil YS, Kang U, Kim SH, Nam SJ, Seo EK. A new secoiridoid glycoside from the fruits of *Cornus officinalis* (Cornaceae). Nat Prod Res. 2016;30:1504–10.
77. He J, Ye XS, Wang XX, Yang YN, Zhang PC, Ma BZ, Zhang WK, Xu JK. Four new iridoid glucosides containing the furan ring from the fruit of *Cornus officinalis*. Fitoterapia. 2017;120:136–41.
78. Han SY, Pan Y, Yang GM, Cai BC. Research on components of *Cornus officinalis* extracted by supercritical carbon dioxide. Zhongguo Zhong Yao Za Zhi. 2003;28:1148–50, 83.
79. Kim DK, Kwak JY. A furan derivative from *Comus officinalis*. Arch Pharm Res. 1998;21:787–9.
80. Xie X, Wang R, Shi Y. Chemical constituents from the fruits of *Cornus officinalis*. Biochem Syst Ecol. 2012;45:120–3.

81. Yang L, Wang Z, Huang L. Isolation and structural characterization of a polysaccharide FCAP1 from the fruit of *Cornus officinalis*. Carbohydr Res. 2010;345:1909–13.
82. Wang LL, Zhang T, Chen SQ, Shang CL. Study on the correlation between the quality of *Cornus officinalis* and the contents of the inorganic elements in the planting soil. Zhong Yao Cai. 2011;34:1167–72.
83. Hsu JH, Wu YC, Liu IM, Cheng JT. Release of acetylcholine to raise insulin secretion in Wistar rats by oleanolic acid, one of the active principles contained in *Cornus officinalis*. Neurosci Lett. 2006;404:112–6.
84. Gu H, Jiang Z, Wang M, Jiang H, Zhao F, Ding X, Cai B, Zhan Z. 5-Hydroxymethylfurfural from wine-processed *Fructus corni* inhibits hippocampal neuron apoptosis. Neural Regen Res. 2013;8:2605–14.
85. Zhang QC, Zhao Y, Bian HM. Antiplatelet activity of a novel formula composed of malic acid, succinic acid and citric acid from *Cornus officinalis* fruit. Phytother Res. 2013;27:1894–6.

14

Coptidis rhizoma and its main bioactive components: recent advances in chemical investigation, quality evaluation and pharmacological activity

Fan-Cheng Meng[1], Zheng-Feng Wu[1], Zhi-Qi Yin[2], Li-Gen Lin[1], Ruibing Wang[1*] and Qing-Wen Zhang[1*]

Abstract

Background: Coptidis rhizoma (CR) is the dried rhizome of *Coptis chinensis* Franch., *C. deltoidea* C. Y. Cheng et Hsiao or *C. teeta* Wall. (Ranunculaceae) and is commonly used in Traditional Chinese Medicine for the treatment of various diseases including bacillary dysentery, typhoid, tuberculosis, epidemic cerebrospinal meningitis, empyrosis, pertussis, and other illnesses.

Methods: A literature survey was conducted via SciFinder, ScieneDirect, PubMed, Springer, and Wiley databases. A total of 139 selected references were classified on the basis of their research scopes, including chemical investigation, quality evaluation and pharmacological studies.

Results: Many types of secondary metabolites including alkaloids, lignans, phenylpropanoids, flavonoids, phenolic compounds, saccharides, and steroids have been isolated from CR. Among them, protoberberine-type alkaloids, such as berberine, palmatine, coptisine, epiberberine, jatrorrhizine, columamine, are the main components of CR. Quantitative determination of these alkaloids is a very important aspect in the quality evaluation of CR. In recent years, with the advances in isolation and detection technologies, many new instruments and methods have been developed for the quantitative and qualitative analysis of the main alkaloids from CR. The quality control of CR has provided safety for pharmacological applications. These quality evaluation methods are also frequently employed to screen the active components from CR. Various investigations have shown that CR and its main alkaloids exhibited many powerful pharmacological effects including anti-inflammatory, anti-cancer, anti-diabetic, neuroprotective, cardioprotective, hypoglycemic, anti-Alzheimer and hepatoprotective activities.

Conclusion: This review summarizes the recent phytochemical investigations, quality evaluation methods, the biological studies focusing on CR as well as its main alkaloids.

Keywords: Coptidis rhizoma, *Coptis* genus, Phytochemistry, Quality evaluation, Pharmacological effects

Background

Coptidis rhizoma (CR) is the dried rhizome of *Coptis chinensis* Franch., *C. deltoidea* C. Y. Cheng et Hsiao or *C. teeta* Wall. (Ranunculaceae). The rhizomes of *C. japonica* Makino and *C. japonica var. dissecta* are also used as CR in Japan. CR has a long history of usage for clearing heat, eliminating dampness, purging fire and detoxification in Traditional Chinese Medicine (TCM). CR, also called goldthread, was frequently used for the treatment of bacillary dysentery, typhoid, tuberculosis, epidemic cerebrospinal meningitis, empyrosis, pertussis, and other diseases.

Chemical investigations have led to the discovery of multiple secondary metabolites including alkaloids, lignans, phenylpropanoids, flavonoids, phenolic acids,

*Correspondence: rwang@umac.mo; qwzhang@umac.mo
[1] State Key Laboratory of Quality Research in Chinese Medicine, Institute of Chinese Medical Sciences, University of Macau, Macao SAR, People's Republic of China
Full list of author information is available at the end of the article

saccharides and steroids in CR. Protoberberine-type alkaloids, such as berberine, palmatine, coptisine, epiberberine, jatrorrhizine and columamine, are the main bioactive components of CR.

Achieving a high degree of quality control is very important to ensure the safety and efficacy of TCM. Recent technological advances have made great progress in the quantitative and qualitative analysis of the main alkaloids extracted from CR. The applications of High Performance Liquid Chromatography (HPLC) or Ultra Performance Liquid Chromatography (UPLC) combined with Mass Spectrometry (MS) or MS^n [1, 2] and quantitative ^1H-NMR [3] are the most attractive strategies of ensuring quality control. Besides, these quality evaluation methods were also frequently employed to screen the pharmaceutically active components derived from CR [4, 5].

Various pharmacological investigations have indicated that CR and its main alkaloids exhibit many biological activities including anti-inflammatory, anti-cancer, hypoglycemic, anti-diabetic, neuroprotective and cardioprotective effects [6–12]. In this paper, we have summarized the phytochemical investigations, quality evaluation methods, and biological studies of CR as well as its main alkaloids that have been developed and conducted in recent years.

Phytochemical investigation

Previous phytochemical investigations on CR have led to the isolation and identification of many types of natural products including alkaloids, lignans, phenylpropanoids, flavonoids, phenolic compounds, saccharides and steroids. Up to this point, phytochemical investigations have focused on *C. chinensis*, *C. Japonica* var. *dissecta*, *C. teeta* and the main components of the plants from *Coptis* genus were found to be similar while the minor constituents differed.

Classic column chromatography utilizing silica gel as the stationary phase was widely used for the isolation of constituents from CR. Column chromatography over Sephadex LH-20, polyamide and octadecylsilane (ODS) was also used as well as preparative HPLC equipped with a reversed phase column or a chiral column. In general, it has often been difficult to isolate alkaloids from CR. However, through the application of suitable solvent systems in high-speed countercurrent chromatography, such as *n*-hexane–ethyl-acetate–methanol–water (2:5:2:5) [13] and chloroform–methanol–water (4:3:3, v/v) with HCl (60 mM) and triethylamine (5 mM) added into the upper aqueous phase and the lower organic phase [14], the highly pure main alkaloids could be readily separated and obtained in considerable yields. Spectroscopic analyses were employed in structural determination.

Alkaloids

Alkaloids are the main components of CR (Fig. 1 and Table 1), of which protoberberine alkaloids are most common in plants from the *Coptis* genus. Most of them are isoquinolines and quaternary iminium type alkaloids. So far, the protoberberine alkaloids reported from CR include berberine-type (**1–9**) [15], oxyberberine-type (**10–16**, **23–24**, **30**), methyl berberine type (**20**), and protoberberine-type (**21**) alkaloids. Benzophenanthridines (**17–19**, **22**), aporphine (**25**), benzylisoquinolines (**26–27**), phenethylamines (**28–29**, **35**) and isoquinolines (**31–34**) were also the main alkaloid components of various species of *Coptis* genus. Additionally, some other nitrogen-containing molecules were also isolated from *C. chinensis* [16–29].

Lignans

Lignans (Fig. 2 and Table 2) are also abundant in CR and have a wide variety of structures which can be classified into several skeletal types, such as benzofurans (**42–48**), furofurans (**49–53**), tetrahydrofurans (**54–60**), arylnaphthanlenes (**61–63**) and others (**64–72**) [18, 20, 26, 27, 30–38].

Simple phenylpropanoids

Simple phenylpropanoids with a mother-nucleus of phenylpropionic acid have been isolated from CR (Fig. 3 and Table 3). The esterified derivatives of these phenylpropionic acids bearing methyl, ethyl, *n*-butyl, quinic acid, etc. moieties were also isolated from the plants of CR [18–20, 22, 26–28, 31–35, 37, 39].

Flavonoids

Plants of the *Coptis* genus also contain flavonoids [33, 34, 36, 40]. Up to now, 8 flavonoids (Fig. 4 and Table 4) have been isolated from CR. Meng [32] reported a 6,8-dimethyl substituted flavonol (**98**) that was isolated from the rhizome of *C. teeta*. Chen et al. [33] purified a flavonol (**99**) and a flavone (**100**) from the rhizome of *C. chinensis*. In earlier chemical studies, a flavanone (**101**) and a dihydrochalcone (**102**) were extracted from the seeds of *C. japonica*, and three flavonoid glycosides (**103–105**) were isolated from the leaves of *C. japonica* and rhizomes of *C. japonica* var. *dissecta* [34, 36, 40].

Others

Phenethyl alcohol and its glycosides (**106–108**), phenols and organic acids (**109–117**), hemiterpenoids (**118–121**), dipeptides (**122–123**), *β*-sitosterol (**124**) and polysaccharides were also isolated from CR [18–20, 22, 26–28, 32, 34, 37, 39]. The structures of these compounds are shown in Fig. 5, while their corresponding references and sources are summarized in Table 5.

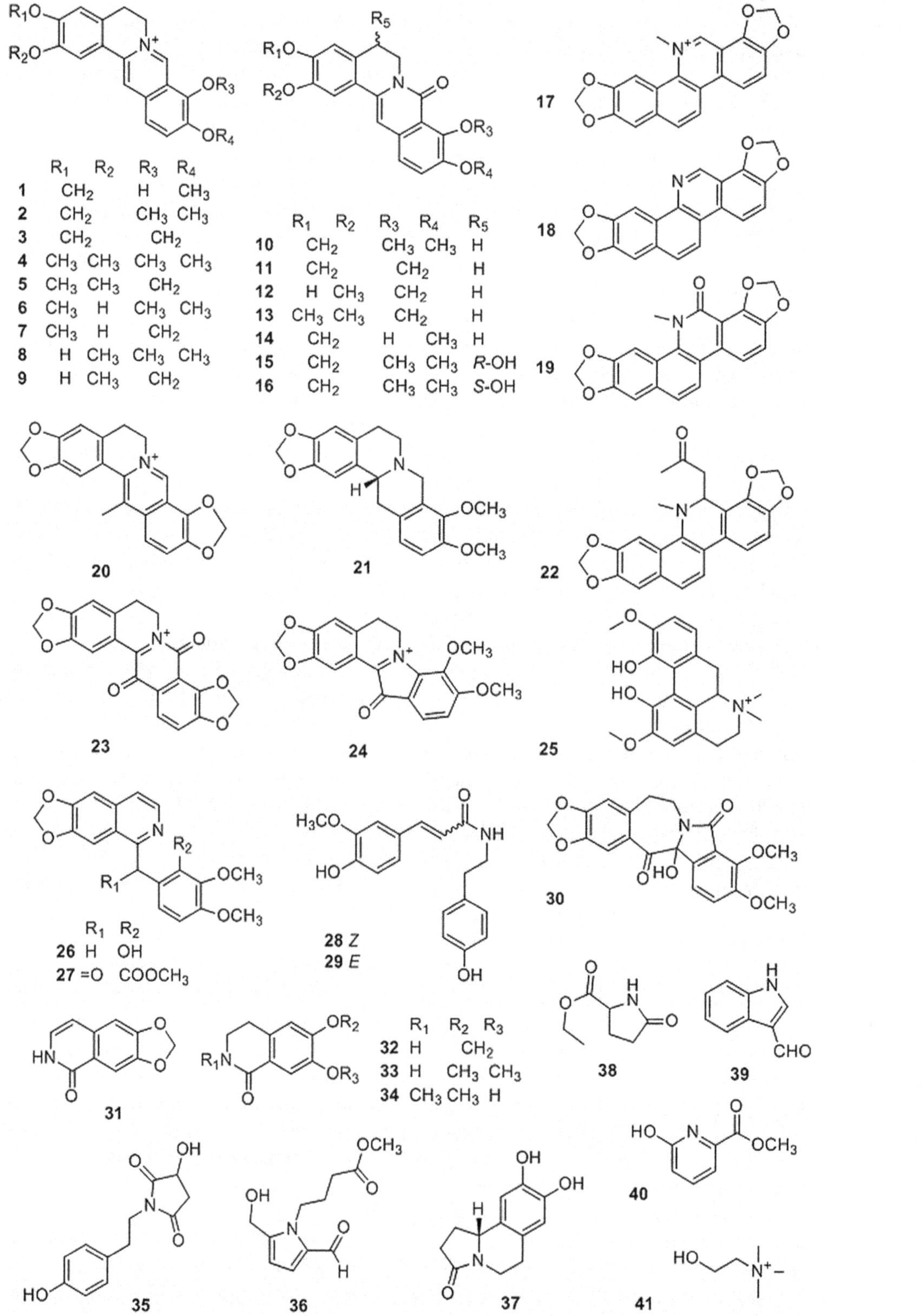

Fig. 1 Structures of alkaloids isolated from *Coptis* genus

Table 1 Alkaloids isolated from *Coptis* genus

No.	Compounds	Source	Rfs.
1	Berberrubine	*C. chinensis*	[15, 16]
2	Berberine	*C. chinensis*	[16–22]
3	Coptisine	*C. chinensis*	[16–18, 21]
4	Palmatine	*C. chinensis*	[15, 17, 18, 21]
5	Epiberberine	*C. chinensis*	[15–18, 21]
6	Columbamine	*C. chinensis*	[15, 17, 18]
7	Tetradehydroscoulerine	*C. chinensis*	[17]
8	Jatrorrhizine	*C. chinensis*	[15, 17, 18]
9	Groenlandicine	*C. chinensis*	[15–18]
10	8-Oxyberberine	*C. chinensis*	[15, 19–24]
11	8-oxo-Coptisine	*C. chinensis*	[15, 18, 19, 21–24]
12	3-Hydroxy-2-methoxy-9,10-methylenedioxy-8-oxo-Protoberberine	*C. chinensis*	[24]
13	8-oxo-Epiberberine	*C. chinensis*	[22, 23]
14	8-Oxyberberrubine	*C. chinensis*	[22]
15	(−)-5-Hydroxyl-8-oxyberberine	*C. chinensis*	[21]
16	(+)-5-Hydroxyl-8-oxyberberine	*C. chinensis*	[21]
17	Sanguinarine	*C. Japonica* var. *dissecta*	[25]
18	Norsanguinarine	*C. Japonica* var. *dissecta*	[25]
19	Oxysanguinarine	*C. Japonica* var. *dissecta*	[25]
20	Worenine	*C. chinensis*	[26]
21	Tetrahydroberberine	*C. chinensis*	[21]
22	6-Acetonyl-5,6-dihydrosanguinarine	*C. Japonica* var. *dissecta*	[25]
23	8,13-Dioxocoptisine hydroxide	*C. chinensis*	[22]
24	Coptisonine	*C. chinensis*	[22]
25	Magnoflorine	*C. chinensis*	[15, 17, 18]
26	Berbithine	*C. chinensis*	[21, 22]
27	6-([1,3]Dioxolo[4,5-g]isoquinoline-5-carbonyl)-2,3-dimethoxy benzoic acid methyl ester	*C. chinensis*	[21, 23]
28	*N-cis*-Ferulyltyramine	*C. chinensis*	[27]
29	*N-tran*-Feruloyltyramine	*C. chinensis*	[20, 28]
30	Chilenine	*C. chinensis*	[22, 28]
31	1,3-Dioxolo[4,5-g]isoquinolin-5(6*H*)-one	*C. chinensis*	[23]
32	Noroxyhydrastinine	*C. chinensis*	[19, 22, 23]
33	Corydaldine	*C. chinensis*	[19, 22, 23]
34	Thalifoline	*C. chinensis*	[27]
35	3-Hydroxy-1-(4-hydroxyphenethyl) pyrrolidine-2,5-dione	*C. chinensis*	[29]
36	4′-[Formyl-5-(hydroxymethyl)-1H-pyrrol-1-yl] butanoate	*C. chinensis*	[28]
37	8,9-Dihydroxy-1,5,6,10b-tetrahydro-2*H*-pyrrolo[2,1-α]-isoquinolin-5-one	*C. chinensis*	[26]
38	Ehyl-2-pyrrolidinone-5(*S*)-carboxylate	*C. chinensis*	[27]
39	Methyl-5-hydroxy-2-pyridinecarboxylate	*C. chinensis*	[27]
40	1*H*-Indole-3-carboxaldehyde	*C. chinensis*	[27]
41	Choline	*C. chinensis*	[15]

Quality evaluation of CR

Quality control will play a key role in the development of TCM industry. Identification of medicinal materials is the first crucial step. DNA barcoding, a technique for species identification using standardized short gene sequences, has played an important role in the authentication herbal medicines [42]. The feasibility of identifying the species sources of CR by DNA barcoding was investigated. It was supposed that ITS2 DNA barcode could be used to identify CR and its adulterants [43]. Li et al. suggested that the combination of nuclear DNA ITS and mitochondrial DNA ycf1 could be the standard barcoding for identification of CR [44].

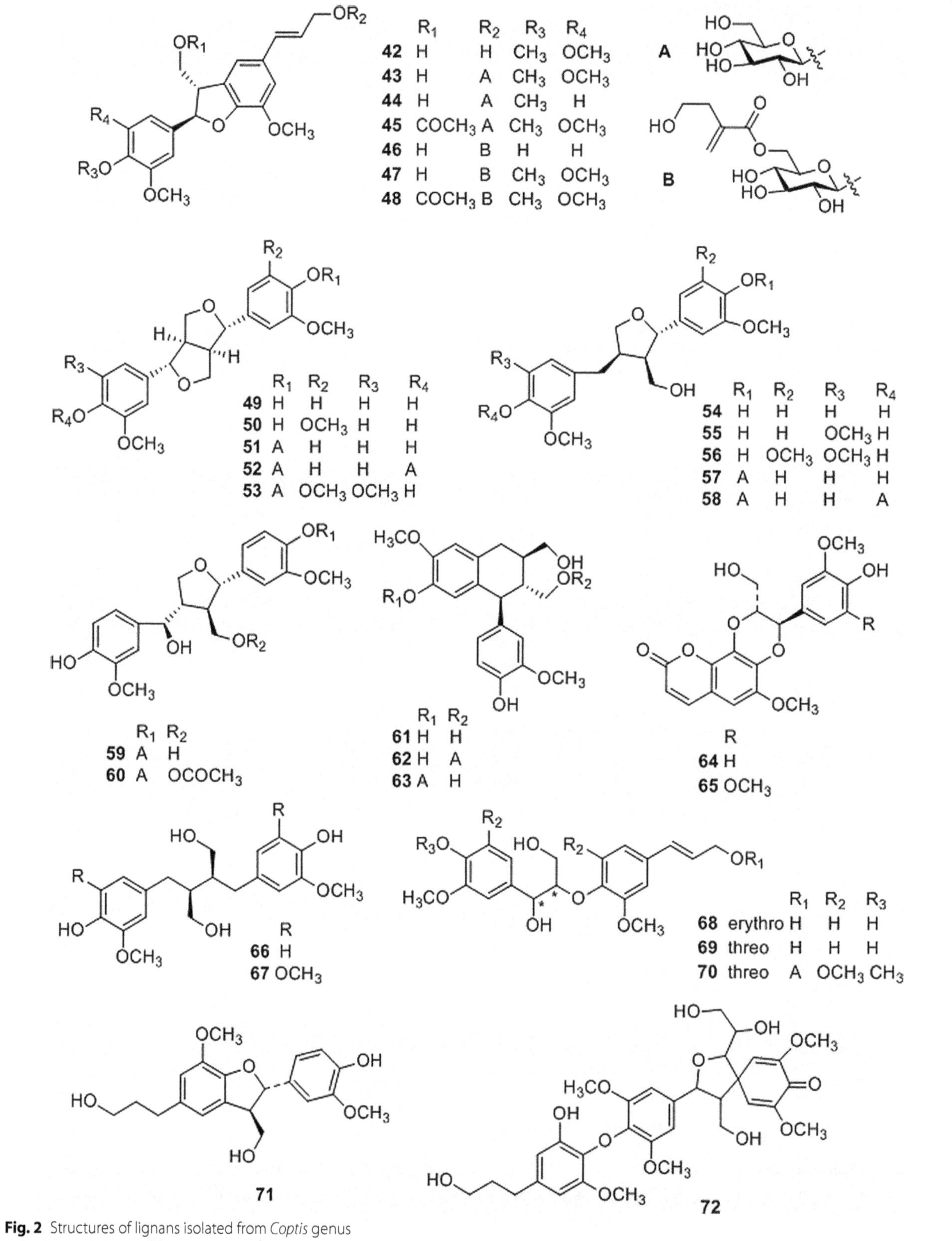

Fig. 2 Structures of lignans isolated from *Coptis* genus

Table 2 Lignans isolated from *Coptis* genus

No.	Compounds	Source	Rfs.
42	Woorenogenin	*C. chinensis; C. japonica* var. *dissecta*	[30, 31]
43	Woorenoside I	*C. japonica* var. *dissecta; C. teeta*	[31, 32]
44	Longifolroside A	*C. teeta*	[32]
45	Woorenoside II	*C. japonica* var. *dissecta; C. teeta*	[31, 32]
46	Woorenoside V	*C. japonica* var. *dissecta*	[31]
47	Woorenoside III	*C. japonica* var. *dissecta*	[31]
48	Woorenoside IV	*C. japonica* var. *dissecta*	[31]
49	(+)-Pinoresinol	*C. chinensis; C. japonica* var. *dissecta*	[31, 33]
50	(+)-Medioresinol	*C. chinensis*	[33]
51	(+)-Pinoresinol glucoside	*C. japonica* var. *dissecta*	[31]
52	(+)-Pinoresinol-4,4′-*O*-β-D-diglucopyranoside	*C. chinensis; C. japonica* var. *dissecta*	[18, 34]
53	(+)-Syringaresinol glucoside	*C. japonica* var. *dissecta; C. teeta*	[32]
54	(+)-Lariciresinol	*C. chinensis; C. teeta*	[20, 32, 33, 35]
55	(±)-5,5′-Dimethoxylariciresinol	*C. chinensis*	[26]
56	(+)-5′-Methoxylariciresinol	*C. chinensis*	[33]
57	(+)-Lariciresinol glucoside	*C. chinensis; C. japonica* var. *dissecta*	[18, 30, 31]
58	7*S*,8*R*,8′*R*-(+)-Lariciresinol-4,4′-*O*-β-D-diglucopyranoside	*C. chinensis; C. japonica* var. *dissecta*	[18, 34]
59	Lanicepside A	*C. chinensis*	[30]
60	9-Acetyl lanicepside B	*C. chinensis*	[30]
61	(+)-Isolariciresinol	*C. chinensis; C. japonica* var. *dissecta*	[30, 31, 33]
62	Isolarisiresinol-9-*O*-β-D-glucopyranoside	*C. chinensis*	[18]
63	Woorenoside XI	*C. japonica* var. *dissecta*	[34]
64	Cleomiscosin A	*C. japonica* var. *dissecta*	[36]
65	Aquillochin	*C. japonica* var. *dissecta*	[36]
66	2,3-bis[(4-Hydroxy-3,5-dimethoxyphenyl)-methyl]-1,4-butanediol	*C. chinensis*	[37]
67	Secoisolariciresinol	*C. chinensis*	[27]
68	*erythro*-Guaiacylglycerol-8-*O*-4′-(coniferyl alcohol) ether	*C. chinensis*	[33]
69	*threo*-Guaiacylglycerol-8-*O*-4′-(coniferyl alcohol) ether	*C. chinensis*	[33]
70	Woorenoside X	*C. japonica* var. *dissecta*	[34]
71	Dihydrodehydrodiconiferyl alcohol	*C. chinensis*	[37]
72	Woorenol	*C. japonica* var. *dissecta*	[38]

The protoberberine-type alkaloids, such as berberine, palmatine, coptisine, epiberberine, jatrorrhizine and columbamine, are the main components of CR [45–53] and also considered as its main bioactive compounds. The quantitative determination of these alkaloids is a very important aspect in the quality evaluation of CR. In recent years, with the advances of isolation and detection technologies, many new instrumental techniques have been employed for the quantitative and qualitative analysis of CR and the screening of the active components isolated from CR.

Achieving as complete of an extraction as possible is crucial for obtaining an accurate determination of the contents of CR. So far, refluxing or ultrasonic extraction are commonly employed in the extraction of the alkaloids from CR [45–49]. Methanol, ethanol or/and water with acid (H_2SO_4 or HCl) have been most frequently used as extraction solvents.

Teng and Choi [45] optimized the ultrasonic-assisted extraction method by investigating three independent variables including ethanol concentration, extraction time and the extraction temperature. Optimal extraction conditions were achieved with an ethanol concentration of 59%, extraction time of 46.57 min, and a temperature of 66.22 °C.

Methods based on HPLC are commonly used and provide a powerful tool for the quality evaluation of natural medicines. Researchers are seeking to develop new methods to extend its range of applications. Quantitative determination, differentiating the species or screening the bioactive components were achieved by thoroughly extracting information from HPLC data by

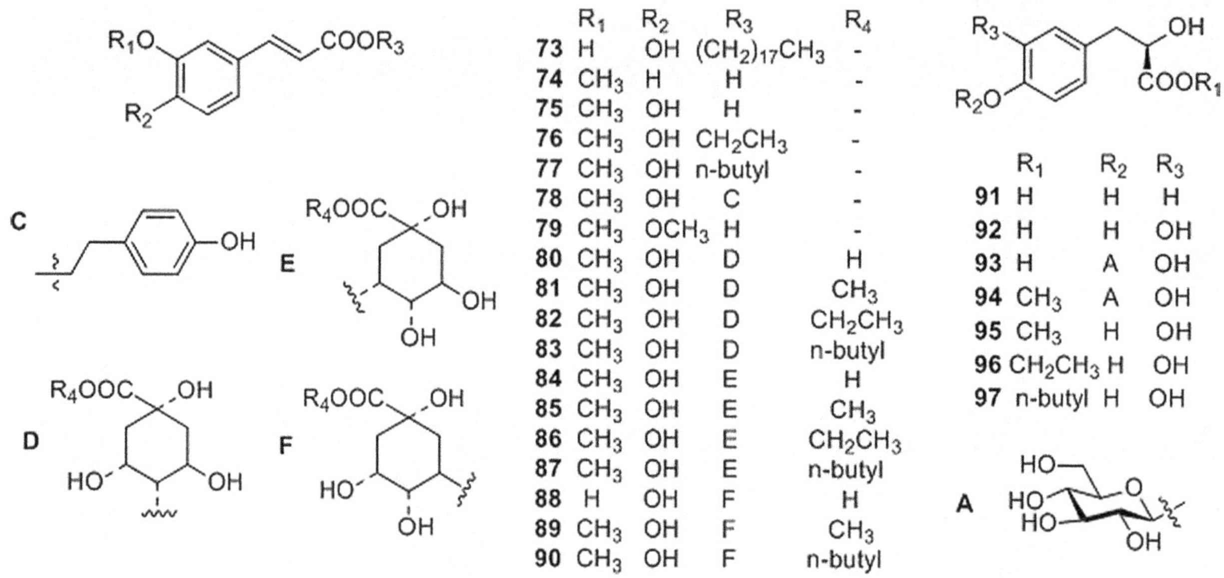

Fig. 3 Structures of phenylpropanoids isolated from *Coptis* genus

Table 3 Phenylpropanoids isolated from *Coptis* genus

No.	Compounds	Source	Rfs.
73	*Z*-Octadecyl caffeate	*C. chinensis*; *C. teeta*	[22, 32, 33]
74	*E*-3-Methoxycinnamic acid	*C. chinensis*	[19]
75	Ferulic acid	*C. chinensis*; *C. teeta*	[18, 32, 33]
76	Ethyl ferulate	*C. chinensis*; *C. japonica* var. *dissecta*	[31]
77	*n*-Butyl ferulate	*C. chinensis*	[19]
78	*p*-Hydroxyphenethyl trans-ferulate	*C. japonica*	[35]
79	*E*-3,4-Dimethoxycinnamic acid	*C. chinensis*	[19]
80	4-*O*-Feruloylquinic acid	*C. chinensis*	[18, 39]
81	Methyl 4-*O*-feruloylquicinate	*C. japonica* var. *dissecta*	[34]
82	Ethyl 4-*O*-feruloylquicinate	*C. chinensis*	[37]
83	4-*O*-Feruloylquinic acid butyl ester	*C. chinensis*	[19]
84	5-*O*-Feruloylquinic acid	*C. chinensis*	[18, 39]
85	Methyl 5-*O*-feruloylquicinate	*C. chinensis*	[26]
86	Ethyl 5-*O*-feruloylquicinate	*C. chinensis*	[26]
87	5-*O*-Feruloylquinic acid butyl ester	*C. chinensis*	[19]
88	Chlorogenic acid	*C. chinensis*	[33]
89	Methyl 3-*O*-feruloylquicinate	*C. chinensis*	[27, 28, 37]
90	*n*-Butyl 3-*O*-feruloylquicinate	*C. chinensis*	[27, 28]
91	3-(4′-Hydroxyphenyl)-(2*R*)-lactic acid	*C. chinensis*	[18]
92	3-(3′,4′-Hydroxyphenyl)-(2*R*)-lactic acid	*C. chinensis*	[18, 39]
93	3-(3′,4′-Dihydroxyphenyl)-(2*R*)-lactic acid-4′-*O*-*β*-D-glucopyranoside	*C. chinensis*	[18, 39]
94	Methyl-3-(4′-O-β-D-glucopyranosyl-3′,4′-dihydroxyphenyl)-lactate	*C. japonica* var. *dissecta*	[34]
95	Methyl-3,4-dihydroxyphenyl lactate	*C. chinensis* *C. teeta*	[18, 20, 28, 32]
96	Ethyl-3,4-dihydroxyphenyl lactate	*C. chinensis*	[28]
97	*n*-Butyl-3,4-dihydroxyphenyl lactate	*C. chinensis*	[19]

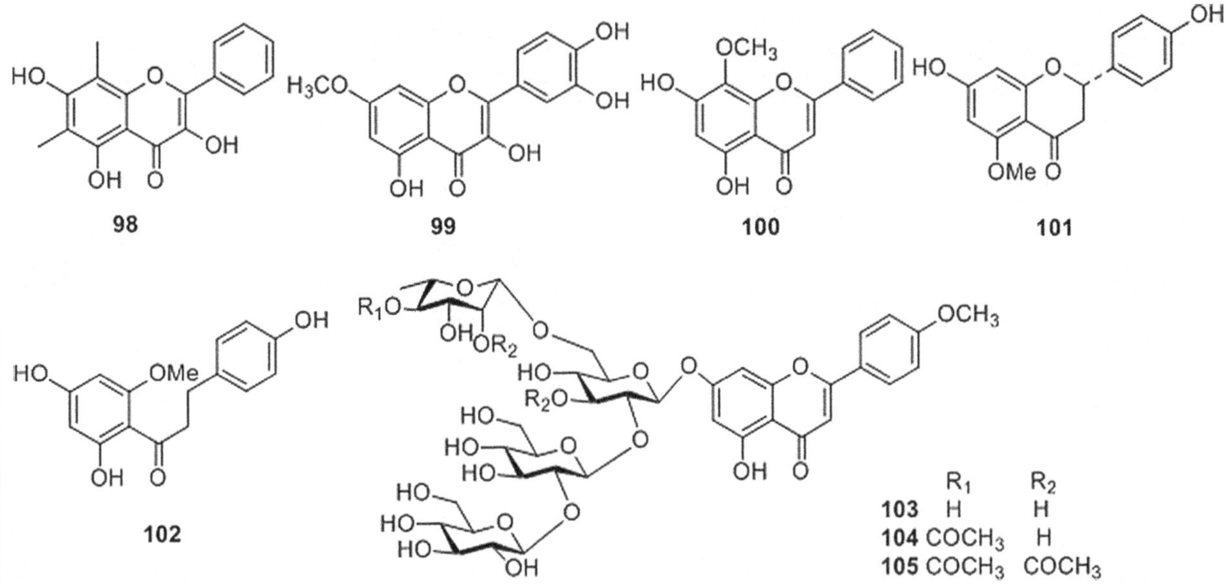

Fig. 4 Structures of flavonoids isolated from *Coptis* genus

Table 4 Flavonoids isolated from *Coptis* genus

No.	Compounds	Source	Rf.
98	6,8-Dimethyl-3,5,7-trihydroxyflavone	*C. teeta*	[32]
99	Rhamnetin	*C. chinensis*	[33]
100	Wogonin	*C. chinensis*	[33]
101	7,4′-Dihydroxy-5-methoxyflavanone	*C. japonica* var. *dissecta*	[36]
102	2′,4,4′-Trihydroxy-6′-methoxy-dihydrochalcone	*C. japonica* var. *dissecta*	[36]
103	Coptiside II	*C. japonica*	[40]
104	Woorenoside XII	*C. japonica* var. *dissecta*	[34]
105	Coptiside I	*C. japonica*	[40]

using different detectors, columns, mobile phases, etc. [4, 46, 47]. Electrochemical detection was employed for the simultaneous determination of four main alkaloids of CR, and the limit of detection achieved with this technique was 80 times lower than that obtained by UV detection [48]. The application of ultra-high performance liquid chromatography greatly reduced the consumption of organic solvents and the amount of injected sample required, which saved detection time and improved the efficiency [49].

Mass spectrometry (MS) in the quality evaluation of CR

Mass spectrometry is one of the most powerful tools for the identification of natural products, including the determination of relative molecular weights and chemical formulas, structural identification, and quantification. GC–MS was used to evaluate the volatile components of CR [50], while LC–MS has been used to detect the alkaloids present in CR [1, 2, 51–53]. An in situ reactive desorption corona beam ionization MS method was developed by Hou [48] for the direct detection of quaternary alkaloids within 1 min. The structures of the compounds were identified by analysis of their retention times, quasi-molecular ion peaks and fragment ion peaks obtained by HPLC with ESI–MS/MS methods [1] and methods for the simultaneous determination of alkaloids by MS were also developed [2]. Laser microdissection in combination with liquid chromatography–mass spectrometry (LC–MS) was employed to quantify six major alkaloids in different sections, tissues and cells of CR [52]. This method could correlate the internal quality and external features of CR from different growing areas.

Nuclear magnetic resonance (NMR) in the quality evaluation of CR

Quantitative ^{1}H-NMR (qH-NMR) has been widely used for the analysis of bioactive components in complex plant extracts in recent years [54–56]. qH-NMR has shown some advantages for quantitative analysis over traditional chromatographic methods, such as simple and easy sample preparation and handling, lower reagent consumption, elimination of the need of expensive standard compounds, and shorter analysis time. Because the C13-H signals of the main alkaloids in ^{1}H NMR can be easily distinguished from each other, the quantitative determination of the main alkaloids from CR could be achieved by qH-NMR and the 3 species of CR could also

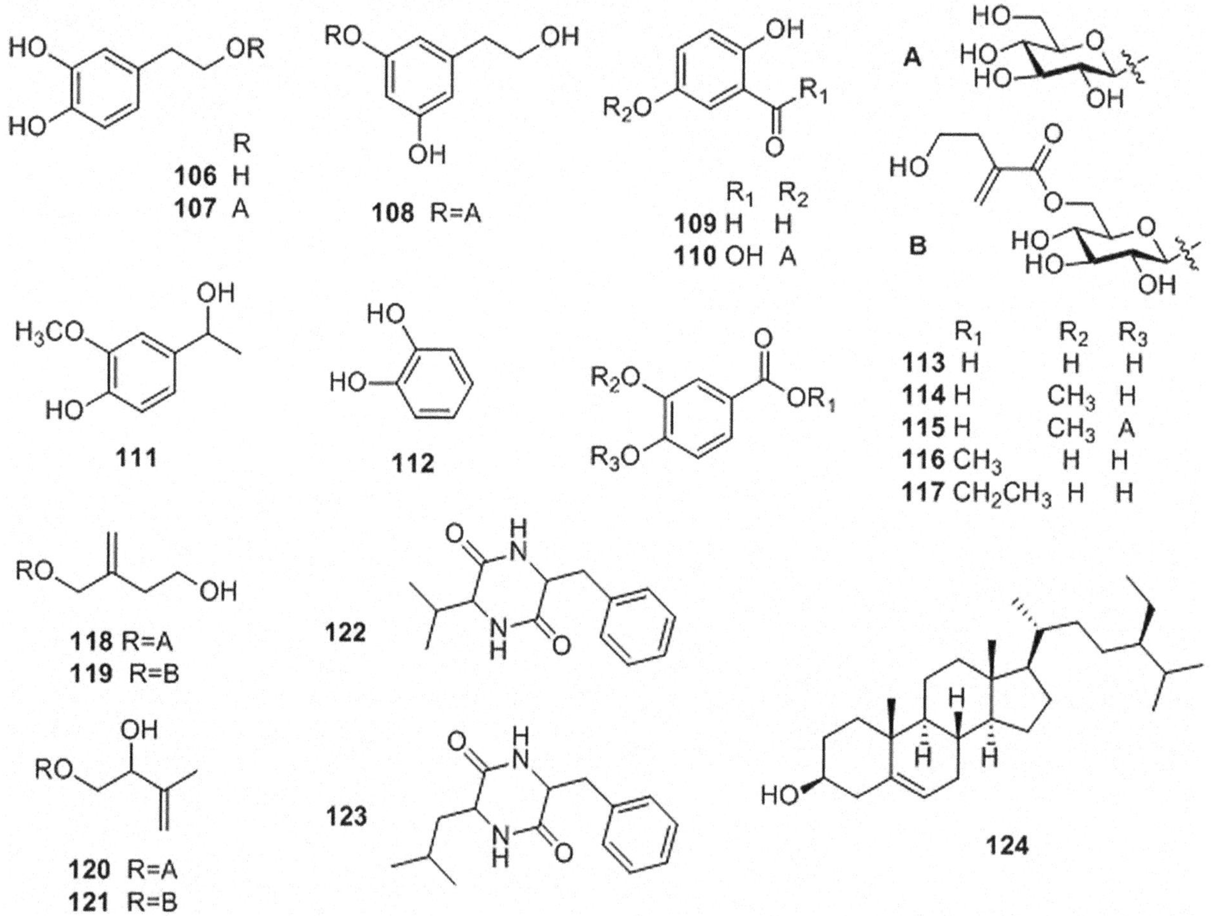

Fig. 5 Structures of other compounds isolated from *Coptis* genus

be differentiated by ^{1}H NMR and principal component analysis [3, 56–58].

Others methods for quality evaluation of CR

Many other instruments and approaches have been developed for the quality evaluation of CR, such as capillary electrophoresis, ultraviolet-near infrared (UV–NIR) spectroscopy [59], Fourier transform infrared (FT-IR) spectroscopy, Raman scattering spectroscopy, as well as other methods.

A stable and reliable nanospray technique was developed by Liu et al. [60] which facilitated the differential detection of CR using CE in combination with MS. Hou et al. [61] found that surfactant-coated multi-walled carbon nanotubes, as a novel pseudostationary phase, could improve the separation resolution and selectivity of the tested isoquinoline alkaloids in nonaqueous capillary electrophoresis during the quantitative evaluation of 5 main alkaloids (coptisine, berberine, epiberberine, palmatine, and jatrorrhizine) in CR.

That the peak at 1641/cm in FT-IR of raw CR shifts to lower wave number in that of processed CR associated with second derivative IR and two-dimensional correlation IR are applied for the differentiation of various processed products and different extracts of CR [62]. He et al. [63] developed a novel method using surface enhanced Raman scattering spectroscopy to identify the geographic origins of the *C. chinensis* by analysis of the main characteristics of the Raman peaks. This method did not require elaborate separation protocols or complex data preprocessing.

Pharmacological effects

CR, a traditional Chinese herbal medicine with potent anti-inflammatory activity, was frequently used for the treatment of bacillary dysentery, typhoid, tuberculosis, epidemic cerebrospinal meningitis, empyrosis, bronchocephalitis and other diseases [64, 65]. In recent pharmacological studies, CR and its main bioactive components, alkaloids especially berberine, have been reported to exhibit various pharmacological effects, such

Table 5 Other compounds isolated from *Coptis* genus

No.	Compounds	Source	Rfs.
106	3,4-Dihydroxyphenylethyl alcohol	*C. chinensis; C. teeta*	[26, 32]
107	3′,4′-Dihydroxyphenethyl alcohol 1-*O*-*β*-D-glucopyranoside		[39]
108	3,5-Dihydroxyphenethyl alcohol-3-*O*-*β*-D-glucopyranoside	*C. teeta*	[32]
109	Protocatechuic aldehyde	*C. chinensis*	[41]
110	Gentisic acid-5-*O*-*β*-D-glucopyranoside		[39]
111	Apocynol	*C. chinensis*	[26, 41]
112	1,2-Dihydroxy-benzene	*C. chinensis*	[37]
113	Protocatechuic acid	*C. teeta*	[32]
114	Vanillic acid	*C. chinensis*	[18, 20]
115	Vanillic acid-4-*O*-*β*-D-glucopyranoside	*C. chinensis*	[18]
116	Protocatechuic acid methyl ester	*C. chinensis*	[19]
117	Protocatechuic acid ethyl ester	*C. chinensis*	[20]
118	Woorenoside VI	*C. japonica var. dissecta*	[34]
119	Woorenoside VII	*C. japonica var. dissecta*	[34]
120	Woorenoside VIII	*C. japonica var. dissecta*	[34]
121	Woorenoside IX	*C. japonica var. dissecta*	[34]
122	Cyclo-(Phe-Val)	*C. chinensis*	[27]
123	Cyclo-(Phe-Leu)	*C. chinensis*	[27]
124	*β*-Sitosterol	*C. chinensis*	[22]

as anti-bacterial, anti-inflammatory, anti-oxidative, anti-tumor, anti-diabetic, hypolipidemic and neuroprotective activities [20, 22, 66–75].

Pharmacological effects of extracts of CR

CR extracts have been studied for their variety of pharmacological activities. Protoberberine-type alkaloids are the main bioactive components of CR extracts, while other unknown ingredients may also exhibit pharmacological activities. Due to its anti-inflammatory effects, pretreatment with CR extract could decrease lipopolysaccharide (LPS)-stimulated interleukin (IL)-6 secretion, inhibit LPS-mediated nuclear factor-κB (NF-κB) activation and restore LPS-induced acute liver injury, and thus attenuate liver histopathological changes in endotoxemic mice [68]. CR could also enhance immunity by activating MOLT-4 cells and Type I helper T cells, increasing the production of Type I helper T cell cytokines including IFN-γ, IL-1β, IL-2, and IL-6 as well as by activating the mitogen-activated protein kinase (MAPKs) signaling pathways [74].

The hypolipidemic effect of CR extract may be attributed to its several functions in lipid metabolism. CR extract could promote the conversion of cholesterol into bile acids by increasing CYP7A1 activity in the liver of high lipid diet-induced hyperlipidemic rats [67]. In 3T3-L1 cells, the lipid accumulation was inhibited via the downregulation of protein levels of the adipocyte markers peroxisome proliferator-activated receptor (PPAR)-γ and C/EBP-α by CR alkaloids [76]. A modulation effect of gut microbiota of CR alkaloids may also contribute to the hypolipidemic potential [72].

CR extract exerts an anti-diabetic effect through several courses of action. CR extract had a α-glucosidase inhibitory activity with a IC_{50} value of 3.528 mg/mL, and its main alkaloids, coptisine, epiberberine, jatrorrhizin and berberine were identified as α-glucosidase inhibitors by in vitro screening [71]. The protein tyrosine phosphatase 1B inhibitory activity of berberine, epiberberine, magnoflorine and coptisine with the IC_{50} values of 16.43, 24.19, 28.14, and 51.04 μM may also contribute to the anti-diabetic effects of CR [69]. Yang [22] found that glucose uptake in differentiated C2C12 cells were increased by dichloromethane and *n*-butanol sub-fractions of CR extract at concentrations of 50 μg/mL.

CR was also reported to exhibit a neuroprotective effect against oxidative stress in human neuroblastoma cells [70] and in MPP^+ and MPTP-induced Parkinson's disease models [77]. The methanol and aqueous extracts of CR showed significant acetylcholinesterase inhibitory activity with IC_{50} values of 0.031 μg/mL and 2.5 μg/mL, respectively [73].

Tjong et al. [75] found that 70% ethanol extract of CR could serve as an analgesic by inhibiting the release of serotonin and cholecystokinin expression in the distal colons of rats. After treatment with an aqueous extract of CR, the elevated MDA contents were reduced and superoxide dismutase (SOD) activities were inhibited in the skin and serum of rats with radiation-induced acute skin injuries [20, 66].

Pharmacological effects of CR-containing formulae

Traditional Chinese medicines are often used in the form of formulae and the medicines in the formulae interact with each other. Many classic formulae which contained CR have been used for 1000 of years, including Huang-Lian-Jie-Du-Decoction (Coptidis rhizoma, Scutellariae Radix, Phellodendri Cortex and Gardeniae Fructus), San-Huang-Xie-Xin-Decoction (Coptidis rhizoma, Scutellariae radix and Rhei rhizoma), Ge-Gen-Qin-Lian-Tang (Puerariae Radix, Scutellariae Radix, Coptidis rhizoma and Glycyrrhizae Radix), etc. Huang-Lian-Jie-Du-Decoction, which was frequently used for the treatment of sepsis [78], could exerted significant anti-inflammatory and anti-allergic effects [79]. It could also improve gastrointestinal motility function [80]. San-Huang-Xie-Xin-Tang has been widely used to ameliorate gastrointestinal disorders [81] and showed protective effect from neurotoxicity [82, 83] and immunomodulatory effects [84]. The traditional Chinese anti-diabetic formula, Jinqi formula (Coptidis rhizoma, *Astragali rhadix* and *Lonicerae japonicae* Flos) could inhibit TG accumulation [85]. Zuojin and Fan-Zuojin formulas with reverse mixture ratios of CR and Euodiae fructus led to different interactions on the in vitro absorption of alkaloids and opposite effects [86, 87]. Ge-Gen-Qin-Lian-Tang could decrease lipid formation [88]. Combination of Mume Fructus, Schizandrae Fructus, and CR exhibited antimicrobial activity on Enterohemorrhagic *Escherichia coli* [89]. CR and Rhei rhizoma mixture showed antioxidant and anti-inflammatory effects in Rats with reflux esophagitis [90].

Pharmacological effects of berberine

Multiple pharmacological effects of berberine have been reported in recent years including anti-inflammatory, anti-oxidant, anti-diabetic, hypolipidemia, anti-tumor, cardiovascular protective, neuroprotective, hepatoprotective, renal protective, gut protective, and other effects [6–9, 11, 91–96]. The anti-inflammatory and anti-oxidant effects of berberine play an important role in its efficacy against various diseases, such as diabetes, hyperlipidemia and cancer by regulating the key kinases and signaling pathways [10, 12, 97, 98].

Inflammatory effects

The expressions of tumor necrosis factor (TNF)-α, IL-1β, IL-6, IL-17 and vascular endothelial growth factor (VEGF) were significantly reduced by berberine in the sera of rats with bovine type II collagen-induced arthritis, and the expression of VEGF and CD34 and the p-ERK, p-p38 and p-JNK activation were also inhibited [6]. Berberine could improve osteoarthritis by modulating the expression of genes and proteins related to cell proliferation, differentiation and apoptosis. In rabbit articular chondrocytes, berberine induced actin cytoskeletal architecture reorganization and dedifferentiation by inhibiting PI3-kinase/Akt as well as p38 kinase activation [99]. In osteoarthritic rat cartilage, berberine promoted cell proliferation, G1/S phase transitions and the proliferation of cell nuclear antigen synthesis via up-regulation of β-catenin, c-Myc, and cyclin D1 expression, and the down-regulation of glycogen synthase kinase-3β (GSK-3β) and matrix metalloproteinase-7 (MMP-7) expression [100]. Berberine could also prevent glucocorticoid-induced osteoporosis by inhibiting bone resorption and improving bone formation [101].

Anti-diabetic effects

The anti-inflammatory and anti-oxidant activities of berberine also play an important role in the treatment of diabetes mellitus. The ameliorating insulin resistance effect of berberine was first discovered, and then berberine was found to promote the synthesis and secretion of insulin [97, 98, 102–104]. Berberine had modulation effects on multiple kinases and signaling pathways, including 5′-adenosine monophosphate-activated protein kinase (AMPK), MAPKs, the nuclear factor erythroid-2-related factor-2 (Nrf2) pathway, and the NF-κB pathway [97, 98, 103, 104]. In the livers of high-fat diet-induced diabetic Sprague–Dawley rats, berberine could directly inhibit gluconeogenesis by decreasing the expression of gluconeogenic genes, phosphoenolpyruvate carboxykinase and glucose-6-phosphatase. Hepatic steatosis, expression of fatty acid synthase, activities of Forkhead transcription factor O1, sterol regulatory element-binding protein 1c and carbohydrate responsive element-binding protein were also inhibited in the liver by berberine [7].

Hypolipidemia effects

Studies indicated that the lipid-lowering effect of berberine via inhibition of cholesterol absorption, promotion of bile acid synthesis and decreasing lipid peroxidation. Berberine could significantly inhibit increases in body weight and reduce blood lipid levels in human subjects and rats [8]. It was found that treatment with berberine could up-regulate LDLR mRNA and protein expression, thus inhibiting cellular lipid accumulation in Hep G2 cells. Berberine could inhibit AMPK activity, promote brown adipose tissue formation and thereby increase energy expenditure in white and brown adipose tissue [105]. In a study conducted by Zhou et al. [106], they considered that the metabolites of berberine were the active forms due to its poor absorption and rapid metabolism.

Anti-tumor effects

Berberine exhibited anti-tumor activities in various cancer cell lines through inducing cell cycle arrest and apoptosis [9, 91, 107–110], inhibiting angiogenesis [109], anti-inflammation, anti-invasion and anti-metastasis [10] etc.

Cardiovascular protective effects

The cardiovascular protective effects of berberine were reflected by its beneficial effects in myocardial ischemia reperfusion (I/R), myocardial ischemia injury and apoptosis, cardiomyocyte hypertrophy, as well as other effects [11, 12, 92, 111–113]. In addition, berberine treatment reduced I/R induced excessive autophagy via the inhibition of SIRT1, BNIP3, and Beclin-1 expression [114].

Neuroprotective effects

Berberine exerts a cardiovascular protective effect by regulating the synthesis and secretion of neurotransmitters in the central nervous system. Therefore, it has a potent effect on various neurological diseases including apoplexy, depression and Alzheimer's disease [93, 115, 116].

Hepatoprotective effects

Berberine has an efficacy in non-alcoholic fatty liver patients. A significant reduction of hepatic fat content and better improvement in body weight, HOMA-IR, and serum lipid profiles were displayed in patients treated with berberine and lifestyle intervention [94]. This efficacy may be related to the lipid metabolism regulatory effect of berberine. Pretreatment of berberine L02 hepatic cell lines exposed to hydrogen peroxide could increase cell viability and reduce apoptosis via the upregulation of sirtuin 1 and downregulation of apoptosis-related proteins [117].

Renal protective effects

Berberine could increase expressions of nephrin and podocin and exert an ameliorative effect on renal damage in high-fat diet and streptozotocin induced diabetic rats [95]. Berberine could ameliorate diabetic nephropathy via the suppression of high glucose-induced TGF-β1 and fibronectin synthesis in mesangial cells through an inhibition of the sphingosine kinase 1/AP-1 pathway [118].

Gut protective effects

In the sennoside A-induced diarrhoea mice, treatment with berberine enhanced the absorption of Na^+ and water by improving the Na^+/H^+ exchanger 3 and aquaporin 4 expression, and thus ameliorated the diarrhea [96]. Berberine could also reduce the sensitivity to rectal distension and defecation of inflammatory bowel disease model rats. Berberine had an anti-nociceptive effect on visceral hypersensitivity [119]. In addition, berberine markedly elevated the activities of SOD and GSH-Px and prevented MDA, NO and villi injuries in ileum [120]. Berberine ameliorated COX-2 overexpression in the small intestinal mucosa of rats during acute endotoxemia [121].

Other effects

Human retinal endothelial cells (HRECs) apoptosis induced by leukocytes from diabetic patients was inhibited by berberine through a decrease in the integrin beta-2 expression of leukocytes [122]. Berberine also inhibited *Microcystis aeruginosa* growth by inducing oxidative damage [123]. Berberine acted as an efflux inhibitor and improved aminoglycoside resistance of *P. aeruginosa* [124].

Pharmacological effects of other alkaloids from CR

Besides berberine, the main protoberberine-type alkaloids, such as palmatine, jatrorrhizine, coptisine, epiberberine, columbamine also exhibited various biological activities similar with that of berberine [125–141].

Palmatine

Research has shown that palmatine has modulatory effects on various cytokines and exhibits various biological activities. Ning [125] found that palmatine upregulated the mRNA and protein expressions of LDLR, CYP7A1 and downregulated ASBT mRNA and protein expressions while exhibiting a lipid-lowering effect in hamsters fed with a high-fat diet. Palmatine could regulate serum mRNA expression of TNF-α and IL-10, and inhibit apoptosis in mice with D-galactosamine/LPS-induced fulminant hepatic failure [126]. In osteoblast cells, palmatine could inhibit receptor activator of NF-κB ligand expression and attenuate osteoclast differentiation and function [127]. Gene reporter assays indicated that palmatine significantly activated aryl hydrocarbon receptors and elevated CYP1A1 gene promoter expression in transiently transfected HepG2 cells, which was validated in a HepG2 monolayer culture. However, no similar effects were observed in HepG2 spheroids or primary cultures of human hepatocytes [128].

Palmatine could ameliorate ischemia–reperfusion-mediated acute myocardial injuries in rats by reducing oxidative stress and modulating inflammatory mediators [129]. Among the five main alkaloids isolated from CR, palmatine showed the best AChE inhibitory activities, as demonstrated by in vitro AChE inhibition assays with IC_{50} values of 36.6 μM [130]. Jia et al. reported that West Nile virus NS2B–NS3 protease activity was inhibited by palmatine in an uncompetitive manner, with an IC_{50}

value of 96 μM without detectable cytotoxicity; Furthermore, palmatine also exhibits inhibitory effects on dengue virus and yellow fever virus [131].

Coptisine

Coptisine could inhibit the mRNA expression of inflammatory cytokines, including nitric oxide, IL-1β, and IL-6 in LPS-stimulated RAW 264.7 murine macrophage cells by blocking the activation of NF-κB, MAPK and PI3K/Akt in macrophages [132]. Obesity-related inflammation was attenuated by coptisine in high fat and high cholesterol induced obese Syrian golden hamsters through LPS/TLR-4-mediated signaling pathways. Treatment with coptisine could significantly ameliorate the body weight, plasma lipid levels of TC, TG, LDL-c, VLDL-c, APoB and pro-inflammatory cytokines (TNF-α, IL-6, LPS) of obese hamsters. The TLR-4 in visceral fat and CD14 expression in the livers of hamsters were also suppressed [133].

The neuroprotective effect of coptisine was achieved by strengthening the thioredoxin defense system against oxidative stress and inhibition of apoptosis [134]. Coptisine could reduce myocardial injuries by attenuating the infarct size and release of MDA and increasing SOD activity. In vitro, coptisine could decrease apoptosis and protect cardiomyocytes [135].

Jatrorrhizine

Jatrorrhizine exhibited an inhibitory effect on the proliferation and neovascularization of metastatic melanoma cells by inducing the overexpression of cell cycle-suppressive genes p21 and p27, and cell cycle arrest at the G0/G1 transition [136]. After treatment with jatrorrhizine, the body weight of high-fat diet-induced diabetic mice was reduced, glucose tolerance and insulin sensitivity were improved and the levels of serum lipid components were ameliorated to various degrees [137]. These effects were realized by inhibiting lipogenesis and increasing lipid oxidation through the downregulation of SREBP-1c and FAS mRNA expression and induction of PPAR-α and CPT1A mRNA expression.

Jatrorrhizine could offset delayed gastric purging and intestinal transit via the cholinergic pathway, which was not affected by pretreatment with SB204070 in postoperative ileus rats [138]. Jatrorrhizine also had a neuroprotective effect through its anti-oxidative activity in primary rat cortical neurons [139].

Epiberberine

Epiberberine could inhibit 3T3-L1 adipocyte differentiation and lipid accumulation by regulating differentiation-mediated phosphorylation of factors in the Raf/MEK1/2/EREK1/2 and AMPKα/Akt pathways [140].

Columbamine

Columbamine had an anti-proliferative effect on metastatic osteosarcoma U2OS cells with an IC_{50} value of 21.31 ± 0.38 μM and low cytotoxicity. It could induce cyclic arrest of metastatic osteosarcoma U2OS cells at the G2/M transition by inhibiting CDK6 gene expression and STAT3 phosphorylation. Columbamine could also inhibit neovascularization of metastatic osteosarcoma U2OS cells through a down-regulation of MMP 2 expression and reduction of cell migration, adhesion, and invasion [141].

Pharmacological effects of CR polysaccharide

Polysaccharides are polymeric carbohydrate molecules composed of more than ten monosaccharide units joined by glycosidic bonds. Natural polysaccharides are important sources of active substances. It was reported that the polysaccharides isolated from CR exhibited modest hypoglycemic effects. The *C. chinensis* polysaccharides (CCP) could increase glucose uptake in high-fat diet-induced diabetic C57bl/6J mice through lowering fasting plasma glucose levels, recovering impaired glucose tolerance and regulating the expression of glucose metabolism related genes [142]. The CCP could also inhibit the formation of advanced glycation end product (AGE) formation in vitro and in streptozotocin-induced diabetic mice. The bodyweight and serum insulin levels of streptozotocin-induced diabetic mice were significantly ameliorated and fasting blood glucose and glycated serum protein concentrations decreased. Meanwhile, the AGE accumulations and morphological abnormalities in the pancreas and liver were also improved [143]. It was also reported that the anti-diabetic effect of a water-soluble polysaccharide isolated from CR was achieved through its anti-oxidative effect involving the JNK pathway [144, 145]. This water-soluble polysaccharide CCPW-1 could increase glutathione peroxidases, SOD, catalase activities and decrease glutathione and MDA contents while inhibiting JNK expression in high-fat with streptozotocin diet induced diabetic mice. CCP also presented a protective effect against UV-induced oxidative damage [146].

Safety and toxicity of CR

CR is usually relatively safe at normal dosages. Studies have indicated that the toxic constituents of CR were the alkaloids, and mainly berberine [147]. However, research has suggested that CR and its alkaloids could exhibit beneficial activities at low concentrations due to their increased plasma exposures [148] and enhanced intestinal absorption [149] by naturally occurring proteinaceous nanoparticles in CR extract [150]. Although CR was banned in Singapore because berberine has been associated with the aggravating effects of jaundice and kernicterus in neonates with glucose-6-phosphate dehydrogenase deficiency, in a study on 20 patients with chronic cytopenic haematological conditions, RC was administered for 1055 patient-days and no organ toxicity or electrolyte imbalance were observed [151]. Acute toxicity assays of mice showed that the LD_{50} values of berberine, coptisine, palmatine and epiberberine were 713.57, 852.12, 1533.68 and 1360 mg/kg, respectively. Their IC_{50} values in HepG2 cells were 48.17, 64.81, 112.80 and 120.58 mg/mL, and the values were 41.76, 56.48, 84.32 and 104.18 mg/mL in 3T3-L1 cells [152]. However, its toxic and adverse effects cannot be ignored. There are still many challenges in treating various diseases with CR or the alkaloids isolated from CR. Diarrhea was the most frequent toxicity effect of treatment at high dosages of CR treatment due to disturbance in the normal gut microbiota [153]. Liver and lung injuries were attributed to the fibrous root of CR at a dose of 3.76 g/kg [154]. Berberine could also act as human ether-a-go-go-related gene inhibitor which may lead to sudden death [155].

Conclusion

Coptidis rhizoma is widely used as herbal medicine in TCM with various significant bioactivities. Until now, numerous phytochemical investigations have been carried out on CR and many types of secondary metabolites including alkaloids, lignans, phenylpropanoids, flavonoids, phenolic compounds, saccharides, steroids were reported. However, the multi-component composition of Chinese herbs and their multi-functional activities that may have greater effectiveness and more complex behavior than a single compound are also reflected in CR. Studies on the chemical components of CR are still needed to thoroughly elucidate its chemical composition and to provide a firm basis for quality control and pharmacological research. As technology has developed, more advanced instrumental methods were introduced for the quality evaluation of CR in recent years. In particular, the application of quantitative MS and quantitative NMR has provided more potential for achieving high degrees of quality control for herbal medicine. These methods will still need to be improved further to extend their applicability. Many studies have revealed that CR is a relatively safe medicine with multiple activities. The various pharmacological effects of CR and its active components also present researchers with a significant challenge to thoroughly understand their mechanisms of action. Research reveals that CR has promising potential: the bioactivities of CR were achieved by the synergistic action of multiple ingredients in the complex composition of CR. Many mechanisms underlying these pharmacological effects are still unknown and need to be discovered. To better understand the complex mechanisms that underlie the complex behavior of CR, novel research ideas and methods need to be introduced.

Abbreviations

CR: Coptidis rhizoma; MS: mass spectrometry; HPLC: high performance liquid chromatography; UPLC: ultra high performance liquid chromatography; NMR: nuclear magnetic resonance; ODS: octadecylsilane; ESI: electrospray ionization mass spectrometry; FT-IR: Fourier transform infrared; UV: ultraviolet; ECD: electrochemical detection; QTOF: quadrupole-time of flight; GC: gas chromatography; CE: capillary electrophoresis; LPS: lipopolysaccharide; NF-Kb: nuclear factor-κB; MAPK: mitogen-activated protein kinase; SOD: superoxide dismutase; TNF: tumor necrosis factor; VEGF: vascular endothelial growth factor; MMP-7: matrix metalloproteinase-7; AMPK: 5′-adenosine monophosphate-activated protein kinase; P-TEFb: positive transcription elongation factor b; I/R: ischemia reperfusion; NOS: NO synthase; CCP: *C. chinensis* polysaccharides; AGE: advanced glycation end product.

Authors' contributions

FCM drafted the manuscript and prepared tables and figures. ZFW conducted the literature searches, extracted and analyzed data and drafted the manuscript. LGL contributed to the critical revisions of the manuscript. ZQY co-designed the study and co-developed the full text of the review. RW and QWZ designed the study, developed the manuscript and are the corresponding authors. All authors read and approved the final manuscript.

Author details

[1] State Key Laboratory of Quality Research in Chinese Medicine, Institute of Chinese Medical Sciences, University of Macau, Macao SAR, People's Republic of China. [2] Department of Traditional Chinese Medicines Pharmaceuticals, China Pharmaceutical University, Nanjing 210009, People's Republic of China.

Acknowledgements

Dr. Ian Wyman from Queen's University, Kingston, Canada, is acknowledged for providing technical support and assistance with the proofreading of this manuscript.

Competing interests

The authors declare that they have no competing interests.

Consent for publication

Not applicable.

Funding

This work was supported by University of Macau (MYRG2014-00162-ICMS-QRCM).

References

1. Ren L, Xue X, Liang X. Characterization of protoberberine alkaloids in Coptidis rhizoma (Huanglian) by HPLC with ESI–MS/MS. J Sep Sci. 2013;36:1389–96.
2. Qian XC, Zhang L, Tao Y, Huang P, Li JS, Chai C, Li W, Di LQ, Cai BC. Simultaneous determination of ten alkaloids of crude and wine-processed

rhizoma Coptidis aqueous extracts in rat plasma by UHPLC–ESI–MS/MS and its application to a comparative pharmacokinetic study. J. Pharm Biomed. 2015;105:64–73.
3. Fan G, Zhang MY, Zhou XD, Lai XR, Yue QH, Tang C, Luo WZ, Zhang Y. Quality evaluation and species differentiation of rhizoma Coptidis by using proton nuclear magnetic resonance spectroscopy. Anal Chim Acta. 2012;747:76–83.
4. Chen X, Wang J, Hu S, Bai X. Hollow-fiber double-solvent synergistic microextraction with high-performance liquid chromatography for the determination of antitumor alkaloids in *Coptis chinensis*. J Sep Sci. 2016;39:827–34.
5. Liu X, Hu S, Chen X, Bai X. Hollow fiber cell fishing with high-performance liquid chromatography for rapid screening and analysis of an antitumor-active protoberberine alkaloid group from *Coptis chinensis*. J Pharm Biomed. 2014;98:463–75.
6. Wang Z, Chen Z, Yang S, Wang Y, Huang Z, Gao J, Tu S, Rao Z. Berberine ameliorates collagen-induced arthritis in rats associated with anti-inflammatory and anti-angiogenic effects. Inflammation. 2014;37:1789–98.
7. Xia X, Yan J, Shen Y, Tang K, Yin J, Zhang Y, Yang D, Liang H, Ye J, Weng J. Berberine improves glucose metabolism in diabetic rats by inhibition of hepatic gluconeogenesis. PLoS ONE. 2011;6:e16556.
8. Hu Y, Ehli EA, Kittelsrud J, Ronan PJ, Munger K, Downey T, Bohlen K, Callahan L, Munson V, Jahnke M, Marshall LL, Nelson K, Huizenga P, Hansen R, Soundy TJ, Davies GE. Lipid-lowering effect of berberine in human subjects and rats. Phytomedicine. 2012;19:861–7.
9. Zhang L, Miao XJ, Wang X, Pan HH, Li P, Ren H, Jia YR, Lu C, Wang HB, Yuan L, Zhang GL. Antiproliferation of berberine is mediated by epigenetic modification of constitutive androstane receptor (CAR) metabolic pathway in hepatoma cells. Sci Rep. 2016;6:28116.
10. Liu X, Ji Q, Ye N, Sui H, Zhou L, Zhu H, Fan Z, Cai J, Li Q. Berberine inhibits invasion and metastasis of colorectal cancer cells via COX-2/PGE2 mediated JAK2/STAT3 signaling pathway. PLoS ONE. 2015;10:e0123478.
11. Zhu QW, Li YG. Berberine attenuates myocardial ischemia reperfusion injury by suppressing the activation of PI3K/AKT signaling. Exp Ther Med. 2016;11:978–84.
12. Liu X, Zhang X, Ye L, Yuan H. Protective mechanisms of berberine against experimental autoimmune myocarditis in a rat model. Biomed Pharmacother. 2016;79:222–30.
13. Zhang S, Wang M, Wang C. Preparative separation and purification of alkaloids from rhizoma Coptidis by high-speed counter-current chromatography. Sep Purif Technol. 2011;76:428–31.
14. Sun C, Li J, Wang X, Duan W, Zhang T, Ito Y. Preparative separation of quaternary ammonium alkaloids from Coptis chinensis Franch by pH-zone-refining counter-current chromatography. J Chromatogr A. 2014;1370:156–61.
15. Chen HY, Ye XL, Cui XL, He K, Jin YN, Chen Z, Li XG. Cytotoxicity and antihyperglycemic effect of minor constituents from rhizoma Coptis in HepG2 cells. Fitoterapia. 2012;83:67–73.
16. Kobayashi Y, Yamashita Y, Fujii N, Takaboshi K, Kawakami T, Kawamura M, Mizukami T, Nakano H. Inhibitors of DNA topoisomerase I and II. isolated from the Coptis Rhizomes. Planta Med. 1995;61:414–8.
17. Chen J, Wang F, Liu J, Lee FS, Wang X, Yang H. Analysis of alkaloids in *Coptis chinensis* Franch by accelerated solvent extraction combined with ultra performance liquid chromatographic analysis with photodiode array and tandem mass spectrometry detections. Anal Chim Acta. 2008;613:184–95.
18. Li XG, Yang LG, Chen LX, Qiu F. Chemical constituents from the decoction of *Coptis chinensis* Franch. J Shenyang Pharm Univ. 2012;29(193–198):226.
19. Ma HM, Chen G, Li W, Fan XM, Li ZF, Pei YH. Isolation and identification of chemical constituents from rhizoma of *Coptis chinensis*. J Shenyang Pharm Univ. 2011;28:695–9.
20. Wang Q, Li ZF, Chen G, Feng YL, Fan MM, Pei YH. Chemical constituents from *Coptis Chinensis* Franch. Chin J Exp Tradit Med Form. 2012;18:74–6.
21. Wang L, Zhang SY, Chen L, Huang XJ, Zhang QW, Jiang RW, Yao F, Ye WC. New enantiomeric isoquinoline alkaloids from *Coptis chinensis*. Phytochem Lett. 2014;7:89–92.
22. Yang TC, Chao HF, Shi LS, Chang TC, Lin HC, Chang WL. Alkaloids from *Coptis chinensis* root promote glucose uptake in C2C12 myotubes. Fitoterapia. 2014;93:239–44.
23. Wang W, Zhang QW, Ye WC, Wang YT. Isoquinoline alkaloids from the rhizoma of *Coptis chinensis*. Chin J Nat Med. 2007;5:348–50.
24. Zhao M, Xian YF, Ip SP, Fong HH, Che CT. A new and weakly antispasmodic protoberberine alkaloid from rhizoma Coptidis. Phytother Res. 2010;24:1414–6.
25. Mizuno M, Kojima H, Tanaka T, Iinuma M. Benzophenanthridine alkaloids from the seeds of *Coptis japonica var. dissecta*. J Nat Prod. 1987;50:326.
26. Li ZF, Wang Q, Feng YL, Luo XJ, Fan MM, Yang SL. Chemical constituents from *Coptis chinensis*. Chin Med Mat. 2012;35:1438–41.
27. Li ZF, Wang Q, Feng YL, Rao Y, Yang SL, Pei YH. Chemical constituents from rhizomes of *Coptis chinensis*. Chin Tradit Herbal Drugs. 2012;43:1273–5.
28. Ma HM, Chen G, Pei YH. Isolation and identification of chemical constituents from rhizoma of *Coptis chinensis* and their cytotoxic activities. J Shenyang Pharm Univ. 2013;30(759–763):828.
29. Li ZF, Wang Q, Chen G, Hua HM, Yang SL, Feng YL, Pei YH. A new pyrrolidine derivative from the rhizome of *Coptis chinensis*. Chem Nat Compd. 2013;49:493–4.
30. Chen GC, Li XL, Chen G. Isolation and identification of lignans chemical constituents from *Coptis chinensis* and their inhibitory activity to protein tyrosine phosphatase-1B. Chin Pharm. 2016;27:2197–200.
31. Yoshikawa K, Kinoshita H, Kan Y, Arihara S. Neolignans and phenylpropanoids from the rhizomes of *Coptis japonica var. dissecta*. Chem Pharm Bull. 1995;43:578–81.
32. Meng FC, Wang L, Zhang J, Yin ZQ, Zhang QW, Ye WC. Non-alkaloid chemical constituents from the rhizome of *Coptis teeta*. J Chin Pharm Univ. 2013;44:307–10.
33. Chen L, Wang L, Zhang QW, Zhang SY, Ye WC. Non-alkaloid chemical constituents from *Coptis chinensis*. Chin Mat Med. 2012;37:1241–4.
34. Yoshikawa K, Kinoshita H, Arihara S. Non-basic components of Coptis rhizoma. II. Four new hemiterpenoid glucosides, two new phenylpropanoid glucosides and a new lavonoid glycoside from *Coptis japonica var. dissecta*. Nat Med. 1997;51:244–8.
35. Hirano H, Satoshiro M, Nishioka I, Shingu T. Isolation of free radical scavenger from Coptidis rhizoma. Nat Med. 1997;51:539–40.
36. Mizuno M, Kojima H, Tanaka T, Iinuma M, Kimura R, Min ZD, Murata H. Phenolic constituents from seeds of *Coptis japonika var. dissecta*. Phytochemistry. 1987;26:2071–4.
37. Li ZF, Wang Q, Feng YL, Yan YB, Fan MM, Yang SL. Chemical constituents in *Coptis chinensis* Franch. Chin New Drug J. 2012;21:1551–3.
38. Yoshikawa K, Kinoshita H, Arihara S. Woorenol, a novel Sesquineolignan with a unique spiro skeleton from the rhizomes of *Coptis japonica var. dissecta*. J Nat Prod. 1997;60:511–3.
39. Yahara S, Satoshiro M, Nishioka I, Nagasawa T, Oura H. Isolation and characterization of phenolic compounds from Coptidis rhizoma. Chem Pharm Bull. 1985;32:527–31.
40. Fujiwara H, Nonaka G, Yagi A, Nishioka I. Studies on the components of the leaves of *Coptis japonica* makino. I. the structures of coptiside I and II. Chem Pharm Bull. 1976;24:407–13.
41. Ma B, Zhu L, Zang X, Chen Y, Li D, Wang Y. *Coptis chinensis* inflorescence and its main alkaloids protect against ultraviolet-B-induced oxidative damage. J Funct Foods. 2013;5:1665–72.
42. Chen SL, Song JY, Yao H, Shi LC, Luo K, Han JP. Strategy and key technique of identification of Chinese herbal medicine using DNA barcoding. Chin J Nat Med. 2009;7(5):322–7.
43. Sun T, Sun DY, Teng SN, Lu LH, Deng CH, Li YG. Identification of rhizoma Coptidis and its adulterants based on ITS2 DNA barcode. Guizhou Agric Sci. 2013;41(9):20–2.
44. Li B, Liu J, Min DZ, He XH, Li BC, Zhu CL, Zhang ZY, Yuan QJ, Wu D. DNA barcoding evaluation in the genus *Coptis salisb*. Acta Agriculturae Universitatis Jiangxiensis. 2017;39(6):1089–95.
45. Teng H, Choi YH. Optimization of ultrasonic-assisted extraction of bioactive alkaloid compounds from rhizoma Coptidis (*Coptis chinensis* Franch.) using response surface methodology. Food Chem. 2014;142:299–305.
46. Lv X, Li Y, Tang C, Zhang Y, Zhang J, Fan G. Integration of HPLC-based fingerprint and quantitative analyses for differentiating botanical species and geographical growing origins of rhizoma Coptidis. Pharm Biol. 2016;54:3264–71.

47. Dai SY, Xu B, Zhang Y, Li JY, Sun F, Shi XY, Qiao YJ. Establishment and reliability evaluation of the design space for HPLC analysis of six alkaloids in *Coptis chinensis* (Huanglian) using Bayesian approach. Chin J Nat Med. 2016;14:697–708.
48. Liu L, Chen Z. Analysis of four alkaloids of *Coptis chinensis* in rat plasma by high performance liquid chromatography with electrochemical detection. Anal Chim Acta. 2012;737:99–104.
49. Jiang X, Huang LF, Wu LB, Wang ZH, Chen SL. UPLC–QTOF/MS analysis of alkaloids in traditional processed *Coptis chinensis* Franch. Evid Based Complement Altern. 2012;2012:942384.
50. Gao X, Yang X, Mitrevski BS, Marriott PJ. Headspace solid-phase microextraction combined with GCxGC–TOFMS for the analysis of volatile compounds of *Coptis* species rhizomes. J Sep Sci. 2011;34:1157–66.
51. Hou Y, Wu T, Liu Y, Wang H, Chen Y, Chen B, Sun W. Direct analysis of quaternary alkaloids by in situ reactive desorption corona beam ionization MS. Analyst. 2014;139:5185–91.
52. Yi L, Liang ZT, Peng Y, Guo P, Wong LL, Wan XJ, Ho HM, Yi T, Zhao ZZ. Histochemical evaluation of alkaloids in rhizome of *Coptis chinensis* using laser microdissection and liquid chromatography/mass spectrometry. Drug Test Anal. 2015;7:519–30.
53. Liu Q, Qiu S, Yu H, Ke Y, Jin Y, Liang X. Selective separation of structure-related alkaloids in rhizoma Coptidis with "click" binaphthyl stationary phase and their structural elucidation with liquid chromatography–mass spectrometry. Analyst. 2011;136:4357–65.
54. Pauli GF, Jaki BU, Lankin DC. Quantitative ^{1}H NMR: development and potential of a method for natural products analysis. J Nat Prod. 2005;68:133–49.
55. Tanaka R, Inagaki R, Sugimoto N, Akiyama H, Nagatsu A. Application of a quantitative ^{1}H-NMR (^{1}H-qNMR) method for the determination of geniposidic acid and acteoside in *Plantaginis semen*. J Nat Med. 2017;71:315–20.
56. Fan G, Tao LH, Yue QH, Kuang TT, Tang C, Yang YD, Luo WZ, Zhou XD, Zhang Y. Metabolic discrimination of rhizoma Coptidis from different species using ^{1}H NMR spectroscopy and principal component analysis. Planta Med. 2012;78:641–8.
57. Hasada K, Yoshida T, Yamazaki T, Sugimoto N, Nishimura T, Nagatsu A, Mizukami H. Application of ^{1}H-NMR spectroscopy to validation of berberine alkaloid reagents and to chemical evaluation of Coptidis rhizoma. J Nat Med. 2011;65:262–7.
58. Ding PL, Chen LQ, Lu Y, Li YG. Determination of protoberberine alkaloids in rhizoma Coptidis by ERETIC ^{1}H NMR method. J Pharm Biomed. 2012;60:44–50.
59. Dai X, Song H, Liu W, Yao S, Wang G. On-line UV–NIR spectroscopy as a process analytical technology (PAT) tool for on-line and real-time monitoring of the extraction process of Coptis Rhizome. RSC Adv. 2016;6:10078–85.
60. Liu JX, Zhang YW, Yuan F, Chen HX, Zhang XX. Differential detection of rhizoma Coptidis by capillary electrophoresis electrospray ionization mass spectrometry with a nanospray interface. Electrophoresis. 2014;35:3258–63.
61. Hou J, Li G, Wei Y, Lu H, Jiang C, Zhou X, Meng F, Cao J, Liu J. Analysis of five alkaloids using surfactant-coated multi-walled carbon nanotubes as the pseudostationary phase in nonaqueous capillary electrophoresis. J Chromatogr A. 2014;1343:174–81.
62. Xu B, Zhang G, Xu C, Sun S. Analysis of fingerprints features of infrared spectra of various processed products of rhizoma Coptidis and their different extracts. J Mol Struct. 2015;1096:147–56.
63. He S, Liu X, Zhang W, Xie W, Zhang H, Fu W, Liu H, Liu X, Xu Y, Yang D, Gao Y. Discrimination of the *Coptis chinensis* geographic origins with surface enhanced Raman scattering spectroscopy. Chemometr Intell Lab. 2015;146:472–7.
64. Chinese Materia Meidca. Editional committee of Chinese Materia Medica SAoTCM. Shanghai: Chinese Materia Meidca; 1999.
65. Editional committee of flora of China CAoS. Flroa of China. Beijing: Scence Press; 2004.
66. Wang XJ, Lin S, Kang HF, Dai ZJ. The effect of rhizoma Coptidis and *Coptis Chinensis* aqueous extract on radiation-induced skin injury in a rat model. BMC Complem Altern M. 2013;13:105.
67. Cao Y, Bei W, Hu Y, Cao L, Huang L, Wang L, Luo D, Chen Y, Yao X, He W, Liu X, Guo J. Hypocholesterolemia of rhizoma Coptidis alkaloids is related to the bile acid by up-regulated CYP7A1 in hyperlipidemic rats. Phytomedicine. 2012;19:686–92.
68. Choi YY, Kim MH, Cho IH, Kim JH, Hong J, Lee TH, Yang WM. Inhibitory effect of *Coptis chinensis* on inflammation in LPS-induced endotoxemia. J Ethnopharmacol. 2013;149:506–12.
69. Choi JS, Ali MY, Jung HA, Oh SH, Choi RJ, Kim EJ. Protein tyrosine phosphatase 1B inhibitory activity of alkaloids from rhizoma Coptidis and their molecular docking studies. J Ethnopharmacol. 2015;171:28–36.
70. Friedemann T, Otto B, Klatschke K, Schumacher U, Tao Y, Leung AK, Efferth T, Schroder S. *Coptis chinensis* Franch. exhibits neuroprotective properties against oxidative stress in human neuroblastoma cells. J Ethnopharmacol. 2014;155:607–15.
71. Ge AH, Bai Y, Li J, Liu J, He J, Liu EW, Zhang P, Zhang BL, Gao XM, Chang YX. An activity-integrated strategy involving ultra-high-performance liquid chromatography/quadrupole-time-of-flight mass spectrometry and fraction collector for rapid screening and characterization of the α-glucosidase inhibitors in Coptis chinensis Franch. (Huanglian). J Pharm Biomed. 2014;100:79–87.
72. He K, Hu Y, Ma H, Zou Z, Xiao Y, Yang Y, Feng M, Li X, Ye X. Rhizoma Coptidis alkaloids alleviate hyperlipidemia in B6 mice by modulating gut microbiota and bile acid pathways. BBA Mol Basis Dis. 2016;1862:1696–709.
73. Kaufmann D, Kaur Dogra A, Tahrani A, Herrmann F, Wink M. Extracts from traditional chinese medicinal plants inhibit acetylcholinesterase, a Known Alzheimer's disease target. Molecules. 2016;21:1161.
74. Kim E, Ahn S, Rhee HI, Lee DC. *Coptis chinensis* Franch. extract up-regulate type I helper T-cell cytokine through MAPK activation in MOLT-4 T cell. J Ethnopharmacol. 2016;189:126–31.
75. Tjong Y, Ip S, Lao L, Fong HH, Sung JJ, Berman B, Che C. Analgesic effect of *Coptis chinensis* rhizomes (Coptidis Rhizoma) extract on rat model of irritable bowel syndrome. J Ethnopharmacol. 2011;135:754–61.
76. Choi JS, Kim JH, Ali MY, Min BS, Kim GD, Jung HA. *Coptis chinensis* alkaloids exert anti-adipogenic activity on 3T3-L1 adipocytes by down-regulating C/EBP-*α* and PPAR-*γ*. Fitoterapia. 2014;98:199–208.
77. Friedemann T, Ying Y, Wang W, Kramer ER, Schumacher U, Fei J, Schroder S. Neuroprotective effect of *Coptis chinensis* in MPP$^+$ and MPTP-induced Parkinson's disease models. Am J Chin Med. 2016;44:907–25.
78. Xu DQ, Lv Y, Yang MH, Wang JS, Kong LY. Deciphering the mechanism of Huang-Lian-Jie-Du-Decoction on the treatment of sepsis by formula decomposition and metabolomics: enhancement of cholinergic pathways and inhibition of HMGB-1/TLR4/NF-κB signaling. Pharmacol Res. 2017;121:94–113.
79. Chen YL, Xian YF, Lai ZQ, Loo S, Lin ZX, Chan WY. Anti-inflammatory and anti-allergic effects and underlying mechanisms of Huang-Lian-Jie-Du extract: Implication for atopic dermatitis treatment. J Ethnopharmacol. 2016;185:41–52.
80. Kim H, Kim I, Lee MC, Kim HJ, Lee GS, Kim H, Kim BJ. Effects of Hwangryunhaedok-tang on gastrointestinal motility function in mice. World J Gastroenterol. 2017;23(15):2705–15.
81. Kim BJ, Kim H, Lee GS, So I, Kim SJ. Effects of San-Huang-Xie-Xin-tang, a traditional Chinese prescription for clearing away heat and toxin, on the pacemaker activities of interstitial cells of Cajal from the murine small intestine. J Ethnopharmacol. 2014;155(1):744–52.
82. Lo YC, Shih YT, Tseng YT, Hsu HT. Neuroprotective effects of San-Huang-Xie-Xin-Tang in the MPP(+)/MPTP models of Parkinson's disease in vitro and in vivo. Evid-based Compl Alt. 2012;2012:501032. https://doi.org/10.1155/2012/501032.
83. Shih YT, Chen IJ, Wu YC, Lo YC. San-Huang-Xie-Xin-Tang protects against activated microglia- and 6-OHDA-induced toxicity in neuronal SH-SY5Y cells. Evid Based Complement Altern. 2011;2011:429384. https://doi.org/10.1093/ecam/nep025.
84. Li CY, Hou YC, Lee CPD, Shia CS, Hsu IC, Fang SH. Potential ex vivo immunomodulatory effects of San-Huang-Xie-Xin-Tang and its component herbs on mice and humans. J Ethnopharmacol. 2010;127(2):292–8.
85. Qian Q, Liu X, He W, An Y, Chen Q, Wu J, Deng Y, Guo L, Zhang Y, Wang T. TG accumulation inhibitory effects of Jinqi formula by AMPK signaling pathway. J Ethnopharmacol. 2012;143(1):41–8.
86. Yang YF, Zhou QL, Yang XW. Elucidation of compatibility interactions of Traditional Chinese Medicines: in vitro absorptions across caco-2 monolayer of Coptidis rhizoma and Euodiae fructus in Zuojin and Fanzuojin formulas as a case. Phytother Res. 2017;31(8):1220–9.

87. Qian P, Zhang YB, Yang YF, Xu W, Yang XW. Pharmacokinetics studies of 12 alkaloids in rat plasma after oral administration of Zuojin and Fan-Zuojin Formulas. Molecules. 2017;22(2):214/1–18.
88. Ho FM, Liao YH, Yang AJ, Lee CPD, Hou YC, Huang CT, Lin SR, Lee KR, Huang KC, Lin WW. Anti-atherosclerotic action of Ger-Gen-Chyn-Lian-Tang and AMPK-dependent lipid lowering effect in hepatocytes. J Ethnopharmacol. 2012;142(1):175–87.
89. Lee JH, Stein BD. Antimicrobial activity of a combination of Mume Fructus, Schizandrae Fructus, and Coptidis rhizoma on enterohemorrhagic *Escherichia coli* O26, O111, and O157 and its effect on shiga toxin releases. Foodborne Pathog Dis. 2011;8(5):643–6.
90. Kwon OJ, Kim MY, Shin SH, Lee AR, Lee JY, Seo BI, Shin MR, Roh SS, Choi HG, Kim JA, Min BS, Kim GN, Noh JS, Rhee MH, Roh SS. Antioxidant and anti-inflammatory effects of Rhei rhizoma and Coptidis rhizoma mixture on reflux esophagitis in Rats. Evid Based Complement Altern. 2016;2016:2052180. https://doi.org/10.1155/2016/2052180.
91. Tsang CT, Cheung YC, Lui VWY, Yip YL, Zhang GT, Lin VWT, Cheung KCP, Feng YB, Tsao SW. Berberine suppresses tumorigenicity and growth of nasopharyngeal carcinoma cells by inhibiting STAT3 activation induced by tumor associated fibroblasts. BMC Cancer. 2013;13:619.
92. Chang W, Zhang M, Li J, Meng Z, Xiao D, Wei S, Chen L, Wang C, Hatch GM. Berberine attenuates ischemia-reperfusion injury via regulation of adenosine-5′-monophosphate kinase activity in both non-ischemic and ischemic areas of the rat heart. Cardiovasc Drug Ther. 2012;26:467–78.
93. Sun S, Wang K, Lei H, Li L, Tu M, Zeng S, Zhou H, Jiang H. Inhibition of organic cation transporter 2 and 3 may be involved in the mechanism of the antidepressant-like action of berberine. Prog Neuro Psychoph. 2014;49:1–6.
94. Yan HM, Xia MF, Wang Y, Chang XX, Yao XZ, Rao SX, Zeng MS, Tu YF, Feng R, Jia WP, Liu J, Deng W, Jiang JD, Gao X. Efficacy of berberine in patients with non-alcoholic fatty liver disease. PLoS ONE. 2015;10:e0134172.
95. Wu D, Wen W, Qi CL, Zhao RX, Lu JH, Zhong CY, Chen YY. Ameliorative effect of berberine on renal damage in rats with diabetes induced by high-fat diet and streptozotocin. Phytomedicine. 2012;19:712–8.
96. Zhang Y, Wang X, Sha S, Liang S, Zhao L, Liu L, Chai N, Wang H, Wu K. Berberine increases the expression of NHE3 and AQP4 in sennoside A-induced diarrhoea model. Fitoterapia. 2012;83:1014–22.
97. Chatuphonprasert W, Nemoto N, Sakuma T, Jarukamjorn K. Modulations of cytochrome P450 expression in diabetic mice by berberine. Chem Biol Interact. 2012;196:23–9.
98. Lo SN, Chang YP, Tsai KC, Chang CY, Wu TS, Ueng YF. Inhibition of CYP1 by berberine, palmatine, and jatrorrhizine: selectivity, kinetic characterization, and molecular modeling. Toxicol Appl Pharm. 2013;272:671–80.
99. Yu SM, Cho H, Kim GH, Chung KW, Seo SY, Kim SJ. Berberine induces dedifferentiation by actin cytoskeleton reorganization via phosphoinositide 3-kinase/Akt and p38 kinase pathways in rabbit articular chondrocytes. Exp Biol Med. 2016;241:800–7.
100. Zhou Y, Tao H, Li Y, Deng M, He B, Xia S, Zhang C, Liu S. Berberine promotes proliferation of sodium nitroprusside-stimulated rat chondrocytes and osteoarthritic rat cartilage via Wnt/beta-catenin pathway. Eur J Pharmacol. 2016;789:109–18.
101. Xu D, Yang W, Zhou C, Liu Y, Xu B. Preventive effects of berberine on glucocorticoid-induced osteoporosis in rats. Planta Med. 2010;76:1809–13.
102. Zhou JY, Zhou SW. Protective effect of berberine on antioxidant enzymes and positive transcription elongation factor b expression in diabetic rat liver. Fitoterapia. 2011;82:184–9.
103. Ma X, Egawa T, Kimura H, Karaike K, Masuda S, Iwanaka N, Hayashi T. Berberine-induced activation of 5′-adenosine monophosphate-activated protein kinase and glucose transport in rat skeletal muscles. Metabolism. 2010;59:1619–27.
104. Li ZQ, Zuo DY, Qie XD, Qi H, Zhao MQ, Wu YL. Berberine acutely inhibits the digestion of maltose in the intestine. J Ethnopharmacol. 2012;142:474–80.
105. Zhang Z, Zhang H, Li B, Meng X, Wang J, Zhang Y, Yao S, Ma Q, Jin L, Yang J, Wang W, Ning G. Berberine activates thermogenesis in white and brown adipose tissue. Nature Comm. 2014;5:5493.
106. Zhou Y, Cao S, Wang Y, Xu P, Yan J, Bin W, Qiu F, Kang N. Berberine metabolites could induce low density lipoprotein receptor up-regulation to exert lipid-lowering effects in human hepatoma cells. Fitoterapia. 2014;92:230–7.
107. Lo TF, Tsai WC, Chen ST. MicroRNA-21-3p, a berberine-induced miRNA, directly down-regulates human methionine adenosyltransferases 2A and 2B and inhibits hepatoma cell growth. PLoS ONE. 2013;8:e75628.
108. Yip NK, Ho WS. Berberine induces apoptosis via the mitochondrial pathway in liver cancer cells. Oncol Rep. 2013;30:1107–12.
109. Zhang J, Cao H, Zhang B, Cao H, Xu X, Ruan H, Yi T, Tan L, Qu R, Song G, Wang B, Hu T. Berberine potently attenuates intestinal polyps growth in ApcMin mice and familial adenomatous polyposis patients through inhibition of Wnt signalling. J Cell Mol Med. 2013;17:1484–93.
110. Kim JB, Yu JH, Ko E, Lee KW, Song AK, Park SY, Shin I, Han W, Noh DY. The alkaloid berberine inhibits the growth of Anoikis-resistant MCF-7 and MDA-MB-231 breast cancer cell lines by inducing cell cycle arrest. Phytomed Int J Phytother Phytopharmacol. 2010;17:436–40.
111. Huang Z, Han Z, Ye B, Dai Z, Shan P, Lu Z, Dai K, Wang C, Huang W. Berberine alleviates cardiac ischemia/reperfusion injury by inhibiting excessive autophagy in cardiomyocytes. Eur J Pharmacol. 2015;762:1–10.
112. Lv XX, Yu XH, Wang YY, Wang FQ, Li HM. Wang Yp, Lu DX, Qi RB, Wang HD. Berberine inhibits doxorubicin-triggered cardiomyocyte apoptosis via attenuating mitochondrial dysfunction and increasing Bcl-2 expression. PLoS ONE. 2012;7:e47351.
113. Wang M, Wang J, Tan R, Wu Q, Qiu H, Yang J, Jiang Q. Effect of berberine on PPAR α/NO activation in high glucose- and insulin-induced cardiomyocyte hypertrophy. Evid Based Complement Altern. 2013;2013:285489.
114. Zhang T, Yang S, Du J. Protective effects of berberine on isoproterenol-induced acute myocardial ischemia in rats through regulating HMGB1-TLR4 axis. Evid Based Complement Altern. 2014;2014:849783.
115. Durairajan SSK, Liu LF, Lu JH, Chen LL, Yuan Q, Chung SK, Huang L, Li XS, Huang JD, Li M. Berberine ameliorates β-amyloid pathology, gliosis, and cognitive impairment in an Alzheimer's disease transgenic mouse model. Neurobiol Aging. 2012;33:2903–19.
116. Liu YQ, Cheng MC, Wang LX, Xiao HB. Rhizoma Coptidis and berberine-induced activation of murine microglia N9 cells. J Ethnopharmacol. 2010;129:121–6.
117. Zhu X, Guo X, Mao G, Gao Z, Wang H, He Q, Li D. Hepatoprotection of berberine against hydrogen peroxide-induced apoptosis by upregulation of Sirtuin 1. Phytother Res. 2013;27:417–21.
118. Lan T, Liu W, Xie X, Huang K, Peng J, Huang J, Shen X, Liu P, Yang H, Huang H. Berberine suppresses high glucose-induced TGF-beta1 and fibronectin synthesis in mesangial cells through inhibition of sphingosine kinase 1/AP-1 pathway. Eur J Pharmacol. 2012;697:165–72.
119. Tang QL, Lai ML, Zhong YF, Wang AM, Su JK, Zhang MQ. Antinociceptive effect of berberine on visceral hypersensitivity in rats. World J Gastroenterol. 2013;19:4582–9.
120. Zhang Q, Piao XL, Piao XS, Lu T, Wang D, Kim SW. Preventive effect of *Coptis chinensis* and berberine on intestinal injury in rats challenged with lipopolysaccharides. Food Chem Toxicol. 2011;49:61–9.
121. Feng AW, Yu C, Mao Q, Li N, Li QR, Li JS. Berberine hydrochloride attenuates cyclooxygenase-2 expression in rat small intestinal mucosa during acute endotoxemia. Fitoterapia. 2011;82:976–82.
122. Tian P, Ge HY, Liu HT, Kern TS, Du LL, Guan LN, Su S, Liu P. Leukocytes from diabetic patients kill retinal endothelial cells: effects of berberine. Mol Vision. 2013;19:2092–105.
123. Zhang S, Zhang B, Dai W, Zhang X. Oxidative damage and antioxidant responses in *Microcystis aeruginosa* exposed to the allelochemical berberine isolated from golden thread. J Plant Physiol. 2011;168:639–43.
124. Morita Y, Nakashima K, Nishino K, Kotani K, Tomida J, Inoue M, Kawamura Y. Berberine is a novel type efflux inhibitor which attenuates the MexXY-mediated aminoglycoside resistance in *Pseudomonas aeruginosa*. Front Microbiol. 2016;7:1223.
125. Ning N, He K, Wang Y, Zou Z, Wu H, Li X, Ye X. Hypolipidemic effect and mechanism of palmatine from *Coptis chinensis* in hamsters fed high-fat diet. Phytother Res. 2015;29:668–73.
126. Lee WC, Kim JK, Kang JW, Oh WY, Jung JY, Kim YS, Jung HA, Choi JS, Lee SM. Palmatine attenuates D-galactosamine/lipopolysaccharide-induced fulminant hepatic failure in mice. Food Chem Toxicol. 2010;48:222–8.

127. Lee JW, Mase N, Yonezawa T, Seo HG. Palmatine attenuates osteoclast differentiation and function through inhibition of receptor activator of nuclear factor-kB ligand expression in Osteoblast Cells. Biol Pharm Bull. 2010;33:1733–9.
128. Vrba J, Havlikova M, Gerhardova D, Ulrichova J. Palmatine activates AhR and upregulates CYP1A activity in HepG2 cells but not in human hepatocytes. Toxicol In Vitr. 2014;28:693–9.
129. Kim YM, Ha YM, Jin YC, Shi LY, Lee YS, Kim HJ, Seo HG, Choi JS, Kim YS, Kang SS, Lee JH, Chang KC. Palmatine from Coptidis rhizoma reduces ischemia-reperfusion-mediated acute myocardial injury in the rat. Food Chem Toxicol. 2009;47:2097–102.
130. Zhao H, Zhou S, Zhang M, Feng J, Wang S, Wang D, Geng Y, Wang X. An in vitro AChE inhibition assay combined with UF-HPLC–ESI-Q-TOF/MS approach for screening and characterizing of AChE inhibitors from roots of *Coptis chinensis* Franch. J Pharm Biomed. 2016;120:235–40.
131. Jia F, Zou G, Fan J, Yuan Z. Identification of palmatine as an inhibitor of West Nile virus. Arch Virol. 2010;155:1325–9.
132. Wu J, Zhang H, Hu B, Yang L, Wang P, Wang F, Meng X. Coptisine from *Coptis chinensis* inhibits production of inflammatory mediators in lipopolysaccharide-stimulated RAW 264.7 murine macrophage cells. Eur J Pharmacol. 2016;780:106–14.
133. Zou ZY, Hu YR, Ma H, Wang YZ, He K, Xia S, Wu H, Xue DF, Li XG, Ye XL. Coptisine attenuates obesity-related inflammation through LPS/TLR-4-mediated signaling pathway in Syrian golden hamsters. Fitoterapia. 2015;105:139–46.
134. Friedemann T, Schumacher U, Tao Y, Leung AK, Schroder S. Neuroprotective activity of coptisine from *Coptis chinensis* (Franch). Evid Based Complement Altern. 2015;2015:827308.
135. Yue Y, Dou L, Wang X, Xue H, Song Y, Li X. Screening β_1AR inhibitors by cell membrane chromatography and offline UPLC/MS method for protecting myocardial ischemia. J Pharm Biomed. 2015;115:339–44.
136. Liu RF, Cao ZF, Pan YY, Zhang GC, Yang P, Guo PD, Zhou QS. Jatrorrhizine hydrochloride inhibits the proliferation and neovascularization of C8161 metastatic melanoma cells. Anti Cancer Drug. 2013;24:667–76.
137. Yang WW, She LP, Yu K, Yan S, Zhang XF, Tian XY, Ma SR, Zhang XW. Jatrorrhizine hydrochloride attenuates hyperlipidemia in a high-fat diet-induced obesity mouse model. Mol Med Rep. 2016;14:3277–84.
138. Zhang B, Cao A, Zhou J, Hu Z, Wu D. Effect of jatrorrhizine on delayed gastrointestinal transit in rat postoperative ileus. J Pharm Pharmacol. 2012;64:413–9.
139. Luo T, Shen XY, Li S, Ouyang T. The protective effect of jatrorrhizine against oxidative stress in primary rat cortical neurons. CNS Neurol Disord DR. 2016;16(5):617–23.
140. Choi JS, Kim JH, Ali MY, Jung HJ, Min BS, Choi RJ, Kim GD, Jung HA. Anti-adipogenic effect of epiberberine is mediated by regulation of the Raf/MEK1/2/ERK1/2 and AMPKalpha/Akt pathways. Arch Pharm Res. 2015;38:2153–62.
141. Bao M, Cao Z, Yu D, Fu S, Zhang G, Yang P, Pan Y, Yang B, Han H, Zhou Q. Columbamine suppresses the proliferation and neovascularization of metastatic osteosarcoma U2OS cells with low cytotoxicity. Toxicol Lett. 2012;215:174–80.
142. Cui L, Liu M, Chang X, Sun K. The inhibiting effect of the Coptis chinensis polysaccharide on the type II diabetic mice. Biomed Pharmacother. 2016;81:111–9.
143. Yang Y, Li Y, Yin DK, Chen S, Gao XD. *Coptis chinensis* polysaccharides inhibit advanced glycation end product formation. J Med Food. 2016;19:593–600.
144. Jiang S, Du P, An L, Yuan G, Sun Z. Anti-diabetic effect of *Coptis Chinensis* polysaccharide in high-fat diet with STZ-induced diabetic mice. Int J Biol Macromol. 2013;55:118–22.
145. Jiang S, Wang Y, Ren D, Li J, Yuan G, An L, Du P, Ma J. Antidiabetic mechanism of *Coptis chinensis* polysaccharide through its antioxidant property involving the JNK pathway. Pharm Biol. 2015;53:1022–9.
146. Yan H, Sun X, Sun S, Wang S, Zhang J, Wang R, An P, Yang F, Kang W. Anti-ultraviolet radiation effects of *Coptis chinensis* and *Phellodendron amurense* glycans by immunomodulating and inhibiting oxidative injury. Int J Biol Macromol. 2011;48:720–5.
147. Ma BL, Ma YM, Shi R, Wang TM, Zhang N, Wang CH, Yang Y. Identification of the toxic constituents in rhizoma Coptidis. J Ethnopharmacol. 2010;128:357–64.
148. Yu S, Yu Y, Liu L, Wang X, Lu S, Liang Y, Liu X, Xie L, Wang G. Increased plasma exposures of five protoberberine alkaloids from Coptidis rhizoma in streptozotocin-induced diabetic rats: is P-GP involved? Planta Med. 2010;76:876–81.
149. Ma BL, Yao MK, Zhong J, Ma YM, Gao CL, Wu JS, Qiu FR, Wang CH, Wang XH. Increased systemic exposure to rhizoma coptidis alkaloids in lipopolysaccharide-pretreated rats attributable to enhanced intestinal absorption. Drug Metab Dispos. 2012;40:381–8.
150. Ma BL, Yin C, Zhang BK, Dai Y, Jia YQ, Yang Y, Li Q, Shi R, Wang TM, Wu JS, Li YY, Lin G, Ma YM. Naturally occurring proteinaceous nanoparticles in Coptidis rhizoma extract act as concentration-dependent carriers that facilitate berberine absorption. Sci Rep. 2016;6:20110.
151. Linn YC, Lu J, Lim LC, Sun H, Sun J, Zhou Y, Ng HS. Berberine-induced haemolysis revisited: safety of rhizoma Coptidis and Cortex phellodendri in chronic haematological diseases. Phytother Res. 2012;26:682–6.
152. Yi J, Ye X, Wang D, He K, Yang Y, Liu X, Li X. Safety evaluation of main alkaloids from rhizoma Coptidis. J Ethnopharmacol. 2013;145:303–10.
153. Zhou YT, Liao QF, Lin MN, Deng XJ, Zhang PT, Yao MC, Zhang L, Xie ZY. Combination of ^{1}H NMR- and GC–MS-based metabonomics to study on the toxicity of Coptidis Rhizome in rats. PLoS ONE. 2014;9:e88281.
154. Ning N, Wang YZ, Zou ZY, Zhang DZ, de Wang Z, Li XG. Pharmacological and safety evaluation of fibrous root of rhizoma Coptidis. Environ Toxicol Pharmacol. 2015;39:53–69.
155. Schramm A, Baburin I, Hering S, Hamburger M. HERG channel inhibitors in extracts of Coptidis rhizoma. Planta Med. 2011;77:692–7.

15

A network pharmacology approach to explore the mechanisms of Erxian decoction in polycystic ovary syndrome

Lihong Liu[1,2], Bo Du[1,2], Haiying Zhang[3], Xiaofei Guo[1,2], Zheng Zhou[1,2], Aihui Xiu[4], Chang Liu[1,2], Shiyu Su[1,2] and Hao Ai[2,4*]

Abstract

Background: Polycystic ovary syndrome (PCOS) significantly affects women's health and well-being. To explore the pharmacological basis of the Erxian decoction (EXD) action in PCOS therapy, a network interaction analysis was conducted at the molecular level.

Methods: The active elements of EXD were identified according to the oral bioavailability and drug-likeness filters from three databases: traditional Chinese medicine system pharmacology analysis platform, TCM@taiwan and TCMID, and their potential targets were also identified. Genes associated with PCOS and established protein–protein interaction networks were mined from the NCBI database. Finally, significant pathways and functions of these networks were identified using Gene Ontology and Kyoto Encyclopedia of Genes and Genomes analyses to determine the mechanism of action of EXD.

Results: Seventy active compounds were obtained from 981 ingredients present in the EXD decoction, corresponding to 247 targets. In addition, 262 genes were found to be closely related with PCOS, of which 50 overlapped with EXD and were thus considered therapeutically relevant. Pathway enrichment analysis identified PI3k-Akt, insulin resistance, Toll-like receptor, MAPK and AGE-RAGE from a total of 15 significant pathways in PCOS and its treatment.

Conclusions: EXD can effectively improve the symptoms of PCOS and our systemic pharmacological analysis lays the experimental foundation for further clinical applications of EXD.

Keywords: System pharmacology, Erxian decoction, Polycystic ovary syndrome, Pharmacological mechanism, Targets

Background

Polycystic ovary syndrome (PCOS) affects 5–20% of all reproductive aged women around the world, and is characterized by hyper-androgenism, infertility, irregular menstrual cycle and polycystic ovarian morphology (PCOM) due to abnormal production of androgens by the ovaries [1]. In addition, metabolic disruptions like hyperinsulinemia and abnormal adipokine secretion from the adipose tissue is also seen [2]. PCOS not only compromises women's physical and mental health, but also increases the risk of type 2 diabetes mellitus (T2DM), atherosclerosis, cardiovascular disease, endometrial cancer, breast cancer and other long-term complications. Currently, PCOS treatment mostly relies on anti-androgen drugs, insulin sensitizers, and ovulation-promoting drugs [3]. Studies show that PCOS is frequently associated with insulin signaling [4], PI3K-Akt Signaling Pathway [5], FoxO 1 Signaling [6], and non-alcoholic fatty liver disease (NAFLD) [7], but the underlying mechanisms are not clear.

Traditional Chinese medicine (TCM) has been continually practiced since 2000 years. The Erxian decoction

*Correspondence: fcaihao@163.com
[4] Department of Gynecological Ward, The First Affiliated Hospital, Jinzhou Medical University, Jinzhou, China
Full list of author information is available at the end of the article

(EXD) consists of six herbs: *Epimedium brevicornum* (Yinyanghuo), *Curculigo orchioides* (Xianmao), *Morinda officinalis* (Bajitian), *Angelica sinensis* (Danggui), *Anemarrhena asphodeloides* (Zhimu) and *Phellodendron chinense* (Huangbo), and is used to mitigate menopausal side effects [8], osteoporosis [9], and ovarian failure [10]. One study showed that EXD upregulated estrogen receptor, enhanced ovarian function, reduced serum FSH and LH levels, increased E2 and progesterone levels, decreased malonic dialdehyde (MDA) in ovarian tissues, increased total anti-oxidative capacity (T-AOC), reduced follicular atresia by increasing follicle count, and reduced cell stromal hyperplasia [11]. Another study found that EXD could restore menstrual cycle, regulate hypothalamic-pituitary-ovarian axis function, increase steroid hormone secretion, restore primordial follicle recruitment and superior follicle selection, and improve ovulation rate and ovarian function [12]. Although EXD has been used clinically for gynecological diseases for more than 60 years, its mechanism of action is unclear due to its complex composition. In order to enhance their therapeutic efficacy, it is essential to elucidate the molecular and biological basis of TCM preparations. Systems pharmacology (SP) has recently emerged as a technique to decipher complex pharmacological problems [13]. Recently, the traditional Chinese medicine systems pharmacology database and analysis platform (TCMSP) was developed as a digital repository of traditional medicines. In addition, it can predict pharmacological targets and specific maladies of every dynamic compound, and is a major analytical tool in network pharmacology that helps determine the complex interactions between drugs and targets [14]. Since TCM formulations have multiple targets and complex ingredients, SP can even predict novel compounds based on existing formulations [15]. Network pharmacology has helped elucidate the mechanism of several TCM formulations so far [16, 17]. In this study, we used the SP approach to determine the potential mechanism of EXD action in treating PCOS. We first screened the TCMSP database for active compounds of EXD and identified its targets, followed by mining for disease-related genes, and network analysis of those genes (Fig. 1).

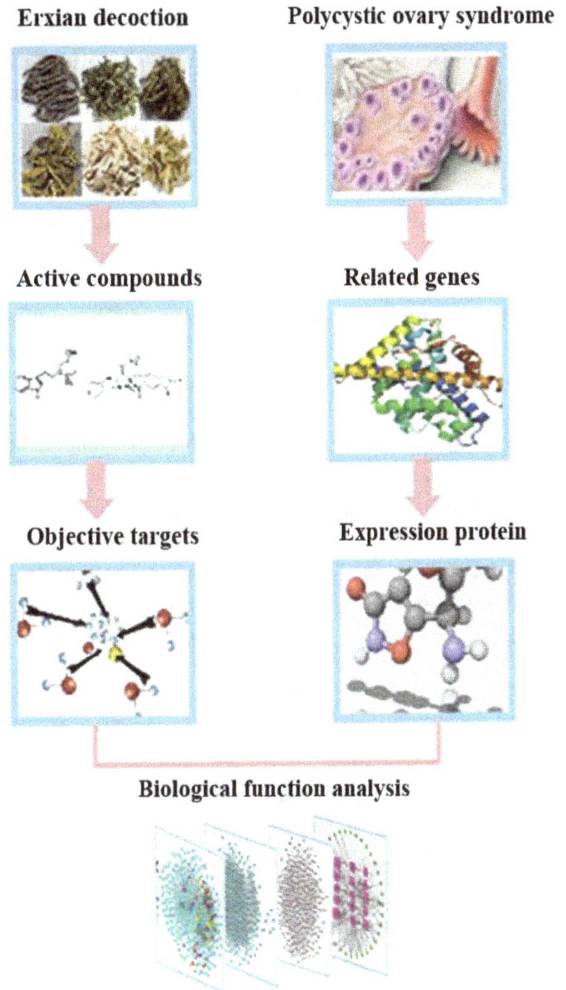

Fig. 1 A schematic diagram of the systems biology-based methodologies for unraveling the pharmacological basis of EXD action in PCOS

Methods

Identification of active EXD compounds

TCMSP (http://lsp.nwu.edu.cn/tcmsp.php) is a Chinese medicine pharmacology database containing information about the herbs used in TCM, and absorption, distribution, metabolism and excretion (ADME) characteristics of the individual compounds, their targets, related diseases, and pathways. The database search for EXD revealed its constituent herbs (*E. brevicornum, C. orchioides, M. officinalis, A. sinensis, A. asphodeloides, P. chinense*). In drug research and development, approximately 90% of the novel candidates fail the tests due to unexpected toxicity, poor absorption or bioavailability (in addition to other biopharmaceutical/metabolic issues), or poor efficacy [18]. Although the drug ADME characteristics are highly significant, biological testing of each and every candidate drug is impractical due to the high-costs and time involved. In recent years, the focus has therefore shifted to bioinformatics to determine the pharmacokinetic properties of candidate drugs. In order to maximize the chances of finding the fully active compounds, we set two conditions as the criteria for screening these active compounds—oral bioavailability (OB) and drug-likeness (DL), which are the two most important indicators for evaluating ADME characteristics via bioinformatics.

Orally administered drugs must pass some obstructions, like P-glycoprotein (P-gp) [19] and cytochrome P450 s [20], before reaching their target site. The OB of candidate drugs can be predicted with QSAR modeling using linear [multiple linear regression (MLR) and partial least squares regression (PLS)] and nonlinear [support-vector machine regression (SVR)] methods, and the OBioavail 1.2 program [21]. The compounds with OB $\geq$ 30% were filtered for further analysis. DL, i.e. similarities with the physiochemical or/and structural properties of existing drugs is used to filter out compounds with undesirable qualities [22]. The Dragon program was used to determine the DL index based on parameters like molecular weight, one-dimensional descriptors (e.g. logP, H-donors and H-acceptors), two-dimensional profiles (e.g. extremity number, worldwide topological charge file), three-dimensional variables (average geometric distance degree and radius of gyration), and total positive and negative charges. The DL index of any new molecule is calculated based on Tanimoto similarity [23] as per the formula:

$$f(A, B) = \frac{A \cdot B}{|A|^2 + |B|^2 - A \cdot B}$$

where A represents the descriptor of the new numerator and B represents all the 6511 molecules selected from the Drug Bank database. The average of all descriptors was calculated by Dragon and the compounds with DL index $\geq$ 0.18 were selected.

Prediction of EXD targets and compound-target network establishment

An essential step following the discovery of active molecules is to identify their molecular targets that trigger the biological effects [24]. Bioinformatics methodologies like chemometrics and chemogenomics are often used to mine and integrate information, in order to identify the molecular targets [25]. The Chinese chemical databases and PubChem were mined for the compounds, and their physicochemical properties and biological targets were determined. The genetic information of the targets were obtained from the UniProt Online Resources (http://www.uniprot.org) [26]. Random Forest and Support Vector Machine (SVM) method and prediction models were used for large scale chemical simulation of the drug targets [27, 28]. A compound-target network refers to a mathematical and computable expression of different associations between TCM formulae and diseases, especially in complex natural frameworks [29]. Target interactions were obtained from the STITCH protein database (http://stitch.embl.de/) [30]. The relationship between the above candidate compounds and potential targets were determined with EXCEL as the input source, and the Cytoscape program was used to form a compound-target visual interaction network (CT network) [31]. The nodes in the network are compounds, proteins, enzymes, and targets, and the relationship between them is represented by the lines between the nodes [32].

PCOS-EXD gene network establishment

Genes related to PCOS were downloaded from the NCBI Gene database (http://www.ncbi.nlm.nih.gov/quality) [33]. The database was searched using the keyword 'Polycystic ovary syndrome', which yielded 296 known PCOS-related genes of *Homo sapiens*. The CT network was then mapped to the PCOS-related gene network to establish a PCOS-drug interaction network based on overlapping genes, to determine the mechanism of EXD action in PCOS. In such a network, a node can represent a herb, a compound, or a gene/protein, and an "edge" is an association between the nodes. The "degree" of a hub is the number of edges associated with it, and the "betweenness" of a hub is the number of closest associations. The nodes whose connectivity was greater than twice the median of all nodes are selected as the hub nodes in the network. The hubs with high centrality are considered the key hubs in a network.

Biological function analysis

Gene Ontology (GO, http://www.geneontology.org/) and Kyoto Encyclopedia of Genes and Genomes (KEGG, http://www.genome.jp/kegg/) pathway analysis were used to analyze the primary pharmacological units. GO

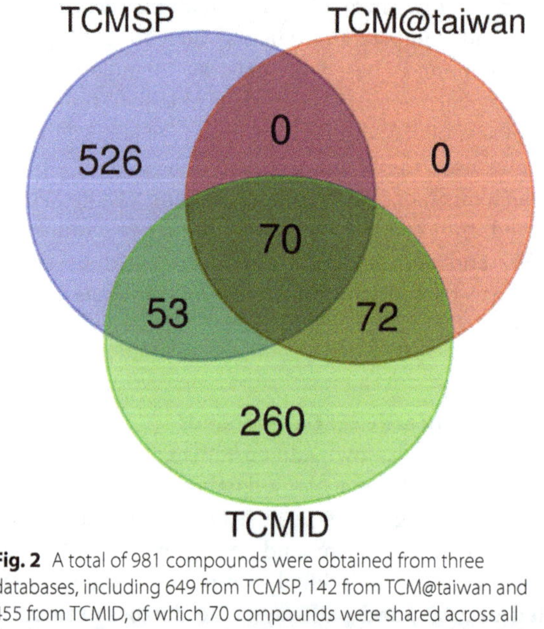

Fig. 2 A total of 981 compounds were obtained from three databases, including 649 from TCMSP, 142 from TCM@taiwan and 455 from TCMID, of which 70 compounds were shared across all databases

Table 1 Active compounds properties

Compound	Herb	Chemical	OB	DL	Degree
C01	CR01	ZINC03982454	36.91	0.76	2
C02	CR02	Cycloartenol	38.69	0.78	1
C03	CR03 MO13 AS01 PC14	Beta-sitosterol	36.91	0.75	38
C04	CR04	3,2′,4′,6′-Tetrahydroxy-4,3′-dimethoxy chalcone	52.69	0.28	11
C05	CR05	Curculigoside B_qt	83.36	0.19	5
C06	CR06 AS02 AR07 PC10	Stigmasterol	43.83	0.76	31
C07	EH01	24-Epicampesterol	37.58	0.71	2
C08	EH02	Linoleyl acetate	42.1	0.2	4
C09	EH03 PC22	Poriferast-5-en-3beta-ol	36.91	0.75	2
C10	EH04	DFV	32.76	0.18	11
C11	EH05	Chryseriol	35.85	0.27	18
C12	EH06 MO12	Sitosterol	36.91	0.75	3
C13	EH07 AR02	Kaempferol	41.88	0.24	63
C14	EH08	Olivil	62.23	0.41	4
C15	EH09 AR03	Anhydroicaritin	45.41	0.44	37
C16	EH10	C-Homoerythrinan,1,6-didehydro-3,15,16-trimethoxy-,(3.beta.)-	39.14	0.49	38
C17	EH11	Yinyanghuo A	56.96	0.77	9
C18	EH12	Yinyanghuo C	45.67	0.5	11
C19	EH13	Yinyanghuo E	51.63	0.55	11
C20	EH14	6-Hydroxy-11,12-dimethoxy-2,2-dimethyl-1,8-dioxo-2,3,4,8-tetrahydro-1H-isochromeno[3,4-h]isoquinolin-2-ium	60.64	0.66	6
C21	EH15	8-(3-Methylbut-2-enyl)-2-phenyl-chromone	48.54	0.25	30
C22	EH16	Anhydroicaritin-3-O-alpha-L-rhamnoside	41.58	0.61	1
C23	EH17	1,2-bis(4-Hydroxy-3-methoxyphenyl)propan-1,3-diol	52.31	0.22	11
C24	EH18	Icariin	41.58	0.61	1
C25	EH19	Icariside A7	31.91	0.86	3
C26	EH20	Luteolin	36.16	0.25	57
C27	EH21 PC15	Magnograndiolide	63.71	0.19	4
C28	EH22 PC19	Quercetin	46.43	0.28	153
C29	MO01	Ethyl oleate (NF)	32.4	0.19	1
C30	MO02	Alizarin-2-methylether	32.81	0.21	13
C31	MO03	1-Hydroxy-6-hydroxymethylanthracenequinone	81.77	0.21	12
C32	MO04	(2R,3S)-(+)-3′,5-Dihydroxy-4,7-dimethoxydihydroflavonol	77.24	0.33	9
C33	MO05	1,6-Dihydroxy-5-methoxy-2-(methoxymethyl)-9,10-anthraquinone	104.54	0.34	12
C34	MO06	Americanin A	46.71	0.35	11
C35	MO07	2-Hydroxy-1,8-dimethoxy-7-methoxymethylanthracenequinone	112.3	0.37	11
C36	MO08	2-Hydroxy-1,5-dimethoxy-6-(methoxymethyl)-9,10-anthraquinone	95.85	0.37	14
C37	MO09	1,5,7-Trihydroxy-6-methoxy-2-methoxymethylanthracenequinone	80.42	0.38	10
C38	MO10	Diop	43.59	0.39	3
C39	MO11	3beta,20(R),5-alkenyl-stigmastol	36.91	0.75	1
C40	MO14	Isoprincepin	49.12	0.77	2
C41	MO15	3beta-24S(R)-butyl-5-alkenyl-cholestol	35.35	0.82	1
C42	MO16	Ohioensin-A	38.13	0.76	3
C43	AR01	Asperglaucide	58.02	0.52	5
C44	AR04	Anemarsaponin F_qt	60.06	0.79	1
C45	AR05	Hippeastrine	51.65	0.62	11
C46	AR06	Timosaponin B III_qt	35.26	0.87	2
C47	AR08	Icariin I	41.58	0.61	1
C48	AR09	(Z)-3-(4-hydroxy-3-methoxy-phenyl)-N-[2-(4-hydroxyphenyl)ethyl]acrylamide	118.35	0.26	8
C49	AR10	Diosgenin	80.88	0.81	16

Table 1 (continued)

Compound	Herb	Chemical	OB	DL	Degree
C50	AR11	Coumaroyltyramine	112.9	0.2	10
C51	PC01	Berberine	36.86	0.78	17
C52	PC02	Coptisine	30.67	0.86	9
C53	PC03	Phellavin_qt	35.86	0.44	3
C54	PC04	Delta 7-stigmastenol	37.42	0.75	1
C55	PC05	Phellopterin	40.19	0.28	12
C56	PC06	Dehydrotanshinone II A	43.76	0.4	21
C57	PC07	Rutaecarpine	40.3	0.6	18
C58	PC08	Skimmianin	40.14	0.2	5
C59	PC09	Chelerythrine	34.18	0.78	6
C60	PC11	Worenine	45.83	0.87	7
C61	PC12	Cavidine	35.64	0.81	28
C62	PC13	Hericenone H	39	0.63	1
C63	PC16	Palmatine	64.6	0.65	19
C64	PC17	Fumarine	59.26	0.83	28
C65	PC18	Isocorypalmine	35.77	0.59	36
C66	PC20	Phellamurin_qt	56.6	0.39	10
C67	PC21	(S)-Canadine	53.83	0.77	32
C68	PC23	Berberrubine	35.74	0.73	13
C69	PC24	Campesterol	37.58	0.71	1
C70	PC25	Thalifendine	44.41	0.73	14

is a database that functionally annotates genes and proteins into three main terms—cellular components (CC), molecular functions (MF), and biological processes (BP) [34] and pathway analysis reveals the possible biological processes with key hub genes. KEGG is a database for determining the high-level functions and biological relevance of a large set of genes [35]. The molecular action of mechanism of EXD could be elucidated by analyzing the significant GO terms and pathways of the overlapping genes. The ClueGO plugin of Cytoscape was used to integrate the GO terms with KEGG pathways [36].

Results

OB prediction and DL calculation

We obtained 981 active compounds from the initial search of three databases: 649 from TCMSP, 142 from TCM@taiwan, and 455 from TCMID. There were 123 common compounds between the TCMSP and TCMID databases, while TCM@taiwan and TCMID had 142 common compounds amongst them, and 70 compounds were shared across the three databases (Fig. 2). Seventy compounds passed the OB and DL filters and had favorable pharmacokinetic profiles, and a total of 247 targets were identified for these compounds. The pharmacokinetic properties of the compounds and the corresponding number of targets are shown in Table 1.

Network analysis

To determine the relationship between the active compounds of EXD with their putative targets, a compound-target (CT) network was first built (Fig. 3). In such a network, nodes with degree greater than twice the median are considered key nodes; accordingly, 71 hub targets and 13 central compounds were obtained. The protein–protein interaction (PPI) network was constructed using the 247 drug targets, which revealed 238 nodes and 3880 edges. The network radius, diameter and characteristic path length were 3, 5 and 2.2, respectively. The greatest degree was of AKT1 (125), followed by JUN (121), TP53 (118), FOS (113), and EGFR (101). A total of 58 central targets were obtained that had values greater than twice the median (Fig. 4). In addition, the potential targets associated with PCOS were retrieved from the NCBI Gene database, and a network of related genes was built using STITCH, which showed 262 nodes and 3428

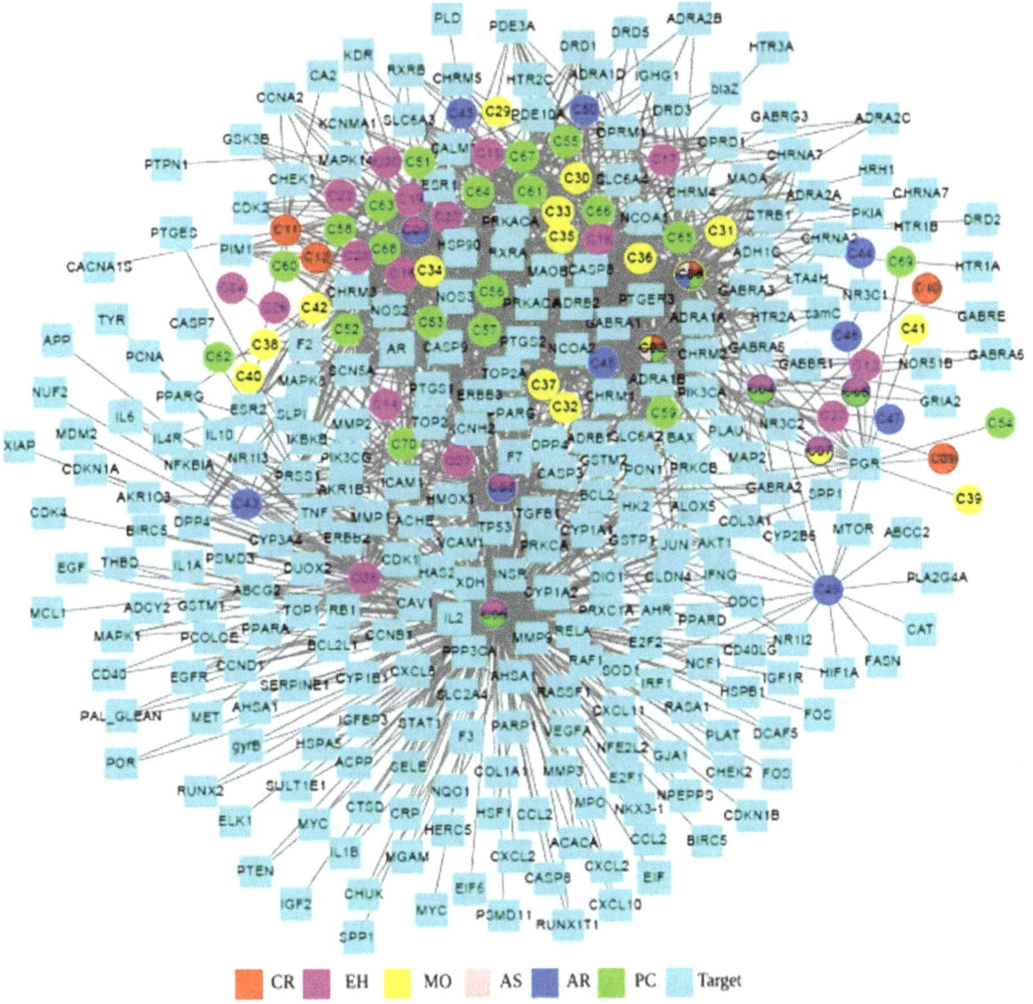

Fig. 3 C-T network, The multi-colored circles represent different herbs and squares represent the targets. (red for *Curculigo*, dark pink for *Epimedium*, yellow for *Morinda*, light pink for *Angelica*, dark blue for *Anemarrhena*, and green for Cork). The blue squares represent the targets of each compound. One target can have multiple compounds and vice versa

edges (Fig. 5). We mapped the drug interaction network to the PCOS-related gene interactions network to obtain the drug-PCOS interaction network (Fig. 6). Pink nodes represent genes associated with PCOS, blue nodes represent EXD targets, green nodes represent co-acting genes, and the edges between nodes represent inter-nodal relationships. A total of 50 targets were identified which are likely the key drug targets in PCOS.

Biological functional analysis

Biological functions of the PCOS specific drug targets were annotated to clarify the mechanism of action of EXD in PCOS. GO enrichment analysis was performed on the 50 targets using ClueGO, and the top five BP terms were extrinsic apoptotic signaling pathway, positive regulation of reactive oxygen species metabolic process, protein kinase B signaling, positive regulation of sequence-specific DNA binding transcription factor activity, and response to corticosteroids. The top five MF terms were growth factor receptor binding, cytokine activity, ion channel regulator activity, nitric-oxide synthase regulator activity and steroid binding, while the main CC terms were plasma membrane raft, nuclear transcription factor complex, caveola RNA polymerase

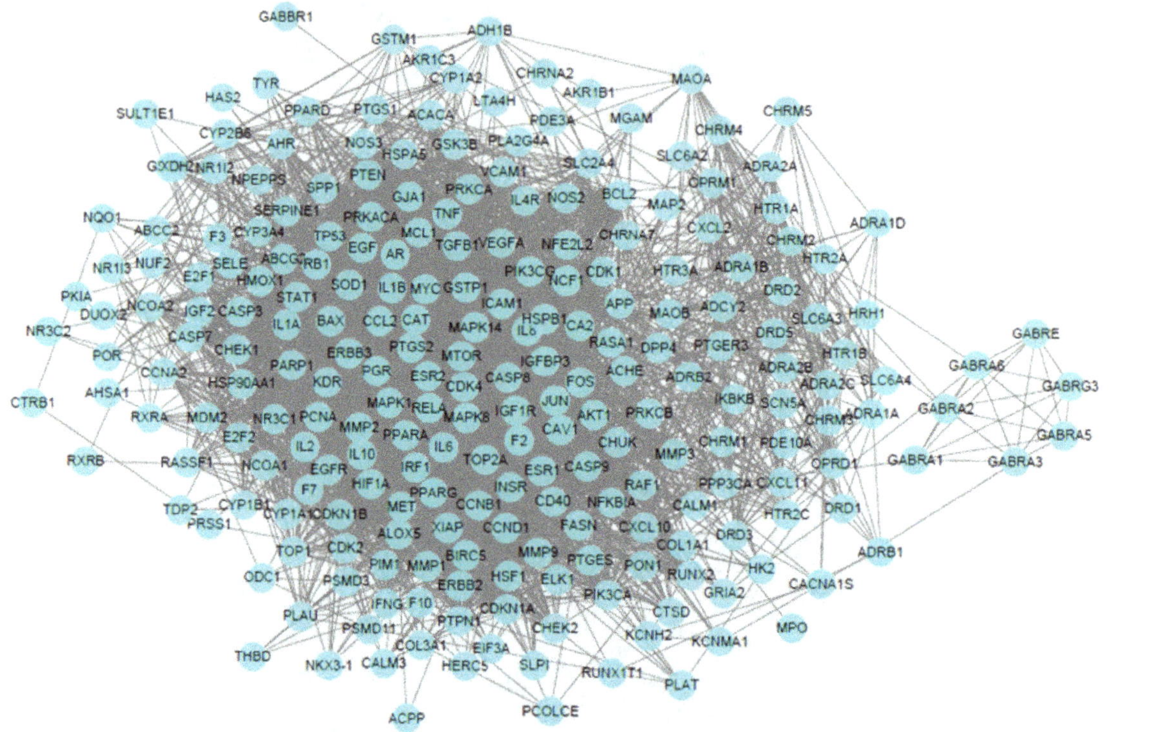

Fig. 4 PPI-target interaction network. Nodes represent targets, proteins, and genes of EXD. The edges represent the links between nodes. There are 238 nodes and 3880 edges in this network

II transcription factor complex, platelet alpha granule and platelet alpha granule lumen (Fig. 7). The significant KEGG pathways were AGE-RAGE in diabetic complications, fluid shear stress and atherosclerosis, PI3K-Akt, MAPK and FoxO, among a total of 15 pathways (Fig. 8).

Discussion

Traditional Chinese medicine (TCM) consists of complex formulations which have hitherto been difficult to characterize, thus limiting their widespread clinical use. In this study, we combined systems pharmacology (SP), pharmacokinetics (PK) and bioinformatics to identify the individual compounds of the EXD formula and their specific PCOS-related targets. EXD is a formulation of six herbs with known ameliorative effects in gynecopathy.

After screening EXD for OB and DL, 70 compounds were obtained, of which the most effective were C28 (quercetin, 153 targets) and C13 (kaempferol, 63 targets). Two constituent herbs of EXD contain these compounds. Quercetin, a polyphenol derived from many plants species, is known for its anti-carcinogenic, anti-inflammatory and antiviral activities, in addition to its active roles in platelet aggregation, lipid peroxidation and capillary permeability [37], cellular uptake, and free radical quenching [38]. Rezvan et al. found that oral quercetin supplementation enhanced AMPK levels to improve the metabolic features of PCOS in a randomized placebo-controlled double-blind trial [39]. Wang et al. showed that quercetin inhibited the Toll-like receptor/NF-kB signaling pathway and improved the inflammatory microenvironment of the ovarian tissue in a PCOS rat model [40]. Kaempferol, a dietary flavonoid, has anti-oxidant, anti-inflammatory, anti-apoptotic, anticancer, estrogenic, and anti-estrogenic activities [41]. It regulates the MAPK pathway to protect against IR injury by attenuating inflammation and apoptosis [42]. Nevertheless, since each herb of EXD contains multiple compounds, they act on multiple targets via several mechanisms.

The drug target network and the PCOS network had 50 overlapping genes, of which 37 were enriched in 15 pathways, and are likely the key genes involved in PCOS treatment. The significant pathways involving the candidate

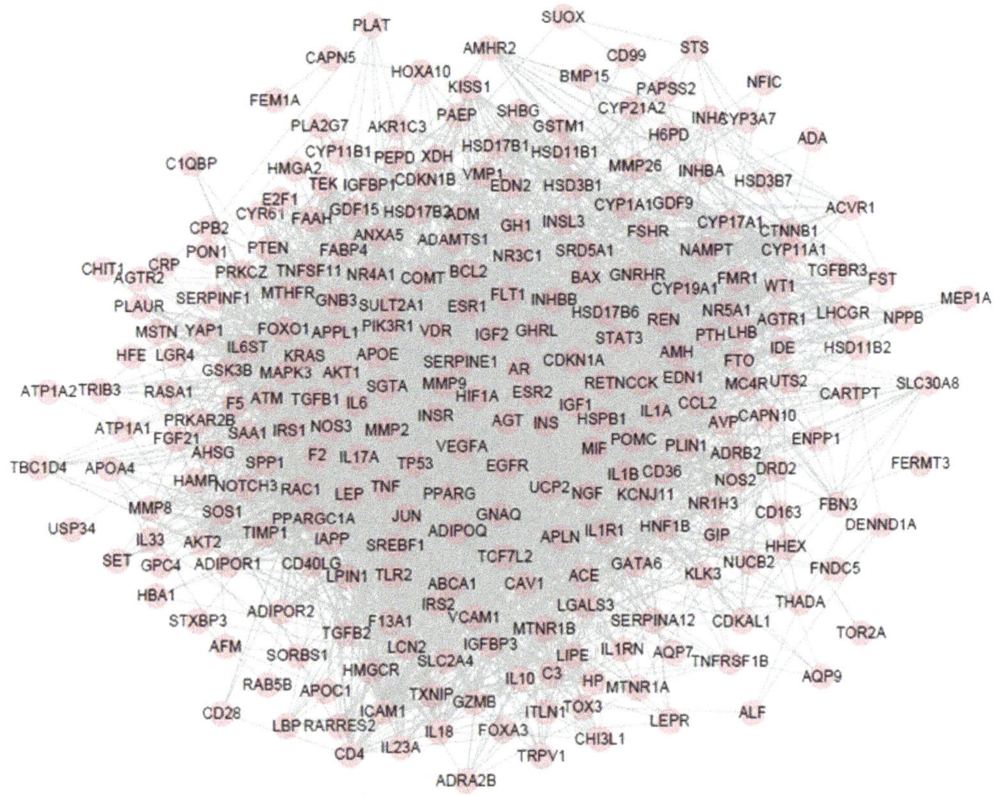

Fig. 5 A PPI interaction network of PCOS-related genes. Dots represent genes associated with PCOS, and edges represent interactions between genes. There are 262 nodes and 3428 edges in this network

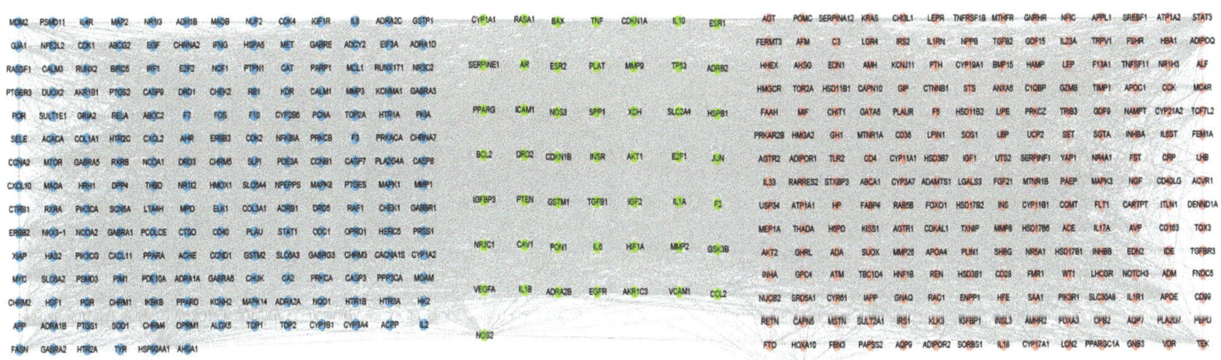

Fig. 6 PCOS-related drug targets. Pink nodes represent genes associated with PCOS, blue nodes represent EXD targets, green nodes represent co-acting genes, and the edges represent inter-nodal relationships

compounds targeting PCOS can be classified as prototypes, direct and indirect pathways depending on their functions. Based on the network analysis, we obtained three proteins of interest—AKT1, IL6 and INSR. In the hyper-androgenic PCOS patients, high levels of AKT1 have been associated with GCs dysfunction [43]. In addition, IL6, IL1B1 and TNF are associated with increased susceptibility to PCOS [44], and INSR plays a role in compensatory hyperinsulinemia [45]. EXD can regulate the expression of these genes via the AGE-RAGE,

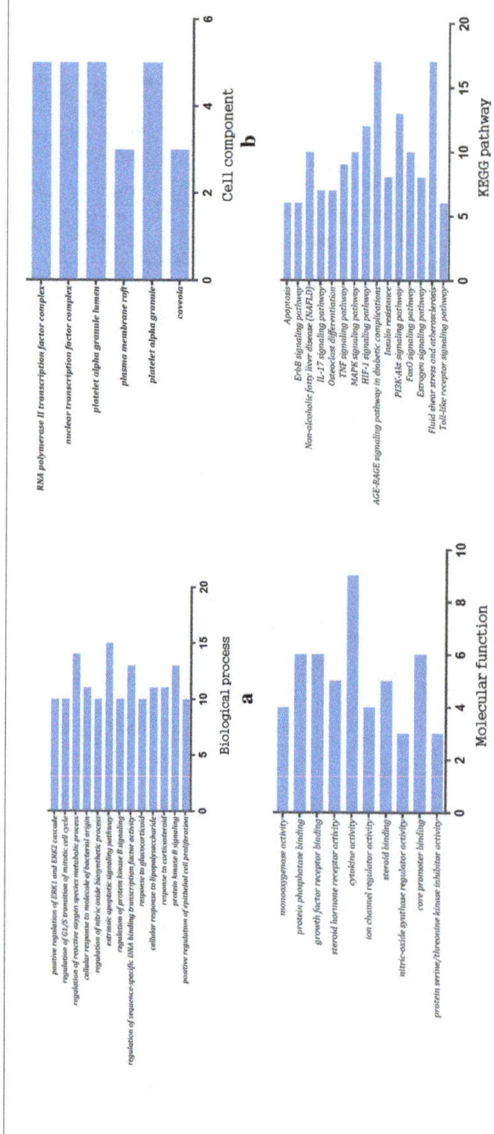

Fig. 7 GO functional analysis. **a** Biological processes terms were extrinsic apoptotic signaling pathway, positive regulation of reactive oxygen species metabolic process, protein kinase B signaling, positive regulation of sequence-specific DNA binding transcription factor activity, and response to corticosteroids etc. **b** Cell component terms included plasma membrane raft, nuclear transcription factor complex, caveola RNA polymerase II transcription factor complex, platelet alpha granule, platelet alpha granule lumen etc. **c** Molecular function terms were growth factor receptor binding, cytokine activity, ion channel regulator activity, nitric-oxide synthase regulator activity, steroid binding etc. **d** Significant KEGG pathways were AGE-RAGE in diabetic complications, fluid shear stress, atherosclerosis, PI3K-Akt, MAPK, and FoxO signaling pathway etc

PI3K-Akt, and MAPK signaling pathways. The PI3K-Akt signaling pathway [46], non-alcoholic fatty liver disease (NAFLD) [47], MAPK signaling pathway [48], FoxO signaling pathway [6], insulin resistance [4], apoptosis, and Toll-like receptor signaling pathway [46] are strongly correlated with the occurrence and development of PCOS. Therefore, they are mechanistically important for PCOS and may play a role in its treatment as well. Studies show that one pathway contains multiple targets, and each target can act on the multiple pathways, thereby creating an intricate network.

Conclusions

Systems pharmacology and genomics were combined to identify the PCOS relevant targets of the EXD formula. Our findings indicate that 6 of the constituent herbs in EXD act synergistically on certain putative PCOS targets.

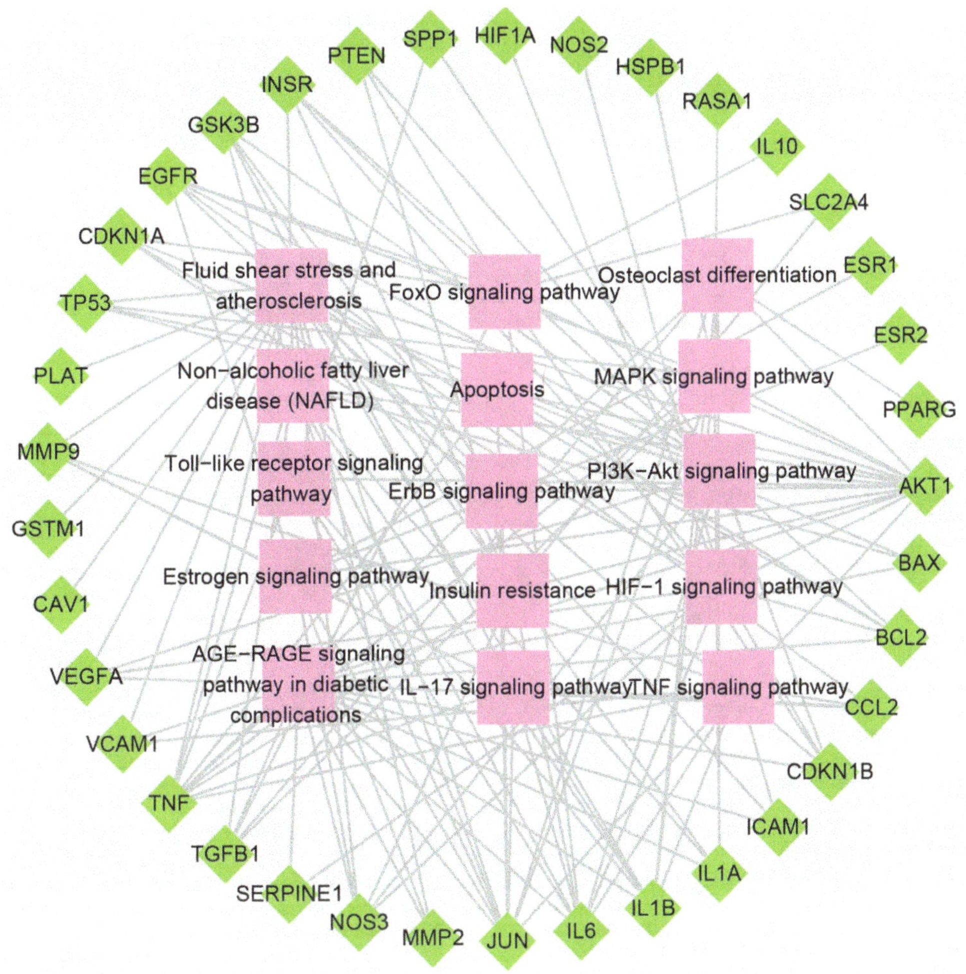

Fig. 8 Analysis of Biological Function of KEGG Pathways (Pathway-Target network). The green points represent the key targets of PCOS relevant to EXD action, and the pink points represent the path of action related to the targets

This study presents a high throughput and economic method of identifying drug targets, and may have significant clinical utility.

Abbreviations

PCOS: polycystic ovary syndrome; PCOM: polycystic ovarian morphology; EXD: Erxian decoction; TCMSP: traditional Chinese medicine system pharmacology analysis platform; GO: Biological Network Gene Ontology tools; KEGG: Kyoto Encyclopedia of Genes and Genomes; TCM: traditional Chinese medicine; CC: cellular components; MF: molecular functions; BP: biological processes; FSH: follicle stimulating hormone; LH: luteinizing hormone; E2: estradiol; P: progesterone; MDA: malonic dialdehyde; T-AOC: total anti-oxidative capacity; ADME: absorption, distribution, metabolism, excretion; OB: oral bioavailability; DL: drug-likeness; NAFLD: non-alcoholic fatty liver disease.

Authors' contributions

LLH, and AH conceived and designed the study. ZHY and DB collected the data. LLH, AH, GXF and ZZ performed the data analysis, LLH and AH wrote the manuscript. All authors are responsible for reviewing data. All authors read and approved the final manuscript.

Author details

[1] Department of Gynecological Ward, The Third Affiliated Hospital, Jinzhou Medical University, Jinzhou, China. [2] Liaoning Provincial Key Laboratory of Follicle Development and Reproductive Health (Office of Science and Technology), Jinzhou, China. [3] Library Department, Jinzhou Medical University, Jinzhou, China. [4] Department of Gynecological Ward, The First Affiliated Hospital, Jinzhou Medical University, Jinzhou, China.

Acknowledgements

Not applicable.

Competing interests

The authors declare that they have no competing interests.

Consent for publication

Not applicable.

Funding

Project supported by the Natural Science Foundation of Liaoning province, China (Grant No. 20170540373).

Project supported by the Jinzhou Foundation for Science and Technology, China (Grant No. 16B1G35).

References

1. Azziz R, Carmina E, Chen Z, Dunaif A, Laven JS, Legro RS, Lizneva D, Natterson-Horowtiz B, Teede HJ, Yildiz BO. Polycystic ovary syndrome. Nat Rev Dis Primers. 2016;2:16057.
2. Utiger RD. Insulin and the polycystic ovary syndrome. N Engl J Med. 1996;335(9):657–8.
3. Ouyang X. Drug treatment of clinical application development of polycystic ovary syndrome. J Mod Med Health Care. 2017;33(11):1667–9 **(in Chinese)**.
4. Wang F, Wang SB, Zhang ZH, Lin QQ, Liu YP, Xiao YJ, Xiao KJ, Wang Z. Defective insulin signaling and the protective effects of dimethyldiguanide during follicular development in the ovaries of polycystic ovary syndrome. Mol Med Rep. 2017;16(6):8164–70.
5. Li TT, Mo H, Chen WF. Role of the PI3K-Akt signaling pathway in the pathogenesis of polycystic ovary syndrome. Reprod Sci. 2017;24(5):646–55.
6. Li N, Wang XY, Wang XJ, Yu HN, Lin L, Sun CM, Liu P, Chu YL, Hou JQ. Upregulation of FoxO 1 signaling mediates the proinflammatory cytokine upregulation in the macrophage from polycystic ovary syndrome patients. Clin Lab. 2017;63(2):301–11.
7. Anzai A, Marcondes RR, Gonçalves TH, Carvalho KC, Simões MJ, Garcia N, Soares JM Jr, Padmanabhan V, Baracat EC, Silva IDCG, Maciel GAR. Impaired branched-chain amino acid metabolism may underlie the nonalcoholic fatty liver disease-like pathology of neonatal testosterone-treated female rats. Sci Rep. 2017;7(1):13167.
8. Sze SC, Cheung HP, Ng TB, Zhang ZJ, Wong KL, Wong HK, Hu YM, Yow CM, Tong Y. Effects of Erxian decoction, a Chinese medicinal formulation, on serum lipid profile in a rat model of menopause. Chin Med. 2011;6(1):40.
9. Sze SC, Ip CW, Ng TB, Zhang KY, Zhang ZJ, Cheung HP, Cheng CL, Tong Y. Compatibility of multiple herbal components in Erxian Decoction, a Chinese medicinal formula, for treating osteoporosis. Eur J Integr Med. 2012;4(2):187–96.
10. Wang FY, Xie C, Cheng WW, Han W, Lai DM. Establishment of mouse model of cyclophosphamide-induced ovarian failure. J Shanghai Jiaotong Univ. 2011;31(10):1398–402.
11. Ai H, Zhang HY, Zhang YL, Xue XO. Effect of Er Xian decoction on ovary function after injury of cisplatin in mic. Tianjin J Tradit Chin Med. 2013;30(5):498–500 **(in Chinese)**.
12. Mao XL, Bao WQ, Zhao PW, Niu JZ, Zhao FJ, Tao SY. Influence of Erxian Decoction on ovarian reserve of rats suffered from premature ovarian failure. Chin J Tradit Chin Med. 2017;32(2):771–3 **(in Chinese)**.
13. Berger SI, Iyengar R. Network analyses in systems pharmacology. Bioinformatics. 2009;25(19):2466–72.
14. Ru JL, Li P, Wang JN, Zhou W, Li BH, Huang C, Li PD, Guo ZH, Tao WY, Yang YF, Xu X, Li Y, Wang YH, Yang L. TCMSP: a database of systems pharmacology for drug discovery from herbal medicines. J Cheminform. 2014;6(1):13.
15. Li S, Zhang B, Jiang D, Wei Y, Zhang N. Herb network construction and co-module analysis for uncovering the combination rule of traditional Chinese herbal formulae. BMC Bioinform. 2010;11(S11):1–12.
16. Wang S, Tong Y, Ng TB, Lao L, Lam JK, Zhang KY, Zhang ZJ, et al. Network pharmacological identification of active compounds and potential actions of Erxian decoction in alleviating menopause-related symptoms. Chin Med. 2015;10:19.
17. Wu L, Wang Y, Li Z, Zhang B, Cheng Y, Fan X. Identifying roles of "Jun-Chen-Zuo-Shi" component herbs of QiShenYiQi formula in treating acute myocardial ischemia by network pharmacology. Chin Med. 2014;9(1):24.
18. Baertschi SW, Olsen BA, Alsante KM, Ree RA. Stress testing: relation to the development timeline. Boca Raton: CRC Press; 2011.
19. Fromm MF. P-glycoprotein: a defense mechanism limiting oral bioavailability and CNS accumulation of drugs. Int J Clin Pharmacol Ther. 2000;38:69–74.
20. Van Waterschoot RA, Lagas JS, Wagenaar E, Wagenaar E, van der Kruijssen CM, van Herwaarden AE, et al. Absence of both cytochrome P450 3A and P-glycoprotein dramatically increases docetaxel oral bioavailability and risk of intestinal toxicity. Cancer Res. 2009;69(23):8996–9002.
21. Xu X, Zhang W, Huang C, Li Y, Yu H, Wang Y, Duan J, Ling Y. A novel chemometric method for the prediction of human oral bioavailability. Int J Mol Sci. 2012;13(6):6964–82.
22. Jadhav PB, Yadav AR, Gore MG. Concept of drug likeness in pharmaceutical research. Int J Pharm Biol Sci. 2015;6:142–54.
23. Ma C, Wang L, Xie XQ. GPU accelerated chemical similarity calculation for compound library comparison. J Chem Inf Model. 2011;51(7):1521–7.
24. Schenone M, Dančík V, Wagner BK, Clemons PA. Target identification and mechanism of action in chemical biology and drug discovery. Nat Chem Biol. 2013;9(4):232–40.
25. Yue SJ, Liu J, Feng WW, Zhang FL, Chen JX, Xin LT, Peng C, Guan HS, Wang CY, Yan D. System pharmacology-based dissection of the synergistic mechanism of Huangqi and Huanglian for diabetes mellitus. Front Pharmacol. 2017;8:694.
26. Apweiler R, UniProt Consortium. UniProt: the universal protein knowledgebase. Nucleic Acids Res. 2018;35(Database issue):2699.
27. Svetnik V, Liaw A, Tong C, Culberson JC, Sheridan RP, Feuston BP. Random forest: a classification and regression tool for compound classification and QSAR modeling. J Chem Inf Comput Sci. 2003;43(6):1947–58.
28. Tong S, Koller D. Support vector machine active learning with applications to text classification. J Mach Learn Res. 2002;11(2):45–66.
29. Li S, Zhang B. Traditional Chinese medicine network pharmacology: theory, methodology and application. Chin J Nat Med. 2013;11(2):110–20.
30. Kuhn M, Szklarczyk D, Franceschini A, von Mering C, Jensen LJ, Bork P. STITCH 3: zooming in on protein–chemical interactions. Nucleic Acids Res. 2012;40(Database issue):876–80.
31. Shannon P, Markiel A, Ozier O, Baliga NS, Wang JT, Ramage D, Amin N, Schwikowski B, Ideker T. Cytoscape: a software environment for integrated models of biomolecular interaction networks. Genome Res. 2003;13(11):2498–504.
32. Smoot ME, Ono K, Ruscheinski J, Wang PL, Ideker T. Cytoscape 2.8: new features for data integration and network visualization. Bioinformatics. 2011;27(3):431–2.
33. Maglott D, Ostell J, Pruitt KD, Tatusova T. Entrez Gene: gene-centered information at NCBI. Nucleic Acids Res. 2005;33(S1):54–8.
34. Ashburner M, Ball CA, Blake JA, Botstein D, Butler H, Cherry JM, The Gene Ontology Consortium, et al. Gene ontology: tool for the unification of biology. Nat Genet. 2000;25:25–9.
35. Ogata H, Goto S, Sato K, Fujibuchi W, Bono H, Kanehisa M. KEGG: Kyoto Encyclopedia of Genes and Genomes. Nucleic Acids Res. 1999;1(1):27–30.
36. Bindea G, Mlecnik B, Hackl H, Charoentong P, Tosolini M, Kirilovsky A, Fridman WH, Pagès F, Trajanoski Z, Galon J. ClueGO: a Cytoscape plug-into decipher functionally grouped gene ontology and pathway annotation networks. Bioinformatics. 2009;25(8):1091–3.
37. Li Y, Yao J, Han C, Yang J, Chaudhry MT, Wang S, Liu H, Yin Y. Quercetin, inflammation and immunity. Nutrients. 2016;8(3):167.
38. Roubalová L, Purchartová K, Papoušková B, Vacek J, Křen V, Ulrichová J, Vrba J. Sulfation modulates the cell uptake, antiradical activity and biological effects of flavonoids in vitro: an examination of quercetin, isoquercitrin and taxifolin. Bioorg Med Chem. 2015;23(17):5402–9.
39. Rezvan N, Moini A, Gorgani-Firuzjaee S, Hosseinzadeh-Attar MJ. Oral quercetin supplementation enhances adiponectin receptor transcript expression in polycystic ovary syndrome patients: a randomized placebo-controlled double-blind clinical trial. Cell J. 2018;19(4):627–33.
40. Wang ZZ, Zhai DX, Zhang DY, Bai LL, Yao RP, Yu J, et al. Quercetin decreases insulin resistance in a polycystic ovary syndrome rat model by improving inflammatory microenvironment. Reprod Sci. 2017;24(5):682–90.

41. Calderónmontaño JM, Burgosmorón E, Pérezguerrero C, López-Lázaro M. A review on the dietary flavonoid kaempferol. Mini Rev Med Chem. 2011;11(4):298–344.
42. Suchal K, Malik S, Gamad N, Malhotra RK, Goyal SN, Chaudhary U, et al. Kaempferol attenuates myocardial ischemic injury via inhibition of mapk signaling pathway in experimental model of myocardial ischemia-reperfusion injury. Oxid Med Cell Longev. 2016;2016(9):1–10.
43. Nekoonam S, Naji M, Nashtaei MS, Mortezaee K, Koruji M, Safdarian L, Amidi F. Expression of AKT1 along with AKT2 in granulosa-lutein cells of hyperandrogenic PCOS patients. Arch Gynecol Obstet. 2017;295(4):1041–50.
44. de Alencar JB, Alves HV, Elpidio LN, Visentainer JE, Sell AM. Polymorphisms of cytokine genes and polycystic ovary syndrome: a review. Metab Syndr Relat Disord. 2016;14(10):468–74.
45. Chiofalo B, Laganà AS, Palmara V, Granese R, Corrado G, Mancini E, Vitale SG, Ban Frangež H, Vrtačnik-Bokal E, Triolo O. Fasting as possible complementary approach for polycystic ovary syndrome: Hope or hype? Med Hypotheses. 2017;105:1–3.
46. Zhang HY, Zhang YF, Han YK, Xue FX, Zhao XH, Zhang XL. Activation and significance of the PI3K/Akt pathway in endometrium with polycystic ovary syndrome patients. Zhonghua Fu Chan Ke Za Zhi. 2012;47(1):19–23.
47. Kelley CE, Brown AJ, Diehl AM, Setji TL. Review of nonalcoholic fatty liver disease in women with polycystic ovary syndrome. World J Gastroenterol. 2014;20(39):14172–84.
48. Makker A, Goel MM, Das V, Agarwal A. PI3K-Akt-mTOR and MAPK signaling pathways in polycystic ovarian syndrome, uterine leiomyomas and endometriosis: an update. Gynecol Endocrinol. 2012;28(3):175–81.

16

HPLC–ICP-MS speciation analysis and risk assessment of arsenic in *Cordyceps sinensis*

Tian-Tian Zuo[†], Yao-Lei Li[†], Hong-Yu Jin, Fei Gao, Qi Wang, Ya-Dan Wang and Shuang-Cheng Ma[*]

Abstract

Background: *Cordyceps sinensis*, one of the most valued traditional herbal medicines in China, contains high amount of arsenic. Considering the adverse health effects of arsenic, this is of particular concern. The aim of this study was to determine and analyze arsenic speciation in *C. sinensis*, and to measure the associated human health risks.

Methods: We used microwave extraction and high-performance liquid chromatography coupled with inductively coupled plasma mass spectrometry to determine and analyze the arsenic content in *C. sinensis*, and measured the associated human health risks according to the hazard index (HI), lifetime cancer risk (CR), and target hazard quotient (THQ).

Results: The main arsenic speciation in *C. sinensis* were not the four organic arsenic compounds, including dimethyl arsenic, monomethyl arsenic, arsenobetaine, and arsenocholine, but comprised inorganic arsenic and other unknown risk arsenic compounds. HI scores indicated that the risk of *C. sinensis* was acceptable. CR results suggested that the cancer risk was greater than the acceptable lifetime risk of 10^{-5}, even at low exposure levels. THQ results indicated that at the exposure level < 2.0 months/year, the arsenic was not likely to harm human health during a lifetime; however, if the exposure rate was > 3.0 months/year, the systemic effects of the arsenic in *C. sinensis* was of great concern.

Conclusion: The arsenic in *C. sinensis* might not be free of risks. The suggested *C. sinensis* consumption rate of 2.0 months/year provided important insights into the ways by which to minimize potential health risks. Our study not only played the role of "cast a brick to attract jade" by which to analyze arsenic speciation in *C. sinensis* but also offered a promising strategy of risk assessment for harmful residues in traditional herbal medicines.

Keywords: Arsenic, Speciation, Inductively coupled plasma mass spectrometry (HPLC–ICP-MS), Risk assessment, Hazard index (HI), Lifetime cancer risk (CR), Target hazard quotient (THQ)

Background

Cordyceps sinensis (Berk.) Sacc. is the Chinese caterpillar fungus that consists of the stromata of the fungus. This fungus is also known as "winter worm summer grass" because of its appearance during different seasons [1]. *C. sinensis* is distributed mostly in Tibet and in the Qinghai, Sichuan, Yunnan, and Gansu Provinces in China at an altitude of 3500–5000 m. With various biological activities, *C. sinensis* has been considered as one of the most well-known and valued traditional medicinal herbs and has been used extensively for ailing patients in China and other Asian countries over the past 300 years. It is also officially listed in Pharmacopoeia of the People's Republic of China (PPRC) [2]. Its proposed therapeutic benefits include antitumor, antioxidant, antidiabetic, hepatoprotective, nephroprotective, diuretic, anti-inflammatory, and soothing asthma effects [3–9].

Heavy metals are ubiquitous environmental pollutants resulting from natural or anthropogenic activities such as waste disposal, coal combustion, mining, pesticides application and chemical fertilizer use, which can lead to the contamination of traditional herbal medicines,

*Correspondence: masc@nifdc.org.cn
[†]Tian-Tian Zuo and Yao-Lei Li contributed equally to this work
National Institutes for Food and Drug Control, No. 2 Tiantan Xili, Dongcheng District, Beijing 100050, China

including *C. sinensis*. Prolonged exposure to toxic heavy metals is responsible for a variety of detrimental effects on the health of the human body [10]. Recent studies have demonstrated the high content of heavy metals, specifically arsenic, in *C. sinensis* [11, 12].

Arsenic is a ubiquitous metalloid and is considered to be one of the most significant pollutants in the world, existing in both organic and inorganic forms. Different arsenic speciation displays different toxicity; therefore, it is important to identify this speciation in *C. sinensis*. It was reported that organic arsenic, found mainly as arsenobetaine (AsB), arsenosugars, and arsenolipids, presents often in seafood and is relatively nontoxic [13, 14]; however, inorganic arsenic, including As III and As V, has been demonstrated to be a human group I carcinogen without threshold [15]. Although the carcinogenic mechanisms of inorganic arsenic are not clear, it has been proposed that because of the interaction of inorganic arsenic with cysteine residues in zinc finger domains, the formation of complexes with inorganic arsenic results in the substitution of zinc and consequently DNA damage and the loss of protein function [16, 17]. Other health effects of inorganic arsenic include skin lesions, cardiovascular problems, diabetes, kidney dysfunction, respiratory infection, and immune system diseases [17–22]. For pregnant women, chronic inorganic arsenic exposure has caused excessive stillbirth, spontaneous abortion, and preterm birth rates [23]. In the previous study, the contents of high toxic elements including lead, cadmium, total mercury and total arsenic in *C. sinensis* were determined. The results displayed that except arsenic, the levels of other three types of heavy metals in *C. sinensis* were far below the limit for herbal medicines in PPRC [2]. However, the contents of total arsenic in *C. sinensis* were about four times higher than the arsenic limit for herbal medicines recorded in PPRC [2]. Considering the increase in the popularity of *C. sinensis* use in China in recent years and considering public health safety, it is crucial to determine the level of arsenic speciation in *C. sinensis* and the associated risks to human health. The objectives of our study are as follows: (1) determine the concentrations of total arsenic in *C. sinensis*; (2) develop method by which to determine the concentration levels of different speciation of arsenic in *C. sinensis* and compare them with total arsenic; (3) assess the associated potential risks to human health using hazard index (HI), cancer risk (CR), and target hazard quotient (THQ) scales by the rule of risk maximization and protecting most people, and provide consumption suggestions for *C. sinensis* to minimize these risks.

Methods

The Minimum Standards of Reporting Checklist contains details of the experimental design, and statistics, and resources used in this study (Additional file 1).

Reagents

Doubly deionized water was prepared using the Milli-Q (Millipore, Milford, MA, USA) water purification system. The arsenic mono-element standard solution (100.0 μg/mL), dimethyl arsenic (DMA), monomethyl arsenic (MMA), As III, As V, AsB, and arsenocholine (AsC) standard solution were purchased from National Standard Material Research Center (Beijing, China). The internal standard solution containing germanium (m/z = 74, 100.0 μg/mL) was purchased from Agilent (Agilent Technologies, Folsom, CA, USA). Suprapur trace metal grade concentrated nitric acid (HNO_3, 65.0%) was purchased from Merck (Merck, Munchen, Germany). Analytical grade ammonium carbonate ($[NH_4]_2CO_3$) was purchased from Beijing Chemical Reagent Co. (Beijing, China).

Herbs

Thirty four samples of *C. sinensis* were collected in batches from traditional herbal-medicine markets or retail pharmacies in Tibet and in Qinghai, Yunnan, and Sichuan Provinces, the areas in which *C. sinensis* is the most highly distributed in China (Table 1). All samples were authenticated by Mr. Shuai Kang. The voucher specimens were deposited in National Institutes for Food and Drug Control (NIFDC), Beijing, China.

Analysis of total arsenic in *C. sinensis*

Sample preparation

For total arsenic analysis, all samples were digested following the method officially listed in Pharmacopoeia of the People's Republic of China (PPRC) [2]. Briefly, the tested samples were ground into powder and 0.25 g was placed into microwave digestion vessels (CEM Corporation, Matthews, NC, USA). An additional 8.0 mL HNO_3 was mixed with the samples in the vessel. The microwave digestion procedures are shown in Table 2. After digestion, the samples were cooled to 60.0 °C, and the acid in the vessels was dispelled for 40.0 min. The digestion solution was then transferred into 50.0-mL volumetric flasks and diluted with Milli-Q water to volume.

Inductively coupled plasma mass spectrometry (ICP-MS) analysis of concentrations of total arsenic in C. sinensis

ICP-MS data were obtained using the Agilent 7700X ICP-MS (Agilent Technologies, Folsom, CA, USA). The ICP-MS system was calibrated before each batch of analysis using five point calibration curves ($R^2 > 0.999$). ICP-MS measurements were executed under the following conditions: plasma gas flow rate: 15.0 L/min; peristaltic pump: 0.2 r/s; atomizing chamber temperature: 2.0 °C; auxiliary gas flow rate: 0.8 L/min; He gas flow rate: 5.0 mL/min; carrier gas flow rate: 0.8 L/min; RF power: 1550 W; 100 sweeps; three replicates; sampling depth: 10.0 mm.

Table 1 Sample collection information in present study

Code	Collecting time	Location	Source
01	2016, 06	Yushu, Qinghai	Production site
02	2016, 06	Yushu, Qinghai	Production site
03	2016, 05	Guoluo, Qinghai	Production site
04	2016, 05	Guoluo, Qinghai	Production site
05	2016, 06	Guoluo, Qinghai	Production site
06	2016, 06	Guoluo, Qinghai	Production site
07	2016, 05	Hainan, Qinghai	Production site
08	2016, 06	Hainan, Qinghai	Production site
09	2016, 06	Hainan, Qinghai	Production site
10	2016, 05	Huangnan, Qinghai	Production site
11	2016, 05	Huangnan, Qinghai	Production site
12	2016, 06	Huangnan, Qinghai	Production site
13	2016, 06	Huangnan, Qinghai	Production site
14	2016, 06	Changdu, Tibet	Production site
15	2016, 06	Changdu, Tibet	Production site
16	2016, 06	Biru, Tibet	Production site
17	2016, 06	Suo, Tibet	Production site
18	2016, 06	Maqu, Gansu	Production site
19	2016, 06	Shiping, Yunnan	Production site
20	2016, 06	Ganzi, Sichuan	Production site
21	2016, 05	Litang, Sichuan	Production site
22	2016, 06	Gannan, Qinghai	Production site
23	2016, 06	Shannan, Tibet	Production site
24	2016, 06	Naqu, Tibet	Production site
25	2016, 06	Guoluo, Qinghai	Market
26	2016, 06	Guoluo, Qinghai	Market
27	2016, 06	Guoluo, Qinghai	Market
28	2016, 06	Biru, Tibet	Market
29	2016, 06	Maqu, Gansu	Market
30	2016, 06	Ganzi, Sichuan	Market
31	2016, 06	Yushu, Qinghai	Market
32	2016, 06	Guoluo, Qinghai	Pharmacy
33	2016, 06	Yushu, Qinghai	Pharmacy
34	2016, 06	Ganzi, Sichuan	Pharmacy

Table 2 Microwave digestion program

	Step		
	I	II	III
Power (%)	100	Parameter	100
Time (min)	3	3	12
Temperature (°C)	120	150	200

For quality control, blanks and duplicate samples were analyzed during the procedure. Germanium (m/z 74) was used as the internal standard and added to the blanks, samples, and calibration standards to compensate for matrix effects and signal drift. The mean percent recovery of the internal standard solution was 102.6%; the mean percent recovery of total arsenic was 116.3% (n = 34).

Concentration levels of arsenic speciation

Preparation of mixed arsenic reference standard solution

The mixed arsenic standard solution of six speciations comprising DMA, MMA, AsIII, AsV, AsB, and AsC was diluted to a series concentrations of 10.0, 20.0, 50.0, 100.0, 250.0, and 500.0 μg/L by Milli-Q water that was prepared for speciation analysis.

Sample preparation

The samples were ground into powder and 0.25 g was placed into the 50.0-mL glass tubes that were matched with the microwave extraction system (CEM Corporation, Matthews, NC, USA), after which 10.0 mL HNO_3 (1.4 mol/L) were added to the glass tubes. The samples were extracted using the microwave extraction system at 70.0 °C for 10.0 min. After cooling to room temperature, the samples were filtrated through 0.22-μm membranes.

High performance liquid chromatography (HPLC)–ICP-MS analysis of the concentration levels of different speciation of arsenic in C. sinensis

The different speciation of arsenic was analyzed by HPLC–ICP-MS. HPLC conditions included a gradient HPLC system using $(NH_4)_2CO_3$ (mobile phase A) and water (mobile phase B) at a flow rate of 0.5 mL/min to separate the analytes on an anion-exchange column (Agilent AS7 column, 4.6 × 250 mm, 5.0 μm particle size). The analysis was conducted according to the following procedures: for eluent A: 10.0% initial proportion; a linear increase to 50.0% at 3.0 min and to 100.0% at 4.0 min; keep to 11.0 min; linear decrease to 10.0% at 13.0 min; keep equilibrium for 17.0 min. The total acquisition time was 17.0 min. The injection volume was 10.0 μL.

Health risk assessment of arsenic in *C. sinensis*

HI

Hazard index is calculated using the estimated weekly intake (EWI) for a contaminant divided by the provisional tolerable weekly intake (PTWI) [24]. The World Health Organization (WHO) recommended the PTWI for inorganic arsenic to be 15.0 μg/kg body weight (bw) [25]. If HI > 1.0, the risk is unacceptable [26].

$$\text{EWI} = 7 \times \text{maximum daily consumption of } C.\ sinensis \times \text{concentration of inorganic arsenic/W}.$$

According to PPRC, the recommended maximum daily consumption of *C. sinensis* is 9.0 g [2]. The concentration of inorganic arsenic is the average inorganic arsenic concentration detected; W is the average body weight. According to statistical data from the National Health and Family Planning Commission of the People's Republic of China, the average adult female body weight and average adult male body weight in China in 2015 were 57.3 and 66.2 kg, respectively.

CR

Lifetime cancer risk for inorganic arsenic was expressed by the cancer slope factor (CSF) according to the U.S. Environmental Protection Agency (USEPA). If CR risk is larger than the acceptable lifetime risk of 10^{-5} considered by USEPA, there is a probability of a > 1 in 100,000 chance of an individual developing cancer [27]. CR is obtained by the following equation [28]:

$$CR = EF \times Ed \times FIR \times C \times CFS \times 0.001/W \times AT,$$

where EF is the exposure frequency or number of exposure events per year (from 365.0 day/year for people who consumes *C. sinensis* every month to 30.0 day/year for people who consumes *C. sinensis* in only 1.0 month/year); Ed is the exposure duration and is equivalent to the average lifetime. According to the statistical data from WHO, the average lifetime of an adult Chinese female is 77.0 years and the average lifetime of adult Chinese male is 74.0 years; FIR is the *C. sinensis* ingestion rate. In this study, we used PPRC's provision for *C. sinensis*, the maximum daily ingestion rate of which is 9.0 g/day [2]. CSF is the cancer slope factor for inorganic arsenic provided by USEPA, which is 1.5 $(\mu g/g/day)^{-1}$. C is the arsenic concentration in *C. sinensis*; W is the average body weight; AT is the average exposure time for *C. sinensis* (365.0 day/year × Ed).

THQ

Target hazard quotient is calculated using the formula provided by USEPA as follows:

$$THQ = EF \times Ed \times FIR \times C \times 0.001/RfD \times W \times AT,$$

where RfD is the oral reference dose for arsenic recommended as 3.0×10^{-4} µg/g/day. The other parameters in the equation are the same as those for CR. THQ is calculated using the ratio between the exposure and the reference dose. If THQ is < 1, considered by USEPA, no adverse health effects are expected as a result of exposure. If THQ is > 1, meaning that it is higher than the reference dose, the health of the exposed population is of concern [29].

Statistical analysis

A frequency distribution was performed to determine the relationship between the sum contents of As III and As V in *C. sinensis* and their frequencies using SPSS 19.0 (IBM Corporation, Armonk, NY, USA). Statistical analysis was performed to compute the significant differences among the sum contents of As III and As V in the endosclerotium, stroma, and the whole *C. sinensis* by one-way analysis of variance (ANOVA) using GraphPad 5.0 Software (San Diego, CA, USA), applying $p < 0.001$ as the minimum level of significance.

Results

From the results of "Method validation" section in the present study, it was demonstrated that the four organic arsenic speciations (AsB, DMA, MMA, AsC) were not transformed to inorganic arsenic speciations or other organic arsenic compounds. But it is still not clear that except the four organic speciations, whether other organic arsenic speciations with unknown chemical structure, toxicity or risk, which were called "unknown risk arsenic compounds" in the present study, transformed to inorganic arsenic speciations or not. Nevertheless, considering the primary purpose of the study was to evaluate the risk of *C. sinensis* complying with the rule of risk maximization in order to protect most people. Therefore, in the process of health risk assessment, the risks of *C. sinensis* were maximized, and the unknown risk arsenic compounds were assumed as the inorganic arsenic with high toxicity to obtain a relatively conservative conclusion to protect most people. And the AsIII and AsV in the "Results" section in the study represents "AsIII and unknown risk arsenic compounds" and "AsV and unknown risk arsenic compounds", respectively.

Results of total arsenic and arsenic speciation analysis in *C. sinensis*

The contents of arsenic speciation in 34 batches of *C. sinensis* were analyzed using the established HPLC–ICP-MS method. The representative ion chromatograms for typical separation of different arsenics are shown in Fig. 1. The contents of different arsenic speciation in the samples are shown in Table 3.

The analysis results for arsenic speciation (Fig. 1a) showed that different arsenic speciation was well separated. Figure 1b and Table 3 indicate that the dominant speciations in the *C. sinensis* samples were not four organic arsenic (AsB, DMA, AsC, and MMA) but As III and As V. Statistical analysis showed that the frequency distribution of the sum content of As III and As V in 34 batches of samples was normal, and the sum content of As III and As V in most samples (> 50.0%) ranged from 6.50 to 10.50 mg/kg (Fig. 2a). Furthermore, the total arsenic contents in 34 batches of *C. sinensis* were experimentally compared with the different arsenic speciation in the samples. The results showed that the total arsenic contents in *C. sinensis* were within the range of

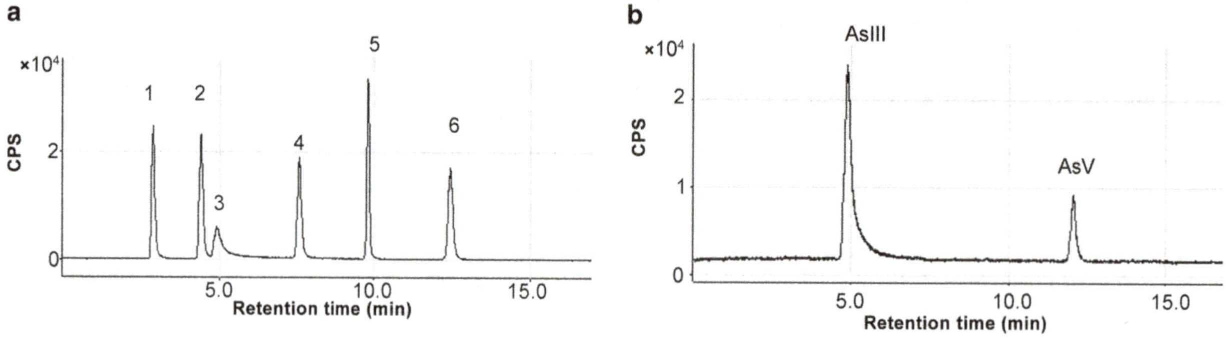

Fig. 1 Representative ion chromatograms for arsenic speciation. **a** Arsenic speciation of mixed arsenic standard solution. 1–6 represented AsB, DMA, AsIII, MMA, AsC, and AsV, respectively. **b** Arsenic speciation in *Cordyceps sinensis*

Table 3 Contents of different arsenic speciation in *Cordyceps sinensis* (mg/kg, n = 34)

AsB	DMA	AsIII[a]	AsC	MMA	AsV	Total arsenic
ND	ND	6.68 ± 2.68	ND	ND	1.84 ± 1.15	8.53 ± 3.49

ND not detected

[a] Data are represented as the mean ± SD

2.12–15.51 mg/kg; the mean content was 8.32 mg/kg. The sum content of As III and As V in 34 batches of samples ranged from 2.31 to 18.71 mg/kg; the mean content was 8.53 mg/kg (Fig. 2b). The average deviation between the total arsenic contents and the sum contents of As III and As V was ~ 0.15%. We found that the extraction efficiency of the optimized procedure was > 99.0%, and the results from the ICP-MS method for the detection of total arsenic contents were in excellent agreement with the results obtained from the HPLC–ICP-MS method for the detection of all of the different speciations (Table 4).

Moreover, arsenic speciation in fungal endosclerotium, stroma, and the whole *C. sinensis* of the five batches were analyzed. Statistical analysis indicated that the sum level of As III and As V in fungal endosclerotium was significantly higher ($p < 0.001$) than that in stroma. But there was no significant difference between the sum level of As III and As V in fungal endosclerotium and in the whole *C. sinensis* ($p > 0.05$). A clear trend was observed that both As III and As V were found mainly in the fungal endosclerotium (Table 5, Fig. 3).

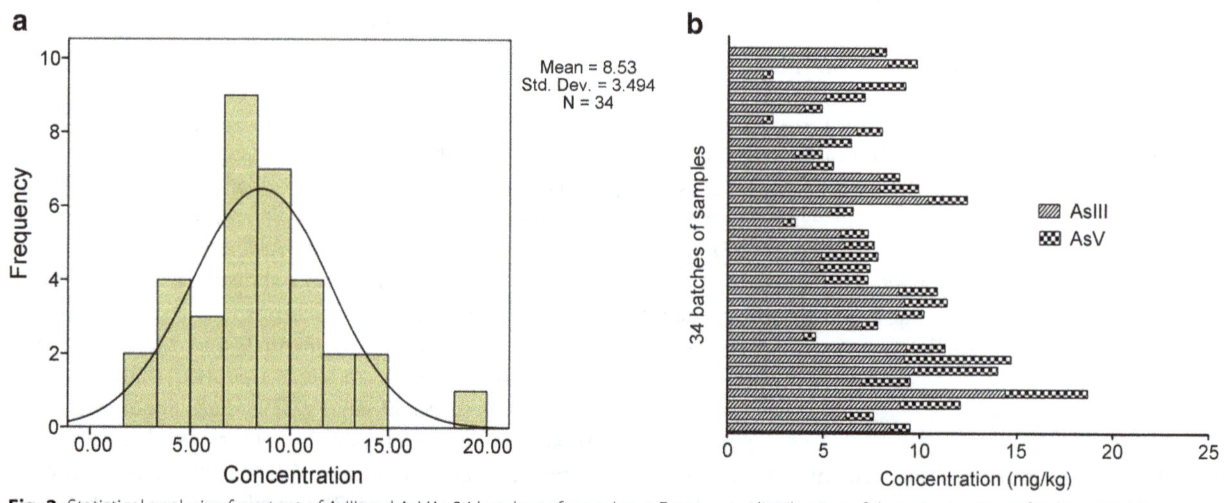

Fig. 2 Statistical analysis of content of AsIII and AsV in 34 batches of samples. **a** Frequency distribution of the sum content of AsIII and AsV in samples. **b** Sum content of AsIII and AsV in samples

Table 4 Extraction efficiency using the optimized method

AsIII (mg/kg)	AsV (mg/kg)	AsIII + AsV (mg/kg)[a]	Total arsenic (mg/kg)[b]	Extraction efficiency (%)[c]
6.67 ± 2.68[d]	1.84 ± 1.15	8.53 ± 3.49	8.32 ± 3.25	99.85 ± 0.007

[a] Sum of AsIII and AsV was determined by high-performance liquid chromatography coupled with inductively coupled plasma mass spectrometer spectrometry (HPLC–ICP-MS)

[b] Total arsenic was determined using ICP-MS after digestion

[c] Ratio of AsIII + AsV to total arsenic

[d] Data are represented as mean value ± standard deviation (n = 34)

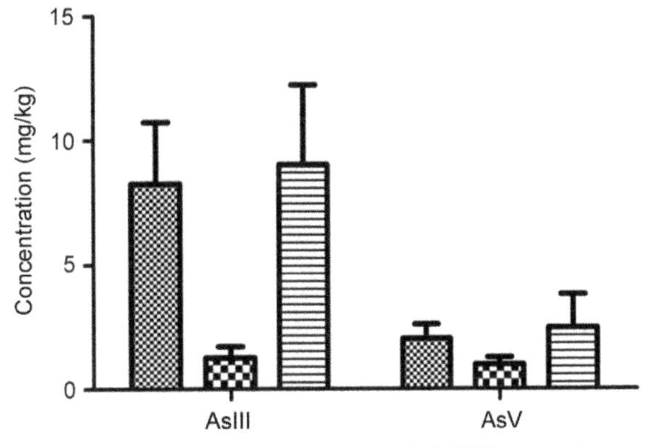

Fig. 3 AsIII and AsV contents analyzed in fungal endosclerotium, stroma, and the whole *Cordyceps sinensis*

Health risk assessment of arsenic in *C. sinensis*

Estimated weekly intake was calculated and compared to PTWI suggested by the Food and Agriculture Organization of the United Nations (FAO)/WHO expert to determine HI of females and males. HI of females and males for inorganic arsenic was 0.6 and 0.5, respectively, which was lower than the critical value of 1; therefore, as seen from HI values, the health risk associated with inorganic arsenic in *C. sinensis* was assumed to be acceptable.

To assess the cancer risk, CR vales were above the acceptable lifetime risk of 10^{-5} for all levels of assumed exposure for *C. sinensis* (Table 6). This indicated that even at the minimum stage of exposure, which was presumed to be 1.0 month/year, the probability of a > 1 in 100,000 chance of an individual developing cancer.

Target hazard quotient proposed by USEPA is a complicated parameter used to estimate the potential health risks associated with long-term exposure to chemical pollutants by comparing the ingested amount of a contaminant with a standard reference dose. The inorganic arsenic THQ values (Table 6) were estimated to be < 1 for *C. sinensis* if the exposure was assumed to be < 2.0 months/year, especially for males; therefore, at exposure levels < 2.0 months/year, it is not likely to cause any deleterious effects to human health during a lifetime. On the contrary, for exposure levels > 3.0 months/year, the systemic effects of arsenic in *C. sinensis* were assumed to be of concern in terms of the health risks for both females and males; therefore, the maximum allowable *C. sinensis* rate for both males and females was stated as 2.0 months/year, which was the suggested THQ value for exposure levels to avoid the harmful systemic effects.

The THQ index used in risk assessment of arsenic offers a better picture than a simple parameter, such as the contents of arsenic in *C. sinensis*. It involves not only the content level of contaminants but also important information of exposure frequency, exposure duration, RfD, and body weight. The method for estimating THQ cannot be translated into a quantitative estimate on the probability of health effects occurring in a given exposed population, and it is unlikely to be proportional to the risk. THQ > 1 does not necessarily suggest that there will be definite adverse effects, but it does indicate that the systemic effects are assumed to be of concern [30, 31]. In our study, because of the differences in body weight, the THQ values were higher for females than males [32–34]. It should not be ignored that factors such as contaminant bioavailability, the uncertainty factor regarding RfD, and contaminant transfer rates from raw herbal medicines to decoction also play important roles in the THQ value [35]; therefore, THQ is designed to be a conservative estimate, and further research is needed to be able

Table 5 Arsenic speciation analysis in *Cordyceps sinensis* from different parts (mg/kg, n = 5)

Part	Concentration						
	AsB	DMA	AsIII[a]	AsC	MMA	AsV	Total
Endosclerotium	ND	ND	8.26 ± 2.47	ND	ND	2.02 ± 0.57	10.26 ± 2.79
Stroma	ND	ND	1.26 ± 0.45	ND	ND	0.98 ± 0.29	2.24 ± 0.48
The whole *C. sinensis*	ND	ND	9.02 ± 3.21	ND	ND	2.46 ± 1.33	11.54 ± 4.33

ND detected

[a] Data are represented as the mean ± SD

Table 6 THQ and CR estimated for inorganic arsenic at different levels of exposure

Level of exposure (months per year)	THQ		CR	
	Female	Male	Female	Male
1	0.36	0.32	1.6×10^{-4}	1.4×10^{-4}
2	0.73	0.63	3.3×10^{-4}	2.8×10^{-4}
6	2.19	1.89	9.9×10^{-4}	8.4×10^{-4}
12	4.38	3.78	2.0×10^{-3}	1.7×10^{-3}

to offer guidance on applicable value choices for the risk assessment of harmful contaminants in traditional herbal medicines, including *C. sinensis.*

Discussion

Optimization of sample preparation for arsenic speciation analysis

The analysis of arsenic speciation in *C. sinensis* is challenging. An acceptable method should extract most of the arsenic from the matrix without altering speciation or producing toxic waste. For determining optimal extraction conditions, a variety of extraction methods have been developed. The extraction method (shaking, enzymolysis, ultrasonic extraction, and microwave extraction), extraction solvents (50.0% methanol; 50.0% acetonitrile; hydrochloric acid of 1.0, 5.0, and 10.0%; 1.4 mol/L HNO_3; artificial gastric juice; and artificial intestinal juice), extraction temperatures (room temperature, 40.0, 50.0, or 70.0 °C) and extraction times (10.0, 20.0, or 120.0 min) were optimized. One of the criterions for selecting extraction method was based on the recovery, for which the degradation of the target analytes was expected to be minimum. The results demonstrated that microwave extraction was the most effective of all extraction methods. Extraction time was another factor that microwave extraction was applied in the present study. It was indicated that the target samples could be extracted completely within 10.0 min. As compared with other methods of extraction, microwave extraction took much less time. And a closed system of microwave extraction guaranteed a sealed experimental environment which prevented contamination [36].

Microwave extraction technology is a new and efficient extraction technology for the extraction of chemicals from food or herbal medicines. A high-frequency electromagnetic wave is necessary to penetrate the medium for extraction and then the heat energy is converted [36]. The cells rupture and the intracellular active ingredients discharge and dissolve in the extraction medium at a relatively low temperature. With these mechanisms, the extraction rate increases several times at a relatively low temperature and guarantees the quality of extraction to the highest extent. It was also observed that 1.4 mol/L HNO_3 was the most efficient of all the solvents. Above all, the sample solutions were prepared by microwave extraction with 1.4 mol/L HNO_3 for 10.0 min.

Optimization of chromatographic condition

A variety of mobile phase systems ($(NH_4)_2CO_3$–water, NH_4HCO_3–water, $(NH_4)_2HPO_4$–water, and $NH_4H_2PO_4$–water) were investigated in order to achieve an appropriate chromatographic behavior. The $(NH_4)_2CO_3$–water system was selected because it offered the best peak shape and resolution of the target analytes. Different concentrations of $(NH4)_2CO_3$ solution and flow rate were also tested. Finally, 0.1 mol/L $(NH_4)_2CO_3$–water eluting solvent system at a flow rate of 0.5 mL/min was preferred, because it produced a satisfactory separation efficiency, good ionization intensity and low baseline noise. Furthermore, the elution gradient programs were then optimized.

Method validation

Linearity, limit of detection (LOD), limit of quantification (LOQ), precision, and the accuracy of the developed HPLC–ICP-MS method for the analysis of arsenic speciation were tested following the criteria for the validation of an analytical method. The precision of the method was tested using relative standard deviation (RSD).

The calibration curves for all the six speciations of arsenic were expressed by plotting the peak area (y) versus concentration (x) of each analyte, as shown in Table 7.

The samples with known contents were diluted to a series of concentrations and prepared and analyzed using the method previously described. LODs and LOQs based on the signal–noise ratios of three and ten times, was 2.0 and 10.0 ng/mL, respectively.

To confirm the repeatability of the developed method, six samples from the same source were extracted and analyzed using the previously mentioned method. The RSD value for inorganic arsenic and unknown risk arsenic compounds, the main speciation found in the target

Table 7 Calibration curves and correlation coefficients of all arsenic speciations

Speciation	Calibration curves	r^2
AsB	$y=1920x-5817.1$	0.9999
DMA	$y=1905x-1457.1$	1.0000
AsIII	$y=1070.7x-5547$	0.9993
AsC	$y=1743.2x-1003.9$	0.9999
MMA	$y=1833.5x+7428.9$	0.9988
AsV	$y=1844.8x+882.21$	0.9998

Table 8 Recovery rates of the developed method (n = 6)

Specifications	Original (ng)[a]	Spiked amount (ng)	Determined amount (ng)	Recovery rate (%)	RSD (%)
AsB	ND[b]	103.75	97.95 ± 2.38	94.41 ± 0.02	2.43
DMA	ND	99.50	106.00 ± 0.70	106.53 ± 0.007	0.66
AsIII	15.96 ± 0.01	100.20	110.29 ± 3.30	94.14 ± 0.03	3.49
MMA	ND	100.12	97.73 ± 2.26	97.61 ± 0.02	2.31
As III[c]	ND	100.02	108.88 ± 1.73	108.86 ± 0.01	1.59
As V[d]	3.39 ± 0.35	100.97	102.43 ± 1.22	98.09 ± 0.01	1.18

[a] Data are represented as the mean ± SD

[b] ND = not detected

[c] AsIII represents AsIII and unknown risk arsenic compounds

[d] AsV represents AsV and unknown risk arsenic compounds

samples, was 3.90%, indicating good repeatability of the method.

The accuracy was determined by the mean recovery rate of the target samples. A known amount of the mixed standard solution was added to 0.25 g of the samples. The spiked samples were then extracted and analyzed using the method described above. As shown in Table 8, the mean recovery rates for different speciations of arsenic were in the range of 94.14–106.53%, with RSD values < 3.50%.

Conclusion

In this study, we developed the HPLC–ICP-MS method to determine the contents of arsenic speciation in *C. sinensis*. The optimized microwave extraction procedures, which were a new technology for pretreatment of traditional herbal medicines, saved time and resulted in a satisfactory extraction efficiency (> 99.0%). It was demonstrated that the main speciation of arsenic in *C. sinensis* were the inorganic arsenic and unknown risk arsenic compounds. We first assessed the health risk using HI, CR, and THQ parameters. HI suggested that the health risk for consumption of *C. sinensis* was acceptable. CR provided that even at the lowest exposure stage of 1.0 month/year, the risk of cancer should not be ignored. THQ indicated that at an exposure level < 2.0 months/year, ingestion was not likely to harm human health during a lifetime; however, if the exposure was > 3.0 months/year, the systemic effects of inorganic arsenic in *C. sinensis* might be of concern. These results indicating the recommended *C. sinensis* consumption rate of 2.0 months/year provided important input on the exposure suggestion or consumption limits to minimize potential health risks.

For *C. sinensis*, arsenic exposure is a significant worldwide environmental and health concern. It was reported that there were a number of organic arsenic compounds, however, the speciation, toxicity or risk were unclear [37]. For further research, there is still a lot to explore in terms of these unknown risk arsenic compounds. I hope our study played the role of "cast a brick to attract jade" to analyze arsenic speciations in *C. sinensis*. Continuous monitoring of arsenic speciation levels and the evaluation of the risks in *C. sinensis* are necessary. Further research is also needed in the interest of public health, including studying the techniques able to reduce heavy metal translocation in traditional herbal medicines. In the meantime, new methods by which to artificially reproduce *C. sinensis* with low arsenic residues are desirable.

The risk assessment methods for traditional herbal medicines are still in the exploration stages. We have focused more on determining contaminant contents in traditional herbal medicines; however, the contents of the contaminants at a high level or even exceeding the legal limits do not always represent risks for human health. Therefore, after obtaining the levels of contaminants by using modern technology, the methods of risk assessment for harmful residues or contaminants in traditional herbal medicines will be a new trend and of great significance. Thus, we hope that our study plays a role in providing new ideas for quality control and evaluation of traditional herbal medicines by the rule of risk maximization. We also hope that the combination of modern instrument analysis and risk assessment methods for traditional herbal medicines can be promoted and developed to scientifically evaluate possible risks regarding human health hazards.

Abbreviations

AsB: arsenobetaine; AsC: arsenocholine; CR: lifetime cancer risk; CSF: cancer slope factor; DMA: dimethyl arsenic; EWI: estimated weekly intake; HI: hazard index; HPLC–ICP-MS: high-performance liquid chromatography coupled with inductively coupled plasma mass spectrometry; ICP-MS: inductively coupled plasma mass spectrometry; LOD: limit of detection; LOQ: limit of quantification; MMA: monomethyl arsenic; PPRC: Pharmacopoeia of the People's Republic of China; PTWI: provisional tolerable weekly intake; RSD: relative standard deviation; THQ: target hazard quotient.

Authors' contributions

SCM and HYJ designed the study. YLL and TTZ conducted the experiments. TTZ and YYL analyzed the data. TTZ wrote the manuscript. SCM, FG, QW, and YDW revised the manuscript. All authors read and approved the final manuscript.

Acknowledgements

We would like to appreciate Dr. Yuanjun Shen from University of Rhode Island and Mr. Shuai Kang from NIFDC for the valuable suggestion on this paper.

Competing interests

The authors declare that they have no competing interests.

Consent for publication

Not applicable.

Funding

This study was supported by the National Major Scientific and Technological Special Project for "Significant New Drugs Development" (2014ZX09304307-002) and Project for Medicine and Medical Instruments Review and Approval System Reform (ZG2016-1).

References

1. Li SP, Yang FQ, Tsim KW. Quality control of *Cordyceps sinensis*, a valued traditional Chinese medicine. J Pharm Biomed Anal. 2006;41:1571–84. https://doi.org/10.1016/j.jpba.2006.01.046.
2. The Pharmacopoeia Commission of PRC. Pharmacopoeia of the People's Republic of China. Beijing: Chinese Medical Science and Technology Press; 2015.
3. Kuo YC, Tsai WJ, Wang JY, Chang SC, Lin CY, Shiao MS. Regulation of bronchoalveolar lavage fluids cell function by the immunomodulatory agents from *Cordyceps sinensis*. Life Sci. 2001;68:1067–82.
4. Chen YC, Huang YL, Huang BM. *Cordyceps sinensis* mycelium activates PKA and PKC signal pathways to stimulate steroidogenesis in MA-10 mouse Leydig tumor cells. Int J Biochem Cell Biol. 2005;37:214–23. https://doi.org/10.1016/j.biocel.2004.05.019.
5. Yamaguchi N, Yoshida J, Ren LJ, Chen H, Miyazawa Y, Fujii Y, et al. Augmentation of various immune reactivities of tumor-bearing hosts with an extract of *Cordyceps sinensis*. Biotherapy. 1990;2:199–205.
6. Kuo CF, Chen CC, Lin CF, Jan MS, Huang RY, Luo YH, et al. Abrogation of streptococcal pyrogenic exotoxin B-mediated suppression of phagocytosis in U937 cells by *Cordyceps sinensis* mycelium via production of cytokines. Food Chem Toxicol. 2007;45:278–85. https://doi.org/10.1016/j.fct.2006.08.017.
7. Lo HC, Hsu TH, Tu ST, Lin KC. Anti-hyperglycemic activity of natural and fermented *Cordyceps sinensis* in rats with diabetes induced by nicotinamide and streptozotocin. Am J Chin Med. 2006;34:819–32. https://doi.org/10.1142/s0192415x06004314.
8. Nakamura K, Konoha K, Yamaguchi Y, Kagota S, Shinozuka K, Kunitomo M. Combined effects of *Cordyceps sinensis* and methotrexate on hematogenic lung metastasis in mice. Receptors Channels. 2003;9:329–34.
9. Lu YL, Wen KM. Study on pharmacological action of *Cordyceps sinensis*. Chin Pharmacist. 2003;6:371–2.
10. Concha G, Vogler G, Lezcano D, Nermell B, Vahter M. Exposure to inorganic arsenic metabolites during early human development. Toxicol Sci. 1998;44:185–90. https://doi.org/10.1006/toxs.1998.2486.
11. Zuo TT, Li YL, Jin HY, Ma SC. Determination of residues of heavy metals and harmful elements in 18 types of animal medicines by ICP-MS and preliminary risk analysis. Chin J Pharm Anal. 2017;37:237–42.
12. Liu J, Li YL, Zan K, Zheng J, Guo LN, Ma SC, et al. A comparative study on the content of Pb, Cd, As, Hg and Cu between cultivated and natural *Cordyceps Sinensis*. Chin Pharm Affa. 2016;30:912–8.
13. Davis MA, Mackenzie TA, Cottingham KL, Gilbert-Diamond D, Punshon T, Karagas MR. Rice consumption and urinary arsenic concentrations in US children. Environ Health Perspect. 2012;120:1418–24. https://doi.org/10.1289/ehp.1205014.
14. Navas-Acien A, Francesconi KA, Silbergeld EK, Guallar E. Seafood intake and urine concentrations of total arsenic, dimethylarsinate and arsenobetaine in the US population. Environ Res. 2011;111:110–8. https://doi.org/10.1016/j.envres.2010.10.009.
15. IARC Working Group on the Evaluation of Carcinogenic Risks to Humans, World Health Organization, International Agency for Research on Cancer. Some drinking-water disinfectants and contaminants, including arsenic. IARC Monogr Eval Carcinog Risks Hum, vol. 84. Lyon: IARC; 2004. p. 1–477.
16. NRC, Committee on Toxicology. Arsenic in drinking water. Washington, DC: The National Academic Press; 2001.
17. Sirot V, Guerin T, Volatier JL, Leblanc JC. Dietary exposure and biomarkers of arsenic in consumers of fish and shellfish from France. Sci Total Environ. 2009;407:1875–85. https://doi.org/10.1016/j.scitotenv.2008.11.050.
18. Barker DJ. The origins of the developmental origins theory. J Intern Med. 2007;261:412–7. https://doi.org/10.1111/j.1365-2796.2007.01809.x.
19. Srivastava S, D'Souza SE, Sen U, States JC. In utero arsenic exposure induces early onset of atherosclerosis in ApoE−/− mice. Reprod Toxicol. 2007;23:449–56. https://doi.org/10.1016/j.reprotox.2007.01.005.
20. Kaltreider RC, Davis AM, Lariviere JP, Hamilton JW. Arsenic alters the function of the glucocorticoid receptor as a transcription factor. Environ Health Perspect. 2001;109:245–51.
21. Rahman A, Vahter M, Ekstrom EC, Persson LA. Arsenic exposure in pregnancy increases the risk of lower respiratory tract infection and diarrhea during infancy in Bangladesh. Environ Health Perspect. 2011;119:719–24. https://doi.org/10.1289/ehp.1002265.
22. Davey JC, Nomikos AP, Wungjiranirun M, Sherman JR, Ingram L, Batki C, et al. Arsenic as an endocrine disruptor: arsenic disrupts retinoic acid receptor-and thyroid hormone receptor-mediated gene regulation and thyroid hormone-mediated amphibian tail metamorphosis. Environ Health Perspect. 2008;116:165–72. https://doi.org/10.1289/ehp.10131.
23. Tofail F, Vahter M, Hamadani JD, Nermell B, Huda SN, Yunus M, et al. Effect of arsenic exposure during pregnancy on infant development at 7 months in rural Matlab, Bangladesh. Environ Health Perspect. 2009;117:288–93. https://doi.org/10.1289/ehp.11670.
24. Antonijevic B, Jankovic S, Curcic M, Durgo K, Stokic E, Srdic B, et al. Risk characterization for mercury, dichlorodiphenyltrichloroethane and polychlorinated biphenyls associated with fish consumption in Serbia. Food Chem Toxicol. 2011;49:2586–93. https://doi.org/10.1016/j.fct.2011.06.078.
25. Evaluation of Certain Food Additives. Seventy-second meeting of the Joint FAO/WHO Expert Committee on Food Additives. World Health Organ Tech Rep Ser. 20101–105, back cover.
26. Özden Ö, Erkan N. Evaluation of risk characterization for mercury, cadmium, lead and arsenic associated with seafood consumption in Turkey. Expo Health. 2016;8:43–52. https://doi.org/10.1007/s12403-015-0181-7.
27. US-EPA. Guidance for assessing chemical contamination data for use in fish advisories. Risk assessment and fish consumption limits, vol. II. Washington, DC: United States Environmental Protection Agency; 2000.
28. US-EPA. Risk assessment guidance for superfund. Human health evaluation manual (Part A), interim final, vol. I. Washington, DC: United States Environmental Protection Agency; 1989.
29. US-EPA. Guidance manual for assessing human health risks from chemically contaminated, fish and shellfish US. Washington, DC: Environmental Protection Agency; 1989.
30. Naughton DP, Petroczi A. Heavy metal ions in wines: meta-analysis of target hazard quotients reveal health risks. Chem Cent J. 2008;2:22. https://doi.org/10.1186/1752-153x-2-22.
31. Harmanescu M, Alda LM, Bordean DM, Gogoasa I, Gergen I. Heavy metals health risk assessment for population via consumption of vegetables grown in old mining area; a case study: Banat County, Romania. Chem Cent J. 2011;5:64. https://doi.org/10.1186/1752-153x-5-64.
32. Hague T, Petroczi A, Andrews PL, Barker J, Naughton DP. Determination of metal ion content of beverages and estimation of target hazard quotients: a comparative study. Chem Cent J. 2008;2:13. https://doi.org/10.1186/1752-153x-2-13.
33. Petroczi A, Naughton DP. Mercury, cadmium and lead contamination in seafood: a comparative study to evaluate the usefulness of target

hazard quotients. Food Chem Toxicol. 2009;47:298–302. https://doi.org/10.1016/j.fct.2008.11.007.

34. Khan S, Farooq R, Shahbaz S, Khan MA, Sadique M. Health risk assessment of heavy metals for population via consumption of vegetables. World Appl Sci J. 2009;6:1602–6.
35. Ting A, Chow Y, Tan W. Microbial and heavy metal contamination in commonly consumed traditional Chinese herbal medicines. J Tradit Chin Med. 2013;33:119–24.
36. Routray W, Orsat V. Microwave-assisted extraction of flavonoids: a review. Food Bioprocess Technol. 2012;5:409–24.
37. Tchounwou PB, Patlolla A, Centeno JA. Carcinogenic and systemic health effects associated with arsenic exposure–a critical review. Toxicol Pathol. 2003;31:575–88.

17

Systems biology approaches in the study of Chinese herbal formulae

Fei-Fei Cai, Wen-Jun Zhou, Rong Wu and Shi-Bing Su*

Abstract

Systems biology is an academic field that attempts to integrate different levels of information to understand how biological systems function. It is the study of the composition of all components of a biological system and their interactions under specific conditions. The core of systems biology is holistic and systematic research, which is different from the manner of thinking and research of all other branches of biology to date. Chinese herbal formulae (CHF) are the main form of Chinese medicine and are composed of single Chinese herbal medicines (CHMs) with pharmacological and pharmacodynamic compatibility. When single CHMs are combined into CHF, the result is different from the original effect of a single drug and can be better adapted to more diseases with complex symptoms. CHF represent a complex system with multiple components, targets and effects. Therefore, the use of systems biology is conducive to revealing the complex characteristics of CHF. With the rapid development of omics technologies, systems biology has been widely and increasingly applied to the study of the basis of the pharmacological substances, action targets and mechanisms of CHF. To meet the challenges of multiomics synthesis-intensive studies and system dynamics research in CHF, this paper reviews the common techniques of genomics, transcriptomics, proteomics, metabolomics, and metagenomics and their applications in research on CHF.

Keywords: Systems biology, Chinese herbal formulae, Chinese medicine, Omics

Introduction

Chinese herbal formulae (CHF) are the main forms of prescription for the clinical application of Chinese medicine (CM) and embody the holistic philosophy of CM and the characteristics of treatment according to syndrome differentiation. The complexity of the chemical compositions and the diversity of the prescription compatibility and therapeutic functions of CHF have long presented great difficulties in the research of CM [1]. In contrast to the single compounds of Western medicine, which have specific targets and definite modes of action, CHF contain many types of components. The effects of these chemical components not only are superimposed but also interact with each other through multiple targets, pathways and mechanisms [2, 3]. Slow progress in the research on the pharmacological mechanisms of CHF has hindered their application and popularization throughout the world, thus becoming one of the key scientific problems to be solved in the modernization of CM.

Systems biology studies the interactions among different parts of a biological system at the cellular, tissue, organ and biological levels, and it quantitatively describes and predicts biological functions, phenotypes and behaviors through bioinformatics and through the computational and mathematical modeling of complex biological systems [4, 5]. Systems biology is an interdisciplinary field of study that focuses on complex interactions within biological systems, using a holistic approach instead of the more traditional reductionism of biological research. Systems biology is characterized by holistic and systematic research and explores the laws of life "from surface to point", corresponding to the holistic view of CM. The process of applying systems biology for CHF research is summarized and illustrated in Fig. 1.

With the development of high-throughput technologies and data analysis methods, such as genomics,

*Correspondence: shibingsu07@163.com
Research Center for Traditional Chinese Medicine Complexity System, Shanghai University of Traditional Chinese Medicine, Shanghai 201203, China

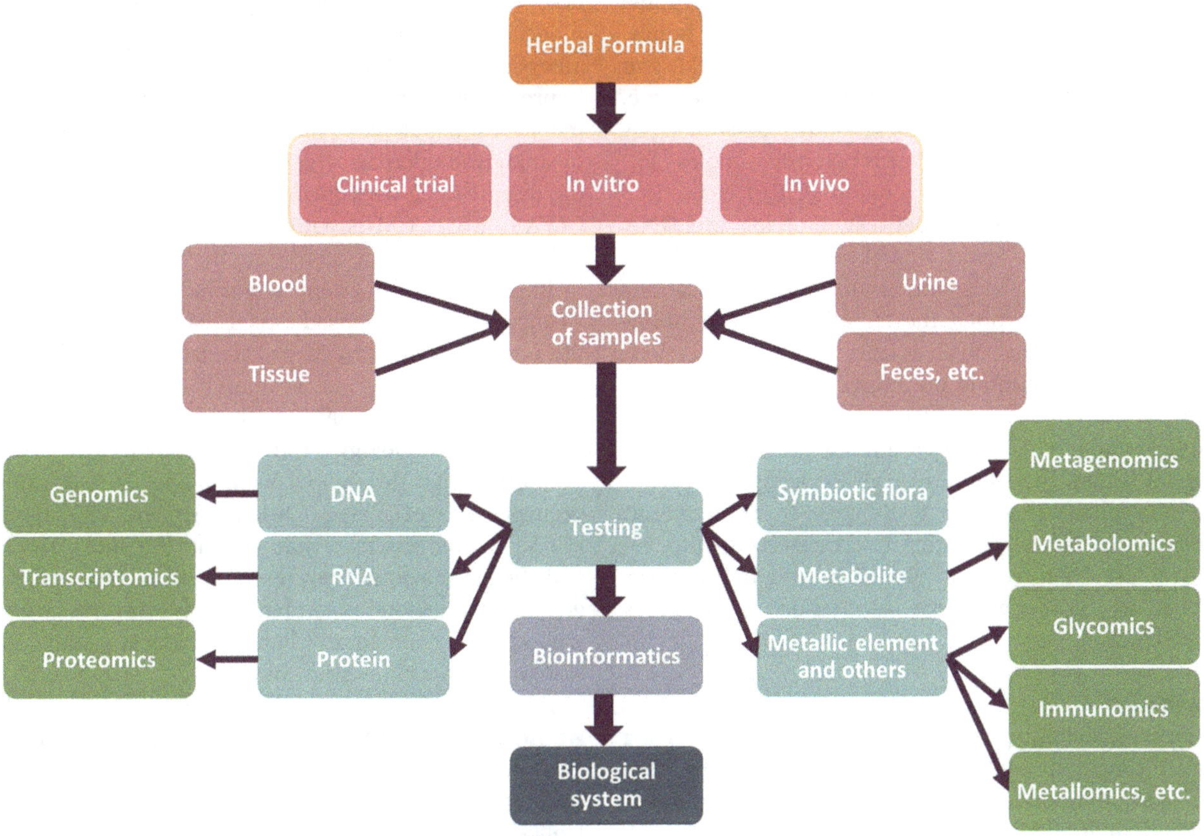

Fig. 1 Overview of the applications of systems biology in CHF research

proteomics, metabolomics and transcriptomics, an increasing number of studies have focused on clarifying complex biological phenomena at the systems level [6, 7]. Large amounts of information from omics technologies and computational studies, including bioinformatics, data mining and machine learning, have been used to understand biological phenomena to predict interactions of biological systems [8, 9]. As a complement to the traditional research mode, a novel CM pharmacological approach through the combination of network pharmacology, omics technologies and computational studies has been established to update the research paradigm from the current "one target, one drug" mode to a new "network target, multicomponents" mode [10]. The approach can discover the combinatorial rules and network regulation effects of CHF from a systems perspective and at the molecular level by prioritizing disease-associated genes, predicting the target profiles and pharmacological actions of herbal compounds, revealing drug-gene-disease comodule associations, screening synergistic multicompounds from CHF in a high-throughput manner [11], analyzing data through computational studies [12], and then clarifying the combinatorial rules and network regulation effects of CHF. Therefore, this article focuses on an overview of systems biology technology and the application of systems biology in CHF studies.

Application of genomics in CHF research

Genomics is an interdisciplinary field of science focusing on genome mapping, nucleotide sequencing and gene function analysis [13]. According to the time of development and research purposes, genomics is divided into the four branches of structural genomics, functional genomics, comparative genomics and pharmacogenomics.

Common techniques in genomics

Commonly used research methods in genomics include DNA sequencing and bioarray technology. According to different sequencing objects, DNA sequencing technology can be divided into the following categories. (1) Genome-wide association study (GWAS) typically focuses on associations between single-nucleotide polymorphisms (SNPs) or copy-number variations (CNVs) and traits [14]. (2) Exome sequencing uses sequence capture technology to capture and enrich genome-wide exon-region DNA for high-throughput sequencing [15], which can be used to find pathogenic and susceptible genes of complex diseases. (3) Methylated DNA immunoprecipitation sequencing (MeDIP-Seq) can quickly and effectively find the methylation regions in the genome, thus enabling a comparison of the differences in DNA methylation modification patterns between samples [16]. (4) Chromatin immunoprecipitation (ChIP) is used to investigate the interaction between proteins and DNA within cells and to determine the specific location in the genome with which various histone modifications are associated, indicating the targets of histone modifiers [17]. Genomics involves chip technology, including the single-nucleotide polymorphism array (SNP-A), array-based comparative genomic hybridization chip (aCGH), and methylated DNA immunoprecipitation chip (MeDIP-Chip). In addition to high-throughput sequencing and microarray chip technology, low-throughput technology, such as real-time fluorescence quantitative polymerase chain reaction (RT-PCR) and the TaqMan probe, are also needed for verification of genomics research.

Application

Genomics technology has the characteristics of being high-throughput, multifactorial, rapid and sensitive [18], and it can be used to systematically study the multicomponent, multipathway and multitarget effects of CHF systematically.

Current studies have reported that genomics is used to evaluate the efficacy of CHF and to reveal the mechanism of action of CHF at multiple levels. Wen et al. [19] used microarray technology to compare the differences in gene expression between the Siwu decoction and estradiol in the human breast cancer cell line MCF-7, using a microarray and a connectivity map to evaluate the efficacy of the Siwu decoction and explore its molecular mechanism of action. The authors found that the Nrf2-mediated oxidative stress pathway might explain the mechanism of Siwu decoction's cancer defense by using IPA software, and RT-PCR confirmed the overexpression of five genes in this pathway. This study demonstrates the feasibility of microarray technology in combination with other techniques for the evaluation of therapeutic efficiencies and mechanism studies of CHF. Wang et al. [20] reported the mechanism of the Danqi pill (DQP) in myocardial ischemia treatment by measuring gene microarrays in a rat model. After evaluating the effects of signaling pathways and metabolism, the authors found that DQP can reverse energy metabolic disorders to recover cardiac function.

In addition, genomics has been used to analyze therapeutic targets of CHF and to predict other potential drugs. Tang et al. [21] examined therapy using Sini decoction (SND) on kidney yang deficiency in a rat model. Using an mRNA microarray with enrichment analysis, Wang et al. found that SND treatment can improve hypothalamic–pituitary–adrenal axis hormones. Kim et al. [22] connected GWAS diseases to CM by analyzing microarray gene expression and constructing disease-gene networks. The authors analyzed 14,713 GWAS disease-CM-target gene pairs to propose potential drugs from CM. Considering that molecular docking technology may lead to omitted or incorrect information, Zhang et al. [23] proposed the GEPSI method to identify the target proteins of CM by calculating the similarities of gene expression.

These reports are promising for the application of DNA microarray technology in the research of CM. However, other high-throughput technologies such as exome sequencing, MeDIP-Seq, ChIP, aCGH and SNP-A have not been used extensively to date in the study of CHF and, hence, need further research. It is expected that genomics or genomics combined with other omics analyses will offer comparatively high practical value with a systematic flow in the study of CHF.

Application of transcriptomics in CHF research

Transcriptomics technologies are techniques used to study gene transcription and transcriptional regulation. Unlike the static genome, the transcriptome is regulated by both exogenous and endogenous factors. Therefore, the transcriptome is a dynamic link between the genome of a species and its external physical characteristics, reflecting the expression level of all genes in a particular organ, tissue or cell at a particular physiological stage. The current methods for obtaining and analyzing transcriptome data can be divided into two categories: targeted and untargeted methods [24].

Targeted methods

Targeted methods are used to analyze the expression of individual RNA sequences, including gene expression profiling chips, mi-RNA microarrays, long noncoding RNA microarrays (LncRNA Microarray), cDNA-amplified fragment length polymorphism (cDNA-AFLP), Northern blotting and in situ hybridization. The advantages of cDNA-AFLP technology are its repeatability, low false-positive rate and ability to detect the expression of mRNA in low abundance, while the associated difficulty is the selection of suitable endonuclease combinations [25]. Northern blotting is mainly applied to studies of the dynamic expression of specific trait genes at the mRNA level. Using in situ hybridization technology to detect the expression of miRNA can provide a more intuitive display of the spatial and temporal expression patterns of miRNA.

Cui et al. [26] identified differentially expressed genes in Buyang Huanwu decoction intracerebral hemorrhage treatment with lncRNA and mRNA microarray technology and verified the results by qRT-PCR. The biological functions and signal transduction pathways of the differentially expressed genes were analyzed and were found to be related to hemoglobin complexes, oxygen transporters, oxygen transporters, and pyruvate metabolism. Wang et al. [27] confirmed that the Jian-Pi-Zhi-Dong decoction could effectively inhibit the abnormal behavior of mice with Tourette syndrome and increase the levels of dopamine transporter proteins and mRNA in striatum by immunohistochemistry and in situ hybridization. Dai et al. [28] identified microRNAs-223-3p as the key microRNAs in Qi-Shen-Yi-Qi dripping pills that regulate the angiogenesis of ischemic myocardial microvascular endothelial cells by miRNA chip and real-time PCR techniques.

Untargeted methods

Untargeted methods analyze the expression of a large number of different RNA sequences and perform extensive screening, including expressed sequence tags (EST), serial analysis of gene expression (SAGE), massively parallel signature sequencing (MPSS), and RNA sequencing (RNA-seq). EST can analyze a large sample number and can be used for cross-species comparative analysis; however, the data volume is large, and the error rate is high. SAGE is not only qualitative but also quantitative for gene differences, but one significant drawback of this technique is that it requires a large amount of mRNA. MPSS is simple and efficient and can provide information on terminal sequences, and it is suitable for any organism; however, the detection cost is high. RNA-seq with digital signaling has high sensitivity and quantitative accuracy.

The transcriptome is characterized by time specificity, tissue specificity and spatial specificity. In a transcriptional analysis of changes in *Candida albicans* gene expression due to treatment with a Huanglian Jiedu decoction (HLJDD) performed by an RNA-seq technique, Yang et al. [29] found that 735 differentially expressed genes were identified through gene expression analysis, including 700 upregulated genes and 35 downregulated genes. Through the functional annotation analysis of differentially expressed genes, 26 important pathways for HLJDD inhibition of *Candida albicans* infection were identified, especially those occurring through DNA replication and transporter activity pathways. However, to enable the transcriptome to play a greater role in the study of CHF, more attention should be paid to the study of gene modification and protein modification to deepen the understanding of the function and structure of functional genes and regulatory genes.

Application of proteomics in CHF research

The term "proteome" was coined in 1994 and is defined as the protein complement of a genome [30]. Proteomics is an extension of the concept of the proteome and generally refers to the large-scale study of proteins and proteomes, including protein expression levels, post-transcriptional modifications and interactions [31].

Separation and detection techniques in proteomics

The separation techniques in proteomics research include two-dimensional gel electrophoresis (2DGE), fluorescence two-dimensional differential gel electrophoresis (2-D DIGE), multidimensional liquid chromatography (MDLC), and capillary electrophoresis (CE). Among these techniques, 2DGE is the most widely used separation technology in proteomics research. The technique can solve the problem of repeatability and reduce the human error associated with gel contrast analysis. 2DGE is suitable for comparing the differences in protein expression between two samples with high sensitivity, but it is expensive [32]. MDLC can be directly linked to mass spectrometry (MS), easily realizing automation and high throughput and avoiding limitations associated with the molecular weight and isoelectric point. However, MDLC is not as intuitive as gel electrophoresis for visualizing protein spots, and its resolution and reproducibility are not as good as those of 2DGE. CE combines electrophoretic separation with chromatographic separation technology. The technique has advantages in sensitivity, separation efficiency and cost, but it is difficult to analyze proteins with high molecular weights using this approach.

Proteomics detection methods include MS, stable isotope labeling, tandem affinity purification (TAP), yeast two-hybrid assays (YTH), protein chips, X-ray crystallography (XRC), and nuclear magnetic resonance (NMR). Among these methods, MS includes matrix-assisted laser desorption ionization (MALDI), surface-enhanced laser desorption ionization (SELDI), and electrospray ionization (ESI). MALDI is suitable for detecting the molecular mass of peptide segments but not peptide sequences. ESI–MS has a shorter detection time and higher sensitivity and resolution than MALDI, but it requires higher sample purity and more complex data acquisition and analysis. SELDI-TOF–MS is a surface-enhanced MS based on MALDI and is an analytical chip used for expression spectrum analysis. Stable isotope labeling includes stable isotope labeling with amino acids in cell culture (SILAC), isotope-coded affinity tags (ICAT), and isobaric tags for relative and absolute quantification (iTRAQ). The limitation of SILAC is that it can only be used for cells. ICAT can only detect cysteine-containing proteins, while iTRAQ can only achieve relative quantification.

Application

According to the occurrence and development of diseases, CHF mostly function at the protein level [33]. Proteomics research overcomes the nonlinear relationship between protein expression and genes and studies the mechanism and target of CHF action directly at the protein level. Proteomics technology, as the main method of large-scale research on proteins, is applied mainly in two respects: to protein expression profile differences and to protein structure, function and interaction analysis.

Analysis of protein profiles in CHF research

Many studies use proteomics to study the changes in protein spectrum before and after intervention of CHF and to evaluate the pharmacodynamics of CHF at the overall level. A study of the Dingxin recipe in rats with ischemia/reperfusion-induced arrhythmias was carried out by Jia et al. [34]. The authors identified differentially expressed proteins using 2DGE and MALDI-TOF–MS and then validated those proteins by immunohistochemistry, qRT-PCR, western blotting and enzyme-linked immunosorbent assays, indicating that the effect of the Dingxin recipe on arrhythmia induced by ischemia/reperfusion may be related to the increase in prohibitin expression inhibiting neutrophil infiltration and IL-6 expression. Fan et al. [35] determined the protein expression profiles of rat mesenchymal stem cells and cardiomyocyte-like cells by the 2DGE technique and found that the Shuanglong formula could induce mesenchymal stem cells to transform into cardiomyocyte-like cells. In the same vein, the determination of protein expression profiles was conducted in research on the effect of the Fuzheng Huayu formula [36] and Yinchenhao decoction [37] on the proteome of fibrotic livers, as well as the effects of the ZiBu PiYin recipe [38] and Tianqi Jiangtang capsule on diabetes, of Yuanshi Shengmai Chenggu tablets on avascular osteonecrosis of the femoral head [39], of Jie-Geng-Tang on lipopolysaccharide-induced acute lung injury in mice [40], and of the Tao Hong Si Wu decoction against ischemia reperfusion injury [41].

Functional analysis of proteins in CHF research

Protein changes in the body may be the result or the cause of disease; therefore, abnormal proteins and their interactions during the disease course may be potential targets for CHF. In research carried out by Tang et al. [42], protein–protein interaction (PPI) networks containing MMP-9 protein data were obtained from proteomic data published in a database and were further analyzed by high-throughput virtual screening, identifying three compounds that bind to the zinc-binding site of MMP-9 with predictable activity. The researchers then proposed three CHFs containing these compounds for increasing the activity of MMP-9 proteins and thus reducing the side effects of tetracycline. Liu et al. [43] coupled iTRAQ with 2-D LC–MS/MS to identify the differentially expressed proteins in serum between Zhibai Dihuang granule-treated rats and yin-deficiency heat syndrome rats and analyzed the differential protein functions via bioinformatics, finding that Zhibai Dihuang granules may alleviate yin-deficiency heat syndrome by regulating complementary activation and inflammation, enhancing the body's ability to recognize antigens.

Application of metabolomics in CHF research

Metabolomics, which emerged in the 1990s, studies the metabolic regulatory networks of organisms by examining their metabolic products and dynamic changes in the course of diseases. Metabolomics is widely used in the study of pathophysiological changes of diseases. By evaluating the differential expression of various endogenous substances, such as blood and urine, much information about disease diagnosis and drug efficacy can be provided [44]. In metabolomics studies, the analytical techniques for samples are mainly ^{1}H-NMR and MS.

NMR

NMR enables noninvasive, unbiased detection of samples and is responsive to hydrogen-containing compounds; thus, the technique can detect as many compounds as possible in a sample. However, the sensitivity of NMR is lower than that of mass spectrometry. Wei et al. [45] studied the therapeutic effect of the HLJDD decoction on acute pancreatitis by comparing two models of cholestasis injury induced by bile duct ligation and thioacetamide. NMR-based metabolomic and pathological studies showed that *Coptis chinensis* and its main alkaloid, berberine, could inhibit inflammatory factors and protect the liver. Combining these methods with ^{1}H-NMR and network analysis, Zhang et al. successfully revealed that the three main compounds in HLJDD, berberine, baicalin and jasmine, can improve metabolic disorders of ischemic stroke by improving metabolic abnormalities and regulating oxidative stress, neuronal autophagy and inflammatory responses [46]. The therapeutic effect of HLJDD and its four variants on a septic cecum ligation and perforation (CLP) model was studied by ^{1}H-NMR, histological examination, biochemical examination and molecular biology. The results showed that HLJDD had a better therapeutic effect in the CLP model than its four variants and that the HMGB-1/TLR4/NF-kappa B signaling pathway may be involved in HLJDD's ability to reduce tissue damage and improve metabolic disorders in septic rats [47].

GS–MS

It is difficult to simultaneously determine the metabolites coexisting in biological systems at very different concentrations. Commonly used separation techniques include gas chromatography (GC), liquid chromatography (LC) and CE. Analytes in metabolomics samples contain highly complex mixtures. By separating some analytes from others, complex mixtures can be simplified before testing. The separation procedure is not mandatory and is usually omitted in NMR. Because existing analytical techniques each have their own advantages and scope of application, the strategy for metabolomics comprehensive analysis is to combine separation and analytical techniques. GC–MS is suitable for the analysis of metabolites with low molecular weights, low polarity and low boiling points or volatile substances after derivatization.

GC–MS is a feasible way to systematically study the therapeutic effect of CHF. The Xuefu Zhuyu Decoction (XFZY) has a distinct therapeutic effect on traumatic brain injury (TBI) in rats. Feng et al. used GC–MS to analyze the plasma metabolomics of sham, vehicle and XFZY groups by univariate and multivariate statistical analysis to illustrate the therapeutic approach of XFZY in TBI. The authors concluded that XFZY treatment can alleviate neurological impairment and cortical lesion volume on the third day after brain injury and reverse the abnormalities of plasma metabolites such as glutamate, lactic acid, 3-hydroxybutyric acid and ribitol [48]. GC-TOF–MS was used to evaluate the efficacy and mechanism of the Shenfu decoction in the treatment of chronic heart failure induced by coronary artery ligation in rats. Unsupervised principal component analysis showed that CHF significantly altered the fingerprint of urinary metabolites. After SFD treatment, the metabolomic profiles of CHF rats were significantly reversed, and the pathways of fatty acid biosynthesis, fatty acid elongation, steroid biosynthesis, galactose metabolism and amino acid metabolism in rats were significantly altered [49].

LC–MS

LC–MS is suitable for the analysis of high-molecular-weight, thermally instable and high-boiling-point compounds. Based on LC-TOF/MS and LC-QqQ/MS, a nontarget metabolomics-driven method for the rapid screening and identification of xenobiotics and related metabolites in vitro was developed. Using this method, Wu et al. [50] found that iridoid glycosides, monoterpenoids, flavonoid glycosides, and anthraquinones are the main absorbed chemical components of the Zhi-Zi-Da-Huang decoction and that hydrolysis, glucuronidation and sulfation are the main metabolic pathways in vivo. Yan et al. [51] applied UHPLC-LTQ-Orbitrap MS combined with a spike-in method to the study of Danqi Tongmai tablets for the preconditioning of acute myocardial ischemia (AMI) rats, which indicated that pretreatment with this CHF can partially regulate disordered TCA circulation and amino acid and nucleotide metabolism, thereby reducing injury from AMI. In addition, the effect and mechanism of Jinxin oral liquid in treating viral pneumonia caused by the respiratory syncytial virus via improving lipid metabolism disorders [52], the protective effect of low-dose Sini decoction against myocardial injury induced by isoproterenol [53], the inhibitory effect of the Yinchenhao decoction toward dimethylnitrosamine-induced liver fibrosis in rats [54], and the improvement from the modified Jiu Wei Qiang Huo decoction on H1N1-virus pneumonia in mice [55] have all been well verified by LC–MS technology.

Regardless of which analytical technology is adopted, no single technique can completely cover all metabolomics compounds [56]. In recent years, researchers have tried to integrate various analytical techniques to give full play to the advantages of various methods. LC–MS and GC–MS analyses were performed to quantitatively evaluate the compatibility of CHF from the perspective of overall metabolic profiles and specific metabolites [57, 58]. These studies suggest that appropriate analytical techniques need to be selected before metabolomics studies on CHF can be carried out so that the results can be more comprehensive and accurate. Metabolites are not confined to the substrates and products of certain enzymes in the metabolic pathway. Instead, metabolites act as structural units, signaling molecules, and regulatory factors and play many other roles and interact in the form of a metabolic network in life activities.

Application of metagenomics in CHF research

Metagenomics is a microbial research method based on the genome of microbial populations in environmental samples, aiming at examining microbial diversity, population structure, evolutionary relationships, functional activities, interactions and environmental relationships. Functional gene screening and sequencing analysis are the research means.

Common techniques in metagenomics

At present, the main application of metagenomics in-clinic is based on gene sequence analysis of microbial species and compositions. 16S rRNA gene cloning and sequencing, PCR-denaturing gradient gel electrophoresis (PCR-DGGE), PCR-temperature gradient gel electrophoresis (PCR-TGGE), terminal restriction fragment length polymorphism (T-RFLP), and next-generation sequencing technology such as 454 and Illumina have been widely used in metagenomics research. High-throughput, large-scale, in-depth sequencing combined with multivariate statistical methods can provide more direct information on the composition and function of microorganisms and identify specific bacterial groups closely related to the physiological and pathological state of the organism. 16S rRNA gene cloning and sequencing can not only analyze the species of bacteria in a sample but can also reflect the proportion of various bacteria and provide relative quantitative analysis [59]. PCR-DGGE has a high resolution and can detect mutant individuals with single-base differences. However, when the length of DNA fragments detected by PCR-DGGE exceeds 500 bp, the resolution will decrease [60]. Similarly to DGGE, TGGE can only analyze DNA fragments shorter than 500 base pairs, and there are only ten to twenty bands in the map reflecting the dominant flora in the community, while the disadvantaged flora cannot be detected. T-RFLP was established based on PCR but without the isolation and cultivation of bacteria. However, when two distinct sequences share a terminal restriction site, they cannot be distinguished and only show one peak on an electropherogram.

Expectations of the application of metagenomics in CHF

One of the main methods for the application of metagenomics in CM research is to construct a 16S rRNA gene library for flora analysis based on the species specificity of the 16S rRNA gene. Another common method is to extract the total nucleic acid from bacteria and amplify the 16S rRNA gene by PCR, then analyze the data by molecular biology techniques such as fingerprinting combined with multivariate statistical analysis. To study the effect of Xiexin Tang on the distribution of intestinal flora in rats with type 2 diabetes mellitus (T2DM), Wei et al. [61] utilized high-throughput 16S rRNA gene sequencing to detect the cecum samples of the rats. Sequencing analysis showed that certain short-chain fatty acid-producing and anti-inflammatory bacteria in the intestinal microflora of T2DM rats were significantly altered after Xiexin Tang intervention, and these microbiotas were closely related to the changes in related indices of T2DM. Tong et al. [62] proved the effect of metformin and a specially designed CHF on T2DM with hyperlipidemia through a randomized clinical trial. Then, Illumina sequencing and multivariate statistical methods were used to analyze the V3 and V4 regions of 16S rRNA genes to evaluate changes in the intestinal microbial structure. The results suggest that the combination of metformin and CHF may improve T2DM with hyperlipidemia by enriching Brucella and fecal bacilli and other beneficial bacteria. To verify that oil tea can induce changes in intestinal microbes and play an antidiabetic role, Lin et al. [63] carried out 16S rRNA gene sequencing on fecal samples of db/db mice fed oral salt, metformin and oil tea. The results showed that Lachnospiraceae were significantly enriched after oil tea treatment and correlated with decrease indicators related to diabetes. Gao et al. [64] studied the effects of S-3-1, a homogeneous polysaccharide purified from the Sijunzi decoction, on human intestinal microflora and short-chain fatty acids by a GC technique, analyzing the V3 and V4 regions of 16S rRNA after Illumina MiSeq sequencing. It appeared that S-3-1 could regulate the abundance of 9 intestinal flora, while S-3-1 incubated in gastric and intestinal juice enhanced the ability to regulate the composition of intestinal flora and regulated 13 types of bacteria genera to play an immunoregulatory role.

The number of microorganisms in the human body is more than ten times that of body cells, and the corresponding genetic code is 100 times the size of the human genome [65]. Most existing studies have focused on the distribution of intestinal microorganisms. We should pay more attention to the impact of intestinal microecological changes on human health and disease; that is, we should pay more attention to the functions of microorganisms. There is a great challenge and opportunity in the deeper and wider application of metagenomics in CHF research to connect the functional changes of intestinal flora with the influence of CHF on microflora.

Comprehensive application of multiple omics methods in CHF research

Considering that the combination of multiple omics methods will enable the comprehensive evaluation of the efficacy and complex mechanisms of CHF, Du et al. [66] used transcriptomics, metabolomics, and pharmacodynamics to observe the therapeutic effect of the Baoyuan decoction on myocardial infarction in rats with left anterior descending coronary artery ligation and investigate its molecular mechanism. Their work successfully revealed the mechanism of multiple pathways regulating the cardioprotective effects of the Baoyuan decoction. Huang et al. [67] established a cold-stagnation and blood-stasis primary dysmenorrhea rat model to investigate the effect and mechanism of the Shaofu Zhuyu decoction. In their work, metabolic profiling was analyzed by LC–MS, and the correlation between biomarkers and biochemical indicators was also analyzed. Meanwhile, peripheral blood mononuclear cells were isolated, and their transcript levels were quantified by RT-PCR. The findings suggested that SFZYD regulated the MAPK pathway and thus improved the metabolic profiles and biochemical parameters in cold-stagnation and blood-stasis primary dysmenorrhea rats. Sun et al. [68] carried out a multilevel evaluation of the Qishe pill by metabolomics, genomics and proteomics. According to their constitutional types, 108 subjects were divided into qi-deficiency, yin-deficiency and blood-stasis groups. ^{1}H-NMR, UHPLC-MS, the Human-CoreExome+v1.1-Psych Array, and Illumina's HT-12 bead chips were used to establish and verify a population pharmacokinetic (PopPK) model for the Qishe pill in the three groups, providing personalized medicine strategies for the application of CHF. Zhao et al. [69] identified a group of short-chain fatty acid-producing bacteria at the strain level that can increase insulin secretion and enhance insulin sensitivity by combining metagenomics analysis with metabolic levels in patients with T2DM. These bacteria can be regarded as a necessary "ecological functional group" for restoring and maintaining human health. The team found that the higher the restored abundance and diversity of these bacteria were, the lower the reduction of HbA1c became, and they established a statistical model to predict the efficacy of these key early bacterial changes.

Perspectives

Clinically effective CHF usually exerts therapeutic effects by regulating multiple targets and affecting multiple pathways. At present, the evaluation system for the clinical efficacy of CHF still needs to be improved. It is difficult to explain the efficacy of CHF systematically and comprehensively by traditional evaluation methods that only use a single index or a few indices. The evaluation of CHF efficacy combined with the integrity and dynamics of systems biology should still be based on CM syndrome differentiation and treatment concepts. In studies of the mechanisms of CHF, in addition to reflecting the pharmacodynamic substance basis of CHF from the aspects of genes, proteins, and metabolites, the bioinformatics method should be used to integrate and construct a biological network map of the mechanism of the CHF therapeutic effects and to clarify the mechanism of CHF therapeutic effects from the perspective of the organism as a whole to replace the study of pharmacodynamic mechanisms from only the molecular perspective. Compared with traditional research techniques, the acquisition and analysis of high-throughput, large-scale data makes the research of systems biology better aligned with the characteristics of CHF. Determining how to carry out system dynamics research of CHF and combine traditional pharmacodynamic and pharmacokinetic methods to assess CHF efficacies and mechanisms remains a big challenge for future research and applications.

Although each omics method exists independently, it reflects biological characteristics from different angles. In specific studies, we should select methods and techniques according to the research objects and purposes. The study of CHF by a single omics method is usually not sufficiently comprehensive. Findings should be mutually validated in combination with multiple -omics methods, and even multicenter, multilevel research strategies should be used to identify changes in gene-protein-metabolite level consistency. Although individualized precision medicine still has a long way to go, CHF treatment based on the molecular subtyping of CM syndrome differentiation as well as holistic evaluation based on systematic pharmacology/network pharmacology are the existing research and application approaches. With the powerful tool of systems biology, CM can rapidly promote the development of personalized medicine.

Abbreviations

CHF: Chinese herbal formulae; CM: Chinese medicine; CHM: Chinese herbal medicine; GWAS: genome-wide association study; SNPs: single-nucleotide polymorphisms; CNVs: copy-number variations; MeDIP-Seq: methylated DNA immunoprecipitation sequencing; ChIP: chromatin immunoprecipitation; aCGH: array-based comparative genomic hybridization chip; MeDIP-Chip: methylated DNA immunoprecipitation chip; RT-PCR: real-time fluorescence quantitative polymerase chain reaction; LncRNA Microarray: long noncoding RNA microarray; cDNA-AFLP: cDNA-amplified fragment length polymorphism; EST: expressed sequence tags; SAGE: serial analysis of gene expression; MPSS: massively parallel signature sequencing; RNA-seq: RNA sequencing; 2DGE: two-dimensional gel electrophoresis; CE: capillary electrophoresis; MS: mass spectrometry; XRC: X-ray crystallography; NMR: nuclear magnetic resonance; ESI: electrospray ionization; iTRAQ: isobaric tags for relative and absolute quantification; GC: gas chromatography; LC: liquid chromatography.

Authors' contributions

CFF wrote manuscript and searched the literature with ZWJ. WR revised the manuscript, and SSB designed and revised the manuscript. All authors read and approved the final manuscript.

Acknowledgements

The authors extend their appreciation for financial support by the Macao Foundation and International Society of Chinese Medicine.

Competing interests

The authors declare that they have no competing interests.

Consent for publication

Not applicable.

Funding

This work was supported by the Key Programme of National Science Foundation of China (81330084), and National Key Research and Development: Special Project for Research on the Modernization of Traditional Chinese Medicine (2018YFC1704204).

References

1. Ma Q, Li PL, Hua YL, Ji P, Yao WL, Zhang XS, et al. Effects of Tao-Hong-Si-Wu decoction on acute blood stasis in rats based on a LC-Q/TOF-MS metabolomics and network approach. Biomed Chromatogr. 2018;32(4):e4144.
2. Zhang Q, Wang J, Liao S, Li P, Xu D, Lv Y, et al. Optimization of Huang-Lian-Jie-Du-decoction for ischemic stroke treatment and mechanistic

study by metabolomic profiling and network analysis. Front Pharmacol. 2017;8:165.
3. Chen S, Wu S, Li W, Chen X, Dong X, Tan G, et al. Investigation of the therapeutic effectiveness of active components in Sini decoction by a comprehensive GC/LC-MS based metabolomics and network pharmacology approaches. Mol BioSyst. 2014;10(12):3310–21.
4. Glaser P, Boone C. Beyond the genome: from genomics to systems biology. Curr Opin Microbiol. 2004;7(5):489–91.
5. Liu L-Y, Zhang H-J, Luo L-Y, Pu J-B, Liang W-Q, Zhu C-Q, et al. Blood and urinary metabolomic evidence validating traditional Chinese medicine diagnostic classification of major depressive disorder. Chin Med. 2018;13(1):53.
6. Lee S. Systems biology—a pivotal research methodology for understanding the mechanisms of traditional medicine. J Pharmacopunct. 2015;18(3):11–8.
7. Duan L, Guo L, Wang L, Yin Q, Zhang C-M, Zheng Y-G, et al. Application of metabolomics in toxicity evaluation of traditional Chinese medicines. Chin Med. 2018;13(1):60.
8. Ulrich-Merzenich G, Zeitler H, Jobst D, Panek D, Vetter H, Wagner H. Application of the "-Omic-" technologies in phytomedicine. Phytomedicine. 2007;14(1):70–82.
9. Zhang Y, Li W, Zou L, Gong Y, Zhang P, Xing S, et al. Metabonomic study of the protective effect of Fukeqianjin formula on multi-pathogen induced pelvic inflammatory disease in rats. Chin Med. 2018;13(1):61.
10. Gong AGW, Duan R, Wang HY, Dong TTX, Tsim KWK. Calycosin orchestrates osteogenesis of Danggui Buxue Tang in cultured osteoblasts: evaluating the mechanism of action by omics and chemical knock-out methodologies. Front Pharmacol. 2018;9:36.
11. Liu L, Du B, Zhang H, Guo X, Zhou Z, Xiu A, et al. A network pharmacology approach to explore the mechanisms of Erxian decoction in polycystic ovary syndrome. Chin Med. 2018;13(1):46.
12. Gupta A, Rawlings JB. Comparison of parameter estimation methods in stochastic chemical kinetic models: examples in systems biology. AIChE J. 2014;60(4):1253–68.
13. Hudson KL. Genomics, health care, and society. N Engl J Med. 2011;365(11):1033–41.
14. Guo J, Yang J, Visscher PM. Leveraging GWAS for complex traits to detect signatures of natural selection in humans. Curr Opin Genet Dev. 2018;53:9–14.
15. Ng SB, Turner EH, Robertson PD, Flygare SD, Bigham AW, Lee C, et al. Targeted capture and massively parallel sequencing of 12 human exomes. Nature. 2009;461(7261):272–6.
16. Weber M, Davies JJ, Wittig D, Oakeley EJ, Haase M, Lam WL, et al. Chromosome-wide and promoter-specific analyses identify sites of differential DNA methylation in normal and transformed human cells. Nat Genet. 2005;37(8):853–62.
17. Collas P. The current state of chromatin immunoprecipitation. Mol Biotechnol. 2010;45(1):87–100.
18. Saqi M, Pellet J, Roznovat I, Mazein A, Ballereau S, De Meulder B, et al. Systems medicine: the future of medical genomics, healthcare, and wellness. Methods Mol Biol. 2016;1386:43–60.
19. Wen Z, Wang Z, Wang S, Ravula R, Yang L, Xu J, et al. Discovery of molecular mechanisms of traditional Chinese medicinal formula Si-Wu-Tang using gene expression microarray and connectivity map. PLoS ONE. 2011;6(3):e18278.
20. Wang Q, Meng H, Zhang Q, Shi T, Zhang X, Shao M, et al. Multitarget effects of Danqi Pill on global gene expression changes in myocardial ischemia. Int J Genomics. 2018;2018:9469670.
21. Tang N, Liu L, Qiu H, Shi W, Mao D. Analysis of gene expression and functional changes of adrenal gland in a rat model of kidney yang deficiency syndrome treated with Sini decoction. Exp Ther Med. 2018;16(4):3107–15.
22. Kim J, Yoo M, Shin J, Kim H, Kang J, Tan AC. Systems pharmacology-based approach of connecting disease genes in genome-wide association studies with traditional chinese medicine. Int J Genomics. 2018;2018:7697356.
23. Zhang B, He S, Lv C, Zhang Y, Wang Y. GEPSI: a gene expression profile similarity-based identification method of bioactive components in traditional Chinese medicine formula. Evid Based Complement Altern Med. 2018;2018:6935350.
24. Pinel G, Weigel S, Antignac JP, Mooney MH, Elliott C, Nielen MWF, et al. Targeted and untargeted profiling of biological fluids to screen for anabolic practices in cattle. TrAC Trends Anal Chem. 2010;29(11):1269–80.
25. Meudt HM, Clarke AC. Almost forgotten or latest practice? AFLP applications, analyses and advances. Trends Plant Sci. 2007;12(3):106–17.
26. Cui H, Liu T, Li P, Yang A, Zhou H, Luo J, et al. An intersectional study of LncRNAs and mRNAs reveals the potential therapeutic targets of Buyang Huanwu decoction in experimental intracerebral hemorrhage. Cell Physiol Biochem. 2018;46(5):2173–86.
27. Wang DH, Li W, Liu XF, Zhang JM, Wang SM. Chinese medicine formula "Jian-Pi-Zhi-Dong Decoction" attenuates Tourette syndrome via downregulating the expression of dopamine transporter in mice. Evid Based Complement Altern Med. 2013;2013:385685.
28. Dai GH, Liu N, Zhu JW, Yao J, Yang C, Ma PZ, et al. Qi-Shen-Yi-Qi dripping pills promote angiogenesis of ischemic cardiac microvascular endothelial cells by regulating MicroRNA-223-3p expression. Evid Based Complement Altern Med. 2016;2016:5057328.
29. Yang Q, Gao L, Tao M, Chen Z, Yang X, Cao Y. Transcriptomics analysis of *Candida albicans* treated with Huanglian Jiedu decoction using RNA-seq. Evid Based Complement Altern Med. 2016;2016:3198249.
30. Wasinger VC, Cordwell SJ, Cerpa-Poljak A, Yan JX, Gooley AA, Wilkins MR, et al. Progress with gene-product mapping of the mollicutes: *Mycoplasma genitalium*. Electrophoresis. 1995;16(7):1090–4.
31. Blackstock WP, Weir MP. Proteomics: quantitative and physical mapping of cellular proteins. Trends Biotechnol. 1999;17(3):121–7.
32. Tonge R, Shaw J, Middleton B, Rowlinson R, Rayner S, Young J, et al. Validation and development of fluorescence two-dimensional differential gel electrophoresis proteomics technology. Proteomics. 2001;1(3):377–96.
33. Ji Q, Zhu F, Liu X, Li Q, Su SB. Recent advance in applications of proteomics technologies on Traditional Chinese medicine research. Evid Based Complement Altern Med. 2015;2015:983139.
34. Jia YH, Zhang YX, Li LJ, Liu YW, Li CH, Fu XQ, et al. Dingxin recipe () prevents ischemia/reperfusion-induced arrhythmias via up-regulating prohibitin and suppressing inflammatory responses. Chin J Integr Med. 2012;18(2):120–9.
35. Fan X, Li X, Lv S, Wang Y, Zhao Y, Luo G. Comparative proteomics research on rat MSCs differentiation induced by Shuanglong Formula. J Ethnopharmacol. 2010;131(3):575–80.
36. Xie H, Tao Y, Lv J, Liu P, Liu C. Proteomic analysis of the effect of fuzheng huayu recipe on fibrotic liver in rats. Evid Based Complement Altern Med. 2013;2013:972863.
37. Sun H, Zhang A, Yan G, Han Y, Sun W, Ye Y, et al. Proteomics study on the hepatoprotective effects of traditional Chinese medicine formulae Yin-Chen-Hao-Tang by a combination of two-dimensional polyacrylamide gel electrophoresis and matrix-assisted laser desorption/ionization-time of flight mass spectrometry. J Pharm Biomed Anal. 2013;75:173–9.
38. Shi X, Lu XG, Zhan LB, Qi X, Liang LN, Hu SY, et al. The effects of the Chinese medicine ZiBu PiYin recipe on the hippocampus in a rat model of diabetes-associated cognitive decline: a proteomic analysis. Diabetologia. 2011;54(7):1888–99.
39. Deng P, Zeng J, Li J, Feng W, Chen J, Zeng Y. Screening of serum protein markers for avascular osteonecrosis of femoral head differentially expressed after treatment with Yuanshi Shengmai Chenggu tablets. Biomed Res Int. 2018;2018:5692735.
40. Tao J, Nie Y, Hou Y, Ma X, Ding G, Gao J, et al. Chemomics-Integrated proteomics analysis of Jie-Geng-Tang to ameliorate lipopolysaccharide-induced acute lung injury in mice. Evid Based Complement Altern Med. 2016;2016:7379146.
41. Qi HY, Li L, Yu J, Chen L, Huang YL, Ning L, et al. Proteomic identification of Nrf2-mediated phase II enzymes critical for protection of Tao Hong Si Wu decoction against oxygen glucose deprivation injury in PC12 Cells. Evid Based Complement Altern Med. 2014;2014:945814.
42. Tang HC, Huang HJ, Lee CC, Chen CYC. Network pharmacology-based approach of novel traditional Chinese medicine formula for treatment of acute skin inflammation in silico. Comput Biol Chem. 2017;71:70–81.
43. Liu CM, Chen J, Yang S, Mao LG, Jiang TT, Tu HH, et al. The Chinese herbal formula Zhibai Dihuang Granule treat Yin-deficiency-heat syndrome rats by regulating the immune responses. J Ethnopharmacol. 2018;225:271–8.

44. Song YN, Chen J, Cai FF, Lu YY, Chen QL, Zhang YY, et al. A metabolic mechanism analysis of Fuzheng-Huayu formula for improving liver cirrhosis with traditional Chinese medicine syndromes. Acta Pharmacol Sin. 2018;39(6):942–51.
45. Wei DD, Wang JS, Duan JA, Kong LY. Metabolomic assessment of acute cholestatic injuries induced by thioacetamide and by bile duct ligation, and the protective effects of Huang-Lian-Jie-Du-decoction. Front Pharmacol. 2018;9:458.
46. Zhang Q, Fu X, Wang J, Yang M, Kong L. Treatment effects of ischemic stroke by berberine, baicalin, and jasminoidin from Huang-Lian-Jie-Du-Decoction (HLJDD) explored by an integrated metabolomics approach. Oxid Med Cell Longev. 2017;2017:9848594.
47. Xu D, Lv Y, Wang J, Yang M, Kong L. Deciphering the mechanism of Huang-Lian-Jie-Du-decoction on the treatment of sepsis by formula decomposition and metabolomics: enhancement of cholinergic pathways and inhibition of HMGB-1/TLR4/NF-kappaB signaling. Pharmacol Res. 2017;121:94–113.
48. Feng D, Xia Z, Zhou J, Lu H, Zhang C, Fan R, et al. Metabolomics reveals the effect of Xuefu Zhuyu decoction on plasma metabolism in rats with acute traumatic brain injury. Oncotarget. 2017;8(55):94692–710.
49. Yang D, Wang X, Wu Y, Lu B, Yuan A, Leon C, et al. Urinary metabolomic profiling reveals the effect of Shenfu decoction on chronic heart failure in rats. Molecules. 2015;20(7):11915–29.
50. Wu H, Li X, Yan X, An L, Luo K, Shao M, et al. An untargeted metabolomics-driven approach based on LC-TOF/MS and LC-MS/MS for the screening of xenobiotics and metabolites of Zhi-Zi-Da-Huang decoction in rat plasma. J Pharm Biomed Anal. 2015;115:315–22.
51. Yan B, Deng Y, Hou J, Bi Q, Yang M, Jiang B, et al. UHPLC-LTQ-Orbitrap MS combined with spike-in method for plasma metabonomics analysis of acute myocardial ischemia rats and pretreatment effect of Danqi Tongmai tablet. Mol BioSyst. 2015;11(2):486–96.
52. Du LN, Xie T, Xu JY, Kang A, Di LQ, Shan JJ, et al. A metabolomics approach to studying the effects of Jinxin oral liquid on RSV-infected mice using UPLC/LTQ-Orbitrap mass spectrometry. J Ethnopharmacol. 2015;174:25–36.
53. Zhou J, Ma X, Shi M, Chen C, Sun Y, Li J, et al. Serum metabolomics analysis reveals that obvious cardioprotective effects of low dose Sini decoction against isoproterenol-induced myocardial injury in rats. Phytomedicine. 2017;31:18–31.
54. Zhang H, Wang X, Hu P, Zhou W, Zhang M, Liu J, et al. Serum metabolomic characterization of liver fibrosis in rats and anti-fibrotic effects of Yin-Chen-Hao-Tang. Molecules. 2016;21(1):E126.
55. Chen L, Fan J, Li Y, Shi X, Ju D, Yan Q, et al. Modified Jiu Wei Qiang Huo decoction improves dysfunctional metabolomics in influenza A pneumonia-infected mice. Biomed Chromatogr. 2014;28(4):468–74.
56. Bedair M, Sumner LW. Current and emerging mass-spectrometry technologies for metabolomics. TrAC Trends Anal Chem. 2008;27(3):238–50.
57. Cui DN, Wang X, Chen JQ, Lv B, Zhang P, Zhang W, et al. Quantitative evaluation of the compatibility effects of Huangqin decoction on the treatment of irinotecan-induced gastrointestinal toxicity using untargeted metabolomics. Front Pharmacol. 2017;8:211.
58. Wang X, Cui DN, Dai XM, Wang J, Zhang W, Zhang ZJ, et al. HuangQin decoction attenuates CPT-11-induced gastrointestinal toxicity by regulating bile acids metabolism homeostasis. Front Pharmacol. 2017;8:156.
59. Oulas A, Pavloudi C, Polymenakou P, Pavlopoulos GA, Papanikolaou N, Kotoulas G, et al. Metagenomics: tools and insights for analyzing next-generation sequencing data derived from biodiversity studies. Bioinform Biol Insights. 2015;9:75–88.
60. Fischer SG, Lerman LS. Length-independent separation of DNA restriction fragments in two-dimensional gel electrophoresis. Cell. 1979;16(1):191–200.
61. Wei X, Tao J, Xiao S, Jiang S, Shang E, Zhu Z, et al. Xiexin Tang improves the symptom of type 2 diabetic rats by modulation of the gut microbiota. Sci Rep. 2018;8(1):3685.
62. Tong X, Xu J, Lian F, Yu X, Zhao Y, Xu L, et al. Structural alteration of gut microbiota during the amelioration of human type 2 diabetes with hyperlipidemia by metformin and a traditional Chinese herbal formula: a multicenter, randomized, open label clinical trial. MBio. 2018;9(3):e02392–417.
63. Lin R, He X, Chen H, He Q, Yao Z, Li Y, et al. Oil tea improves glucose and lipid levels and alters gut microbiota in type 2 diabetic mice. Nutr Res. 2018;57:67–77.
64. Gao B, Wang R, Peng Y, Li X. Effects of a homogeneous polysaccharide from Sijunzi decoction on human intestinal microbes and short chain fatty acids in vitro. J Ethnopharmacol. 2018;224:465–73.
65. Messer JS, Liechty ER, Vogel OA, Chang EB. Evolutionary and ecological forces that shape the bacterial communities of the human gut. Mucosal Immunol. 2017;10(3):567–79.
66. Du Z, Shu Z, Lei W, Li C, Zeng K, Guo X, et al. Integration of metabonomics and transcriptomics reveals the therapeutic effects and mechanisms of Baoyuan decoction for myocardial ischemia. Front Pharmacol. 2018;9:514.
67. Huang X, Su S, Duan JA, Sha X, Zhu KY, Guo J, et al. Effects and mechanisms of Shaofu-Zhuyu decoction and its major bioactive component for Cold-Stagnation and Blood-Stasis primary dysmenorrhea rats. J Ethnopharmacol. 2016;186:234–43.
68. Sun YL, Hou T, Liu SF, Zhang ZL, Zhang N, Yao M, et al. Population pharmacokinetic modeling of the Qishe pill in three major traditional Chinese medicine-defined constitutional types of healthy Chinese subjects: study protocol for a randomized controlled trial. Trials. 2015;16:64.
69. Zhao L, Zhang F, Ding X, Wu G, Lam YY, Wang X, et al. Gut bacteria selectively promoted by dietary fibers alleviate type 2 diabetes. Science. 2018;359(6380):1151–6.

18

Hepatoprotective properties of *Penthorum chinense* Pursh against carbon tetrachloride-induced acute liver injury in mice

Meng Wang[1†], Xiao-Jiao Zhang[1†], Ruibing Feng[1], Yun Jiang[2], Da-Yong Zhang[2], Chengwei He[1], Peng Li[1] and Jian-Bo Wan[1*]

Abstract

Background: *Penthorum chinense* Pursh (Penthoraceae, PCP), a well-known Miao ethnomedicine, has been traditionally used to treat several liver-related diseases, such as jaundice and viral hepatitis. The aims of the present study were to evaluate the probable properties of the aqueous extract of PCP on carbon tetrachloride (CCl_4)—induced acute liver injury in mice.

Methods: C57BL/6 mice were orally administered an aqueous extract of PCP (5.15 and 10.3 g/kg BW) or silymarin (100 mg/kg) once daily for 1 week prior to CCl_4 exposure. Silymarin serves as a positive drug to validate the effectivenes of PCP.

Results: A single dose of CCl_4 exposure caused severe acute liver injury in mice, as evidenced by the elevated serum levels of alanine aminotransferase (ALT), aspartate aminotransferase (AST) and alanine phosphatase (ALP), and the increased TUNEL-positive cells in liver, which were remarkably ameliorated by the pretreatment of PCP. PCP was also found to decrease the levels of malondialdehyde (MDA), restore the glutathione (GSH) and enhance the activities of superoxide dismutase (SOD) and catalase (CAT) in the liver. In addition, the pretreatment of PCP inhibited the degradation of hepatic cytochrome P450 2E1 (CYP2E1), up-regulated the expression of nuclear factor erythroid 2-related factor 2 (Nrf2) and its target proteins in CCl_4-treated mice.

Conclusion: Results indicated that the pretreatment of PCP (10.3 g/kg BW) effectively protected against CCl_4-induced acute liver injury, which was comparable to efficacy of silymarin (100 mg/kg). This hepatoprotective effects might be attributed to amelioration of CCl_4-induced oxidative stress via activating Nrf2 signaling pathway.

Keywords: Carbon tetrachloride, Nuclear factor E2-related factor 2, Hepatotoxicity, Oxidative stress, *Penthorum chinense* Pursh

Background

Oxidative stress is well known to be involved in the pathogenesis of acute or chronic liver injury [1]. The over generation of reactive oxygen species (ROS) may be induced by various hepatotoxicants, including heavy metals, alcohol and carbon tetrachloride (CCl_4) [2]. As a chemical inducer, CCl_4 has been extensively used to assess the protection of natural products on liver injury in experimental cellular and animal models [3]. CCl_4 is metabolized in the liver by cytochrome P450 2E1 (CYP2E1), and mainly yields the highly-reactive trichloromethyl radicals, which disturbs the redox homeostasis and causes oxidative stress. These free radicals may cause cellular DNA damage and the increased lipid peroxidation by reacting with cellular unsaturated lipids, leading to hepatocyte apoptosis and necrosis, which ultimately results in liver injury [4].

*Correspondence: jbwan@umac.mo
†Meng Wang and Xiao-Jiao Zhang contributed equally to this work
[1] State Key Laboratory of Quality Research in Chinese Medicine, Institute of Chinese Medical Sciences, University of Macau, Room 6034, Building N22, Avenida da Universidade, Macao, People's Republic of China
Full list of author information is available at the end of the article

Antioxidant defense system, including non-enzymatic and enzymatic mechanisms, is principally responsible for protecting living organism from oxidative stress [5]. Among them, superoxide dismutase (SOD), catalases (CAT) and glutathione peroxidase (GSH-Px) serve as three main classes of antioxidant defense-related enzymes, which are modulated by nuclear factor-erythroid 2-related factor-2 (Nrf2) [6]. Normally, Nrf2 is restrained in cytosol through interacting with Kelch-like ECH-associated protein 1 (Keap1), a specific repressor [7]. Upon oxidative stress, Nrf2 translocates to the nucleus after the dissociation with Keap1, and regulates the expressions of antioxidant-related genes, including haem oxygenase 1 (HO-1) and glutamate cysteine ligase (GCL) [8]. Thus, chemicals or natural products that can activate Nrf2 signaling pathway might be used to prevent CCl_4-induced liver injury.

Penthorum chinense Pursh (*Penthoraceae*, PCP), has been traditionally used as the Miao ethnomedicine and folk remedy in the treatment of liver-related diseases, including jaundice and viral hepatitis for a long time [9]. PCP is widely cultivated in Gulin county, Sichuan Province, China, around where there are a lot of liquor factories. The tea made from the aerial of PCP became more popular in local residents who often drink liquor, and the bartenders who work in liquor factories. In the recent years, a number of studies have demonstrated that PCP or its ingredients possess the diverse bioactivities, including antioxidant, anti-complement, anti-hyperglycemic, and anti-hepatocarcinoma [10]. Our previous studies have also indicated that the aqueous extract of PCP could protect against both acute [11] and chronic alcohol-induced liver injury [12]. However, the impacts of PCP against CCl_4-induced liver injury has not been adequately addressed. Therefore, in this study, we aimed to evaluate the probable protective properties of PCP against acute liver injury induced by CCl_4, and further elucidate its underlying mechanisms with respect to Nrf2-mediated antioxidant response.

Methods

Materials and sample preparation

Aerial part of PCP was provided by Sichuan New Lotus Traditional Chinese Herb Limited Company (Chengdu, China). Its botanical origin was identified by Dr. Chun-Feng Qiao from our university. The aqueous extract of PCP was prepared as previously described [11, 12]. The dried powder of PCP (150 g) was decocted three times with 1500 mL water for 2 h each. After combination and filtration, the decoction was lyophilized by a freeze dryers (VirTis BenchTop Pro, SP Scientific, Warminster, PA, USA). The freeze-dried extract was re-constructed by the distilled water for the present animal study. To assure the repeatability of the pharmacological study, pinocembrin-7-O-β-D-glucoside, the chemical marker, was measured as 3.49 mg/g in raw PCP by HPLC–UV. The voucher specimen of PCP sample (No. GHX201401) was stored at Institute of Chinese Medical Sciences, University of Macau, Macau.

Animals and treatments

Mice (C57BL/6, 8–9 weeks old) were housed in institutional individually ventilated cage (IVC) system. All animals were assigned randomly to five groups ($n = 10$, half males and half females in each group), i.e. control group, CCl_4 group, silymarin-treated group (100 mg/kg BW, as the positive control), two PCP-treated groups (5.15 and 10.3 g/kg BW). The dose of PCP (10.3 g/kg) was calculated from the usage of *Gan-Su-Ke-Li* (WS3-B-2526-97), a drug approved by China Food and Drug Administration (CFDA), which was made from the aqueous extract of PCP for the management of viral hepatitis. Mice were gavaged silymarin or PCP once daily for 1 week prior to CCl_4 challenge in treatment group. 24 h after last dosing, animals were intraperitoneally injected with 10% CCl_4 diluted in olive oil (*v/v*, 2 mL/kg) to induce acute liver injury [13], mice in the control group were treated with same volume of vehicle (*i.p.*). After fasting for 12 h, all mice were anesthetized, and serum samples and the entire liver tissues were immediately collected. Animal protocol was conducted according to the animal procedure approved by Animal Ethics Committee, Institute of Chinese Medical Sciences, University of Macau (ICMS-AEC-2015-05). The Minimum Standards of Reporting Checklist (Additional file 1) contains details of the experimental design, and statistics, and resources used in this study.

Measurements of haematological parameters

Serum aspartate aminotransferase (AST), alanine aminotransferase (ALT) and alanine phosphatase (ALP) were examined through enzymatic colorimetric methods by their respective commercial assay kits (Nanjing Jiancheng Bioengineering Institute, Nanjing, China) according to the manufacturer's instructions. For the measurements of AST and ALT, serum was mixed well with corresponding matrix solution, and then reacted with 2,4-dinitro-phenylhydrazine for 20 min. NaOH solution (4 mol/L) was added to terminate the reaction. Results were measured by SpectraMax® M5 Multi-Mode Microplate Reader (Waltham, MA, USA).

Histopathological analysis

The right lobe of the liver tissue was fixed in 10% (*v/v*) phosphate-buffered formalin overnight, and embedded in paraffin. The cryostat sections were stained with hematoxylin and eosin according to a standard protocol [14]. The histopathological alterations of liver were observed by an Olympus CX-31 light microscopy with CCD camera (Olympus Crop, Tokyo, Japan).

Parameter measurements for oxidative stress in the liver

Partial liver tissues were homogenized in 9 volumes of cold RIPA (Beyotime Institute of Biotechnology, Nanjing, China) on ice. The liver homogenates (10%) were centrifuged, and the final supernatants were subjected to measure the levels of malondiadehyde (MDA), reduced glutathione (GSH), oxidized glutathione (GSSG), the activities of superoxide dismutase (SOD) and catalase (CAT) by their respective assay kits (Jiancheng Bioengineering). Protein content in the homogenates was determined using a Pierce™ BCA Protein Assay Kit (Thermo Fisher Scientific Inc., Rockford, IL, USA). The results were normalized per gram total protein.

TUNEL assay

The apoptotic cells in liver cryostat section were evaluated by a commercial ApopTag® Plus In Situ Apoptosis Fluorescein Detection Kit (EMD Millipore Corporation, Billerica, MA, USA). Briefly, liver sections (4 μM) were fixed in 1% paraformaldehyde solution, then incubated in green fluorescein labelled dUTP solution at 37 °C for 1 h. After washing, the sections were counterstained with 4,6-diamidino-2-phenylindole (DAPI) (Thermo Fisher Scientific Inc., Rockford, IL, USA). The apoptotic cells were visualized on Zeiss Axio Imager A2 microscope (Carl Zeiss, Oberkochen, Germany).

RT-PCR analysis

The transcriptional expressions of CYP2E1, Keapl, HO-1 and GCLC in liver were determined by qPCR as previously described [5, 11]. In brief, total RNA was extracted from liver by a TRIzol® reagent, and subjected to cDNA synthesis using TaqMan Reverse Transcription Reagents Kit (Life Technologies, Carlsbad, CA). The primers (Table 1) were synthesized by Invitrogen Life Technologies (Shanghai, China). qPCR was conducted on a Mx3005P qPCR system (Agilent Technologies) by SYBR® Green PCR Master Mix (Life Technologies). The mRNA expression was normalized to β-actin.

Immunoblot analysis

The total protein was isolated from the left lobe of the liver tissues by the cold RIPA lysis buffer containing 1% phosphatase inhibitor cocktail (Beyotime Institute of Biotechnology). Approximately 60 μg of total proteins were loaded onto 10% SDS-PAGE, subsequently transblotted onto PVDF membranes (Bio-Rad Laboratories Inc., Hercules, CA, USA). After blocking with 5% nonfat dry milk in TBST (0.1% Tween-20 in Tris-buffered saline), the membranes were incubated with primary antibodies for 24 h at 4 °C, including CYP2E1 (1:1000, Cell Signaling Technology, Danvers, MA, USA), Keap-1 (1:1000, Santa Cruz Biotechnology, Santa Cruz, CA, USA), Nrf2 (1:200, Santa Cruz Biotechnology), HO-1 (1:250, Abcam, Cambridge, MA, USA), GCLC (1:1000, Abcam) and GAPDH (1:1000, Cell Signaling), then incubated with secondary antibodies conjugated to horseradish peroxidase (HRP) for 1 h. The proteins were visualized by Amersham ECL Select Western Blotting Detection Reagent (GE Healthcare BioSciences, Piscataway, NJ, USA).

Table 1 Primers used for the quantitative RT-PCR analysis

Gene	Forward primer	Reverse primer
CYP2E1	5′-CGTTGCCTTGCTTGTC TGGA-3′	5′-AAGAAAGGAATTGGGA AAGGTCC-3′
Keap1	5′-TGCCCCTGTGGTCAAAG TG-3′	5′-GGTTCGGTTACCGTCCT GC-3′
HO-1	5′-AAGCCGAGAATGCTGA GTTCA-3′	5′-GCCGTGTAATATGGTACA AGGA-3′
GCLC	5′-GGGGTGACGAGGTGGAG TA-3′	5′-GTTGGGGTTTGTCCTC TCCC-3′
β-actin	5′-GGCTGTATTCCCCTCCAT CG-3′	5′-GTTGGGGTTTGTCCTC TCCC-3′

Statistical analysis

The value was expressed as mean ± SD. After verifying the distribution of the data by Kolmogorov–Smirnov test, the between-group comparison was conducted by ordinary one-way analysis of variance (ANOVA) using GraphPad 5.0 Software (San Diego, CA, USA).

Results

Effects of PCP on serum parameters

The serum levels of AST, ALT and ALP, the commonly-used biomarkers of liver damage in the clinics [15], were measured by colorimetrical methods. A single dose of CCl_4 exposure caused severe hepatotoxicity in mice (Fig. 1), the serum levels of AST, ALT and ALP in the CCl_4 group were dramatically increased by 11.5-fold (46.6 ± 17.8 vs. 610.0 ± 95.6 U/L), 42.2-fold (6.02 ± 3.61 vs. 260.3 ± 60.0 U/L) and 63.1% (101.2 ± 17.3 vs. 165.1 ± 23.8 U/L), respectively, compared with control group. However, these elevations were decreased significantly ($p < 0.05$) by pre-treatments of PCP at the doses of both 5.15 and 10.3 g/kg BW, and silymarin, a positive control, as well.

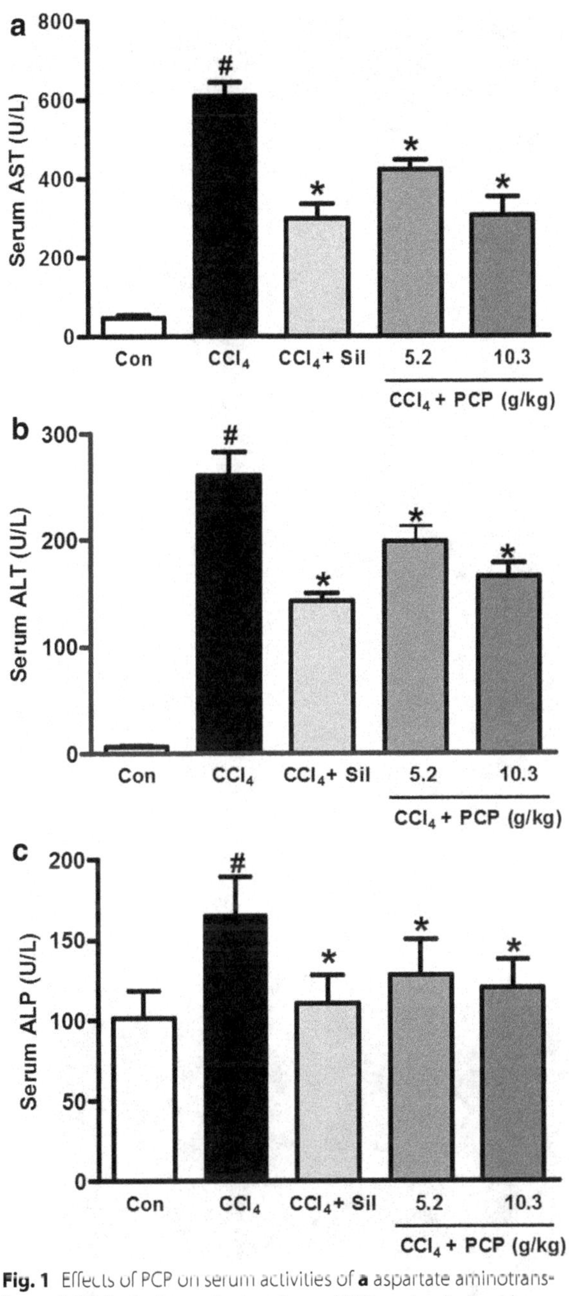

Fig. 1 Effects of PCP on serum activities of **a** aspartate aminotransferase (AST), **b** alanine aminotransferase (ALT), and **c** alanine phosphatase (ALP). Value represents mean ± SD (n = 7–10), $^{\#}p < 0.05$ vs. control group, $^{*}p < 0.05$ vs. CCl_4 group

Effects of PCP on CCl4-induced histopathological alteration

Histological observations were performed to examine the pathological changes in liver. As shown in Fig. 2, the liver tissues from the control group showed normal architectures. CCl_4 challenge caused marked histopathological changes in the liver, characterized by apparent microvesicular and macrovesicular steatosis, massive inflammatory cells infiltration, and extensive hepatocyte necrosis. These histopathological changes were remarkably ameliorated by the pre-treatments of silymarin and PCP (10.3 g/kg BW), which were consistent with the results of serum parameters.

Effects of PCP on CCl4-induced hepatocyte apoptosis

As hepatocyte apoptosis also reflects the extent of CCl_4-induced liver injury [16], a TUNEL assay was performed. As shown in Fig. 3, after 12 h of CCl_4 challenge, the number of TUNEL-positive cells in liver section was obviously increased over the control group, the apoptotic cells were greatly decreased in the pre-treatment of PCP (10.3 g/kg BW) or silymarin.

Effects of PCP on CCl4-induced oxidative stress

To assess the protective effects of PCP on hepatic oxidative stress induced by CCl_4 exposure, the levels of MDA, GSH and GSSG, and the activities of SOD and CAT were examined in liver. As an end-product of lipid peroxidation (LPO), MDA was considered to be a useful marker of oxidative stress [1]. As shown in Fig. 4a, the hepatic MDA level was significantly elevated upon a single dose of CCl_4 exposure, which was decreased in both silymarin and PCP (10.3 g/kg BW)—treated groups. PCP (5.15 g/kg BW) showed a decreased concentration in hepatic MDA, but with no significant difference. CCl_4 exposure also depleted endogenous antioxidants, as indicated by the level of GSH, and the activities of SOD and CAT in CCl_4 group were significantly decreased to 50.5, 22.4 and 58.7%, respectively, compared to control group. These depletions were notably ameliorated by the pretreatment of silymarin and PCP (10.3 g/kg BW) (Fig. 4b–d). Compared to control group, one single dose of CCl_4 challenge significantly elevated the hepatic GSSG level (129 ± 35 vs. 284 ± 48 n mol/mg protein), leading to the decrease in GSH/GSSG ratio (0.77 ± 0.23 vs. 0.25 ± 0.08) (Fig. 4e, f). These alterations were greatly ameliorated by silymarin (100 mg/kg BW) and PCP (10.3 g/kg BW), and their protective efficacies were comparable.

Effects of PCP on CYP2E1 expression

As shown in Fig. 5, CCl_4 challenge dramatically decreased the both mRNA and protein expressions of CYP2E1 in the liver. The pre-treatment of either PCP (10.3 g/kg BW) or silymarin significantly reversed the expression of CYP2E1 in the protein level, but not the transcriptional level.

Effects of PCP on Nrf2-mediated oxidative stress response pathway

To elucidate the molecular mechanisms underlying the protection of PCP against CCl_4-induced oxidative

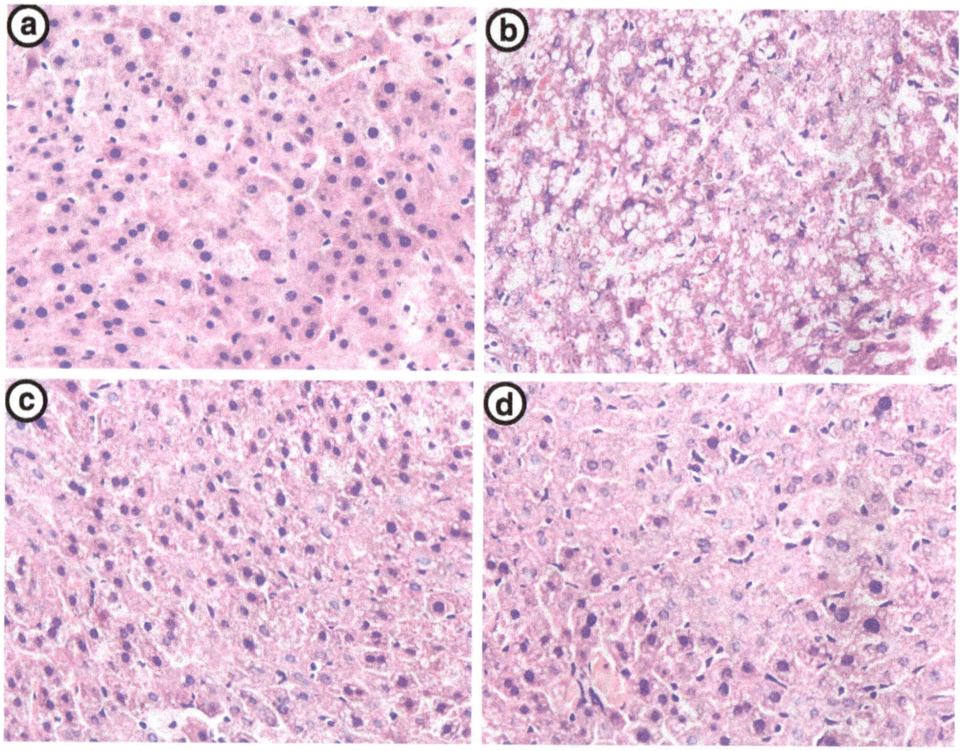

Fig. 2 Representative H&E staining of liver tissues. **a** Control, **b** CCl_4, **c** CCl_4 + Silymarin (100 mg/kg), and **d** CCl_4 + PCP (10.3 g/kg BW)

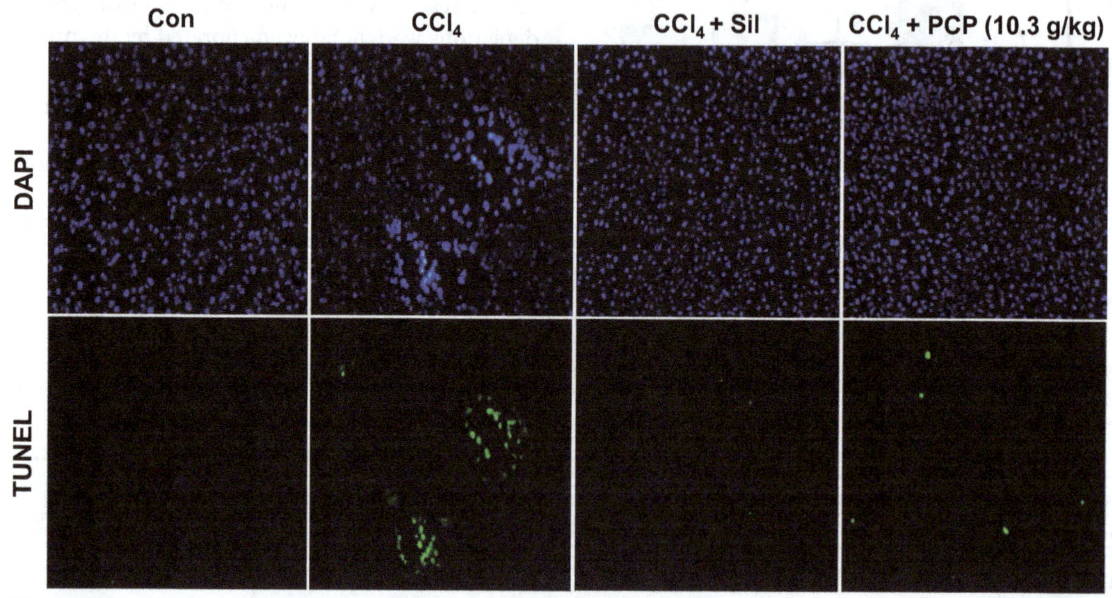

Fig. 3 Effects of PCP on CCl_4-induced hepatocyte apoptosis

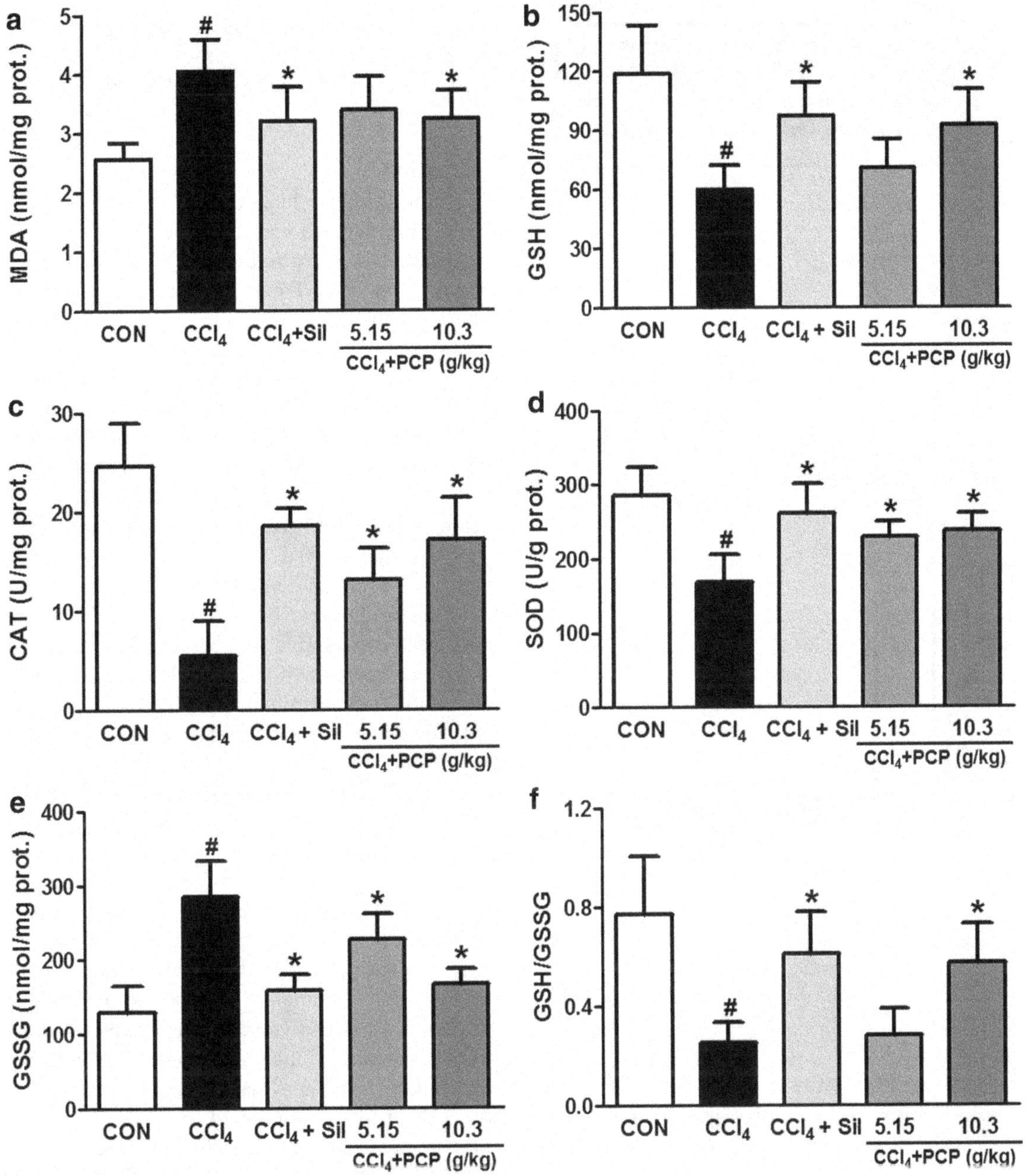

Fig. 4 Effects of PCP on CCl_4-induced oxidative stress in liver. **a** malondialdehyde (MDA); **b** reduced glutathione (GSH); **c** catalase (CAT); **d** superoxide dismutase (SOD); **e** glutathione disulfide (GSSG); **f** the ratio of GSH to GSSG. Value represents mean ± SD (n = 7–10), $^{\#}p < 0.05$ vs. control group, $^{*}p < 0.05$ vs. CCl_4 group

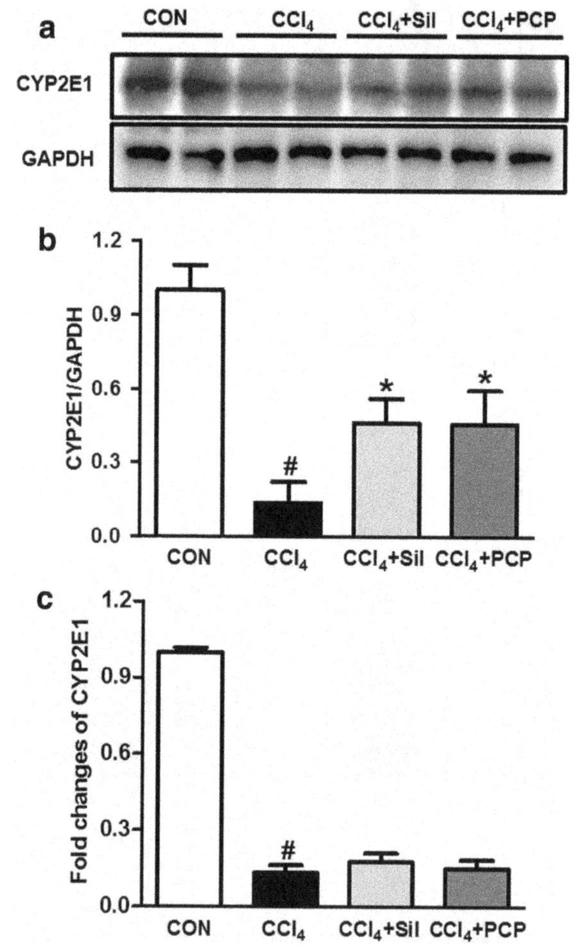

Fig. 5 Effects of PCP (10.3 g/kg BW) on CYP2E1 expression. **a** Immunoblot analysis of CYP2E1; **b** its densitometric analysis; **c** qPCR analysis of CYP2E1. Value represents mean ± SD (n = 3–4), $^{\#}p < 0.05$ vs. control group, $^{*}p < 0.05$ vs. CCl_4 group

stress, the Nrf2 signaling pathway was measured by using immunoblot. Compared to control group, one single dose of CCl_4 exposure decreased the protein expressions of Nrf2 in total, cytosol and nucleus, the pre-treatment of silymarin and PCP (10.3 g/kg BW) significantly normalized these reductions in Nrf2 expressions induced by CCl_4 exposure (Fig. 6). Additionally, Keap-1 and the downstream regulated genes of Nrf2 were also examined in the liver by qPCR and immunoblot analysis. As shown in Fig. 7, the pretreatment of silymarin and PCP (10.3 g/kg BW) remarkably increased the expressions of Keap-1, HO-1 and GCLC in terms of both mRNA and protein levels, over the CCl_4 group. A lower protein expression of Keap-1 in the CCl_4 group was found compared to the control group. However, no significant difference in either mRNA or protein expression of HO-1 and GCLC was observed between the control and the CCl_4 groups.

Discussion

CCl_4, a well-known hepatotoxicant, has been commonly used in cellular and animal models to evaluate the protective effects of natural products on liver injury [17]. Serum levels of AST and ALT are the preferred indicators for evaluation of liver function, they usually reflect the altered permeability of hepatocellular membrane and the damaged structural integrity of hepatocytes [1]. The elevated ALP level in serum was commonly observed in the patients with extrahepatic, intrahepatic biliary obstruction, and infiltrative liver diseases [18]. In our study, CCl_4 challenge induced a profound elevation in serum levels of ALT, AST and ALP, indicating the acute hepatotoxicity caused by CCl_4. However, these increments were effectively alleviated by the pretreatment with PCP and silymarin. The effects of PCP (10.30 g/kg BW) were comparable to silymarin (100 mg/kg BW), a positive control which is a herbal remedy for liver treatment with anti-inflammatory and antioxidant properties [19]. These results demonstrated that PCP effectively protects against acute liver injury induced by a single dose of CCl_4. This observation was also verified by histopathological examination and TUNEL assay as well.

CCl_4 is metabolized by CYP2E1 to produce the CCl_4-derived free radical in the liver [4]. These highly-reactive species can irreversibly oxidize biological macromolecules, such as DNA, proteins and lipids, resulting in lipid peroxidation, oxidative stress, hepatocyte apoptosis, leading ultimately to hepatotoxicity [20, 21]. CCl_4-induced oxidative stress also depletes the endogenous antioxidants, including the non-enzymatic group, such as GSH, and enzymatic antioxidants, such as SOD and CAT. It was documented that GSH is an important antioxidant in eliminating toxic free radicals and reactive toxic CCl_4 metabolites [22, 23]. The sulfhydryl residues of GSH molecule is easily oxidized to GSSG, in turn, GSSG can be converted back to GSH by the aid of glutathione reductase (GR). Thus, the redox ratio of GSH/GSSG is often used as a useful indicator of oxidative stress [24]. In this study, CCl_4 exposure caused severe oxidative stress in the liver where CCl_4 is primarily metabolized, as evidenced by the increased hepatic levels of MDA and GSSG, the decreased GSH level, GSH/GSSG ratio and antioxidant enzyme activities of CAT and SOD. However,

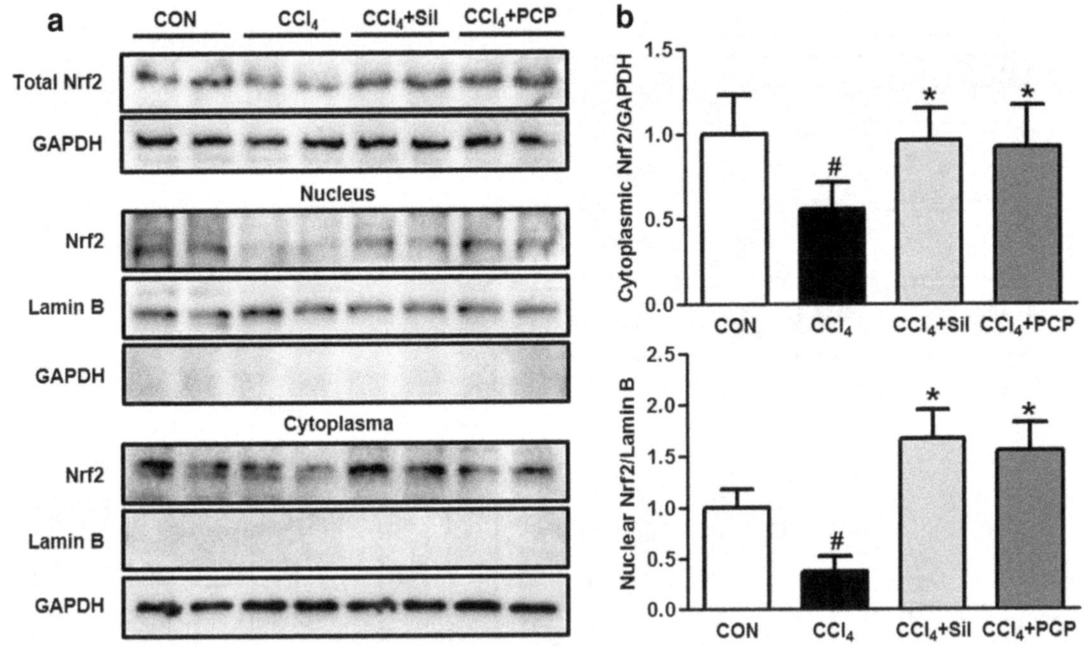

Fig. 6 Effects of PCP (10.3 g/kg BW) on protein expression of Nrf2. **a** Immunoblot analysis of Nrf2 in total, nucleus and cytosol; **b** their results of the densitometric analysis. Value represents mean ± SD (n = 3–4), $^{\#}p < 0.05$ vs. control group, $^{*}p < 0.05$ vs. CCl_4 group

several compounds were identified from PCP, including flavonoids, flavonoid glycosides, polyphenols, steroids [25]. Among these compounds, flavonoids and polyphenols exhibited anti-oxidative effects and other pharmacological bioactivity [26, 27], which may mainly contributed to the hepatoprotection effects of PCP. Our data showed that PCP effectively attenuated CCl_4-induced oxidative stress by not only reducing hepatic MDA level but also enhancing endogenous non-enzymatic and enzymatic antioxidants.

Hepatic CYP2E1 is mainly responsible for the metabolism of CCl_4 to produce highly-reactive trichloromethyl free radicals [28]. Thus, CYP2E1 plays a vital role in the regulation of CCl_4-induced oxidative stress. CYP2E1 deficient mice are resistant to CCl_4-induced hepatoxicity [29], CYP2E1 inhibitors and the antibodies specific for CYP2E1 reduced liver injury induced by CCl_4 exposure in rats [30]. While, CCl_4-induced hepatotoxicity can be enhanced by the pretreatment of alcohol, a CYP2E1 inducer [31]. However, a large body of studies has also indicated that CCl_4 challenge decreased the expression and activity of CYP2E1 [32–34]. A most plausible explanation is that CCl_4 might labilize and inactivate CYP2E1, and enhance its degradation, which reveals ongoing oxidative damage [34]. Our data showed that a remarkable decrease in both mRNA and protein expression of CYP2E1 in the liver was observed after CCl_4 exposure, and the pretreatment of PCP at the doses of either 5.15 or 10.3 g/kg BW significantly elevated the CCl_4-induced decrease of CYP2E1 expression in the protein level, but not in the transcriptional level, suggesting that PCP efficiently reduces the degradation of CYP2E1 induced by CCl_4.

To understand how PCP reduces the oxidative stress induced by CCl_4 exposure, the expressions of Nrf2 and its downstream genes in the liver were measured. Nrf2 plays a critical role in regulating antioxidant defense system in response to oxidative stress [12]. Nrf2-null mice are more susceptible to hepatotoxicity and oxidative stress induced by various chemicals, including CCl_4, ethanol, acetaminophen, pyrazole and arsenic [35]. In response to stress signals, the redox sensitive protein Keap1 undergoes oxidation, leading to the stabilization of Nrf2 and its nuclear translocation [36]. The activation of Nrf2 by binding to ARE triggers the expression of downstream genes, including HO-1 and GCLC. HO-1 is considered

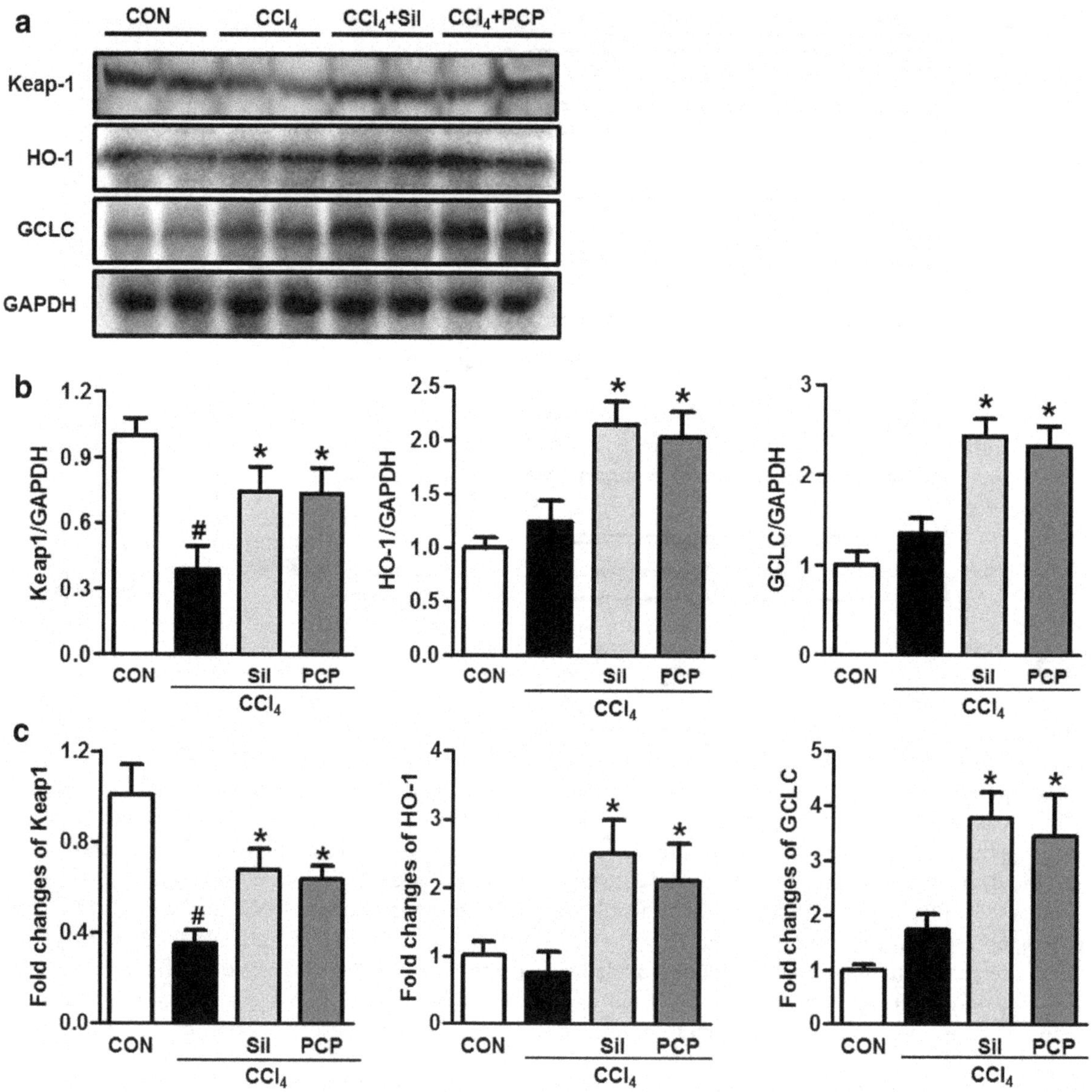

Fig. 7 Effects of PCP (10.3 g/kg BW) on Nrf2-mediated oxidative stress response. **a** Immunoblot analysis of Keap1, HO-1 and GCLC; **b** their results of the densitometric analysis; **c** qPCR analysis of Keap1, HO-1 and GCLC. Value represents mean ± SD (n = 3–4), $^{\#}p < 0.05$ vs. control group, $^{*}p < 0.05$ vs. CCl_4 group

as a strong antioxidant and improves hepatocyte survival. GCLC is a rate-limiting enzyme in GSH biosynthesis in the liver [37]. In the present study, compared with the CCl_4 group, the hepatic Nrf2 expressions in total, cytosol and nucleus were significantly increased in PCP-treated group. As expected, the PCP-treated group showed higher expressions of Keap-1, HO-1 and GCLC in the liver.

Conclusion

Collectively, the pre-treatment of the aqueous extract of PCP (10.3 g/kg BW) can effectively protected against CCl_4-induced acute liver injury, which was closely similar to efficacy of silymarin (100 mg/kg BW). These hepatoprotective effects might be associated with ameliorating CCl_4-induced oxidative stress via activation of Nrf2 signaling pathway (Fig. 8).

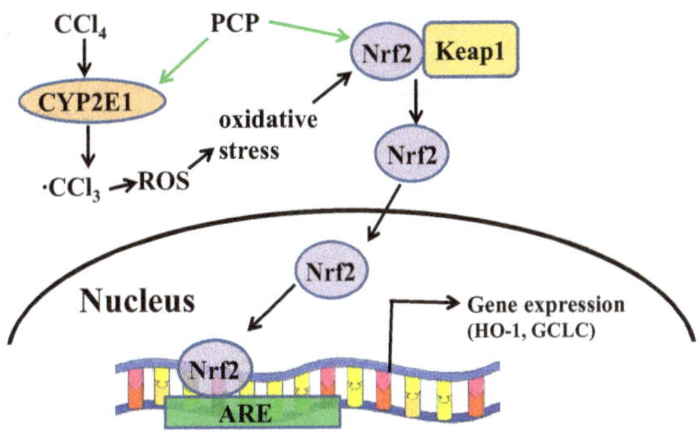

Fig. 8 Schematic diagram of the potential mechanisms underlying the protective effects of PCP on the CCl_4-induced liver injury

Abbreviations

ALP: alanine phosphatase; ALT: alanine aminotransferase; AST: aspartate aminotransferase; CAT: catalase; CCl_4: tetrachloride; CFDA: China Food and Drug Administration; CYP2E1: cytochrome P450 2E1; GCL: glutamate cysteine ligase; GR: glutathione reductase; GSH: reduced glutathione; GSH-Px: glutathione peroxidase; GSSG: oxidized glutathione; HO-1: haem oxygenase 1; IVC: individually ventilated cage; Keap1: Kelch-like ECH-associated protein 1; LPO: lipid peroxidation; MDA: malondialdehyde; Nrf2: nuclear factor erythroid 2-related factor 2; PCP: *Penthorum chinense* Pursh; SOD: superoxide dismutase; ROS: reactive oxygen species.

Authors' contributions

JBW conceived and designed the study; MW and XJZ performed the experiments and drafted the manuscript; RF conducted the western blot of Nrf2; YJ and DYZ. provided the herb; CH and PL revised the manuscript and provided essential comments. All authors read and approved the final manuscript.

Author details

[1] State Key Laboratory of Quality Research in Chinese Medicine, Institute of Chinese Medical Sciences, University of Macau, Room 6034, Building N22, Avenida da Universidade, Macao, People's Republic of China. [2] Sichuan New Lotus Traditional Chinese Herb Limited Company, Chengdu, China.

Acknowledgements

Not applicable.

Competing interests

The authors declare that they have no competing interests.

Consent for publication

All of authors consent to publication of this study in Journal of Chinese Medicine.

Funding

This work was financially supported by the grants from the Research Committee of the University of Macau (MYRG2016-00042-ICMS-QRCM to JB Wan), and from National Natural Science Foundation of China (NSFC, No. 81503288).

References

1. Ding RB, Tian K, Huang LL, He CW, Jiang Y, Wang YT, Wan JB. Herbal medicines for the prevention of alcoholic liver disease: a review. J Ethnopharmacol. 2012;144:457–65.
2. Jadeja RN, Urrunaga NH, Dash S, Khurana S, Saxena NK. Withaferin-A reduces acetaminophen-induced liver injury in mice. Biochem Pharmacol. 2015;97:122–32.
3. Lee IC, Kim SH, Baek HS, Moon C, Kang SS, Kim SH, Kim YB, et al. The involvement of Nrf2 in the protective effects of diallyl disulfide on carbon tetrachloride-induced hepatic oxidative damage and inflammatory response in rats. Food Chem Toxicol. 2014;63:174–85.
4. Su C, Xia X, Shi Q, Song X, Fu J, Xiao C, Chen H, et al. Neohesperidin dihydrochalcone versus CCl4-induced hepatic injury through different mechanisms: the implication of free radical scavenging and Nrf2 activation. J Agric Food Chem. 2015;63:5468–75.
5. Ding RB, Tian K, Cao YW, Bao JL, Wang M, He C, Hu Y, et al. Protective effect of panax notoginseng saponins on acute ethanol-induced liver injury is associated with ameliorating hepatic lipid accumulation and reducing ethanol-mediated oxidative stress. J Agric Food Chem. 2015;63:2413–22.
6. Copple IM, Goldring CE, Kitteringham NR, Park BK. The Nrf2-Keap1 defence pathway: role in protection against drug-induced toxicity. Toxicology. 2008;246:24–33.
7. Taguchi K, Motohashi H, Yamamoto M. Molecular mechanisms of the Keap1-Nrf2 pathway in stress response and cancer evolution. Genes Cells. 2011;16:123–40.
8. Itoh K, Wakabayashi N, Katoh Y, Ishii T, Igarashi K, Engel JD, Yamamoto M. Keap1 represses nuclear activation of antioxidant responsive elements by Nrf2 through binding to the amino-terminal Neh2 domain. Genes Dev. 1999;13:76–86.
9. Lu Q, Jiang M-H, Jiang J-G, Zhang R-F, Zhang M-W. Isolation and identification of compounds from *Penthorum chinense* Pursh with antioxidant and antihepatocarcinoma properties. J Agric Food Chem. 2012;60:11097–103.
10. Wang A, Lin L, Wang Y. Traditional Chinese herbal medicine *Penthorum chinense* Pursh: a phytochemical and pharmacological review. AmJ Chinese Med. 2015;43:601–20.
11. Cao YW, Jiang Y, Zhang DY, Zhang XJ, Hu YJ, Li P, Su H, et al. The hepatoprotective effect of aqueous extracts of *Penthorum chinense* Pursh against acute alcohol-induced liver injury is associated with ameliorating hepatic steatosis and reducing oxidative stress. Food Funct. 2015;6:1510–7.
12. Cao YW, Jiang Y, Zhang DY, Wang M, Chen WS, Su H, Wang YT, et al. Protective effects of *Penthorum chinense* Pursh against chronic ethanol-induced liver injury in mice. J Ethnopharmacol. 2015;161:92–8.
13. Park O, Jeong WI, Wang L, Wang H, Lian ZX, Gershwin ME, Gao B. Diverse roles of invariant natural killer T cells in liver injury and fibrosis induced by carbon tetrachloride. Hepatology. 2009;49:1683–94.
14. Zhang X-J, He C, Li P, Su H, Wan J-B. Ginsenoside Rg1, a potential JNK inhibitor, protects against ischemia/reperfusion-induced liver damage. J Funct Foods. 2015;15:580–92.
15. Wang M, Zhang XJ, Feng K, He C, Li P, Hu YJ, Su H, et al. Dietary alpha-linolenic acid-rich flaxseed oil prevents against alcoholic hepatic steatosis via ameliorating lipid homeostasis at adipose tissue-liver axis in mice. Sci Rep. 2016;6:26826.
16. Feng R, Wang M, Yan C, Li P, Chen M, He C, Wan JB. Endogenous n-3 fatty acids alleviates carbon tetrachloride-induced acute liver injury in fat-1 transgenic mice. Oxid Med Cell Longev. 2016;2016:7962948.
17. Recknagel RO, Glende EA, Dolak JA, Waller RL. Mechanisms of carbon tetrachloride toxicity. Pharmacol Ther. 1989;43:139–54.
18. Field KM, Dow C, Michael M. Part I: liver function in oncology: biochemistry and beyond. Lancet Oncol. 2008;9:1092–101.
19. Surai PF. Silymarin as a natural antioxidant: an overview of the current evidence and perspectives. Antioxidants. 2015;4:204–47.
20. Plaa GL. Chlorinated methanes and liver injury: highlights of the past 50 years. Annu Rev Pharmacol. 2000;40:43–65.
21. Ismail AF, Salem AA, Eassawy MM. Hepatoprotective effect of grape seed oil against carbon tetrachloride induced oxidative stress in liver of gamma-irradiated rat. J Photochem Photobiol B. 2016;160:1–10.
22. Ray G, Husain SA. Oxidants, antioxidants and carcinogenesis. Indian J Exp Biol. 2002;40:1213–32.

23. Boll M, Weber LW, Becker E, Stampfl A. Mechanism of carbon tetrachloride-induced hepatotoxicity. Hepatocellular damage by reactive carbon tetrachloride metabolites. Z Naturforsch C. 2001;56:649–59.
24. Aoyama K, Nakaki T. Glutathione in cellular redox homeostasis: association with the excitatory amino acid carrier 1 (EAAC1). Molecules. 2015;20:8742–58.
25. Wang A, Lin L, Wang Y. Traditional Chinese herbal medicine *Penthorum chinense* Pursh: a phytochemical and pharmacological review. Am J Chin Med. 2015;43:601–20.
26. Roslan J, Giribabu N, Karim K, Salleh N. Quercetin ameliorates oxidative stress, inflammation and apoptosis in the heart of streptozotocin-nicotinamide-induced adult male diabetic rats. Biomed Pharmacother. 2017;86:570–82.
27. Mattera R, Benvenuto M, Giganti MG, Tresoldi I, Pluchinotta FR, Bergante S, Tettamanti G, et al. Effects of polyphenols on oxidative stress-mediated injury in cardiomyocytes. Nutrients. 2017;9:523.
28. Gruebele A, Zawaski K, Kaplan D, Novak RF. Cytochrome P4502E1-and cytochrome P4502B1/2B2-catalyzed carbon tetrachloride metabolism: effects on signal transduction as demonstrated by altered immediate-early (c-Fos and c-Jun) gene expression and nuclear AP-1 and NF-kappa B transcription factor levels. Drug Metab Dispos. 1996;24:15–22.
29. Wong FWY, Chan WY, Lee SST. Resistance to carbon tetrachloride-induced hepatotoxicity in mice which lack CYP2E1 expression. Toxicol Appl Pharm. 1998;153:109–18.
30. Brady JF, Xiao F, Wang MH, Li Y, Ning SM, Gapac JM, Yang CS. Effects of disulfiram on hepatic P450IIE1, other microsomal enzymes, and hepatotoxicity in rats. Toxicol Appl Pharm. 1991;108:366–73.
31. Ray SD, Mehendale HM. Potentiation of CCl4 and CHCl3 hepatotoxicity and lethality by various alcohols. Fundam Appl Toxicol. 1990;15:429–40.
32. Wunjuntuk K, Kettawan A, Charoenkiatkul S, Rungruang T. Parboiled germinated brown rice protects against CCl4-induced oxidative stress and liver injury in rats. J Med Food. 2016;19:15–23.
33. Al-Rasheed N, Faddah L, Al-Rasheed N, Bassiouni YA, Hasan IH, Mahmoud AM, Mohamad RA, et al. Protective effects of silymarin, alone or in combination with chlorogenic acid and/or melatonin, against carbon tetrachloride-induced hepatotoxicity. Pharmacogn Mag. 2016;12:S337–45.
34. Dai Y, Cederbaum AI. Inactivation and degradation of human cytochrome P4502E1 by CCl4 in a transfected HepG2 cell line. J Pharmacol Exp Ther. 1995;275:1614–22.
35. Klaassen CD, Reisman SA. Nrf2 the rescue: effects of the antioxidative/electrophilic response on the liver. Toxicol Appl Pharmacol. 2010;244:57–65.
36. Suzuki T, Motohashi H, Yamamoto M. Toward clinical application of the Keap1-Nrf2 pathway. Trends Pharmacol Sci. 2013;34:340–6.
37. Chen Y, Shertzer HG, Schneider SN, Nebert DW, Dalton TP. Glutamate cysteine ligase catalysis: dependence on ATP and modifier subunit for regulation of tissue glutathione levels. J Biol Chem. 2005;280:33766–74.

19

An innovative anti-cancer Chinese herbal formula exhibited multi-targeted efficacies in metastatic breast cancer mouse model

Grace Gar-Lee Yue[1,2], Julia Kin-Ming Lee[1,2], Ben Chung-Lap Chan[1,2], Hin-Fai Kwok[1,2], Sandy Wan-Heng Hoi[1,2], Daniel Man-Yuen Sze[4], Kwok-Pui Fung[1,2,3], Ping-Chung Leung[1,2] and Clara Bik-San Lau[1,2*]

Abstract

Background: The incidence and mortality of cancer metastasis is high worldwide. Despite of the chemotherapeutic agents, many cancer patients still take traditional Chinese herbal prescriptions as adjuvant treatments. However, most of these herbal formulae/products lack of evidence-based efficacy. Based on our previous investigations on anti-tumor, anti-angiogenic, anti-metastatic, bone protective and immunomodulating activities of various Chinese herbal medicines, four constituent herbs, namely *Andrographis paniculata*, *Acanthopanax senticosus*, *Camellia sinensis*, and *Hedyotis diffusa* were eventually selected to form an innovative herbal formula.

Methods: The anti-tumor efficacies of the formula were evaluated in metastatic breast cancer mice model. The bone protective and immunomodulatory effects were also assessed after formula treatment.

Results: Our results showed that the breast tumor weight as well as lung and liver metastasis in mice could be reduced after herbal formula treatment for 4 weeks. The breast tumor-induced osteolysis in mice was restored by herbal formula treatment, in which the bone volume in treated mice tibia was comparable to that in the non-tumor bearing normal mice. The IL-12 level was augmented and the survival of mice with metastatic breast tumors was prolonged after treatment. Furthermore, combination of herbal formula with chemotherapeutic agent doxorubicin resulted in better anti-tumor efficacy and increased life span in tumor-bearing mice, when compared with doxorubicin alone treatment.

Conclusions: In summary, our innovative Chinese herbal formula was demonstrated to possess anti-tumor, anti-metastatic and bone-protective activities in metastatic breast tumor-bearing mice. The preclinical data generated in this study would lead to the development of evidence-based supplement as adjuvant therapy for metastatic breast cancer.

Keywords: Metastatic breast cancer, Chinese herbal medicines, Metastasis, *Andrographis paniculata*, *Acanthopanax senticosus*, *Camellia sinensis*, *Hedyotis diffusa*

*Correspondence: claralau@cuhk.edu.hk
[1] Institute of Chinese Medicine, E205, Science Centre East Block, The Chinese University of Hong Kong, Shatin, New Territories, Hong Kong
Full list of author information is available at the end of the article

Background

Metastatic cancer is a cancer that has spread from the original site to other tissues and organs. Certain types of cancer are more likely to spread to certain areas than others [1]. Once cancer spreads, the improvement of prognosis continues to provide challenges for patients and healthcare providers. There are treatments for some types of metastatic cancer but not all these treatments are effective enough to control the spread of cancer as well as to relieve symptoms. Limitations of the conventional treatments over their benefits occur.

The increasing use of Chinese herbal medicines (CHM) by cancer patients and survivors can be seen worldwide [2–4]. Cancer patients used CHM to improve their physical and emotional well-beings and to reduce cancer therapy-induced toxicities [5–7]. We have previously proposed that cancer treatment approach needs to be modified from a single target and eliminative direction to a multiple target and holistic direction, which might be achieved by using Chinese herbal medicines as adjuvant therapy [8]. This anticipation has long been pursued by our research team in developing a novel Chinese herbal formula for multi-target therapy approaches [9]. We have also made attempts on establishment of cancer research platforms for modern research of herbal medicines and natural products. One of our focused area is breast cancer treatment.

Breast cancer affects approximately 1.67 million women worldwide in 2012 [10] and it is the 2nd leading causes of cancer death in US [11]. In China, estimated incidence was around 11 out of 100,000 in 2013 [12] and the incidence rate is still increasing [13]. In Chinese community, including Hong Kong, many breast cancer patients take traditional Chinese herbal prescriptions as adjuvant treatments. In view of the high incidence rate of metastatic breast cancer worldwide, the efficacies of CHM were initially investigated in our pre-clinical breast cancer research platform.

In the past decade, our research team has carried out a series of investigations on the anti-tumor activities of various Chinese medicinal herbs and their isolated compounds. Among these herbs, *Andrographis paniculata* (AP, 穿心蓮), *Acanthopanax senticosus* (AS, 刺五加), *Camellia sinensis* (CS, 綠茶), and *Hedyotis diffusa* (HD, 白花蛇舌草) were shown to have promising anti-cancer-related bioactivities. Aqueous extract of AP has been shown to potently inhibit tumor growth and metastasis in esophageal cancer mice in our previous studies [14–16]. *Acanthopanax senticosus* (AS) was investigated for its anti-tumor and immunomodulatory activities in breast cancer cells and immuno-competent mice models [17], unpublished data]. Besides, the anti-tumor, anti-metastatic and bone protective effects of *Camellia sinensis* (CS) have been elucidated thoroughly in a series of studies [18–20]. In addition, both the aqueous extract and the active component from *Hedyotis diffusa* (HD), 4-vinylphenol, have also been demonstrated for their potent anti-angiogenic activities in animal models [21]. The optimal dosages of each herb have been validated in the corresponding in vivo experiments mentioned above. Based on these results, an innovative herbal formula of these four constituent herbs with particular reference to the properties was formed using their corresponding optimal dosages, hence, the ratio of each herb in the formula was AP:AS:CS:HD = 1.7:1:1:8. This formula was designed for cancer patients as it was expected to augment and to relieve the discomfort from the conventional cancer treatment as well as prevent recurrence. The present study aimed at evaluating the efficacies of the herbal formula in our breast tumor-bearing mice model. Promising results showed the anti-metastatic effects of the formula. Furthermore, the adjuvant activities of the formula to chemotherapeutic agent doxorubicin in metastatic breast cancer mice were illustrated for the first time.

Materials and methods

Information of experimental design and resources

The information regarding the experimental design, statistics, and resources used in this study is attached in the minimum standards of reporting checklist (Additional file 1).

Herbal materials and extraction

The dried herbs of *Andrographis paniculata* (AP), *Acanthopanax senticosus* (AS), *Camellia sinensis* (CS) and *Hedyotis diffusa* (HD) were purchased in a single lot from herbal suppliers in Hong Kong. Morphological and chemical authentication were accomplished in accordance with the Chinese Pharmacopoeia 2010 [22] or herbal medicine reference book (since no monograph was found in Chinese Pharmacopoeia for *Hedyotis diffusa*) [23]. The chemical profiles were compared qualitatively using thin layer chromatography (TLC) with the reference herb provided by National Institute for the Control of Pharmaceutical and Biological Products. In addition, the representative chemical markers (andrographolide and dehydroandrographolide for AP; syringin for AS; caffeine, epigallocatechin gallate for CS; asperuloside for HD) were determined quantitatively using UPLC. Authenticated voucher specimens were deposited in the museum of the Institute of Chinese Medicine, the Chinese University of Hong Kong.

Dried herbs were extracted individually under reflux using water for 1 h and the extraction were repeated once. The extracts were filtrated, centrifuged to remove undissolved particles and then freeze-dried into powder. The formula composed of 4 types of aqueous extracts of the above-mentioned herbs, with the ratio (AP:AS:CS:HD = 1.7:1:1:8). The optimal dosages of each herb were mixed (i.e. 1000 mg/kg for AP; 600 mg/kg for AS; 600 mg/kg for CS; 4800 mg/kg for HD, 7000 mg/kg in total). The mixed formula extract powder was dissolved in water for animal studies.

UPLC-QTOF analysis of the herbal formula

Stock solutions

Stock solutions of syringin, asperuloside, caffeine, epigallocatechin gallate, andrographolide and dehydroandrographolide were prepared individually in distilled water at 1 mg/mL. They were stored at −20 °C until use.

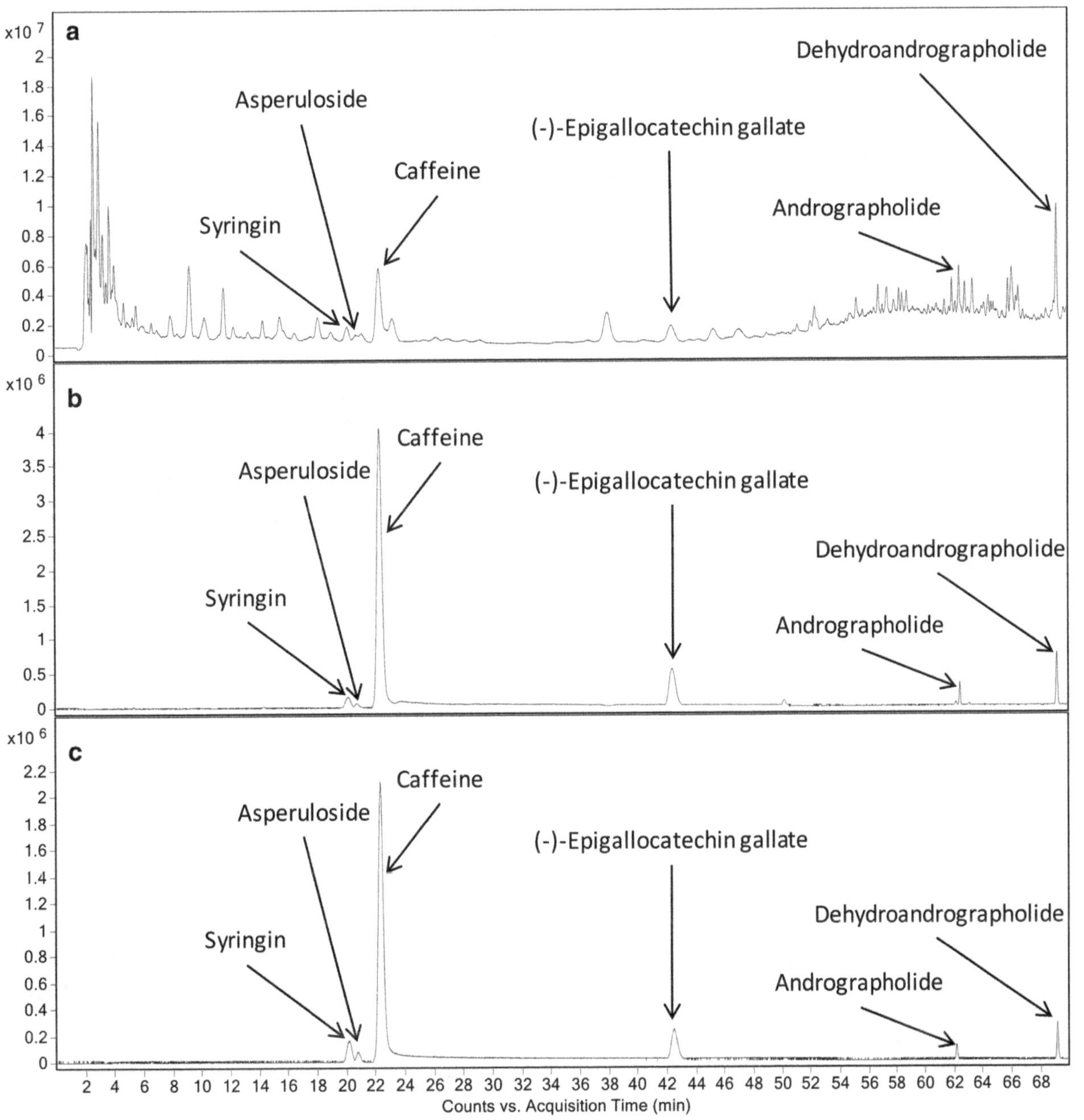

Fig. 1 UPLC chromatograms of the herbal formula. **a** Total ion chromatogram of sample; **b** Base peak chromatogram of sample; **c** Base peak chromatogram of standard markers. 395.1318 m/z (Syringin), 437.1049 m/z (Asperuloside), 195.0874 (Caffeine), 459.0913 (Epigallocatechin gallate), 315.1956 m/z (Andrographolide) and 297.1855 m/z (Dehydroandrographolide) were extracted for the base peak chromatogram

Table 1 Contents of chemical markers (syringin, asperuloside, caffeine, epigallocatechin gallate, andrographolide and dehydroandrographolide) in formula extract

Chemical markers	Content in formula extract (%)
Syringin	0.043 ± 0.005
Asperuloside	0.044 ± 0.003
Caffeine	0.596 ± 0.018
Epigallocatechin gallate	0.817 ± 0.021
Andrographolide	0.475 ± 0.033
Dehydroandrographolide	0.115 ± 0.008

Preparation of standard solution

100 μL of each stock solution were mixed and marked up to 1 mL by distilled water to give a standard solution.

Sample preparation

140 mg of dry sample powder were dissolved in 5 mL distilled water as the sample solution.

UPLC-QTOF analysis

The analysis was conducted using an Agilent 1290 UHPLC with 6530 QTOF system (CA, USA). The column used was GRACE Alltima C18, 5 μm, 4.6 × 250 mm. The chromatographic separation was conducted at room temperature under gradient conditions at a flow rate of 1 mL/min. The LC profile was as follows: Mobile phase: (A) (0.1% formic acid, in deionized and distilled water) and (B) acetonitrile; Gradient: 0–5 min, 8% B; 5–10 min, 8–10% B; 10–30 min, 10% B; 30–42 min, 10–13% B; 42–49 min, 13–18% B; 49–69 min, 18–55% B; 69–70 min, 55% B. High purity nitrogen was used as the curtain and

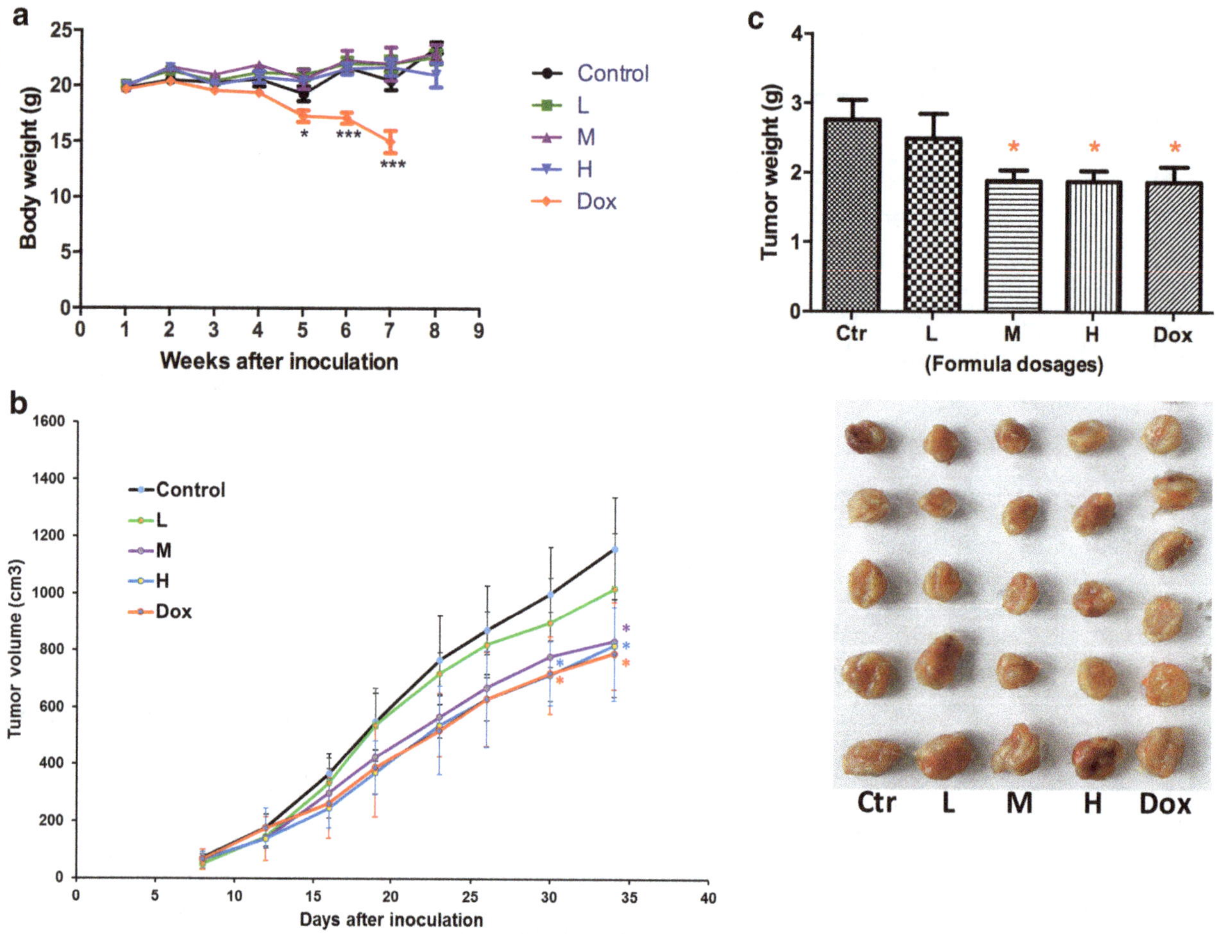

Fig. 2 Effects of formula or doxorubicin (Dox) treatments on the 4T1 breast tumor-bearing mice. **a** Body weight in different treatment groups (L: 231 mg/kg; M: 770 mg/kg; H: 2310 mg/kg, daily). Each point represented mean ± SEM (n = 12). **b** Tumor volume of mice were recorded during treatments. **c** Effects of different treatments on final tumor weight were compared. Results were expressed as mean + SEM (n = 12). *$p < 0.05$, ***$p < 0.005$ when treatment groups compared with control group at the same time point by one-way ANOVA followed by Tukey's multiple comparisons test. Photograph at lower panel showed the representative tumors in different treatment groups

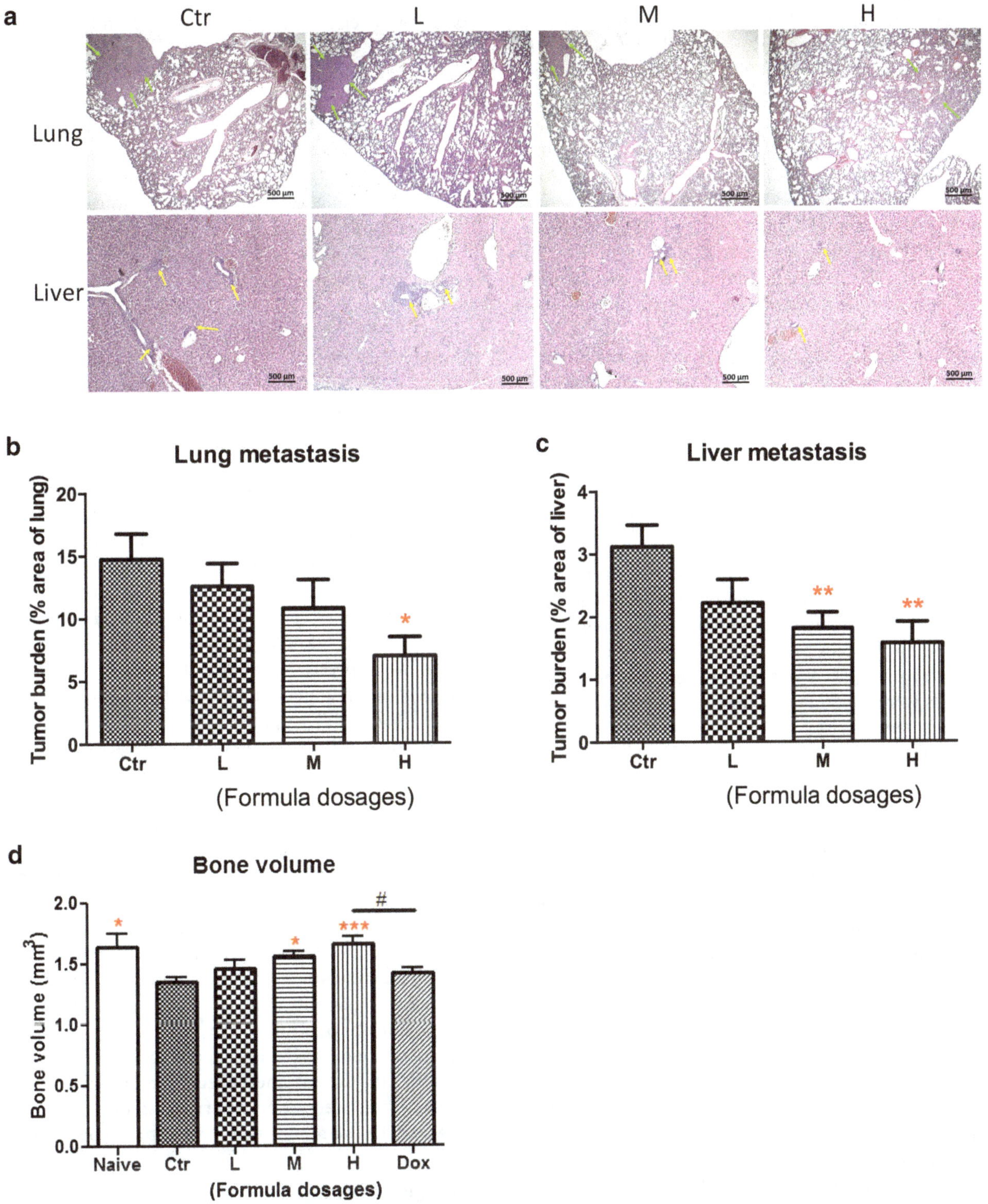

Fig. 3 The paraffin-embedded sections of the lungs and livers were photographed and used to measure metastatic loci area and total lung or liver area. **a** Representative photographs of lungs and livers were shown. Arrows indicated the tumor nodules. The histograms showed the tumor burden in **b** lungs and **c** livers according to the tumor area as a percentage of whole lung or liver area per group (n = 12). **d** Effects of formula treatments on bone volume of tumor-bearing mice. Quantitative assessment of bone structure in mouse tibias after formula or doxorubicin treatments. The graph showed the bone volume of tibias from different groups (n = 10). Data were expressed as mean + SEM. Differences among the treated and control groups were determined by one-way ANOVA followed by Tukey's multiple comparisons test. *$p < 0.05$, **$p < 0.01$, ***$p < 0.005$ as compared to control group. $^{\#}p < 0.05$ when compared among treatment groups

collision gas with a flow rate of 12 L/min. The drying gas temperature was set at 350 °C, and the nebulizer pressure was set at 60 psi. Spectra were recorded in positive ion mode at spray voltage of 3500 V. The mass scan range was between 100 and 1100 m/z. Data analysis was performed using Agilent MassHunter Workstation Qualitative Analysis Software (CA, USA, version B.06.00). Syringin was determined at 395.1318 m/z $[M+Na]^+$, asperuloside was determined at 437.1049 m/z $[M+Na]^+$, caffeine was determined at 195.0874 m/z $[M+H]^+$, epigallocatechin gallate was determined at 459.0913 m/z $[M+H]^+$, andrographolide was determined at 315.1956 m/z $[M\text{-}2H_2O+H]^+$ and dehydroandrographolide was determined at 297.1855 m/z $[M\text{-}2H_2O+H]^+$. The chemical profile of the formula extract was shown as chromatograms in Fig. 1. The contents of these chemical markers in the formula extract were listed in Table 1.

Cell culture

Mouse breast tumor cells (4T1) were purchased from American Type Culture Collection (MD, USA) and maintained in RPMI medium. Culture media were supplemented with 10% (v/v) heat-inactivated FBS, 100 units/mL penicillin–streptomycin. The cells were incubated at 37 °C in a humidified atmosphere of 5% CO_2. When the cells reached 80% confluence in culture flasks, trypsin–EDTA was used to remove the cells and the cells were used in experiments or reseeded in flask. Culture medium, fetal bovine serum (FBS), penicillin–streptomycin, trypsin–EDTA, were obtained from Life Technologies (NY, USA).

Mouse breast tumor model

Female BALB/c mice (6–8 weeks old) were supplied and maintained by Laboratory Animal Services Center, the Chinese University of Hong Kong. All experimental procedures in mice complied with the standards specified by the Animal Experimentation Ethics Committee of the Chinese University of Hong Kong (Ref No. 10/051/MIS).

Mouse breast tumor cells 4T1 (4×10^5) resuspended in 0.1 mL PBS, were subcutaneously inoculated at the mammary fat pad of each mouse. Treatments were initiated 8 days after tumor cell implantation and lasted for 4 weeks. After 4T1 cell implantation, the tumor-bearing mice were randomly assigned into different treatment groups (n = 12). In the pilot study, mice were orally administered with formula at 7000 mg/kg (mixed 4 herbal extract at optimal dosage); however, the efficacy of 7000 mg/kg of formula reached plateau and the solubility of the herbal formula powder was not good at such dosage (i.e. ≥ 7000 mg/kg). Hence, the testing dosage was reduced around 3-, 10-, 30-folds to 2310, 770 and 231 mg/kg, respectively. Tumor-bearing mice were orally administered with formula at 3 different dosages (L: 231 mg/kg; M: 770 mg/kg; H: 2310 mg/kg, daily) and/or treated with doxorubicin (5 mg/kg, once a week) for 4 weeks. The mixed formula powder was dissolved in distilled water. Chemotherapeutic agent doxorubicin at 5 mg/kg was dissolved in saline and administered intraperitoneally to mice. The body weights and tumor sizes of mice were measured once a week during the treatment period. At the end of treatment (8 weeks), mice were sacrificed and blood was collected. The cytokines levels in plasma isolated from mice were determined by ELISA (BD Biosciences, NJ, USA). Lungs and livers were removed for histological analysis. Tibias of mice from different groups were removed for micro-computed tomography analysis.

Immunological responses in breast tumor-bearing mice

The immunomodulatory effects of the formula on breast tumor-bearing mice were further determined. Cells harvested from thymus, spleen and lymph nodes were subjected to population determination of T cells, regulatory T cells (Treg) or myeloid-derived suppressor cells (MDSC) by flow cytometry. In brief, the excised organs were pressed through the nylon membranes using syringe plungers and the cells were washed and blocked using PBS supplemented with 5% FBS. Cells were stained with a cocktail of fluorescence-conjugated anti-CD3, anti-CD4 and anti-CD8 IgG for T cells, or a cocktail of anti-CD4, anti-CD25 and anti-FOXP3 antibodies for regulatory T cells, or a cocktail of anti-Ly6G and anti-CD11b antibodies for MDSC. All stained cells were analyzed using a FACSCanto™ II Flow Cytometer (BD Biosciences, NJ, USA).

Lymphocytes harvested from spleens of mice were cultured ex vivo as described previously [27]. Lymphocytes were resuspended in RPMI 1640 medium, seeded in 24 well-plates at a density of 3×10^6 cells/mL and incubated with phytohemagglutinin (PHA) at 10 mg/mL for 24 h. After incubation, the culture supernatants were collected and subjected to enzyme-linked immunosorbent assay (ELISA) for concentration determination of IL-2, IL-12, IFN-γ and TNF-α according to the kit protocols.

Histological analysis

Lungs and livers were fixed in 10% buffered formalin, paraffin embedded and sectioned at 5 μm. Then the sections were stained with hematoxylin & eosin and examined and photographed as described previously [28]. Tumor burden, defined as the tumor area, was calculated from the section of the lung or liver in a double-blind manner

(See figure on next page.)

Fig. 4 Effects of formula treatments on immune responses of tumor-bearing mice. Populations of T lymphocytes, myeloid-derived suppressor cells (MDSC) and regulatory T cells (Treg) in spleen, thymus and lymph node were determined by flow cytometry. Cells were stained with fluorochrome conjugated antibodies as mentioned in Materials and Methods section. **a**, **b** The proportions of $CD4^+$ and $CD8^+$ T cells in lymphocytes were analyzed using flow cytometry analyses by gating $CD3^+$ population. Populations of **c** regulatory T cells ($CD4^+CD25^+FOXP3^+$) in lymph node and **d** MDSC ($CD11b^+Ly6G^+$) in spleen were analyzed from the 10,000–20,000 viable isolated cells. Results were expressed as mean concentration ± SEM (n = 4–8). **e** Level of IL-12 in plasma of mice from different treatment groups were determined by ELISA. **f** Production of IL-2, IL-12, IFN-γ and TNF-α by isolated spleen lymphocytes from formula-treated mice. The concentrations of cytokines were determined by ELISA. Results were expressed in box and whisker plots of 4–8 mice each group. Statistical difference was determined by one-way ANOVA, followed by Tukey's multiple comparisons test. *$p < 0.05$, **$p < 0.01$, ***$p < 0.005$ as compared with the control group. #$p < 0.05$, ##$p < 0.01$ when compared among treatment groups

using Image J software (NIH, USA). The section photos taking and assessment using Image J software were performed by two investigators. Tumor burden expressed as an average percentage of tumor area to lung or liver area in each treatment group.

Micro-computed tomography (μ-CT) analysis

Tibias removed from tumor-bearing mice were scanned with a high resolution microtomographic system, μ-CT 40 (Scanco Medical AG, Switzerland). Each three-dimensional image data consisted of approximately 500 μ-CT slide image (8 μm/slide) starting from the growth plate of tibial interface and moving down the tibia. Bone volume (mm^3) was generated from μ-CT analysis and compared with the control tibia for each animal [24].

Statistical analysis

Data were expressed as mean + SEM. Statistical analyses and significance were analyzed by one-way ANOVA followed by post hoc test using GraphPad PRISM software version 6.0 (GraphPad Software, USA). In all comparisons, $p < 0.05$ was considered as statistically significant.

Results

Herbal formula treatment significantly reduced weight of breast tumors without affecting body weight

Tumor-bearing mice were orally administered with formula at 3 different dosages (L: 231 mg/kg; M: 770 mg/kg; H: 2310 mg/kg, daily) or treated with doxorubicin (5 mg/kg, once a week) for 4 weeks. During the treatments, no body weight loss was observed in formula-treated groups while there was significant decrease in doxorubicin-treated group since the 4th week after treatment started (Fig. 2a). The tumor volume was shown to be lowered in formula-treated (M and H dosages) and doxorubicin-treated groups (Fig. 2b) when compared with untreated control group. The tumor weights of mice after treatments with formula (at M and H dosages) or doxorubicin were significantly lowered than those of untreated control mice ($p < 0.05$, Fig. 2c).

Herbal formula treatment significantly reduced lung and liver metastasis and restored breast tumor-induced osteolysis

Lungs and livers from each mouse were removed for histological analysis and assessment of lung and liver metastasis. Large tumors were found in untreated control group, while the tumor area and nodules were decreased in formula treatment groups (Fig. 3a). Tumor burden in lung was found to decrease by formula treatment (Fig. 3b). Tumor burden in lung decreased by 52.8% (from 14.74 to 6.96%) in H-dosage formula-treated group. Similar results were also found in liver metastasis. Liver metastasis was decreased significantly after formula treatments (both M- & H-dosages) ($p < 0.01$) (Fig. 3c). Tumor burden in liver decreased by 42.0% and 49.7% in M- and H-dosages formula-treated groups.

As mentioned, breast cancer cells metastasize to bone and induce severe bone destruction. For assessing the efficacy of formula treatment against breast cancer-induced bone destruction, micro-computed tomography (μ-CT) analysis was employed. Tumor-bearing mice with formula treatments showed increased bone volume in a dose-dependent manner. As shown in Fig. 3d, the bone volume (BV) in control group was 1.35 mm^3, lost nearly 18% of BV when compared to the BV of naive group, indicating severe bone destruction in control group. In contrast, treatments with formula (at dosages M & H) resulted in remarkable increase of BV in tumor-bearing mice. No significant difference was shown between doxorubicin-treated and control groups, but there was significant difference between doxorubicin-treated and formula dosage H groups ($p < 0.05$).

Herbal formula treatment modulated immune responses

Since one of the component herbs within the formula possess potent immuno-stimulating activities, the overall modulatory effects of the formula were further determined. Immune cells of immunocompetent tumor-bearing mice will play crucial roles in tumor progression and hence, the effects of formula treatment on the populations of various immune cells were studied. As shown in Fig. 4a, b, $CD8^+$ T cell

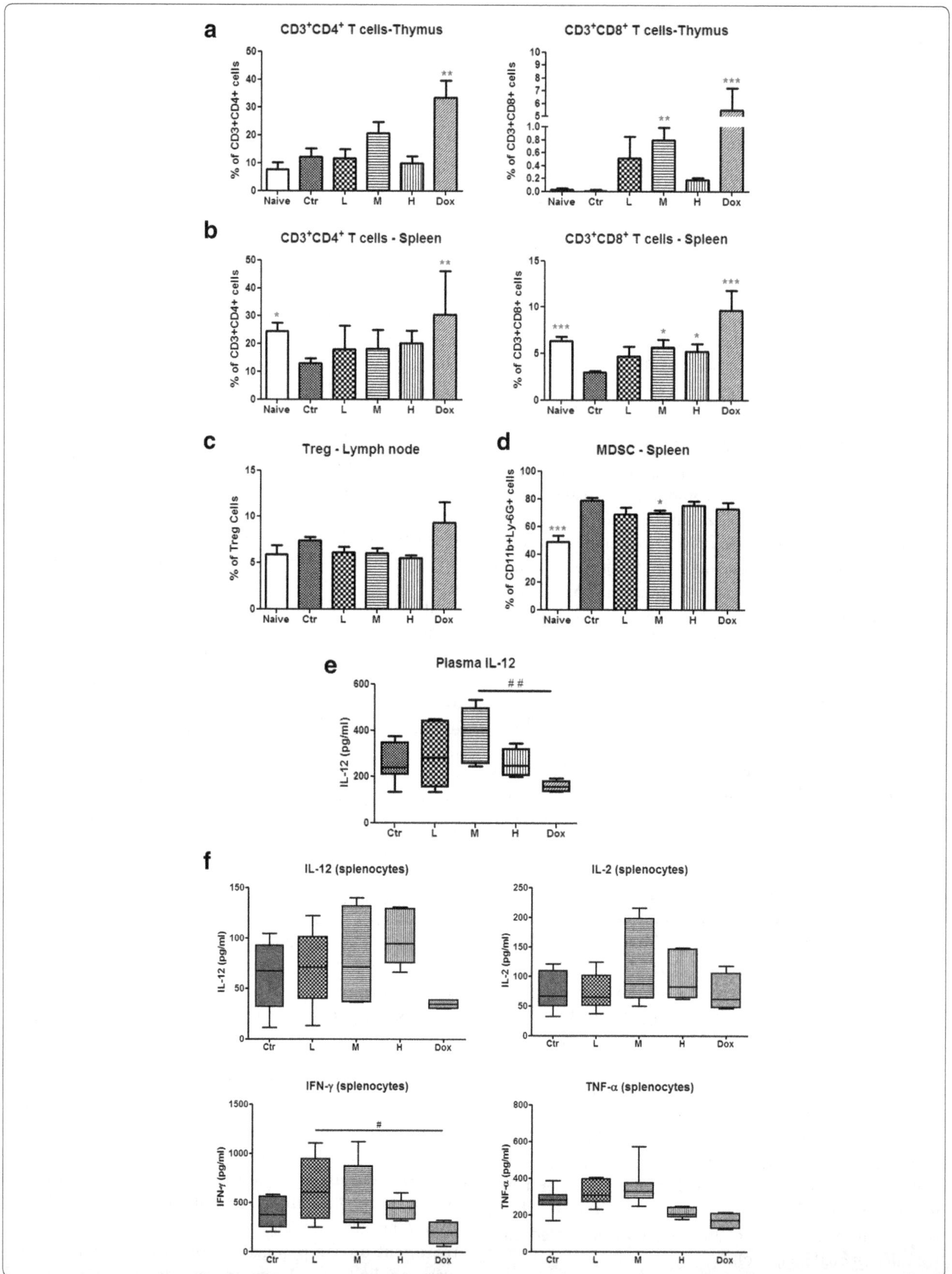
a
CD3+CD4+ T cells-Thymus
% of CD3+CD4+ cells
CD3+CD8+ T cells-Thymus
% of CD3+CD8+ cells
Naive Ctr L M H Dox
b
CD3+CD4+ T cells - Spleen
% of CD3+CD4+ cells
CD3+CD8+ T cells - Spleen
% of CD3+CD8+ cells
c
Treg - Lymph node
% of Treg Cells
d
MDSC - Spleen
% of CD11b+Ly-6G+ cells
e
Plasma IL-12
IL-12 (pg/ml)
Ctr L M H Dox
f
IL-12 (splenocytes)
IL-12 (pg/ml)
IL-2 (splenocytes)
IL-2 (pg/ml)
IFN-γ (splenocytes)
IFN-γ (pg/ml)
TNF-α (splenocytes)
TNF-α (pg/ml)

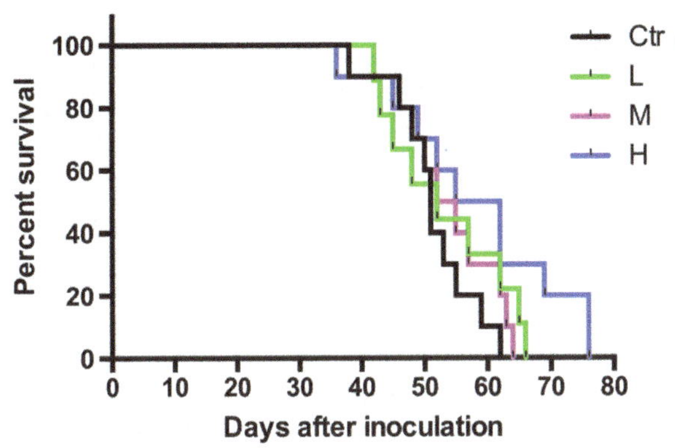

Fig. 5 Survival curves of mice in each treatment group (n = 10). Data were shown in Kaplan–Meier survival curves

population in thymus and spleen in formula dosage M, as well as doxorubicin groups were significantly increased when compared with the untreated control group ($p < 0.05$). Besides, the interference from regulatory T cells (Treg cells) and myeloid-derived suppressor cells (MDSC) on the activation of T cells against cancer were demonstrated in previous studies [28]. Results showed that formula treatment (especially at dosage M) could reduce the populations of Treg cells ($CD4^+CD25^+FOXP3^+$ cells) in lymph node and MDSC ($CD11b^+Ly6G^+$ cells) in spleen (Fig. 4c, d).

On the other hand, the plasma IL-12 level in formula (at dosage M) treatment group was shown to be higher than that of control and doxorubicin-treated groups (Fig. 4e). Furthermore, spleen lymphocytes were isolated from tumor-bearing mice treated with formula activated by PHA for 24 h. The concentrations of Th-1 cytokines (IL-2, IL-12, IFN-γ and TNF-α) released by spleen lymphocytes ex vivo were higher in those from formula-treated groups than those from control group, although the differences were not statistically significant (Fig. 4f). In contrast, the levels of these cytokines were not increased in doxorubicin-treated group. These results suggested that the immune responses against tumor could be modulated by formula treatment.

Herbal formula treatment significantly prolonged survival of breast tumor-bearing mice

The survival rate of mice in the treatment groups were further studied. The death number of mice was recorded in either natural death from tumor-bearing or euthanasia due to the large tumor (diameter exceeded 15 mm). As shown in Fig. 5, the mice treated with formula (at dosage H) lived for the longest period as there were still 20% of mice alive until 76 days after tumor cell inoculation. Median survival days of mice in formula dosage H group was 58.5 days, which was longer than that in control (51 days) group. These results showed that formula treatment could prolong the median survival time (or increased the life span) of the metastatic breast tumor-bearing mice.

Combined treatment of herbal formula with chemotherapeutic agent exhibited better anti-tumor effects

Further investigation on the combined effect of herbal formula and chemotherapeutic agent was conducted in the 4T1 metastatic breast tumor-bearing mice. Mice were administered with herbal formula at the M dosage (770 mg/kg, orally daily) plus doxorubicin (5 mg/kg, intraperitoneally weekly) for 4 weeks. As shown in Fig. 6a, the tumor volume of combined treatment group was significantly lowered than that of control group from the 25th day after inoculation. The final tumor volume of combined treatment group was significantly lowered than that of doxorubicin alone treatment group ($p < 0.01$) and control group ($p < 0.001$). In the other set of experiment, the survival rate of combined treatment group was higher than those of control and doxorubicin alone treatment group (Fig. 6b). The median survival of control, formula at M dosage alone, doxorubicin alone and combined treatment groups were 49, 54.5, 56.5 and 64 days, respectively.

Discussion

In this study, the efficacies in terms of anti-tumor, anti-metastasis, immuno-modulating and bone protective activities of the herbal formula have been evaluated in metastatic breast tumor mouse model. The composition of the herbal formula was based on our hypothesis that combining herbs with the above-mentioned bio-activities to observe synergistic effect. As shown in the results, the herbal formula exhibited remarkable bio-activities in the breast tumor-bearing mice, which was demonstrated for the first time.

As we have been suggesting to develop a novel Chinese herbal formula for multi-target therapy approaches for years [9], the efficacies of various anti-cancer herbs have been examined in our in vivo platforms as mentioned above. Here we demonstrated that treatment with two dosages (770 and 2310 mg/kg) of herbal formula resulted in tumor growth and metastasis inhibition in metastatic breast tumor-bearing mice. In fact, higher dosages (i.e. > 2310 mg/kg) have been tested in our pilot study; however, the efficacy of 7000 mg/kg (threefold of the highest dosage in present study) of formula reached plateau and the solubility of the herbal formula powder was not good for the higher dosage (i.e. ≥ 7000 mg/kg). Hence, the activities

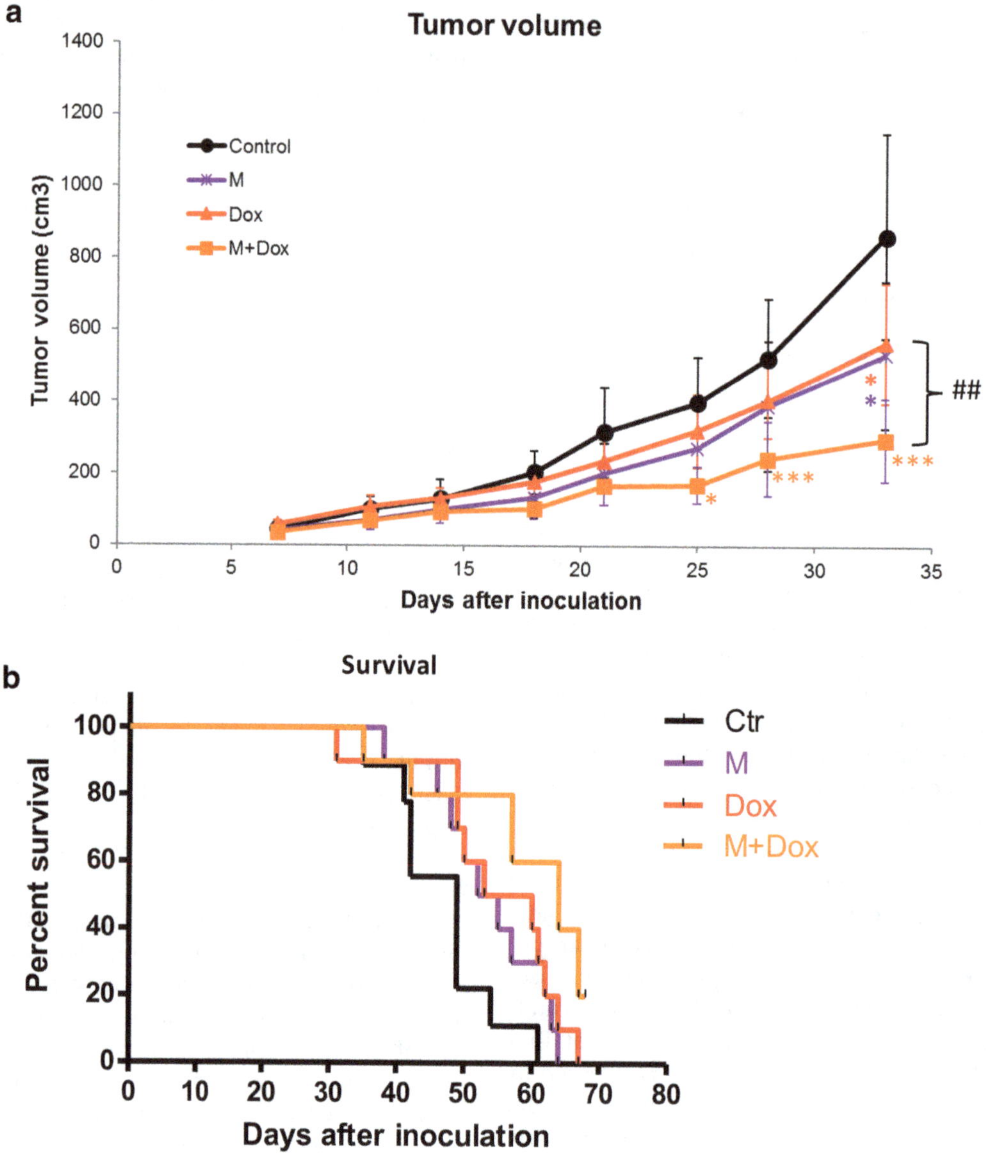

Fig. 6 Effects of combined formula and doxorubicin (Dox) treatments on the mouse breast tumor growth and the survival of tumor-bearing mice. **a** Tumor volume in different treatment groups. Each point represented mean of 10 mice. Results were expressed as mean + SEM (n = 10). $^{*}p < 0.05$, $^{***}p < 0.005$ when treatment groups compared with control group; $^{\#\#}p < 0.01$ when compared among treatment groups. **b** Survival curves of mice in each treatment group (n = 10). Data were shown in Kaplan–Meier survival curves

of the herbal formula at 231, 770 and 2310 mg/kg were reported here.

Metastatic breast cancer is a heterogeneous disease that has a variety of different clinical conditions [24]. It remains a major challenge in cancer treatment that the median survival is 2–3 years [25]. The development of our novel herbal formula aimed to provide an alternative/adjuvant choice for breast cancer patients. To provide pre-clinical evidences of efficacy, the metastatic breast tumor-bearing mouse model with spontaneous metastases to lungs, livers, and bones [26] was adopted. Another characteristic of metastatic breast cancer is the high incidence of bone metastases causing significant morbidity including pain, fracture and spinal cord compression [29]. Recent survey data showed that 62.5% of patients with initial metastatic breast cancer had bone involvement [30]. These patients may require additional medical care from orthopaedics specialists, other than receiving anti-cancer treatments alone. In this regards, multi-targeted anti-metastatic agents which also target for bone metastasis are desired. The bone protective activities showed in the present study could certainly provide a rationale of clinical use of the herbal formula.

On the other hand, the systemic effects of the herbal formula, including immunomodulation, could be evaluated in this syngeneic tumor-bearing model. Our results showed that the herbal formula was effective in inhibiting the metastasis to lungs and livers, which may be contributed by the potent anti-metastatic effects of AP and CS. In addition, herbal formula could modulate the $CD8^+$ T cells, regulatory T cells and MDSC population as well as increase the levels of anti-tumor cytokine IL-12 (in plasma and secreted by splenocytes) [31]. The outcome of herbal formula treatment was the prolong life span of the metastatic breast tumor-bearing mice.

Furthermore, in our previous review on the role of Chinese herbal medicines in cancer management, we suggested that the potential beneficial adjuvant therapies can be attained by combining CHM and chemotherapeutics [9]. The superior anti-tumor and life prolonging effects of the combined herbal formula and chemotherapeutic treatment have demonstrated here. The synergistic effects of the combined treatment as well as the efficacies of the formula in other types of cancer are worth further investigations.

Nowadays, the use of herbal medicines by patients as adjuvant to conventional cancer treatment is common while there were concerns from the users on the efficacy and safety. Some of the herbal prescriptions or supplements for cancer patients are short of evidence-based confirmation of efficacy. In addition, their multi-targeted efficacy and bioavailability may be virtually non-existing. We aimed to apply innovative concepts of evidence-based, multi-targeted and quality-assured for developing a herbal formula targeting on metastatic breast cancer. Our findings provided scientific evidences on this hypothetically created herbal formula in breast tumor-bearing mice. We are ready to go for a clinical trial using this herbal formula and the promising outcome from the trial may provide alternative treatment option for metastatic breast cancer patients in the future.

Conclusions

The innovative herbal formula was shown to possess anti-tumor, anti-metastatic and bone protective effects in metastatic breast tumor animal model, which would lead to the future development of adjuvant therapy for metastatic breast cancer.

Authors' contributions

GY, PL and CL designed the study. GY, JL, BC, HK, SH performed the animal studies. GY and JL analyzed and interpreted the data. DS and KF provided advices on study design and technical support. CL in-charge and supervised the project. GY and CL were major contributors in writing the manuscript. All authors read and approved the final manuscript.

Author details

[1] Institute of Chinese Medicine, E205, Science Centre East Block, The Chinese University of Hong Kong, Shatin, New Territories, Hong Kong. [2] State Key Laboratory of Research On Bioactivities and Clinical Applications of Medicinal Plants, The Chinese University of Hong Kong, Shatin, New Territories, Hong Kong. [3] School of Biomedical Sciences, The Chinese University of Hong Kong, Shatin, New Territories, Hong Kong. [4] Department of Health Technology and Informatics, The Hong Kong Polytechnic University, Hung Hom, Kowloon, Hong Kong.

Acknowledgements

The authors would like to thank Dr. Erik Ko, Mr. Eric Chun-Wai Wong, Mr. Ching-Po Lau, Ms. Ling Cheng, Ms. Anita Shum and Ms. Si Gao for their technical support.

Competing interests

The authors declare that they have no competing interests.

Consent for publication

Not applicable.

Funding

This study was partially supported by Focused Innovations Scheme (Major Area Scheme A—Phase 2) and Vice-Chancellor's One-off Discretionary Fund of The Chinese University of Hong Kong.

References

1. Lambert AW, Pattabiraman DR, Weinberg RA. Emerging biological principles of metastasis. Cell. 2017;168(4):670–91.
2. Chen Z, Gu K, Zheng Y, Zheng W, Lu W, Shu XO. The use of complementary and alternative medicine among Chinese women with breast cancer. J Altern Complement Med. 2008;14(8):1049–55.
3. Deng G, Cassileth B. Complementary or alternative medicine in cancer care-myths and realities. Nat Rev Clin Oncol. 2013;10(11):656–64.
4. Wong KY, Tan EY, Chen JJ, Teo C, Chan PM. The use of traditional Chinese medicine among breast cancer patients: implications for the clinician. Ann Acad Med Singapore. 2014;43(2):74–8.
5. Wong LY, Leung PC, Tang JL, Mercer SW. Use of dietary supplements by breast cancer patients undergoing conventional cancer treatment. Patient Prefer Adherence. 2010;4:407–14.
6. Wang Z, Li J, Ji Y, An P, Zhang S, Li Z. Traditional herbal medicine: a review of potential of inhibitory hepatocellular carcinoma in basic research and clinical trial. Evid Based Complement Alternat Med. 2013;2013:268963.
7. Zhao L, Zhao AG, Zhao G, Xu Y, Zhu XH, Cao HD, Zheng J, Yang JK, Xu JH. Survival benefit of traditional Chinese herbal medicine (a herbal formula for invigorating spleen) in gastric cancer patients with peritoneal metastasis. Evid Based Complement Alternat Med. 2014;2014:625493.
8. Yue GGL, Lau CBS, Leung PC. Creating an appropriate modern herbal formula for the adjuvant treatment of cancer. In: Motoo Yoshiharu, editor. Traditional medicine: new research. New York: Nova Science Publishers; 2012. p. 19–28.
9. Lau CBS, Yue GGL, Fung KP, Tan NH, Leung PC. The potential role of Chinese herbal medicines in cancer management. Science. 2015;347(6219 Suppl):S45–7.
10. Who Health Organization International Agency for Research on Cancer, GLOBOCAN 2012 Cancer fact sheet. http://globocan.iarc.fr/factsheets/cancers/all.asp. Accessed 28 March 2018.

11. American Cancer Society, About Breast Cancer. https://www.cancer.org/cancer/breast-cancer/about.html. Accessed 28 March 2018.
12. National Health Commission of the PRC. Annual Statistical Report 2013. 《2013中国卫生统计年鉴》. http://www.nhfpc.gov.cn/zwgkzt/tjnj/list.shtml. Accessed 25 Oct 2017.
13. Liu S, Yang L, Yuan Y, Li H, Tian J, Lu S, Wang N, Ji J. Cancer incidence in Beijing. Chin J Cancer Res. 2014;30(1):13–20.
14. Yue GGL, Lee JKM, Li L, Chan KM, Wong ECW, Chan JY, Fung KP, Lui VW, Chiu PW, Lau CBS. *Andrographis paniculata* elicits anti-invasion activities by suppressing TM4SF3 gene expression and by anoikis-sensitization in esophageal cancer cells. Am J Cancer Res. 2015;5(12):3570–87.
15. Li L, Yue GGL, Lee JK, Wong EC, Fung KP, Yu J, Lau CBS, Chiu PW. The adjuvant value of *Andrographis paniculata* in metastatic esophageal cancer treatment—from preclinical perspectives. Sci Rep. 2017;7(1):854.
16. Li L, Yue GGL, Lee JK, Wong EC, Fung KP, Yu J, Lau CBS, Chiu PW. Gene expression profiling reveals the plausible mechanisms underlying the antitumor and antimetastasis effects of *Andrographis paniculata* in esophageal cancer. Phytother Res. 2018;32(7):1388–96.
17. Wan CT. Study on the in vitro anti-tumor effect of *Acanthopanax senticosus*. M.Phil. Thesis, The Chinese University of Hong Kong Graduate School. Division of Biochemistry; 2008.
18. Luo KW, Ko CH, Yue GGL, Lee JK, Li KK, Lee M, Li G, Fung KP, Leung PC, Lau CBS. Green tea (*Camellia sinensis*) extract inhibits both the metastasis and osteolytic components of mammary cancer 4T1 lesions in mice. J Nutr Biochem. 2014;25(4):395–403.
19. Luo KW, Ko CH, Yue GGL, Gao S, Lee JK, Li G, Fung KP, Leung PC, Evdokiou A, Lau CBS. The combined use of *Camellia sinensis* and metronomic zoledronic acid in a breast cancer-induced osteolysis mouse model. J Cancer Res Clin Oncol. 2015;141(6):1025–36.
20. Luo KW, Yue GGL, Ko CH, Gao S, Lee JK, Li G, Fung KP, Leung PC, Lau CBS. The combined use of *Camellia sinensis* and metronomic zoledronate in 4T1 mouse carcinoma against tumor growth and metastasis. Oncol Rep. 2015;34(1):477–87.
21. Yue GGL, Lee JK, Kwok HF, Cheng L, Wong EC, Jiang L, Yu H, Leung HW, Wong YL, Leung PC, Fung KP, Lau CBS. Novel PI3 K/AKT targeting anti-angiogenic activities of 4-vinylphenol, a new therapeutic potential of a well-known styrene metabolite. Sci Rep. 2015;5:11149.
22. Chinese Pharmacopoeia Commission. Chinese pharmacopoeia. Shanghai: Commercial Press; 2010.
23. Zhuang ZX, Li NH. *Hedyotis diffusa*. In: Chinese medicinal herbs of Hong Kong, vol. 2. Hong Kong: Commercial Press; 1981. p. 146–9.
24. Pagani O, Senkus E, Wood W, Colleoni M, Cufer T, Kyriakides S, Costa A, Winer EP, Cardoso F, ESO-MBC Task Force. International guidelines for management of metastatic breast cancer: can metastatic breast cancer be cured? J Natl Cancer Inst. 2010;102(7):456–63.
25. Ayoub JP, Verma SH, Verma S. Advances in the management of metastatic breast cancer: options beyond first-line chemotherapy. Curr Oncol. 2012;19(2):91–105.
26. Pulaski BA, Ostrand-Rosenberg S. Reduction of established spontaneous mammary carcinoma metastases following immunotherapy with major histocompatibility complex class II and B7.1 cell-based tumor vaccines. Cancer Res. 1998;58(7):1486–93.
27. Yue GGL, Wong LS, Leung HW, Gao S, Tsang JYS, Lin ZX, Tse GMK, Lau CBS. Evaluation of the safety profiles of estrogenic Chinese herbal medicines in breast cancer. Phytomedicine. 2019;56:103–17.
28. Bates GJ, Fox SB, Han C, Leek RD, Garcia JF, Harris AL, Banham AH. Quantification of regulatory T cells enables the identification of high-risk breast cancer patients and those at risk of late relapse. J Clin Oncol. 2006;24(34):5373–80.
29. Coleman RE. Metastatic bone disease: clinical features, pathophysiology and treatment strategies. Cancer Treat Rev. 2001;27(3):165–76.
30. Xiong Z, Deng G, Huang X, Li X, Xie X, Wang J, Shuang Z, Wang X. Bone metastasis pattern in initial metastatic breast cancer: a population-based study. Cancer Manag Res. 2018;10:287–95.
31. Yang SX, Wei WS, Ouyan QW, Jiang QH, Zou YF, Qu W, Tu JH, Zhou ZB, Ding HL, Xie CW, Lei QM, Zhong CR. Interleukin-12 activated CD8+T cells induces apoptosis in breast cancer cells and reduces tumor growth. Biomed Pharmacother. 2016;84:1466–71.

Chinese herbal medicine for constipation: *zheng*-based associations among herbs, formulae, proprietary medicines, and herb–drug interactions

Linda L. D. Zhong[1,2†], Guang Zheng[1,5†], Li Da Ge[3], Cheng Yuan Lin[1,2], Tao Huang[1,2], Ling Zhao[1,2], Cheng Lu[1,4], Ai Ping Lu[1,2,4] and Zhao Xiang Bian[1,2*]

Abstract

Background: As current symptomatic treatments of constipation are still unsatisfactory, an increasing number of patients seek help from Chinese medicine (CM), particularly Chinese herbal medicine (CHM). This study aimed to review the most frequently used CHM herbs and formulae, proprietary CHMs, and herb–drug interactions for functional constipation using *zheng* (syndrome)-based differentiation, and to determine the current practice of *zheng*-based CHM treatments for functional constipation.

Methods: We developed a search strategy to include all the related clinical studies of CHM for constipation and set inclusion and exclusion criteria as studies on subjects with constipation of all ages and both sexes, using objective measures from laboratory or imaging techniques. The interventions included single herbs, CM classical formulae, CM new formulae, and Chinese herb-derived products and combination products. The clinical study types included were quasi- or randomized controlled trials, observational clinical studies, case series or case reports, and other types of appropriate research methods. The data concerning study design, sample size, mode of recruitment, sampling and diagnostic procedure, inclusion and exclusion criteria, and participants' characteristics (including age, sex, and duration of constipation). CM patterns, CM treatment principles, treatment regimen, and CM treatment outcomes were recorded.

Results: A total of 29,832 relevant records were found, of which 8541 were duplicate records and 20,639 were excluded for reasons of irrelevance. The full text of 965 articles was retrieved for detailed assessment, following which 480 articles were excluded for various reasons. From the included articles, we retrieved 190 different CM *zheng* diagnoses from 485 individual studies. The most common *zheng* was *dual deficiency of qi and blood (N = 48)*, which was diagnosed in 948 out of 15,740 subjects. The most frequently used classical formula was *Ma-Zi-Ren-Wan* (MZRW) (N = 75) and the most frequently used proprietary CHM was *Run-Chang-Wan (N = 87)*. The most frequently used combined medication was *Da Huang* with sodium bicarbonate tablets (frequency across all studies, n = 23), followed by *Fan Xie Ye* with lactulose oral solution (n = 8), *Ma-Ren-Ruan-Jiao-Nang* with lactulose oral solution (n = 6) and *Liu-Wei-An-Xiao-Jiao-Nang* (n = 6) with mosapride citrate tablets.

*Correspondence: bzxiang@hkbu.edu.hk
†Linda LD Zhong and Guang Zheng contributed equally to this work and should be considered co-first authors
[1] School of Chinese Medicine, Hong Kong Baptist University, 7 Baptist University Road, Kowloon Tong, Hong Kong, China
Full list of author information is available at the end of the article

Conclusion: This study examined the use of CHM for constipation and summarized the herbs, formulae, proprietary medicines, and herb–drug interactions application. These data indicated there were limited information about herb-drug interactions and adverse effects of CHM and further randomized controlled trials with strict design are necessary.

Background

Constipation is a common functional bowel disorder that affects many people; 14.7 % of the United States population [1], and 15.6 % of the adult population in Hong Kong [2] experienced this problem in a large sampled cross-sectional survey published in 2014. Treatments for constipation usually include fiber supplements, osmotic and stimulant laxatives, stool softeners, and sometimes enemas for refractory constipation [3]. As current symptomatic treatments produce unsatisfactory responses [4], many patients seek help from Chinese medicine (CM), particularly Chinese herbal medicine (CHM).

Many CM interventions have been used to treat constipation. A recent review [5] listed the current clinical research findings from CM interventions for functional constipation. However, there have been no analysis of the benefits of individual interventions (or individual types of interventions) or of the qualities of individual study designs. Our research team conducted a systematic review of CHM for functional constipation [6] and showed that CHM or CHM combination therapy was more effective than some single conventional medicines [6]. However, these findings did not accurately reflect all clinical practice, as most clinical research on constipation has involved observational studies or case series, and clinical practice has mostly been limited to personal experiences and based on CM theory and *zheng* (syndrome) differentiation [7–9].

We aimed to investigate CHM applications for constipation based on *zheng* differentiation, especially the use of single herbs, CM formulae, proprietary CHMs, and herb–drug interactions. Therefore, we systematically reviewed all the available data from current databases, including clinical trials, clinical observational studies, case series, case reports, and case control studies. Because we examined large data sets from both conventional Western and CM literature, we used a data slicing algorithm for text mining [10].

This study aimed to review the most frequently used CHM herbs and formulae, proprietary CHMs, and herb–drug interactions for functional constipation using *zheng*-based differentiation, and to determine the current practice of *zheng*-based CHM treatments for functional constipation.

Methods

Literature search

The review was performed in accordance with the Preferred Reporting Items for Systematic Reviews and Meta-Analyses (PRISMA) guidelines. We used the following databases to search the conventional medicine literature: PubMed, Ovid, Evidence-Based Medicine Reviews (EBMR), and Embase. The following databases were used to search the traditional CM literature: SinoMed, Chinese National Knowledge Infrastructure (CNKI), Chinese biomedical literature (CBM) CD, and China Journals Full-text Database. From the electronic database records and bibliographic references, we identified relevant primary sources and secondary sources (such as textbooks, review articles, and meta-analyses) as follows. We selected all EBM reviews, including Cochrane DSR, ACP Journal Club, DARE, CCTR, CMR, HTA, and NHSEED from inception to April 2014; EMBASE from 1980 to April 2014; EMBASE Classic from 1947 to 1979; PubMed from inception to April 2014; Ovid MEDLINE(R) from 1950 to April 2014; Ovid OLDMEDLINE(R) from 1948 to 1965; SinoMed from 1978 to April 2014; China Journals Full-text Database from 1994 to April 2014 and CBM disc from 1979 to April 2014. The search strategy was (1) (constipation) OR (chronic constipation) OR (functional constipation); (2) (herb*) OR (herbal medicine) OR (traditional Chinese medicine) OR (Chinese medicine) OR (Complementary medicine) OR (Naturopathy); (3) (case*) OR (clinical observation*) OR (clinical trial) OR (clinical study); (1) AND (2) AND (3) (*was used for truncation).

Study selection

We included interventions using single herbs, CM classical formulae, CM new formulae, and Chinese herb-derived products and combination products. The clinical study types included were quasi- or randomized controlled trials, observational clinical studies, case series or case reports, and other types of appropriate research methods. We included studies on subjects with constipation of all ages and both sexes, studies using objective measures from laboratory or imaging techniques, and studies using measurement from nursing staff, patients, or other informants.

Data extraction

Two authors (LLDZ and GZ) independently searched the databases and selected relevant publications. If the two authors disagreed about a study's eligibility, they would check the study against the selection criteria, discuss its eligibility, and make a further decision (ZXB). One author (LLDZ) extracted the data and the other (GZ) checked the extracted data. For each study, the following information was extracted: study design, sample size, mode of recruitment, sampling and diagnostic procedure, inclusion and exclusion criteria, and participants' characteristics (including age, sex, and duration of constipation). CM patterns, CM treatment principles, treatment regimen, and CM treatment outcomes were recorded.

Quality assessment

The methodological quality of relevant studies was assessed using the Jadad scale (Additional file 1; [11]). The Jadad scale evaluates a study in terms of the description of randomization, blinding, and dropouts. The scale ranges from 1 to 5; randomized controlled trials with a score between 3 and 5 are regarded as better quality trials. Points were awarded if the study was described as randomized (1 point), had an appropriate randomization method (1 point), was described as double-blind (1 point), used an appropriate blinding method (1 point), and had a description of withdrawals and dropouts (1 point) [11].

Identification of herb-*zheng* associations

Classification based on keyword co-occurrence was conducted on the 18,272 items of constipation literature downloaded from SinoMed [12]. We also applied a dictionary-based data slicing algorithm constructed on the principle of keyword co-occurrence. We filtered the downloaded data using CM associated keywords, such as "Chinese herbal medicine," "Chinese patent medicine," and "CM syndrome/*zheng*," which were obtained from textbooks and the Internet. The keyword co-occurrence classification was a good supplement to the literature search, as it provided insights into the quantitative relationship between the individual herbs and formulae used to treat constipation. We used a wheel-shaped network to indicate the association between different types of single herbs and their *zheng* indications [10]. The wheel-shaped network was a visualized graph that showed the frequencies and correlations among the same categories [10].

Translation of terminology

All Chinese-to-English translations were deduced primarily from the *World Health Organization (WHO) Evidence-Based Complementary and Alternative Medicine International Standard Terminologies on Traditional Medicine in the Western Pacific Region* [13].

Results

We accessed 29,832 records that fit the search criteria, of which 8541 were duplicate records and 20,639 were excluded for reasons of irrelevance. The full text of 965 articles was retrieved for detailed assessment; 480 of these were excluded for various reasons (Fig. 1). Of the 485 studies that fulfilled the inclusion and exclusion criteria, 289 were on CM formulae, 91 were on proprietary CM, and 105 were on a combination of CHM and conventional treatment. The sample size of the 485 studies ranged from 35 to 250. Among all the studies, 289 (59.6 %) were case series or reports, 125 (25.8 %) were controlled trials, and 71 (14.6 %) were randomized controlled trials. For the randomized controlled trials, the mean Jadad scores were 2.06 and their average quality was quite low (Additional file 1).

CM *zheng* category and treatment criteria

From the included articles, we retrieved 190 different CM *zheng* diagnoses from 485 individual studies. The most common pattern was *dual deficiency of qi and blood (Qi Xue Liang Xu)*, which was diagnosed in 948 of the 15,740 subjects (frequency = 48, percentage among the top 10 diagnosis = 16.8 %); this was followed by *dual deficiency of qi and yin (Qi Yin Liang Xu)* (subjects = 795, frequency = 45, percentage among the top 10 diagnosis = 15.7 %), *excessive heat and qi stagnation (Qi Zhi Shi Re)* (subjects = 726, frequency = 41, percentage among the top 10 diagnosis = 14.3 %), *yang*

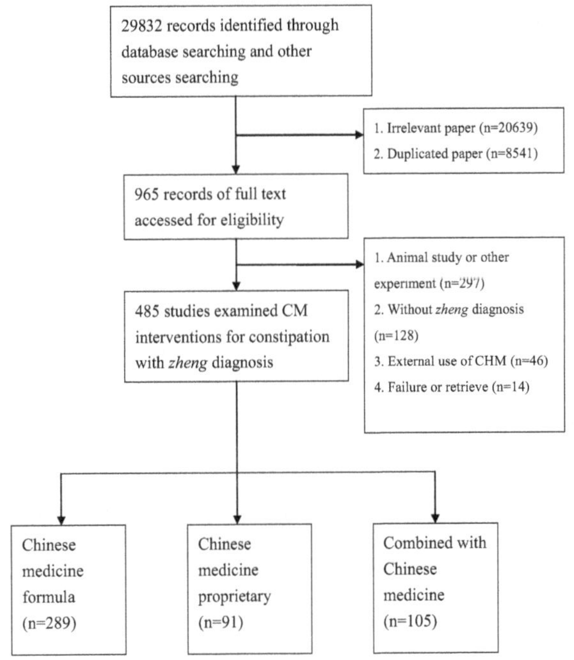

Fig. 1 Flowchart of literature selection logistics

deficiency of spleen and kidney (Pi Shen Yang Xu) (subjects = 636, frequency = 32, percentage among the top 10 diagnosis = 11.2 %), *deficiency of qi and blood (Qi Xue Liang Xu)* (subjects = 595, frequency = 26, percentage among the top 10 diagnosis = 9.1 %), *cold–heat complex (Han Re Cuo Za)* (subjects = 513, frequency = 21, percentage among the top 10 diagnosis = 7.3 %), *liver depression and spleen deficiency (Gan Yu Pi Xu)* (subjects = 495, frequency = 20, percentage among the top 10 diagnosis = 7.0 %), *deficiency–excess complex (Xu Shi Jia Za)* (subjects = 483, frequency = 20, percentage among the top 10 diagnosis = 7.0 %), *dual yin deficiency of liver and kidney (Gan Shen Yin Xu)* (subjects = 410, frequency = 17, percentage among the top 10 diagnosis = 5.9 %) and *intestinal dryness and yin deficiency (Yin Xu Chang Zao)* (subjects = 223, frequency = 16, percentage among the top 10 diagnosis = 5.6 %). Subjects diagnosed with the top 10 CM *zheng* accounted for 37 % of the 15,740 subjects (Table 1). Table 1 lists the therapeutic principles for the CM *zheng*.

CM herbs and their relationships

We identified 296 herbs from 485 clinical studies and analyzed their relationships using the wheel-shaped network (Fig. 2). In this figure, red and green nodes represent different single herbal medicines. The edges represent co-occurrence frequency in clinical studies. The edge label numbers represent the number of clinical studies demonstrating a connection between two single herbal medicines. There was a high concentration of one classical Chinese herbal formula, *Ma-Zi-Ren-Wan*, whose composition of six herbs occupied 42.5 % (1754/4127) of the total frequency of usage. Based on this, the green nodes represent CHMs in the formula *Ma-Zi-Ren-Wan* and the red nodes represent other CHMs used in clinical prescriptions [10]. Node size was calculated with the formula

$$Node\,size = LOG\left(node\_frequency\right) + Degree\,(node)$$

where *node_frequency* is the literature record number of the associated keyword calculated in text mining, *LOG* is the logarithm calculation with a base set to 10, and *Degree (node)* is the number of connections/edges each node has with other nodes. The edge line width was calculated through *LOG (edge_co-occurrent)* where *edge_co-occurrent* was the number of node/keyword pairs that co-occurred in the associated literature.

Table 2 lists the top 10 most frequently used herbs and their actions. The most frequently used herbs were further categorized and analyzed to determine their combinations in classical formulae. The most frequently used classical formulae were *Ma-Zi-Ren-Wan* [14] and *Zeng-Ye-Tang* [15].

CM *zheng*-based Chinese herbal formulae

Among the 289 studies on Chinese herbal formulae, the most frequently used formulae based on *zheng* diagnosis

Table 1 Top ten most commonly used CM *zheng* for constipation

CM *zheng*	Therapeutic principle	Number of subjects diagnosed by the diagnosis	Number of frequency among all the studies	Percentage among the total *zheng* (190)/top 10 *zheng* diagnosis (%)
Dual deficiency of qi and blood qi-xue-liang-xu	Tonify *qi* and replenish *blood*	948	48	16.8/6.2
Dual deficiency of qi and yin qi-yin-liang-xu	Tonify *qi* and replenish *yin*	795	45	15.7/5.9
Excessive heat and qi stagnation qi-zhi-shi-re	Soothe the *liver* and regulate *qi*	726	41	14.3/5.3
Yang deficiency of spleen and kidney pi-shen-yang-xu	Warm the *kidney* and fortify the spleen	636	32	11.2/4.2
Deficiency of qi and blood pi-xue-kui-xu	Tonify *qi* and engender *blood*	595	26	9.1/3.4
Cold-heat complex han-re-cuo-za	Treat *cold* with *heat* and *heat* with *cold*	513	21	7.3/2.7
Liver depression and spleen deficiency gan-yu-pi-xu	Soothe the *liver* and fortify the *spleen*	495	20	7.0/2.6
Deficiency-excess complex xu-shi-jia-za	Treat *deficiency* by tonification and excess by purgation	483	20	7.0/2.6
Dual yin deficiency of liver and kidney gan-shen-yin-xu	Enrich the *kidney* and nourish the *liver yin*	410	17	5.9/2.2
Intestinal dryness and yin deficiency yin-xu-chang-zao	Replenish *yin* and moisten dryness	223	16	5.6/2.1

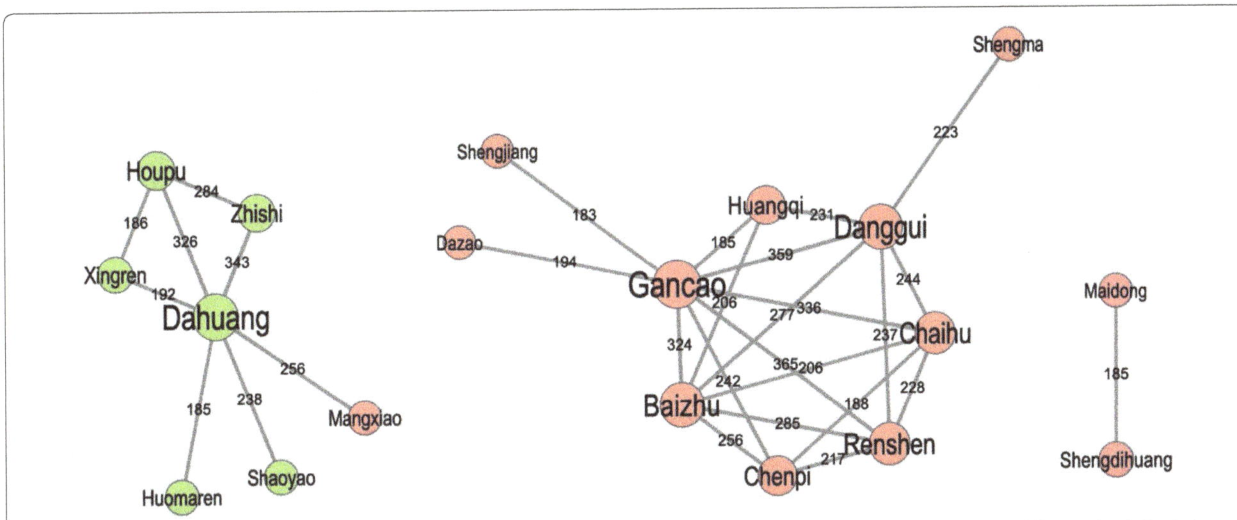

Fig. 2 Network relationship of Chinese herbal medicine in the treatment of constipation. *Red* and *green* nodes represent different single herbal medicines. The *edges* represent co-occurrence frequency in clinical studies. The *edge label numbers* represent the number of clinical studies demonstrating a connection between two single herbal medicines

were *Ma-Zi-Ren-Wan* and its modifications (frequency among all the studies, n = 75, percentage among the top 10 formulae, 33.07 %). This was followed by *Bu-Zhong-Yi-Qi-Tang* (n = 56, 22.58 %), *Ji-Chuan-Jian* (n = 51, 20.56 %), *Zeng-Ye-Tang* (n = 40, 13.84 %), and *Ba-Zhen-Tang* (n = 26, 10.48 %). The five most frequently used CM *zheng*-based Chinese herbal formulae and their indications are summarized in Table 3.

Proprietary CHMs

After the classical herbal decoctions, the next most frequently used clinical treatments for constipation were proprietary CHMs, because of their standard quality control and more convenient administration. We analyzed the most commonly used proprietary CHMs and their dosage (Table 4). The manufacturers of the proprietary CHMs are also shown, to indicate the quality and composition of the medicines. The most commonly used proprietary CHM was *Run-Chang-Wan* (frequency, n = 87), followed by *Ma-Ren-Ruan-Jiao-Nang* (n = 62), *Ma-Ren-Run-Chang-Wan* (n = 52), *Liu-Wei-An-Xiao-Jiao-Nang* (n = 50), *Fu-Fang-Lu-Hui-Jiao-Nang* (n = 35), *Si-Ni-San* (n = 32), *Liu-Wei-Neng-Xiao-Jiao-Nang* (n = 27), and *Bu-Zhong-Yi-Qi-Wan* (n = 17).

CM combined with Western medicine and adverse effects

Few clinical studies reported the combined use of CM and Western medicine for constipation. Table 5 summarized the herb–drug interactions identified. Although most studies did not mention the adverse effects associated with combined administration of herbs and drugs, or proprietary CHMs and drugs, there were 43 reported trials of the integrative use of single herbs or proprietary CHMs. Among these studies, the most frequent adjunctive use was *Da Huang* (*Radix et Rhizoma Rhei*) with *sodium bicarbonate tablets* (n = 23), followed by *Fan Xie Ye* (*Folium Sennae*) with *lactulose oral solution* (n = 8), *Ma-Ren-Ruan-Jiao-Nang* with *lactulose oral solution* (n = 6) and *Liu-Wei-An-Xiao-Jiao-Nang with mosapride citrate tablets* (n = 6).

Discussion

To our knowledge, this is the first study to examine the use of single herbs, classical CM formulae, proprietary CHMs, and the combined use of CM and Western medicine (and its adverse effects) for constipation. The classification of single herbs and CM formulae was generally based on the CM diagnostic *zheng* system. As we pointed out in our commentary paper, *zheng* diagnosis is a critical stage of CM treatment; it is the basis of CM's effectiveness and the main feature that distinguishes it from Western medicine [16]. In this review, we focused on *zheng* diagnosis, in accord with current clinical CM practice. Although we identified 190 different CM *zheng* diagnoses, only 57.9 % (281/485) of studies used the diagnosis system of *zheng* differentiation. The most commonly diagnosed *zheng* for constipation was *dual deficiency of qi and blood* (16.8 %) followed by *dual deficiency of qi and yin* (15.7 %) and *excessive heat and qi stagnation* (14.3 %). As Table 1 showed, among the top 10 CM *zheng*, five belonged to *deficiency zheng* and the others could be categorized as a combination of *deficiency* and *sufficiency* or *sufficiency* syndrome. These results are consistent with those of our previous study [16] and with other research

Table 2 Action and indication of the most ten frequently used herbs

Chinese name in pinyin	Latin name	Frequency of usage	Action	Indication
Da Huang	Radix *et Rhizoma Rhei*	428	Drains *heat* and purges accumulations; clears *heat*, transforms *dampness* and promotes urination; drains *heat* from the *blood*; invigorates the *blood* and dispels blood stasis	Intestinal *heat excess* with high fever, profuse sweating, thirst, constipation, abdominal distention and pain, delirium, a yellow tongue coat and a full pulse; blood stasis with amenorrhea, fixed abdominal masses or fixed pain
Huo Ma Ren	*Semen Cannabis*	247	Nourishes, moistens and lubricates the intestines; nourishes the *yin;* clears *heat* and promotes healing of sores; moistens dryness and benefits the hair	Constipation in the elderly; constipation after a warm febrile disease; postpartum constipation; constipation due to blood and *yin deficiency;* sores and ulcerations (auxiliary-internal and topical); promotes hair growth and treats dry hair
Fan Xie Ye	*Folium Sennae*	232	Drains downward and guides out stagnation; eliminates excess *heat* and drains *summer heat*	*Heat* in the stomach and intestines with constipation and abdominal fullness; *summer heat*
Bai Zhu	Rhizoma *Atractylodis Macrocephalae*	198	Tonifies the *spleen* and augments *qi*; dries *dampness* and promotes water metabolism; stabilizes the exterior and stops sweating	*Spleen* and *stomach deficiency* with diarrhea, fatigue; *spleen damp* or accumulation of fluids affecting the digestion; edema and reduced urination due to *spleen deficiency; qi deficiency* with spontaneous sweating
Dang- Gui	Radix *Angelicae Sinensis*	132	Tonifies the *blood* and regulates the menses; invigorates and harmonizes the *blood* and disperses cold; moistens the intestines and unblocks the bowels	Blood deficiency with pale, ashen complexion, lusterless nails, tinnitus; *blood deficiency* associated irregular menstruation, amenorrhea and dysmenorrhea; dry Intestines due to blood deficiency
Huang Qi	Radix *Astragali*	126	Tonifies *qi* and *blood*; strengthens the *spleen* and raises the *yang qi* of the *spleen* and *stomach*; tonifies *wei qi*, stabilizes the exterior and tonifies the *lungs*	Postpartum fever due to *qi* and *blood deficiency; spleen qi deficiency* with anorexia, fatigue and diarrhea; excessive sweating with *qi*, *yang* or *yin deficiency; dampness* in the head
Gan Cao	Radix *Glycyrrhizae*	112	Tonifies the *spleen* and augments *qi*; moistens the *lungs*, resolves phlegm and stops cough; moderates spasms and alleviates pain; clears *heat* and relieves *fire* toxicity	Spleen *qi deficiency* with shortness of breath, lassitude and loose stools; *qi* and *blood deficiency* with an irregular pulse and/or palpitations; productive or non-productive cough; raw for toxic *heat* with sore throat or carbuncles and sores
Sheng Di	Radix *Rehmanniae*	99	Clears *heat* and cools the *blood*; nourishes *yin*, generates fluids, increases saliva and treats wasting and thirsting; cools heart fire	*Ying*-stage *heat* with high fever, thirst and a scarlet tongue; hemorrhage due to *blood heat;* throat pain due to *yin deficiency*
Bai Shao	Radix *Paeoniae Alba*	94	Nourishes the *blood* and regulates menstruation; astringes *yin* and adjusts the *ying* and *wei*; calms *liver yang* and *liver wind* and alleviates pain	*Liver blood deficiency* with menstrual dysfunction, vaginal discharge and uterine bleeding; anemia; breast distention and pre-menstrual syndrome
Lu Hui	Aloe	93	Purges, drains *fire* and guides out accumulations; clears *heat* and cools the *liver*; kills parasites and strengthens the *stomach*	*Heat* accumulation with constipation, dizziness, red eyes, and irritability; chronic constipation; heat in the liver channel or liver fire with epigastric discomfort, dizziness, headache, irritability, tinnitus, constipation and fever

Table 3 Summary of top five most frequently used Chinese herbal formulae based on *zheng* diagnosis

Chinese name in pinyin	Composition in pinyin	CM *zheng*	Number of frequency among all the studies	Actions in Chinese medicine
Ma-Zi-Ren-Wan	*Huo Ma Ren* *Xing Ren* *Bai Shao* *Zhi Shi* *Hou Pu* *Da Huang*	Excessive *qi* and *heat*	75	Invigorates *Blood* Dispels *Blood* Stasis Moves *qi* Lubricates the intestines Moves the bowels Purges *heat* Alleviates pain
Bu-Zhong-Yi-Qi-Tang	*Huang Qi* *Ren Shen* *Bai Zhu* *Zhi Gan Cao* *Dang Gui* *Chen Pi* *Shen Ma* *Chai Hu*	*Qi deficiency* of *spleen* and *stomach/Sunken middle qi*	56	Tonifies *middle jiao qi* Benefits *qi* Regulates *qi* Raises *sunken yang* Lifts prolapsed organs
Ji-Chuan-Jian	*Dang Gui* *Niu Xi* *Rou Cong Rong* *Ze Xie* *Shen Ma* *Zhi Qiao*	*Yang deficiency* of *spleen* and *kidney*	51	Warms up the *kidney* Replenishes vital essence Lubricates the intestines Induces defecation
Zeng-Ye-Tang	*Xuan Shen* *Mai Dong* *Sheng Di*	*Fluid-humor deficiency*	40	Generates Fluids Moistens dryness Unblocks the bowels Nourishes *yin* Clears *heat*
Ba-Zhen-Tang	*Ren Shen* *Bai Zhu* *Fu Ling* *Zhi Gan Cao* *Shu Di* *Bai Shao* *Chuan Xiong* *Dang Gui*	*Dual deficiency* of *qi* and *blood*	26	Nourishes *qi* Benefits *blood*

on syndrome distribution among constipation patients [8, 17], which indicated that almost half of patients, especially older individuals and postpartum women, had *deficiency* syndromes [18, 19].

Of the 10 most frequently used herbs, the top three were traditional purgatives; the other herbs were *tonifying* and *replenishing* medicines, except *Lu Hui* (*Aloe vera*) [20, 21]. It is interesting that the top five CM *zheng* were *deficiency zheng*; this seemed inconsistent with the fact that the five most frequently used single herbs were purgatives. This was mainly because only 50.26 % of studies used CM *zheng* differentiation, and purgatives are mostly used for general constipation in the absence of any CM *zheng* diagnosis. Table 3 shows that the most commonly used Chinese herbal formula was *Ma-Zi-Ren-Wan*, which suggested that it formed the basis of the most commonly prescribed formulae for constipation according to both CM syndrome differentiation and Western medicine diagnosis.

Many studies of Chinese herbal formulae or proprietary CHM did not provide standard or complete criteria for syndrome diagnosis. The lack of detail and consistency in diagnosis makes these studies difficult to replicate and their findings difficult to compare with other results [22]. Most studies provided only the main composition of the formulae without any indication of dosage or quality control standards (Table 4). Although proprietary CHMs are rapidly gaining attention in the West as sources of new drugs, dietary supplements, and functional foods, the lack of consistent manufacturing processes, quality standards, scientific evidence, and validation of efficacy and safety impede worldwide acceptance of CHM [23].

Currently, herb–drug interactions are of growing concern as a clinical safety issue to clinicians and researchers [24, 25]. Proprietary CHMs are prescribed by Western medical doctors who may not fully understand the indications and actions of these medicines [26]. Although herbal medicines are natural, they are not always safe [27]. Table 5 showed the concomitant use and the adverse effects of herb–drug combinations or proprietary CHM–drug combinations based on the limited literature. These limited data showed that the incidence of adverse effects

Table 4 Summary of top ten most frequently used Chinese herbal medicine proprietary

Chinese name in pinyin (manufacturer)	Composition in pinyin	Oral dosage	Number of frequency among all the studies	Indication
Run-Chang-Wan (Shang Dong Hua Yang Pharmaceutical Co. Ltd.)	*Tao Ren* *Da Hua* *Qiang Huo* *Dang Gui* *Huo Ma Ren*	4 pills t. i. d. for oral administration	87	Constipation with CM *zheng* of *excessive qi* and *heat*, and constipation for elderly people and postpartum women
Ma-Ren-Ruan-Jiao-Nang (Actavis (Foshan) Pharmaceutical Co., Ltd.)	*Huo Ma Ren* *Xing Ren* *Bai Shao* *Zhi Shi* *Hou Pu* *Da Huang*	2 capsules t. i. d. for oral administration	62	Constipation with CM *zheng* of *excessive qi* and *heat*
Ma-Ren-Run-Chang-Wan (Bei Jing Tong Ren Tang Co., Ltd.)	*Huo Ma Ren* *Xing Ren* *Da Hua* *Bai Shao* *Mu Xiang* *Chen Pi*	1–2 big honey pills b. i. d. for oral administration	52	Constipation with CM *zheng* of *heat* in *stomach* and *intestines*
Liu-Wei-An-Xiao-Jiao-Nang (Gui Zhou Xin Bang Pharmaceutical Co., Ltd.)	*Tu Mu Xiang* *Da Huang* *Shan Nai* *Han Shui Shi* *Ke Zi* *Jian Hua*	3–6 pills b. i. d. for oral administration	50	Constipation due to indigestion and bloating; stomachache; dyspepsia
Fu-Fang-Lu-Hui-Jiao-Nang (He Bei Wan Bang & Folon Pharmaceutical Co., Ltd.)	*Lu Hui* *Qing Dai* *Zhu Sha* *Hu Po*	1–2 capsules b. i. d. for oral administration	35	Constipation with CM *zheng* of intense *fire* in *heart* and *liver*
Ma-Ren-Zi-Pi-Wan (Bao Tou Chinese Medicine Pharmaceutical Co., Ltd.)	*Huo Ma Ren* *Xing Ren* *Bai Shao* *Zhi Shi* *Hou Pu* *Da Huang* *Yu Li Ren* *Dang Gui*	1 big honey pills b. i. d. for oral administration	34	Constipation with CM *zheng* of dryness and heat in large intestine

Table 4 continued

Chinese name in pinyin (manufacturer)	Composition in pinyin	Oral dosage	Number of frequency among all the studies	Indication
Si-Ni-San (Fu Zhou Neptunus Futao Pharmaceutical Co., Ltd.)	*Chai Hu* *Zhi Shi* *Bai Shao* *Zhi Gan Cao*	6–9 g granules b. i. d. for oral administration	32	Constipation with CM *zheng* of disharmony between *spleen* and *liver*
Liu-Wei-Neng-Xiao-Jiao-Nang (Yang Zong Pharmaceutical Co., Ltd.)	*Da Hua* *Ke Zi* *Gan Jiang* *Zang Mu Xiang* *Jian Hua* *Hai Shui Shi*	2 capsules b. i. d. for oral administration	27	Constipation due to indigestion; obesity; hyperlipidemia
Bu-Zhong-Yi-Qi-Wan (Bei Jing Tong Ren Tang Co., Ltd.)	*Huang Qi* *Dang Shen* *Bai Zhu* *Dang Gui* *Shen Ma* *Chai Hu* *Chen Pi* *Zhi Gan Cao*	1–2 big honey pills b. i. d. for oral administration	17	Constipation with CM *zheng* of *qi deficiency* of *spleen* and *stomach/Sunken middle qi*

t.i.d. means ter in die, three times a day; *b.i.d.* means bis in die, twice a day

Table 5 Summary of combination of CHM and Western medicine and the reported adverse effects

	Combined used Western medicine	Frequency of reported in all the trials (n > 5)	Adverse effect (N = , percentage, %)
Single herb			
Da Huang	Sodium bicarbonate tablets	23	Symptoms of the gastrointestinal tract (N = 4, 17.3 %)
			Insomnia (N = 1, 4.3 %)
			Skin rash (N = 1, 4.3 %)
			Headache (N = 1, 4.3 %)
Fan Xie Ye	Lactulose oral solution	8	Symptoms of the gastrointestinal tract (N = 2, 25 %)
			Dizzy and anorexia (N = 1, 12.5 %)
CHM Proprietary			
Ma-Ren-Ruan-Jiao-Nang	Lactulose oral solution	6	Symptoms of the gastrointestinal tract (N = 2, 33.3 %)
			Headache (N = 1, 16.7 %)
Liu-Wei-An-Xiao-Jiao-Nang	Mosapride citrate tablets	6	Symptoms of the gastrointestinal tract (N = 3, 50 %)

was not as low as we expected, ranging from 4.3 to 50 %, although most adverse effects were symptoms of the gastrointestinal tract.

A limitation of this study was that the data were drawn from clinical studies that used several different types of design: case reports, cohort studies, and quasi- or randomized controlled trials. The quality of these studies varied and therefore it is difficult to compare them quantitatively. In addition, most studies did not provide sufficient detail regarding inclusion criteria of diseases and syndromes, quality control procedures for single herbs or proprietary CHMs, or withdrawal rates and reasons. Therefore, the analysis of the data derived from this study is limited and should be treated with caution.

Conclusion

This review examined the use of CHM for constipation and summarized the most frequently used Chinese single herbs, the 10 most frequently used CHM formulae and proprietary CHMs, and the combined use of CHM and Western medicine treatments and their reported adverse effects.

Abbreviations

CHM: Chinese herbal medicine; CM: Chinese medicine; MZRW: *Ma-Zi-Ren-Wan*; PRISMA: Preferred Reporting Items for Systematic Reviews and Meta-Analyses; EBMR: Evidence-Based Medicine Reviews; CNKI: Chinese National Knowledge Infrastructure; CBM: Chinese biomedical literature.

Authors' contributions

ZXB designed the study. LDG and CYL conducted text mining. TH and LZ retrieved the herbs and herb-drug interaction data. LLDZ and GZ searched the literature and wrote the manuscript. LDG, CYL, TH, LZ, LLDZ, GZ, CL, and APL revised the manuscript. All authors read and approved the final manuscript.

Author details

[1] School of Chinese Medicine, Hong Kong Baptist University, 7 Baptist University Road, Kowloon Tong, Hong Kong, China. [2] Hong Kong Chinese Medicine Study Centre, Hong Kong Baptist University, Hong Kong SAR, China. [3] Department of Surgery, The First People's Hospital of Xiaoshan District, Hangzhou, China. [4] Institute of Basic Research in Clinical Medicine, China Academy of Traditional Chinese Medicine, Beijing, China. [5] School of Information Science and Engineering, Lanzhou University, Lanzhou, China.

Acknowledgements

We thank Health and Health Services Research Fund (Project No. 09101501), Hong Kong SAR, and Natural Science Foundation of China Project (NSFC-81173363) for financially support this research. The funding agencies have no role in the design and execution of this project. They will not be involved to the analysis and interpretation of data, or make decision to submit the results.

Competing interests

The authors declare that they have no competing interests.

References

1. Mugie SM, Benninga MA, Di Lorenzo C. Epidemiology of constipation in children and adults: a systematic review. Best Pract Res Clin Gastroenterol. 2011;25(1):3–18.
2. Huang R, Ho SY, Lo WS, Lam TH. Physical activity and constipation in Hong Kong adolescents. PLoS ONE. 2014;9(2):e90193.
3. Pasanen ME. Evaluation and treatment of colonic symptoms. Med Clin North Am. 2014;98(3):529–47.
4. McCarberg BH. Overview and treatment of opioid-induced constipation. Postgrad Med. 2013;125(4):7–17.
5. Lin LW, Fu YT, Dunning T, Zhang AL, Ho TH, Duke M, Lo SK. Efficacy of traditional Chinese medicine for the management of constipation: a systematic review. J Altern Complement Med. 2009;15(12):1335–46.
6. Cheng CW, Bian ZX, Wu TX. Systematic review of Chinese herbal medicine for functional constipation. WJG. 2009;15(39):4886–95.
7. Suo T, Gu X, Andersson R, Ma H, Zhang W, Deng W, Zhang B, Cai D, Qin X. Oral traditional Chinese medication for adhesive small bowel obstruction. Cochrane Database Syst Rev. 2012;5:CD008836.
8. Chen CM, Lin LZ, Zhang EX. Standardized treatment of chinese medicine decoction for cancer pain patients with opioid-induced constipation: A

multi-center prospective randomized controlled study. Chin J Integr Med. 2014;20(7):496–502.
9. Yao YB, Cao YQ, Guo XT, Yi J, Liang HT, Wang C, Lu JG. Biofeedback therapy combined with traditional Chinese medicine prescription improves the symptoms, surface myoelectricity, and anal canal pressure of the patients with spleen deficiency constipation. eCAM. 2013;2013:830714.
10. Zheng G, Jiang M, He X, Zhao J, Guo H, Chen G, Zha Q, Lu A. Discrete derivative: a data slicing algorithm for exploration of sharing biological networks between rheumatoid arthritis and coronary heart disease. BioData Min. 2011;4:18.
11. Moher D, Jadad AR, Tugwell P. Assessing the quality of randomized controlled trials. Current issues and future directions. Int J Technol Assess Health Care. 1996;12(2):195–208.
12. Sinomed database: http://www.sinomed.ac.cn/. Accessed 16 May 2014.
13. WHO Regional Office for the Western Pacific. WHO International Standard Terminologies on Traditional Medicine in the Western Pacific Region; 2007.
14. Zhang S. Examples for clinical use of ma zi ren wan. J Tradit Chin Med. 2002;22(3):216–7.
15. Zeng ZC, Tang ZY, Fan J, Zhou J, Qin LX, Ye SL, Sun HC, Wang BL, Li D, Wang JH, Zeng MS, Guo W, Tan YS. Consideration of the role of radiotherapy for unresectable intrahepatic cholangiocarcinoma: a retrospective analysis of 75 patients. Cancer J. 2006;12(2):113–22.
16. Bian ZX, Xu H, Lu AP, Lee MS, Cheung H. Insights of Chinese medicine syndrome study: from current status to future prospects. Chin J Integr Med. 2014;20(5):326–31.
17. Cheng CW, Kwok AO, Bian ZX, Tse DM. The quintessence of traditional Chinese medicine: syndrome and its distribution among advanced cancer patients with constipation. eCAM. 2012;2012:739642.
18. Ren Z, Wu QM, Li DD, Liu WA, Li XR, Lin XM. Post-stroke constipation treated with acupuncture therapy of regulating qi circulation of fu-organ. Zhongguo zhen jiu. 2013;33(10):893–6.
19. Cherniack EP. Use of complementary and alternative medicine to treat constipation in the elderly. Geriatr Gerontol Int. 2013;13(3):533–8.
20. Wang J, Huang JH, Cheng YF, Yang GM. Banana resistant starch and its effects on constipation model mice. J Med Food. 2014;17(8):902–7.
21. Hou ML, Chang LW, Lin CH, Lin LC, Tsai TH. Determination of bioactive components in Chinese herbal formulae and pharmacokinetics of rhein in rats by UPLC-MS/MS. Molecules. 2014;19(4):4058–75.
22. Wang J, Cui M, Jiao H, Tong Y, Xu J, Zhao Y, Han M, Liu J. Content analysis of systematic reviews on effectiveness of traditional Chinese medicine. J Tradit Chin Med. 2013;33(2):156–63.
23. Xue CC, Zhang AL, Greenwood KM, Lin V, Story DF. Traditional Chinese medicine: an update on clinical evidence. J Altern Complement Med. 2010;16(3):301–12.
24. Ge B, Zhang Z, Zuo Z. Updates on the clinical evidenced herb-warfarin interactions. eCAM. 2014;2014:957362.
25. Rahal A, Ahmad AH, Kumar A, Mahima, Verma AK, Chakraborty S, Dhama K. Clinical drug interactions: a holistic view. PJBS. 2013;16(16):751–8.
26. Chan TY. The prevalence use and harmful potential of some Chinese herbal medicines in babies and children. Vet Hum Toxicol. 1994;36(3):238–40.
27. van Andel T, de Boer HJ, Barnes J, Vandebroek I. Medicinal plants used for menstrual disorders in Latin America, the Caribbean, sub-Saharan Africa, South and Southeast Asia and their uterine properties: a review. J Ethnopharmacol. 2014;155:992.

Permissions

All chapters in this book were first published in CM, by BioMed Central; hereby published with permission under the Creative Commons Attribution License or equivalent. Every chapter published in this book has been scrutinized by our experts. Their significance has been extensively debated. The topics covered herein carry significant findings which will fuel the growth of the discipline. They may even be implemented as practical applications or may be referred to as a beginning point for another development.

The contributors of this book come from diverse backgrounds, making this book a truly international effort. This book will bring forth new frontiers with its revolutionizing research information and detailed analysis of the nascent developments around the world.

We would like to thank all the contributing authors for lending their expertise to make the book truly unique. They have played a crucial role in the development of this book. Without their invaluable contributions this book wouldn't have been possible. They have made vital efforts to compile up to date information on the varied aspects of this subject to make this book a valuable addition to the collection of many professionals and students.

This book was conceptualized with the vision of imparting up-to-date information and advanced data in this field. To ensure the same, a matchless editorial board was set up. Every individual on the board went through rigorous rounds of assessment to prove their worth. After which they invested a large part of their time researching and compiling the most relevant data for our readers.

The editorial board has been involved in producing this book since its inception. They have spent rigorous hours researching and exploring the diverse topics which have resulted in the successful publishing of this book. They have passed on their knowledge of decades through this book. To expedite this challenging task, the publisher supported the team at every step. A small team of assistant editors was also appointed to further simplify the editing procedure and attain best results for the readers.

Apart from the editorial board, the designing team has also invested a significant amount of their time in understanding the subject and creating the most relevant covers. They scrutinized every image to scout for the most suitable representation of the subject and create an appropriate cover for the book.

The publishing team has been an ardent support to the editorial, designing and production team. Their endless efforts to recruit the best for this project, has resulted in the accomplishment of this book. They are a veteran in the field of academics and their pool of knowledge is as vast as their experience in printing. Their expertise and guidance has proved useful at every step. Their uncompromising quality standards have made this book an exceptional effort. Their encouragement from time to time has been an inspiration for everyone.

The publisher and the editorial board hope that this book will prove to be a valuable piece of knowledge for researchers, students, practitioners and scholars across the globe.

List of Contributors

Jiang Xu and Xi-wen Li
Institute of Chinese Materia Medica, China Academy of Chinese Medical Sciences, Dongcheng District, Dongzhimen Nanxiaojie within 16, Beijing 100700, China

Ming-li Wu
Institute of Chinese Materia Medica, China Academy of Chinese Medical Sciences, Dongcheng District, Dongzhimen Nanxiaojie within 16, Beijing 100700, China
Pharmacy Faculty, Hubei University of Chinese Medicine, No. 1, Huangjiahu West Road, Hongshan District, Wuhan 430065, Hubei, China

Qing Li
Department of Pharmacy, Changzheng Hospital, Second Military Medical University, No. 415 Fengyang Road, Huangpu District, Shanghai 200003, China

Min He
Leiden University European Center for Chinese Medicine and Natural Compounds, Institute of Biology, Leiden University, Sylviusweg 72, 2333 BE Leiden, The Netherlands

Mei Wang
Leiden University European Center for Chinese Medicine and Natural Compounds, Institute of Biology, Leiden University, Sylviusweg 72, 2333 BE Leiden, The Netherlands
SU BioMedicine, Postbus 546, 2300 AM Leiden, The Netherlands

Mengmeng Sun
Leiden University European Center for Chinese Medicine and Natural Compounds, Institute of Biology, Leiden University, Sylviusweg 72, 2333 BE Leiden, The Netherlands
Changchun University of Chinese Medicine, No. 1035, Boshuo Rd, Jingyue Economic Development District, Changchun 130117, China

Wen-Te Chang
Department of Chinese Pharmaceutical Sciences and Chinese Medicine Resources, College of Chinese Medicine, China Medical University, 91, Hsueh-Shih Road, Taichung 40402, Taiwan

Eduard Van Wijk and Roeland Van Wijk
Meluna Research, Koppelsedijk 1-a, 4191 LC Geldermalsen, The Netherlands
Sino-Dutch Centre for Preventive and Personalized Medicine, Gasthuislingelaan 33, 4002 AG Tiel, The Netherlands

Jin Wang, Qian Ran, Hai-rong Zeng, Lin Wang, Chang-jiang Hu and Qin-wan Huang
College of Pharmacy, Chengdu University of Traditional Chinese Medicine, No. 1166, Liutai Road, Wenjiang District, Chengdu 611137, China

Mu-Yang Huang, Le-Le Zhang and Jin-Jian Lu
State Key Laboratory of Quality Research in Chinese Medicine, Institute of Chinese Medical Sciences, University of Macau, 7014, N22, Avenida da Universidade, Taipa, Macao, China

Jian Ding
Division of Anti-tumor Pharmacology, State Key Laboratory of Drug Research, Shanghai Institute of Materia Medica, Chinese Academy of Sciences, Shanghai, China

Wei Shen, Hui Luo, Zhifang Wu, Hongtai Chen, Liuchao Hu, Bin Wang and Yiwen Luo
Department of Traumatology, The Third Affiliated Hospital of Guangzhou University of Traditional Chinese Medicine, 22 Jiangnan-Xi Road, Guangzhou 510240, Guangdong, People's Republic of China

Liangliang Xu
Key Laboratory of Orthopaedics & Traumatology, The First Affiliated Hospital of Guangzhou University of Chinese Medicine, Guangzhou 510000, Guangdong, People's Republic of China

Yamei Liu and Lijuan Yu
Department of Diagnostics of Chinese Medicine, School of The Basic Medicine, Guangzhou 510006, Guangdong, People's Republic of China

Shuaibing He
School of Chines Materia Medica, Beijing University of Chinese Medicine, Yangguang South Avenue, Fangshan District, Beijing 102488, China

Zhao Chen, Yanfeng Cao and Yanjiang Qiao
School of Chines Materia Medica, Beijing University of Chinese Medicine, Yangguang South Avenue, Fangshan District, Beijing 102488, China
Research Center of TCM Information Engineering, Beijing University of Chinese Medicine, Yangguang South Avenue, Fangshan District, Beijing 102488, China

Yuan Wei, Linwei Wang, Dujun Wang, Dan Wang, Chongwei Wen and Zhen Ouyang
School of Pharmacy, Jiangsu University, 301 Xuefu Road, Zhenjiang 212013, Jiangsu, China

Bangxin Han
School of Biological and Pharmaceutical Engineering, West Anhui University, Lu'an 237012, China

Wei Sang, Kegang Linghu, Wei Xiong and Wai San Cheang
Institute of Chinese Medical Sciences, State Key Laboratory of Quality Research in Chinese Medicine, University of Macau, Macao, China

Hua Yu
Institute of Chinese Medical Sciences, State Key Laboratory of Quality Research in Chinese Medicine, University of Macau, Macao, China
HKBU Shenzhen Research Center, Shenzhen, Guangdong, China
School of Chinese Medicine, Hong Kong Baptist University, Kowloon Tong, Hong Kong, China
Institute of Chinese Medical Sciences, University of Macau, Room 8008, Building N22, Avenida da Universidade, Taipa, Macao SAR, China

Zhangfeng Zhong
Institute of Chinese Medical Sciences, State Key Laboratory of Quality Research in Chinese Medicine, University of Macau, Macao, China
Guangdong Key Laboratory for Research and Development of Natural Drugs, Guangdong Medical University, Zhanjiang, China

Yitao Wang
Institute of Chinese Medical Sciences, State Key Laboratory of Quality Research in Chinese Medicine, University of Macau, Macao, China
Institute of Chinese Medical Sciences, University of Macau, Room 1050, Building N22, Avenida da Universidade, Taipa, Macao SAR, China

Anfernee Kai Wing Tse
Academy for Advanced Interdisciplinary Studies, Southern University of Science and Technology, Shenzhen, Guangdong, China

Lian-ying Liao, Yi-fan He, Li Li, Hong Meng, Yin-mao Dong and Fan Yi
Key Laboratory of Cosmetics, China National Light Industry, Beijing Technology and Business University, No. 11/33, Fucheng Road, Haidian District, Beijing 100048, People's Republic of China
Beijing Key Laboratory of Plant Resources Research and Development, Beijing Technology and Business University, No. 11/33, Fucheng Road, Haidian District, Beijing 100048, People's Republic of China

Pei-gen Xiao
Institute of Medicinal Plant Development, Chinese Academy of Medical Sciences, Peking Union Medical College, Beijing, 151 Malianwa North Road, Haidian District, Beijing 100193, People's Republic of China

Xiang Zhang and Linfang Huang
Institute of Medicinal Plant Development, Chinese Academy of Medical Sciences and Peking Union Medical College, Beijing 100193, China

Xiangxiao Meng, Jie Wu and Shilin Chen
Institute of Chinese Materia Medica, China Academy of Chinese Medical Sciences, Beijing 100700, China

Qiu Li, Yiming Niu, Panfei Xing and Chunming Wang
State Key Laboratory of Quality Research in Chinese Medicine, Institute of Chinese Medical Sciences, University of Macau, Avenida da Universidade, Macau SAR, China

Xie Jun, Yu Lei and Peng Cheng
Chengdu University of Traditional Chinese Medicine, Chengdu, China

Peng Fu
West China School of Pharmacy, Sichuan University, Chengdu, China

Yu Dong, Zhe-Ling Feng and Jia-Hong Lu
State Key Laboratory of Quality Research in Chinese Medicine, Institute of Chinese Medical Sciences, University of Macau, Room 7015, N22, Avenida da Universidade, Taipa, Macau SAR, People's Republic of China

Hu-Biao Chen
School of Chinese Medicine, Hong Kong Baptist University, Hong Kong, SAR, People's Republic of China

Fu-Sheng Wang
Ulcerous Vascular Surgical Department, Beijing Traditional Chinese Medicine Hospital Affiliated to Capital Medical University, Beijing, People's Republic of China

Fan-Cheng Meng, Zheng-Feng Wu, Li-Gen Lin, Ruibing Wang and Qing-Wen Zhang
State Key Laboratory of Quality Research in Chinese Medicine, Institute of Chinese Medical Sciences, University of Macau, Macao SAR, People's Republic of China

Zhi-Qi Yin
Department of Traditional Chinese Medicines Pharmaceuticals, China Pharmaceutical University, Nanjing 210009, People's Republic of China

Lihong Liu, Bo Du, Xiaofei Guo, Zheng Zhou, Chang Liu and Shiyu Su
Department of Gynecological Ward, The Third Affiliated Hospital, Jinzhou Medical University, Jinzhou, China
Liaoning Provincial Key Laboratory of Follicle Development and Reproductive Health (Office of Science and Technology), Jinzhou, China

Hao Ai
Liaoning Provincial Key Laboratory of Follicle Development and Reproductive Health (Office of Science and Technology), Jinzhou, China
Department of Gynecological Ward, The First Affiliated Hospital, Jinzhou Medical University, Jinzhou, China

Haiying Zhang
Library Department, Jinzhou Medical University, Jinzhou, China

Aihui Xiu
Department of Gynecological Ward, The First Affiliated Hospital, Jinzhou Medical University, Jinzhou, China

Tian-Tian Zuo, Yao-Lei Li, Hong-Yu Jin, Fei Gao, Qi Wang, Ya-Dan Wang and Shuang-Cheng Ma
National Institutes for Food and Drug Control, No. 2 Tiantan Xili, Dongcheng District, Beijing 100050, China

Fei-Fei Cai, Wen-Jun Zhou, Rong Wu and Shi-Bing Su
Research Center for Traditional Chinese Medicine Complexity System, Shanghai University of Traditional Chinese Medicine, Shanghai 201203, China

Meng Wang, Xiao-Jiao Zhang, Ruibing Feng, Chengwei He, Peng Li and Jian-Bo Wan
State Key Laboratory of Quality Research in Chinese Medicine, Institute of Chinese Medical Sciences, University of Macau, Room 6034, Building N22, Avenida da Universidade, Macao, People's Republic of China

Yun Jiang and Da-Yong Zhang
Sichuan New Lotus Traditional Chinese Herb Limited Company, Chengdu, China

Grace Gar-Lee Yue, Julia Kin-Ming Lee, Ben Chung-Lap Chan, Hin-Fai Kwok, Sandy Wan-Heng Hoi, Ping-Chung Leung and Clara Bik-San Lau
Institute of Chinese Medicine, E205, Science Centre East Block, The Chinese University of Hong Kong, Shatin, New Territories, Hong Kong
State Key Laboratory of Research On Bioactivities and Clinical Applications of Medicinal Plants, The Chinese University of Hong Kong, Shatin, New Territories, Hong Kong

Kwok-Pui Fung
Institute of Chinese Medicine, E205, Science Centre East Block, The Chinese University of Hong Kong, Shatin, New Territories, Hong Kong
State Key Laboratory of Research On Bioactivities and Clinical Applications of Medicinal Plants, The Chinese University of Hong Kong, Shatin, New Territories, Hong Kong
School of Biomedical Sciences, The Chinese University of Hong Kong, Shatin, New Territories, Hong Kong

Daniel Man-Yuen Sze
Department of Health Technology and Informatics, The Hong Kong Polytechnic University, Hung Hom, Kowloon, Hong Kong

Index

www.ingramcontent.com/pod-product-compliance
Lightning Source LLC
LaVergne TN
LVHW080910210926
848485LV00004B/623